Mincu · Diabetic Macro- and Microangiopathy

Diabetic Macro- and Microangiopathy

by

Iulian Mincu

W DE G

Walter de Gruyter · Berlin · New York 1975

Title of the original romanian edition:
Julian Mincu, Angiopathia Diabetica

Prof. Dr. Julian Mincu, Chairman of the Department for Nutritional and Metabolic Diseases,
Lecturer in Medical Sciences.
Bucharest · Romania

With 304 illustrations

Translation from the Romanian
language made by
EDITURA ACADEMIEI
REPUBLICII SOCIALISTE
ROMANIA - BUCUREŞTI -

Printed in Germany
Printing: Walter de Gruyter & Co., Berlin
Binding: Lüderitz & Bauer, Berlin

ISBN 3 11 004533 8
Library of Congress Catalog Card Number 73-82434

Preface

Diabetic angiopathies represent some of the most important complications of diabetes mellitus.

The advances in therapeutic approach made within the last 50 years have lead to a complete change in the clinical course and diagnosis of diabetes mellitus. The mortality following diabetic coma which was as high as 80% prior to insulin therapy has now dropped to between 1 and 2% of the cases observed. Although the life expectancy has been considerably increased, macro- and microangiopathies still account for some 70–85% of deaths in diabetics. This problem is considerably worsened by the close involvement of these vessel lesions with, for example, dyslipaemic syndrome, i. e. hyperlipoproteinaemia, arteriosclerosis and obesity.

The present report is based on data from the literature as well as observations and experiments carried out at the Clinic of Metabolic Diseases and Nutrition in Bucharest. It is hoped that this represents a modest contribution to this theme without claiming any degree of completeness.

25,000 patients registered as diabetics in our department have been included in these investigations. Furthermore we have carried out epidemiological studies over the last three years using large groups of healthy Rumanians from both town and country districts. I would like to thank all clinicians and research workers of our department, who have given considerable support in the preparation of this book especially:

Dr. S. Campeanu, Head Physician; Dr. C. Dumitrescu, Head of the Out-patient Laboratory; Dr. N. Mihalache, Head of the Biochemical Laboratory as well as Dr. P. Niculescu and Dr. Al. Petrovici, Heads of the Laboratories for Electron Microscopy at the Institute Babes and Institute Cantacuzino Bucharest.

Moreover I am indebted to Prof. Dr. W. I. H. Butterfield, Vice-Chascellor of the University of Nottingham, whose advise during my visit to Guy's Hospital in 1970 was of profound value to me.

Autumn 1974

I. Mincu

Contents

Chapter I Introduction

Diabetes mellitus is one of the diseases whose seriousness and incidence is becoming ever more manifest as medical scientific research increases and ever larger groups of people can be investigated.

A. Mortality in Diabetes Mellitus

Recent research on diabetic mortality has shown that [13, 20, 27, 37, 39]:

1. diabetics' mortality is higher than that of other people, irrespective of the presence of some complications. It was established that over a ten-year period mortality was 2–5 times higher in diabetics than in non-diabetics. The average life span of diabetics is shorter than in non-diabetics.

2. the excess mortality is greater in the younger patients because of the severe forms of diabetes mellitus encountered in the age group.

3. the causal factors of the majority of deaths in diabetics under the age of 45 are cardiovascular and renal diseases.

4. finally, in similar pathological conditions, mortality is higher in diabetics. Thus, for instance, obesity investigated over a ten-year period [48] was associated with a mortality 2.8 times higher among diabetics, who apparently had no other complication of the disease, as against non-diabetic obese individuals.

B. Morbidity of Diabetes Mellitus

Before tackling the main subject of this work – angiopathy in diabetics – some data is necessary on the incidence of diabetic disease itself. Görig's thesis (1969) provides a review of the studies on the incidence of diabetes mellitus up to that date. The reported figures are quite varied, ranging from 0.19% in Newcastle to 4.19% in Malta. These differences may to a great extent be due to the detection method employed (Fig. 1) [28].

In the determination of the incidence of diabetes mellitus, two methods have been used predominantly:

a) the investigation of postprandial glycosuria, generally followed by a glucose tolerance test in suspect persons. This method usually yields lower values for the incidence of diabetes mellitus.

b) investigation of postprandial glycaemia and glycosuria. This device has the advantage of enabling the tracing of forms of diabetes mellitus in the chemical stage of the disease, raising the percentage values of incidence [40].

The International Diabetes Federation recommends that mass investigations for diabetes should be carried out in the following way:

1. the determination of blood sugar and urine levels 2 hours after a meal containing at least 50 g carbohydrate;

2. a complete glucose tolerance test in those cases when initial tests suggest the possibility of diabe-

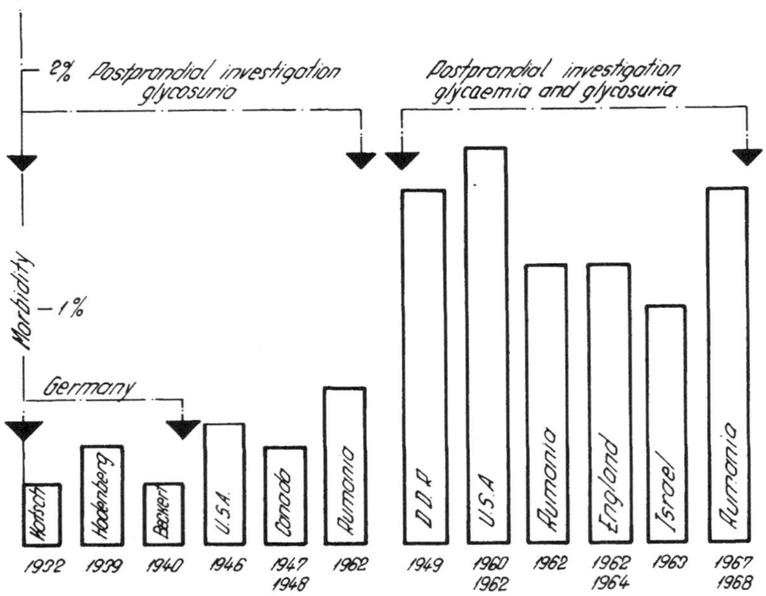

Fig. 1. The morbidity (%) attributed to diabetes mellitus in different lands.

tes. This investigation should be carried out in all subjects having glycosuria as well as a blood sugar level of 130 mg/100 ml or more (Fig. 2).

Most of the researches carried out with the first method (1930–1950) showed a relatively low prevalence [2, 8, 20, 21, 46, 47].

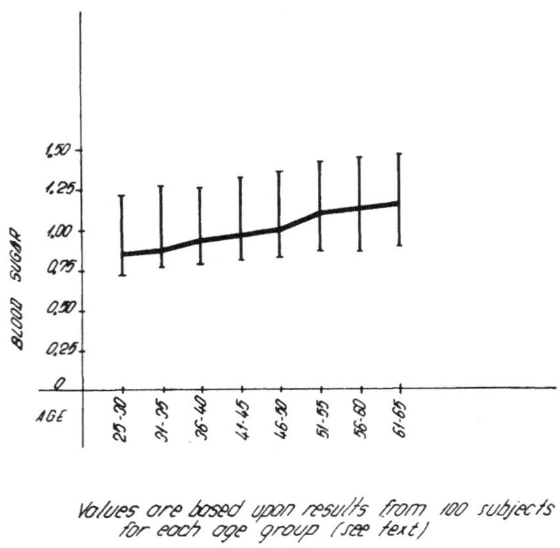

Fig. 2. Normal values for glycaemia according to hours after glucose load.

Such an epidemiological study was also made in Rumania in 1962, estimating the prevalence rate in Bucharest at that time at about 1.1% [46, 47]. The method of active detection based on the postprandial blood sugar measurement represented an important advance. Its application was started in 1950, several variations being used. A 5 to 8 times higher prevalence rate was found by this approach as compared to the first method [8, 9, 10, 14, 45, 60, 62, 66].

The following short summary of a research carried out in Rumania in 1968 and 1970, is a good example both of the influence of the applied detection method on the incidence rate of diabetes and the real state of the latter in this country [41]. This investigation of the entire population in rural and urban areas was carried out be tha Antidiabetic Centre in Bucharest (ACB).

Sex, age, the presence or absence of overweight were considered and their correlation with glycosuria and hyperglycaemia after a standard glucose load was studied (Fig. 3).

This first investigation was carried out in 1968 on 1,314 people aged between 17 and 70 years (728

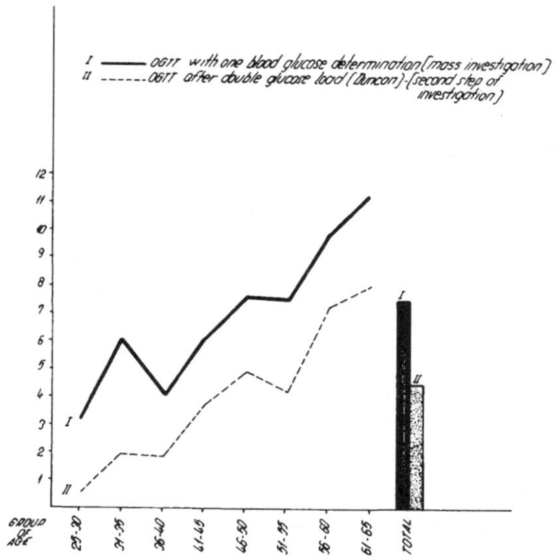

Fig. 3. Age distribution of the incidence of diabetes mellitus.

women and 586 men) representing 88.6% of the whole population of the village of Buda (district of Ilfov). No change in the normal nutrition of the subjects was detected during the few days which preceded the survey.

In the initial screening 75 persons, representing 5.7% of the total investigated, were found to have blood glucose values over 130 mg/100 ml, two hours after the glucose load. All these subjects were subsequently submitted to an oral glucose tolerance test (oGTT).

Abnormal patterns as defined above were obtained in 1.44% of the original population thus exceeding the proportion found for urban areas (Bucharest) in 1962 (see Table I). This investigation was the first to be carried out in Rumania using the shortened oGTT. The results obtained illustrate the value of this method in mass detection researches of diabetes mellitus.

A second search for diabetes mellitus was carried out in Bucharest in 1970 involving 7,113 adults, aged between 25 and 65 years. The study was limited to these groups in view of the rarity of latent diabetes mellitus in the young and the probability of interfering factors in the old.

The results obtained reveal a prevalence of diabetes mellitus which varies with sex and age group, from 0.65% for men, and 0.46% for women in the 25–30 years age group, up to 8.1% for men and 8.4% for women in the 61–65 years age group (Fig. 4).

Within the whole group of 7,113 subjects, 332 diabetics were found representing 4.65% of the whole population. Sex-grouping showed diabetes mellitus in 192 men (5.9%) and 140 women (3.65%) (Fig. 5).

As 74.52% of the population between 25 and 65 years in the respective area was investigated, an estimate of the number of diabetics in the whole population became possible.

A number of diabetics from the investigated district were previously registered at the ACB, they were also included in order to obtain the total prevalence of diabetes (Fig. 4).

AGE GROUP	17-20 yrs.				21-40 yrs.				41-60 yrs.				OVER 60 yrs.			
VALUE	ABNORMAL		NORMAL		ABNORMAL		NORMAL		ABNORMAL		NORMAL		ABNORMAL		NORMAL	
SEXES	MEN	WOMEN	MEN	WOMEN	MEN	WOMEN	MEN	WOMEN	MEN	WOMEN	MEN	WOMEN	MEN	WOMEN	MEN	WOMEN
NUMBER	0	0	0	0	2	0	8	7	4	4	7	18	4	5	10	6
TOTAL	0		0		2		15		8		25		9		16	

Table I. Distribution of the sexes and age groups of the glucose tolerance results of the subjects with blood sugar values over 130 mg % on the first determination

Incidence of diabetes: 1.44 %

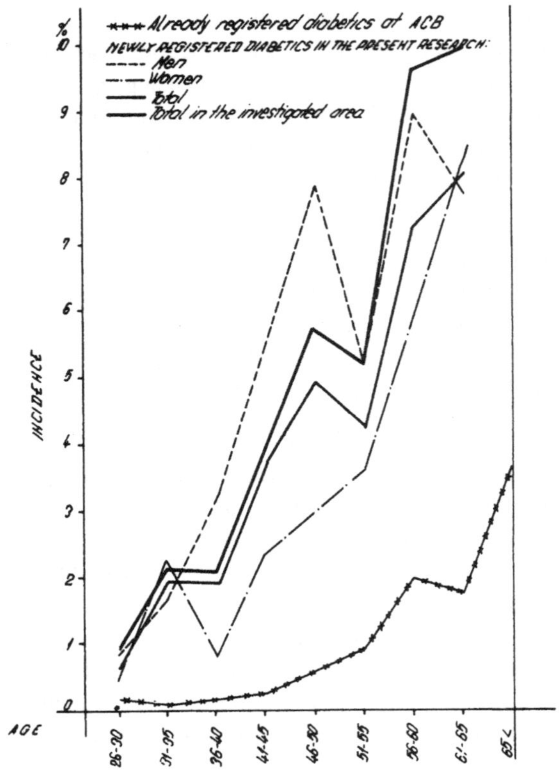

Fig. 4. Incidence of diabetes mellitus.

Thus, for the whole population ranging between 25 and 65 years the prevalence of diabetes mellitus was calculated as 4.9% in the studied area. For the population from 0 to 65 years considering the low prevalence of diabetes mellitus under 25, the calculated prevalence was 3.6%. In the study area there is a prevalence of 3.8% of known diabetes mellitus in persons over 65 years. The number of diabetics over 65 years was added to the total number (known and discovered) of diabetics, under this age, so that the final estimated prevalence of diabetes for the whole population of Bucharest was 3.7% (Fig. 6).

Compared with the previously estimated prevalence (1962) of 1.1% diabetics [46, 47] the newly defined prevalence in the same population group leads to the conclusion that for each known diabetic person, there are two or even three unknown diabetics in the population.

This high prevalence of diabetes mellitus places Rumania, at least when the urban population is considered, among the countries with a high frequency of the disease [8, 14, 22, 24, 28, 29, 30, 31, 57, 60]. These findings strongly suggest that

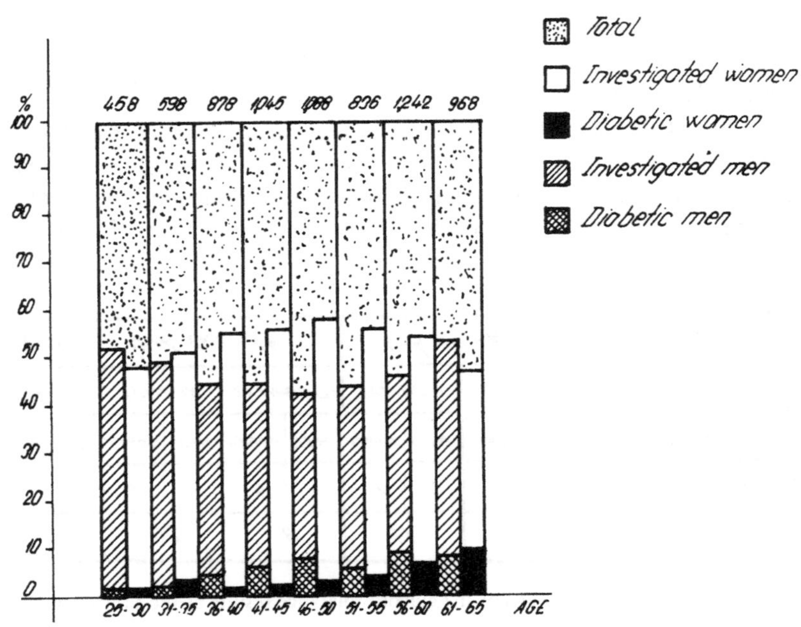

Fig. 5. Distribution of the incidence of diabetes depending on age group and sex.

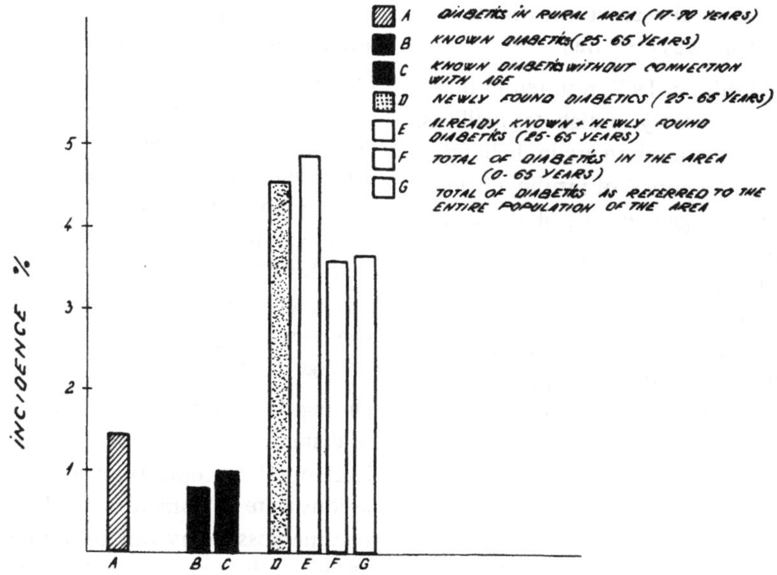

Fig. 6. Epidemiological study on diabetes mellitus in Rumania.

special measures are needed for the management of diabetes and the prevention of the late angiopathic complications of the disease.

C. Angiopathy in Diabetes Mellitus

The acute complications – diabetic comas – were well known even as early as the last century. The late complications of diabetes mellitus, however, began to be studied only in this century, their investigation having led to the notion of "Diabetic Angiopathy", a relatively new concept, therefore, in diabetology. Its true history only begins with the late 19th century, although a description by Jaeger [25, 29] of the symptomatology of diabetic retinopathy, as early as 1855, is usually quoted. It was in fact, only in 1892 that MacKenzie described the morphology of the capillary alterations in diabetes mellitus after having examined the retinal vessels [51] and found, as he put it, their varicose aspect similar to that of aneurysms. Measurements of capillary pressure led Krauss to conclude in 1912 that active dilation of the capillary vessels occurs in diabetes mellitus while von Noorden [7] found that dilation should also be related to diabetic rubeosis.

The typically enlarged aspect of the vessels in the diabetic was described by Weiss in 1916 [7, 51], and confirmed by Jurgensen in 1918 [51]. The preinsulinic era seems to close with the regretful conclusions of Zeller, who confirmed the observations of his forerunners and stated that little is known about the physiology of capillaries and small vessels in general and even less about their fate in diabetes mellitus. Poor information at that time was due, to some extent, to the still rudimentary means of investigation available, but mostly to the fact that before the discovery of insulin, survival in diabetic subjects was too short to permit a full display of the late complications of the disease. In fact mortality during that period (Fig. 7), was chiefly due to the acute complications of the condition, diabetic coma causing 63.8% of the deaths [21]. The importance of diabetic vasculopathy and even of infections, including tuberculosis, was obscured.

The discovery of insulin in 1922 resulted in the first revolution in the history of diabetes mellitus. It is the first period of a modern era in diabetology. We might call it the period of insulin, during which the modern management of diabetes and diabetic coma and precoma have been developed. An impressive fall ensued in mortality due to diabetic coma, rapidly reaching some 10% of deaths, while an equally impressive increase was observed in death rate due to vasculopathy, to around 52% and by infection to around 27% [20] (Fig. 7).

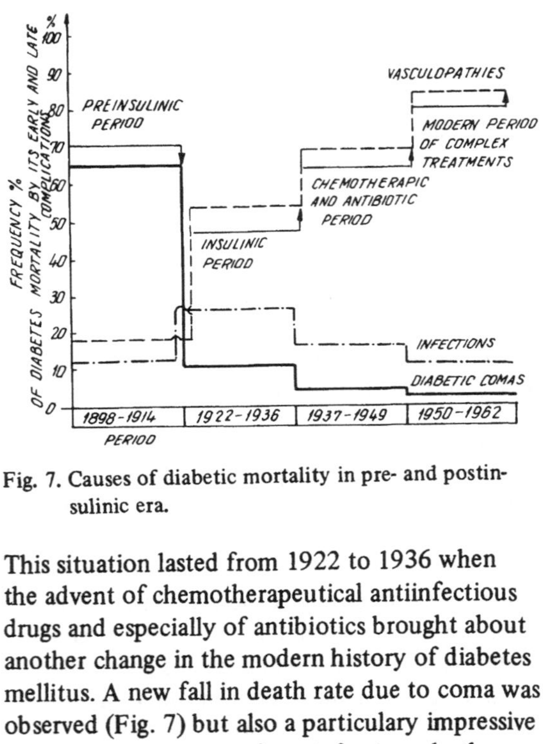

Fig. 7. Causes of diabetic mortality in pre- and postinsulinic era.

This situation lasted from 1922 to 1936 when the advent of chemotherapeutical antiinfectious drugs and especially of antibiotics brought about another change in the modern history of diabetes mellitus. A new fall in death rate due to coma was observed (Fig. 7) but also a particulary impressive reduction of mortality from infections, both resulting in a new increase in deaths due to vasculopathy.

It was this chemotherapeutic and antibiotic period from 1937 to 1949 that enabled Kimmelstiel and Wilson to describe, in 1936, diabetic nephropathy and Balantine and Loewenstein (1944) to substantiate the concept of diabetic retinopathy.

A last period that might be regarded as beginning around 1950, and which is still going on, is featured by the complex and many-sided management of diabetes mellitus, subsequent to the discovery of a wide range of peroral antidiabetic drugs and of the advances in the knowledge of the dysmetabolic states originating in and associated with diabetes. Death rates ascribed to diabetic vasculopathy rose again, reaching 78% [20] while new decreases were noted in deaths by infection (16% on average) and by diabetic coma (1,5% on average) (Fig. 7).

During this latest period the morphological picture of diabetic angiopathy was outlined. The first electronmicroscopic examinations of the vascular lesions were performed around 1950, when it became possible by various bioptic procedures, to obtain fresh human tissue from many organs of the body. It was only in 1956 that Irvine described the thickening of the basement membrane in the glomeruli. During the late fifties diabetic microangiopathy was described in detail and its specificity was claimed [5, 6, 26]. Research in the following decade, including almost every organ of the diabetic demonstrated the ubiquity of microangiopathy.

Thus the concept of a so-called specific [7] or disseminated microangiopathy has gradually taken shape. This has implied differentiation from diabetic arteriopathy or, as it was recently called, diabetic macroangiopathy [54].

The term "diabetic angiopathy" has thus become a wider concept which includes two types of vascular condition occurring in diabetes, namely:

a) arteriopathies, the Mönckeberg medio-calcinosis type, grouped as macroangiopathy and
b) specific or disseminated diabetic microangiopathy.
These two varieties of vasculopathy in diabetes mellitus may occur simultaneously in the same patient or they may follow each other.

The high incidence of death due to vasculopathy in diabetes mellitus suggests that the pathogenesis and the efficient management of this complication are still open problems. The ensuing period in the history of diabetes mellitus will undoubtedly see the incidence of death by late vascular complication follow the example of coma and infection and gradually fall. But the goal requires further knowledge of the pathogenesis of these complications and the advent of efficient prophylactic and therapeutical means able to heal them or capable of arresting their unfavourable course.

D. Some General Epidemiological Factors Involved in Diabetic Angiopathy

It is commonly admitted nowadays that a dyslipaemia generally favours the appearance of degenerative vascular manifestations. Dyslipaemia is one of the most frequent anomalies revealed by laboratory examination. It occurs in approximately 10–25% of the so-called healthy population [34, 58]. Reports in the literature state that the 4th type of dyslipaemia in Frederickson's classification is more often met with in older people, while types 2 and 3 are characteristic of younger people.

We shall further present our epidemiological studies on random populations and upon diabetics with a view to underlining the role played by dyslipaemia in favouring and determining the frequency of diabetic angiopathy.

1. Epidemiology of Dyslipaemia in Random Populations

Epidemiological studies of the disturbances of plasma lipids have been relatively rare [11, 36, 49, 59]. Quite often, the results obtained were not generally relevant owing to the size of the population studied, the method of selecting the subjects, the laboratory methods (table II) [23, 38], the nutritional conditions of the respective group [15] the season [17], the geographic region [35], the duration of the respective investigation [33] as well as to other factors [55]. On the other hand, the importance nowadays given to abnormalities in plasma lipids and other aspects of fat metabolism in the pathogenesis of various degenerative conditions (arteriosclerosis, coronary diseases, complications of diabetes mellitus, etc.) [19], reveals the importance of such studies.

Table II

LIPID FRACTIONS	MEAN BLOOD LEVEL (424 SUBJECTS)	LABORATORY METHOD
CHOLESTEROL	164 ± 44 mg%	RAPPAPORT-EICHORN
TRIGLYCERIDES	133 ± 51 mg%	GALANOS et. al.
NEFA	569 ± 127 mg%	DOLE
β + μ LIPOPROTEINS	65.8 % ± 7.8	PAPER-LIPIDOGRAM

An epidemiological study made in Rumania in 1970 investigated 7,085 apparently healthy persons in a district of Bucharest. The age of the investigated subjects ranged between 25 and 65, and age distribution by decade is to be found in Table III.

3,292 were males and 3,793 females. Fasting blood samples were taken for determination of cholesterol (C) triglycerides (TG), non-esterified fatty acids (NEFA), pre-beta-lipoproteins (pB) and the value of the ratio

$$R = \frac{\text{beta-lipoproteins + chylomicrons}}{\text{alpha-lipoproteins}}$$

With a view to establishing normal values under the above conditions, a previous determination of all these lipid fractions was made on 424 normal individuals, aged between 26–65 of whom 192 were males and 232 females. Table III based on these determinations includes the statistical calculated values considered as normal in the respective epidemiological investigation.

Table III. Normal values for C, TG, NEFA and R

Cholesterol (C)	Triglycerides (TG)	NEFA	R
164 ± 44 mg %	133 ± 51 mg %	569 ± 127 mg %	65.8 ± 7.8

a) Frequency of global dyslipaemia (GD)

Of the 7,085 investigated subjects, 3,271 (46%) had values above those considered as normal (see Table III). These deviations for all the investigated lipid fractions, were denominated global dyslipaemias (GD). (Table IV) They concern one, two,

NORMAL WEIGHTED SUBJECTS

AGE	25-35 years				36-45 years				46-55 years				56-65 years			
TYPE OF FOUND DYSLIPEMIA	M	W	T		M	W	T		M	W	T		M	W	T	
MLD	37	34	71	S	39	41	80	S	35	33	68	S	41	34	75	S
DLD	47	24	71	S	42	35	77	S	30	32	62	S	30	31	61	S
TLD	57	23	80	S	44	17	61	S	38	23	61	S	35	20	55	S
PLD	UNREPRESENTATIVE NUMBER OF SUBJECTS			NS	43	20	63	NS	36	32	68	NS	37	22	59	S

OBESE SUBJECTS

AGE	25-35 years				36-45 years				46-55 years				56-65 years			
MLD	20	9	29	S	9	11	20	S	8	24	32	S	9	16	25	S
DLD	11	18	29	S	6	23	29	S	10	28	38	S	11	28	39	S
TLD	6	14	20	S	17	22	39	S	12	27	39	S	20	25	45	S
PLD	UNREPRESENTATIVE NUMBER OF SUBJECTS				13	24	37	NS	15	17	32	NS	8	33	41	S

MLD = ONE ABNORMAL LIPID FRACTIONS
DLD = TWO " " "
TLD = THREE " " "
PLD = MORE THAN THREE ABNORMAL LIPID FRACTIONS
S = STATISTICALLY SIGNIFICANT; NS = NOT STATISTICALLY SIGNIFICANT
M = MEN; W = WOMEN; T = TOTAL

Table IV. Distribution of differentiated dyslipaemias according to age and weight.

three or all the fractions investigated. Their isolated or partial behaviour will be considered later. Dyslipaemias as a whole display variations in frequency according to age, sex and weight. In order to estimate the influence of these factors, the entire group was divided into 4 subgroups: I 25–35, II 36–45, III 46–55 and IV 56–65 years old. Each decade was examined in relation to sex and weight. Estimation of overweight was made according to Broca, 15% above ideal weight being considered overweight.

For both sexes, decade II is characterised by lower values. Irrespective of sex, in cases of normal weight (NW in Fig. 8) increasing frequency of abnormalities occurs with increasing age. However, the pattern is irregular in the obese (O in Fig. 8). Further in decade IV the obese have a lower frequency than people of normal weight.

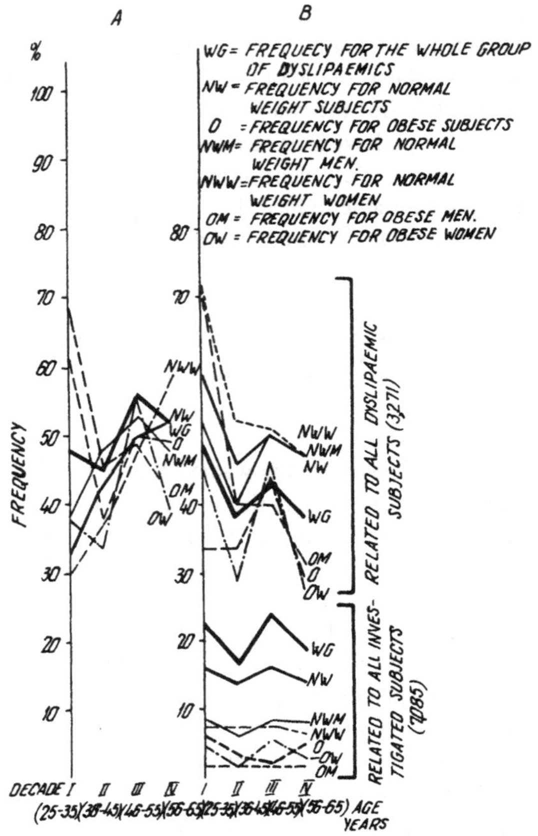

Fig. 8. Frequency of global dyslipaemia according to sex, age and weight in 3,271 subjects.
Frequency of (A) global dyslipaemia and (B) monofractional lipaemic disturbances according to sex, age and weight.

b) Frequency of differentiated dyslipaemias (DD)

A classification of the dyslipaemic subjects into 4 distinct types was made, based on the number of lipid fractions abnormally increased in blood:

- monofractional lipaemic disturbance (MLD)
- difractional " " (DLD)
- trifractional " " (TLD)
- polyfractional " " (PLD).

Out of the total number of lipaemic disturbances detected in 3,271 subjects, 1,463 (45%) displayed abnormally high levels of one of the lipid fractions investigated (MLD), representing 21 % of the entire population investigated (Table V).

AGE DECADE	MEN		WOMEN		TOTAL		TOTAL
	NW	O	NW	O	NW	O	
I 25-35	94	51	85	21	179	72	251
II 36-45	131	30	137	36	268	66	334
III 46-55	163	37	149	107	312	144	456
IV 56-65	175	38	143	66	318	104	422
TOTAL	563	156	514	230	1077	386	1463

NW = NORMAL WEIGHT SUBJECTS
O = OBESE SUBJECTS

Table V. Distribution of MLD according to age and weight.

In summary we may conclude that: (Fig. 9)

- increased blood cholesterol is more frequent in females and in general with more advanced age, except during the last decade in cases of overweight;
- there is a slight tendency for increased blood TG with increasing age. For the last decade, overweight obviously increases the blood TG level for both sexes, particularly in men.
- NEFA level decreases in direct ratio with age, without being influenced by sex. It is influenced by weight, especially in men, in the first decade. In the last decade, the same phenomenon is more obvious in women;
- pre-beta-lipoproteins (pB) frequency decreases with age. Sex has no influence, while overweight determines a remarkable rise in young women (decade I), and in both sexes in the last decade;
- frequency of increased R is the least influenced by age and sex. Overweight determines a decrease in the last decade only in males (Fig. 9).

Of the total number of dyslipaemias detected, 987 (30%) presented abnormally increased levels for two different lipid fractions (DLD) representing 13.9% of the total number of investigated subjects (Table VI).

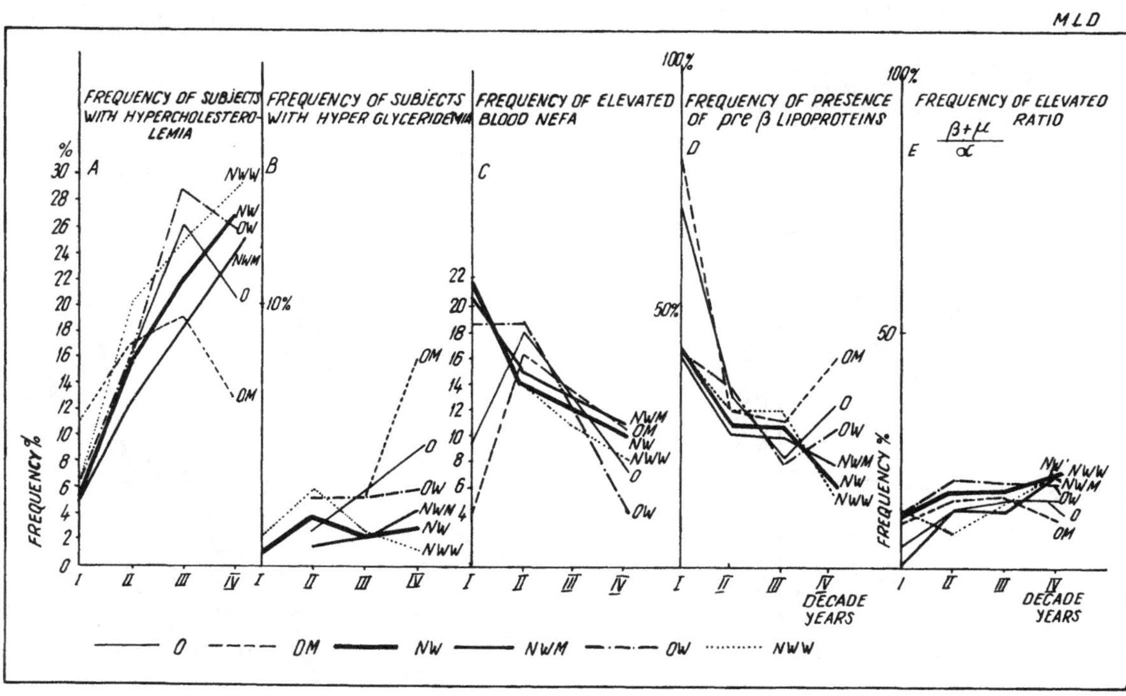

Fig. 9. Frequency of MLD according to sex, age and weight in 1,463 subjects.

A higher frequency of DLD in the last decades is found in the overweight especially in women (Fig. 10).

AGE DECADE	MEN		WOMEN		TOTAL		TOTAL
	NW	O	NW	O	NW	O	
I 25-35	49	11	25	18	74	29	103
II 36-45	110	15	94	47	204	62	266
III 46-55	84	29	87	79	171	108	279
IV 56-65	103	38	104	94	207	132	339
TOTAL	346	93	310	238	656	331	987

NW = NORMAL WEIGHT SUBJECTS
O = OBESE SUBJECTS

Table VI. Distribution of DLD according to age and weight.

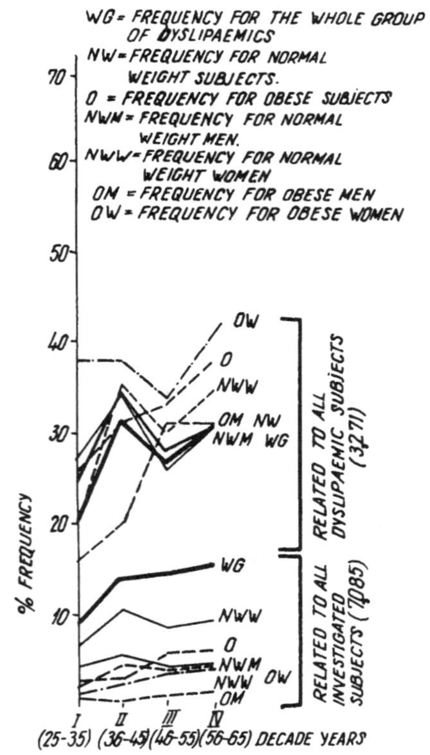

Fig. 10. Frequency of DLD according to sex, age and weight. (NW Fig. 8A, O Fig. 8A)

The association pattern of fractions in DLD is:

– for subjects of normal weight (Fig. 11)
  decade I increased TG + NEFA
  " II " TG + NEFA and pB + R.
  " III see decade II.
  " IV increased C + R, TG + NEFA pB + R.

– for overweight subjects (Fig. 12)
  decade I increased C + R TG + NEFA R + pB.
  " II " R + pB TG + NEFA

– decade III increased R + pB TG + NEFA

– decade IV " TG + NEFA C + pB

As seen from the above, overweight is associated with the frequent appearance of DLD characterised by increased pB associated with either high blood lipoproteins or high blood cholesterol level.

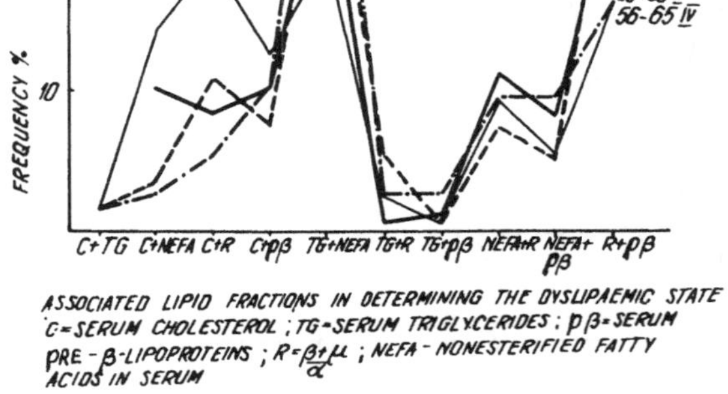

Fig. 11.

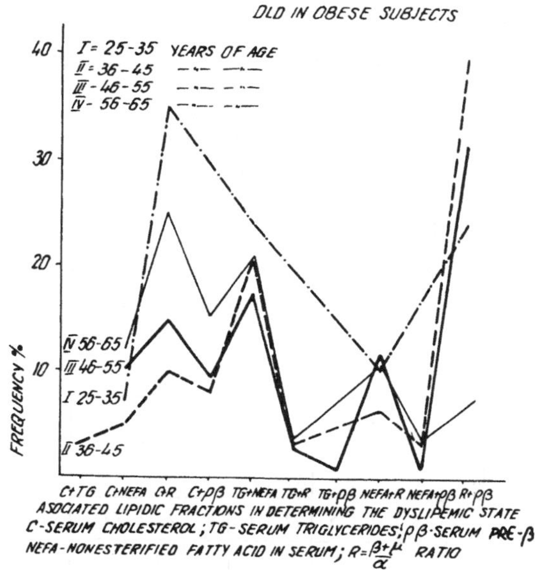

Fig. 12.

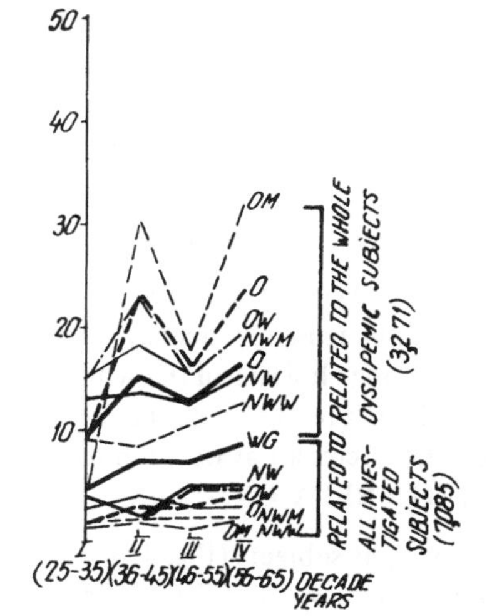

Fig. 13. Frequency of TLD according to age, sex and weight. For legend see fig. 8.

AGE DECADE	MEN		WOMEN		TOTAL		TOTAL
	NW	O	NW	O	NW	O	
I 25-35	28	3	11	7	39	10	49
II 36-45	60	23	23	29	83	52	135
III 46-55	52	17	32	36	84	53	137
IV 56-65	66	39	39	46	105	85	190
TOTAL	206	82	105	118	311	200	511

NW = NORMAL WEIGHT SUBJECTS
O = OBESE SUBJECTS

Table VII. Distribution of TLD according to age and weight.

Of the total number of dyslipaemias, 511 (16%) presented increased values for three of the lipid fractions investigated (TLD), representing 7.2% of the entire population (Table VII).

The investigations showed that TLD frequency increases in direct ratio with age and is more obvious in men of normal weight. Overweight is associated with a TLD increase in both sexes. The 46–55 decade is characterised by a slight tendency of decreasing frequency of TLD (Fig. 13).

The analysis of the association pattern of lipid fractions in TLD shows:

– for subjects of normal weight (Fig. 14):

decade I	increases of	TG	+ NEFA	+ R
		TG	+ NEFA	+ pB.
decade II	" "	TG	+ NEFA	+ R
" III	" "	TG	+ NEFA	+ R and
		more rarely		
		TG	+ NEFA	+ C
		C	+ R	+ pB
		NEFA	+ R	+ C

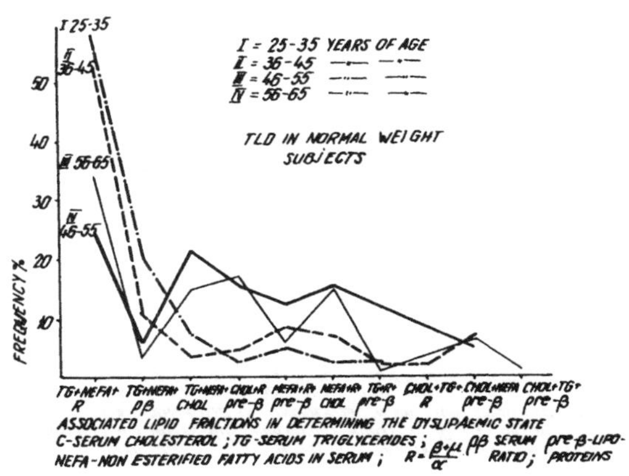

Fig. 14.

" IV " " TG + NEFA + R and
more rarely
TG + NEFA + C
C + R + pB
NEFA + R + pB
NEFA + R + C

The fact may be noticed that, starting with decade III, there is an increased frequency of those associations including cholesterol (C) while in decade IV, pB and C are present in all detected associations. Another frequent association to be found in all ages is TG + NEFA + R.

– for overweight subjects (Fig. 15)
decade I increases of TG + NEFA + R
C + NEFA + TG
" II " " TG + NEFA + R
TG + NEFA + pB and
TG + NEFA + C
" III " " TG + NEFA + R
TG + NEFA + pB
TG + NEFA + C
R + NEFA + C
" IV " " TG + NEFA + R
TG + NEFA + C
C + R + pB
NEFA + R + C

Starting with decade II, pB lipoproteins and cholesterol are always present in highly frequent TLD associations. As in subjects of normal weight the association TG + NEFA + R is frequently present in all decades in obese patients.

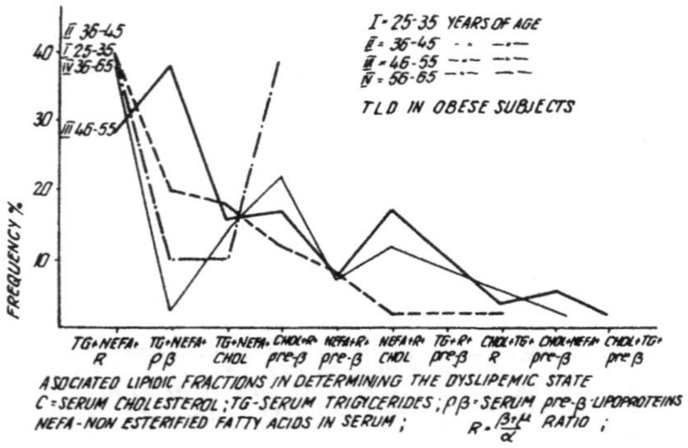

Fig. 15.

It is also worth mentioning that the frequency of each dyslipaemic association increases with age, in both normal and obese subjects.

Of the 3,271 detected dyslipaemias, 223 persons (9%) presented abnormal levels for four or five of the lipid fractions investigated (PLD), representing 3.9% of the entire group (Table VIII).

The PLD frequency, reaches a maximum in decade III. Overweight increases the frequency (Fig. 16).

AGE DECADE	MEN		WOMEN		TOTAL		TOTAL
	NW	O	NW	O	NW	O	
I 25-35	9	5	0	1	9	6	15
II 36-45	23	7	10	11	33	18	51
III 46-55	30	11	23	11	53	22	75
IV 56-65	29	7	19	27	48	34	82
TOTAL	91	40	52	50	143	80	223

NW = NORMAL WEIGHT SUBJECTS
O = OBESE SUBJECTS

Table VIII. Distribution of PLD according to age and weight.

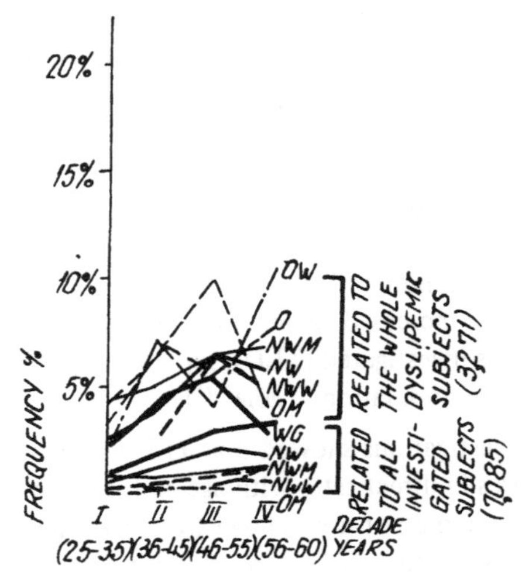

Fig. 16. Frequency of PLD according to sex, age and weight. For legend see Fig. 8.

The analysis of the association pattern of lipid fractions in PLD shows:

– for subjects of normal weight (Fig. 17)
  decade I : the number of subjects with PLD being too small they were eliminated from this study (Table VII)
  decade II increases of TG + NEFA + R + pB
  " III " " R + NEFA + TG + C
  TG + NEFA + R + pB
  " IV " " TG + NEFA + C + R

– for overweight subjects the most frequent association in decades II, III, IV is
  TG + NEFA + C + R
  (Fig. 18)

which frequency is the highest in decade IV. This association is followed, as regards the level of frequency, in decades II and III by

TG + NEFA + R + pB and
C + TG + NEFA + pB for decade II or by
C + NEFA + R + pB for decade III.

In all PLD the associations which include increased blood pB and C are the most frequent.

The high frequency of dyslipaemias and their association pattern may be important in determining

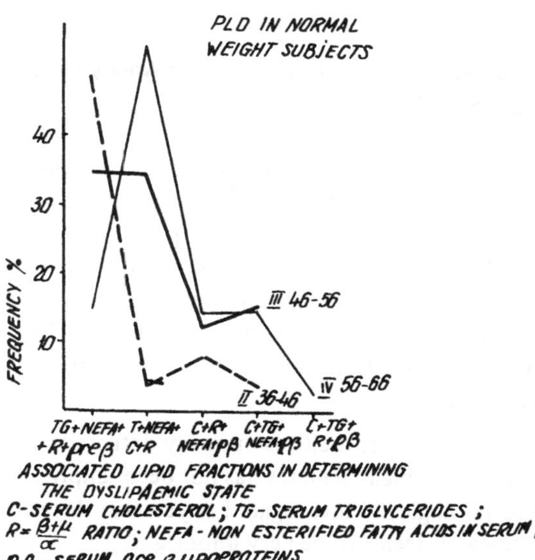

Fig. 17.

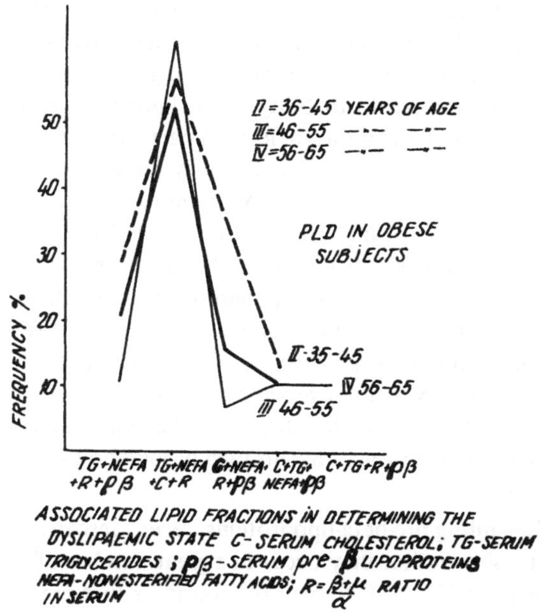

Fig. 18.

vascular complications in both normal and diabetic people. There are other factors, such as age and overweight, which definitely favour the appearance of the dyslipaemic patterns.

c) Age and lipaemic status

Since dyslipaemias represent a risk-factor for arteriosclerosis their early detection is important for a possible prophylaxis. This is also valid for diabetes mellitus.

The diphasic character of the dyslipaemic frequency with age draws the attention to those periods in the life of an individual when the risks become more threatening. The frequency of dyslipaemia is at a minimum between 36 and 45 years and at a maximum between 46–55 and occurs in both GD and in MLD. In the other types of dyslipaemias (DLD, TLD, PLD) a progressive increase in frequency occurs with age.

As far as MLD is concerned, the epidemiological research presented above confirms, completes or refutes some previous observations. Thus, for instance, in 1943 Peters and Man [61] denied all influence of age and even sex on lipaemic status, especially for the blood cholesterol level. Numerous investigations made since have generally proved the great variability of the lipaemic status and of blood cholesterol level in particular. It is generally admitted today that they are somehow dependent on age and sex. Many researchers describe increasing values with age [11, 55] especially in women [16, 49]. This phenomenon was also noticed during the epidemiological investigation in Bucharest, although we could not confirm the finding that the cholesterol level falls after 55 years, except in overweight cases. Our investigation has further disproved the assumption that any overweight means high blood cholesterol [55].

Regarding pre-beta-lipoproteins, recent research has shown that they occur in a great number of persons [32, 38]. Noble [44] considers that pre-beta-lipoproteins can be demonstrated in any adult if the agarose-gel technique is used.

Our research indicates a high percentage of pre-beta-lipoproteins as a single lipaemic disturbance as well as in association with other lipid fractions (DLD, TLD and PLD). With increasing age, pre-beta-lipoproteins are ever more frequently associated with TG or with complex lipoprotein disturbances (R). There is no obvious correlation with sex, while overweight seems to play a certain part in increasing pre-beta-lipoproteins.

The correlation between pre-beta-lipoproteins and TG – those of endogenous origin – is confirmed by the TG behaviour in obese people and by the dyslipaemic association patterns within DLD, PLD and TLD. No correlation could be established between sex and abnormally increased NEFA frequencies.

NEFA are known to vary considerably from the normal level owing to physical activity, activity of the autonomous nervous system, nutritional state and food supply [36]. A certain variation seems to exist in relation to age and weight. NEFA participate in most associated dyslipaemias so that it might seem that their presence should be correlated with the dyslipaemic state itself, rather than with the respective type of dyslipaemia.

d) Overweight and Lipaemic Status

Overweight seems to be a major factor in determining the frequency of dyslipaemias. In MLD, for example, overweight seems to alter the status of lipid fractions for one sex with the status characteristic of the opposite sex. In TG, overweight determines an increased number of individuals with high blood levels (increased frequency of hypertriglyceridaemia).

In DLD, overweight brings about dyslipaemia especially in the last decades, and prevailingly in women. Overweight is also associated with those dyslipaemias where pB lipoproteins are correlated with all blood lipoproteins (R) or hypercholesterolaemia. In both TLD and PLD overweight induces an increased frequency of dyslipaemias in both sexes.

We might conclude that obesity or overweight alongside age is an active factor in altering the lipaemic status. Sex, which plays a less important role in determining the character of dyslipaemias, may aggravate the modifications induced by overweight. All these factors, active in normal individuals, are also present in diabetes mellitus which, itself, induces a certain dyslipaemic state.

2. Epidemiology of Dyslipaemias in Newly Detected Diabetes Mellitus

Dyslipaemias in clinical human diabetes mellitus under treatment, as well as in experimental diabetes have been thoroughly investigated [2, 3, 4, 18, 34, 35, 36, 42, 47, 50, 53, 54, 55, 63]. No doubt exists about the alterations induced by diabetes in lipid status and it is possible that this effect is present from the earliest stages of the diabetic disease.

Chemical diabetes mellitus or newly detected, untreated clinical diabetes has not been amply epidemiologically investigated as yet. But this sort of research seems to be very important.

An investigation on a group of 7,113 adults aged between 25–65 was made in 1970 with a view to detecting clinically untreated chemical diabetes mellitus [41]. The group represented 74.52% of the population of a district in Bucharest.

540 subjects with elevated blood sugar values (above 130 mg % two hours after a glucose meal) were found. These subjects were recalled and a full glucose tolerance test (GTT Duncan) carried out. Within the whole group 332 diabetics were diagnosed in this manner, representing 4.65% of the whole population. After grouping by sex, diabetes mellitus was found in 192 men (5.9%) and 140 women (3.65%). In 328 persons of this group the lipaemic status was investigated. Sex and weight categories of this entire group are presented in Table IX.

Table IX. Distribution of subjects investigated according to illness, age and weight.

SUBJECTS		HEALTHY			DIABETICS			DIABETICS WITH NORMAL WEIGHT			OBESE DIABETICS		
		M	W	TOTAL	M	W	TOTAL	M	W	TOTAL	M	W	TOTAL
AGE BETWEEN 25-66		192	232	424	191	137	328	108	51	159	83	86	169
LIMITS OF AGE (YEARS)	<50	67	80	147	20	12	32	12	9	21	8	3	11
	>50	125	152	277	171	125	296	96	42	138	75	83	158
	TOTAL	192	232	424	191	137	328	108	51	159	83	86	169

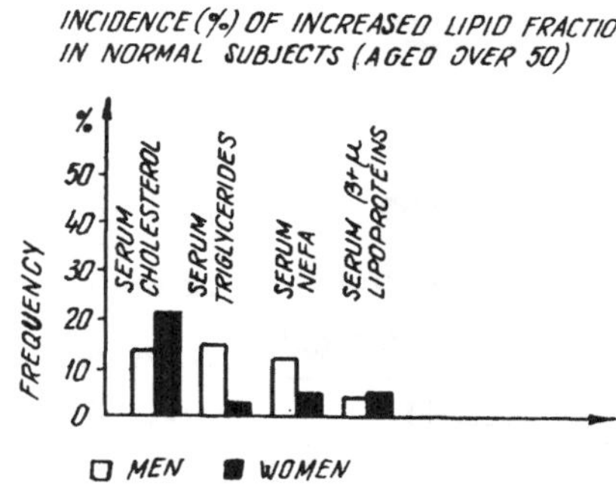

Fig. 19.

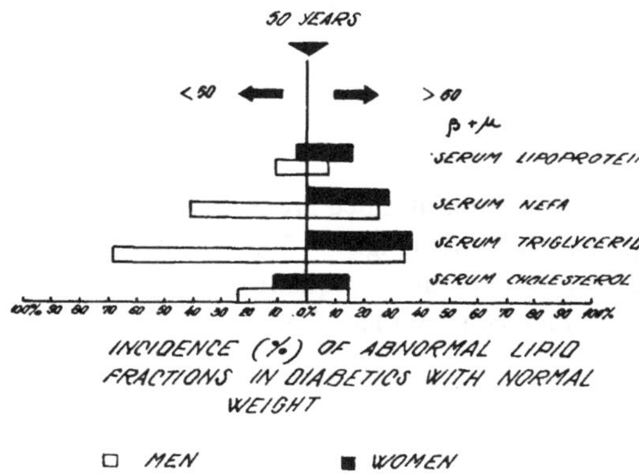

Fig. 20.

The conclusions reached in this investigation are:

a) there is a different incidence of high blood cholesterol level in diabetics compared with healthy persons. In healthy women increased blood cholesterol level is the main modification of the lipaemic status, occurring more frequently than the other lipid fraction over the age of 50. With diabetics, however, there is no difference between men and women as far as the incidence of hypercholesterolaemia is concerned. This is clear in the case of diabetics of normal weight (Fig. 19–20) over the age of 50, while in overweight diabetics the incidence of hypercholesterolaemia is smaller in women over the age of 50 as compared to men of similar age. (Fig. 19, 20, 21). A similar phenomenon occurs with diabetics of normal weight under the age of 50 (Fig. 20).

b) the incidence of hypertriglyceridaemia undergoes important modifications during diabetes mellitus. Its increase was insignificant in healthy women, unlike men of the same age (over 50) (Fig. 19). Normal and overweight diabetics, on the contrary, are characterized by a much increased frequency of hypertriglyceridaemia (Fig. 20), 21). Within the over-50 age-group, hypertriglyceridaemia is more frequent in women, and in the overweight ones, in particular. Increased hypertriglyceridaemia seems to be a characteristic of maturity onset diabetes in females. Age is irrelevant in men (Fig. 20, 21).

c) a very similar behaviour is observed for NEFA (Fig. 19, 20, 21).

d) the status of blood lipoproteins viewed as the ratio "R" undergoes similar variation patterns in both normal and diabetic subjects over the age of

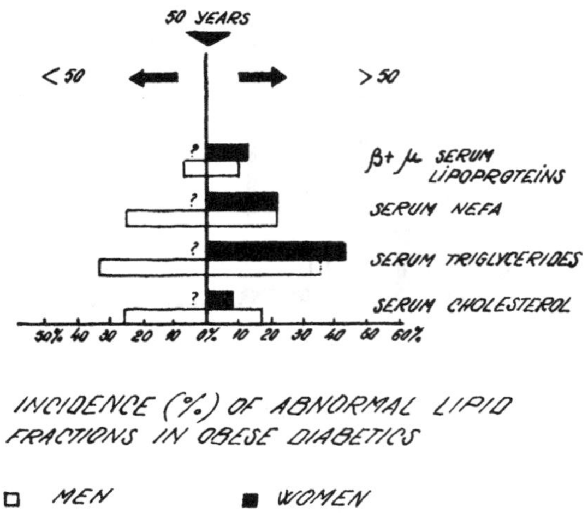

Fig. 21.

50, but the levels attained are different, being higher in diabetics (Fig. 19, 20, 21). Increased NEFA levels are more frequent in men under 50 and women over 50 (Tab. X).

In summary it can be said that:

- there is a difference in the frequency of dyslipaemias in diabetics under 50 compared to those over 50;
- under the age of 50 dyslipaemia is more frequently met with in men: over 50 in women;
- the most frequently abnormal lipid fractions are TG and NEFA in both normal and overweight diabetics, being more obvious in overweight diabetic women.

At the end of these introductory considerations, in which some related general problems have been reviewed, one can state that diabetic angiopathy is becoming a major medical priority because of:

- the great mortality rate among diabetics as compared to the healthy population, especially among the younger people;
- the increased incidence of diabetes mellitus, a phenomenon observed in all investigated areas where there is a rising living standard;

INVESTIGATED GROUP	AGE	CHOLESTEROL MEAN VALUES m %		TRIGLYCERIDES MEAN VALUES m %		NEFA MEAN VALUES mEq ‰		β+μ LIPOPROTEINS %	
		M	W	M	W	M	W	M	W
HEALTHY	< 50	175±4	175±3	124±5	127±4	537±12	545±11	63.8±0.7	62.8±9
	> 50	200±3	212±3	143±5	131±4	600±13	171±10	67.3±6	65.8±6
	% INCREASE	14	21	15	3	12	5	4	5
DIABETES MELLITUS WITH NORMAL WEIGHT	< 50	218±10	191±12	208±17	125±12	766±13	576±18	70.8±2.6	65.2±3
	% INCREASE	24	9	68	0	43	5	11	3
	> 50	228±5	243±9	192±10	179±11	751±12	732±31	72.3±0.9	72.5±19
	% INCREASE	14	14	34	36	25	28	7	10
OBESE DIABETICS	< 50	221±15	–	167±18	–	676±47	–	60.8±3.2	–
	% INCREASE	20	–	34	–	25	–	7	–
	> 50	234±5	231±6	194±11	188±12	763±25	728±23	73.9±1.1	74.0±0.9
	% INCREASE	17	8	35	43	27	27	10	12

Table X. Distribution according to illness, weight, age and sex of the mean values for C, TG, NEFA and β + μ-lipoproteins in serum.

- the remarkably high incidence of dyslipaemic states in the whole population;
- the obvious dyslipaemic effect of diabetes mellitus and the noxious effect of dyslipaemia on the blood vessels;
- therapeutical advances in diabetes, which prevent early deaths from acute complications, making room for the development of late, angiopathic diabetic complications.

There is an urgent requirement for prophylactic measures against diabetic angiopathy, even if, for the time being, its pathogenesis is not fully elucidated.

Chapter II Angiopathy in Diabetics

The importance of the late vascular complications in diabetes is clearly seen if one considers the high mortality associated with them in the post insulin period, as well as the fact that 90 % of diabetics suffering from diabetes mellitus for more than 15 years have one or several angiopathic manifestations [143]. – Certain mortality statistics contain figures over 76 % and the Metropolitan Life insurance reported 80% [71, 145]. Obviously, not all statistical information indicates such high figures. Bell [14], for instance, reported in 1960 the results of postmortem examinations of 2,559 subjects, finding death to be due to vascular lesions in 49.3% of the diabetic, as compared to 24.5% in the non-diabetic subjects. But the distinction must be made between information coming from pathology departments, where only final stages of a given condition are examined and information coming from sources where living individuals are investigated. Figures of the latter origin will always be higher, and most probably, nearer to reality, since not every diabetic angiopathy leads to death and many diabetics die of other causes. There are indications that the incidence of vascular complications in diabetes rises with the duration of the disease. This already appeared from the short historical review of the previous section and is suggested by almost all data reported in recent medical literature [96, 97, 145]. White and Waslow [65] found symptoms in 184 out of 200 subjects who had suffered from diabetes for over 20 years, that is in 92% of the cases.

As for the percentage of the various kinds of vascular lesions, the same authors [145] indicate 85 for retinal sclerosis, 80 for retinal haemorrhage, 75 for arterial calcification, 50 for nephropathy, 40 for arterial hypertension, 8 for coronaropathy and 2.5 for cerebral vascular disorders. It seems obvious, that the two modalities of angiopathy – diabetic micro- and macroangiopathy – are found in fairly similar incidence in diabetic subjects.

The state of metabolic balance of the patient seems to have some importance with regard to the general incidence of diabetic angiopathy, as well as to the moment of its onset, the rate of evolution and perhaps even to its preponderate pattern [145, 171, 177]. Statistical data recorded in various countries during periods when large sections of the population underwent famine have been put forward in favour of this argument. The case of France was quoted during the Franco-German War [32], and that of Germany during the Second World War [171], as well as the statistics recorded over 26 years by the Centre for Diabetes in Bucharest, on 16,676 diabetic subjects registered and under control in the same city. The low incidence of diabetes mellitus in Rumania between 1944 and 1947 is very obvious and coincides with the final period of the war and the subsequent drought. In the following years, increased incidence of diabetes mellitus and ipso facto, of its vascular complications went hand in hand with the improvement in the economic conditions of the population of the country (Fig. 1, 2).

There are also authors [96, 104, 123, 190] who, based on statistical data and long-term observation of patients, have the opposite standpoint, namely that the state of metabolic balance has no significant influence on the incidence and clinical aspect of the late complications of diabetes. When contrasted with the mass of data regarding the

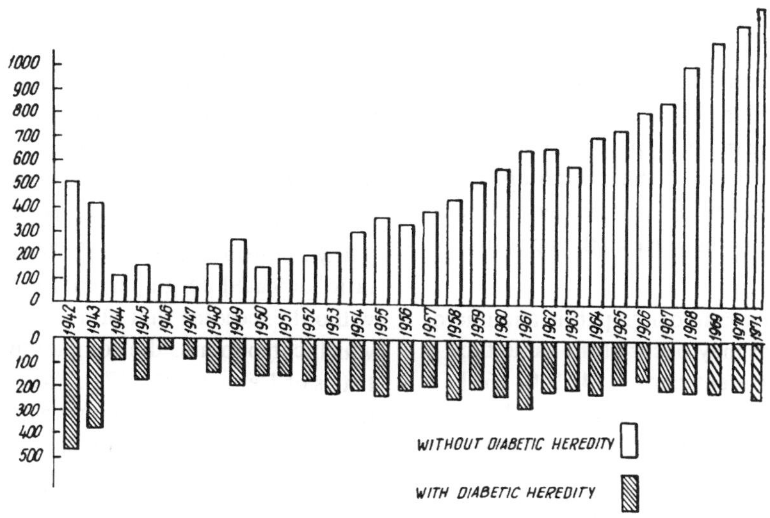

Fig. 1. Number of new diabetics with and without diabetic heredity registered in A.C.B. between 1942–1971.

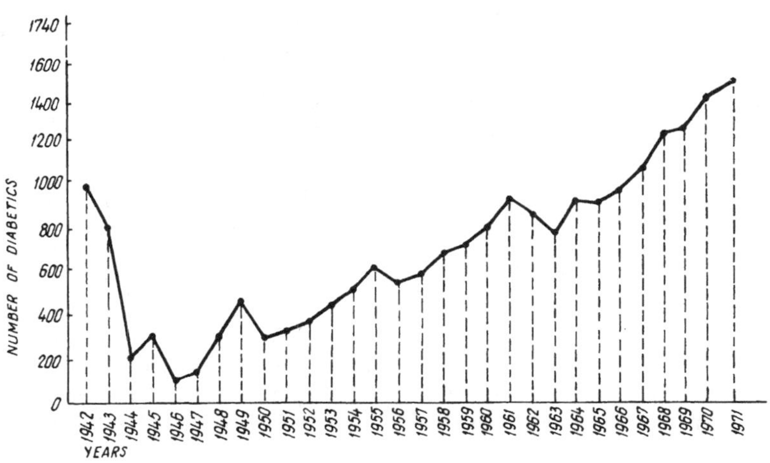

Fig. 2. Number of the newly registered diabetics in the A.C.B. in the period 1942–1971.

evolution of the causes of death in diabetes during the last 70–80 years, this opinion does not appear to be well substantiated.

The relation between diabetic angiopathy and the age and sex of the patients has been much debated in connection with the specificity of vasculopathy in diabetes. The sex distribution, the influence of duration or of a history of permanent or episodic metabolic imbalance and the importance of the patient's age induced some authors to claim that diabetes accelerates the onset and the course of certain common arteriosclerotic processes [14, 112], and others to support a theory in favour of a specific condition secondary to diabetes mellitus [96, 113]. Especially arteriopathy of macroangiopathy has been the object of strong arguments.

A particular feature of macroangiopathy in diabetes consists of its relatively increased frequency in females, a fact which differentiated this complication from the obvious male predominance associated with common arteriosclerosis [53, 138, 171]. But while the almost equal incidence in the two sexes appears to support the theory in favour of a specificity of diabetic arteriopathy, the fact that the condition is more frequent in maturity onset diabetes suggests the opposite [88].

The possibility that macroangiopathic and microangiopathic lesions may occur at the same time and develop at different rates [114, 160, 161], provided another argument in favour of those who attribute diabetic macroangiopathy to common arteriosclerosis.

Numerous observations suggest the existence of a syntropism of arteriosclerosis and diabetes mellitus. Beyond the facts showing an accelerated course of arteriosclerosis in the diabetic, many papers reported on arteriosclerotic phenomena in subjects with no symptoms of diabetes, but in whom biochemical investigations revealed disorders in fat metabolism similar to those found in diabetes and a characteristic diabetic pattern of tests of glucose tolerance [122, 127, 185].

A. Arteriopathy of Diabetic Macroangiopathy

The statistics of the Clinic of Metabolic Diseases and Nutrition in Bucharest, derived from a group of 3,639 diabetic patients admitted between 1964 and 1967, showed in 651 cases clinical, X-ray, electrocardiographic and/or oscillometric signs of diabetic arteriopathy. This group of patients (651) comprised 302 females and 349 males. Distribution according to age, sex and presumed duration of the disease is shown in table I.

The general incidence of diabetic macroangiopathy in our patients was 17.9% (Fig. 3). Sex ratio indicated a high percentage of females, without exceeding that of males, an observation which corroborates the comparatively recent statistics of Dérot (et al. [57]). The preponderence of males is not surprising in our case since the statistics performed at the Antidiabetic Centre in Bucharest on 16,676 diabetic subjects in that city

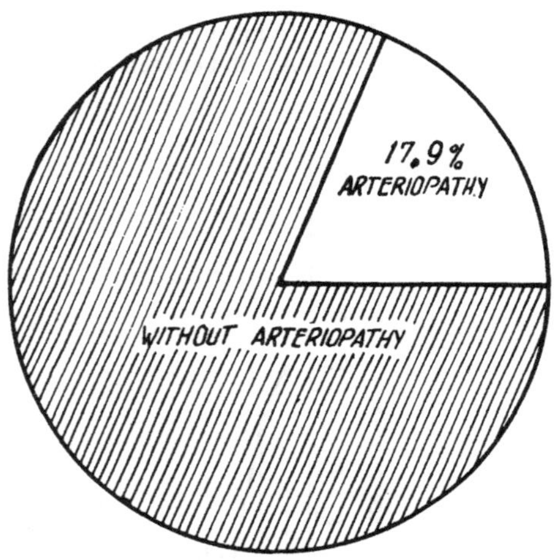

Fig. 3. Incidence of diabetic angiopathy in 3,659 inpatients between 1964–1967 in the Clinic of Metabolic Diseases and Nutrition in Bucharest.

Table I. Distribution of diabetic arteriopathy according to age, sex, and presumed duration of the disease (diabetes).

Year	Number of patients admitted	Number of patients with arteriopathy	Age years		Sex		Presumed diabetes		Duration in years	
			< 40	> 40	F	M	0	5	10	over 10
1964	1084	205	7	198	87	118	20	40	39	106
1965	882	164	4	160	79	85	17	35	40	72
1966	1118	187	7	180	89	98	20	38	43	86
1967	555	95	3	92	47	48	11	18	18	48
Total	3639	651	21	630	302	349	68	131	140	312

show that in all age groups, ranging between 11 and 60 years, males are preponderant. It is only under 10 and over 60 years that female preponderance is found (Fig. 4, 5).

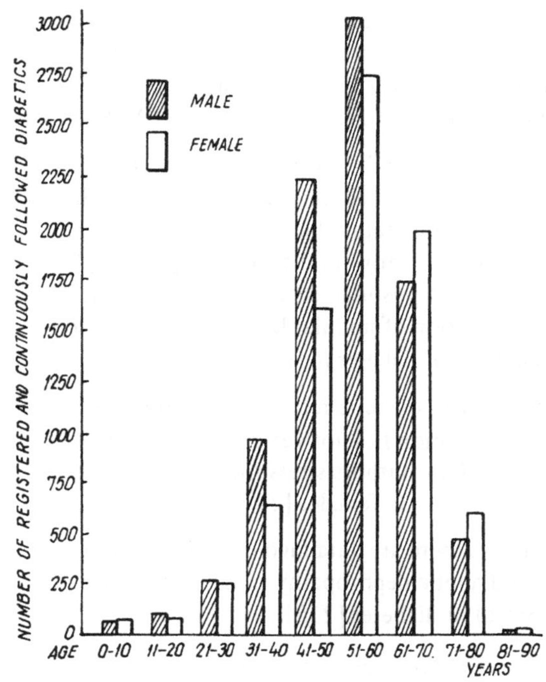

Fig. 4. Statistics of the A.C.B.. Distribution according to the sex and age of the registered diabetics in 1942–1968 period.

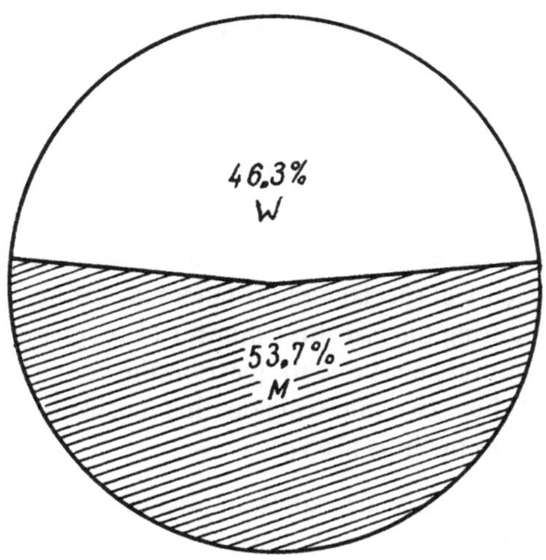

Fig. 5. Percentages of diabetic angiopathy incidence according to sex in 3,659 in-patients (1964–1967).

In a recent report, Pyke [153] was also unable to confirm a higher incidence amongst female diabetics. It must be noted that other series of patients have been reported in the literature, in which diabetic arteriopathy appears predominantly in females [53]. While this controversial circumstance does not permit a firm standpoint on the matter, it suggests that the difference between sexes, a specific feature of common arteriosclerosis, is abolished. In our statistics, diabetic arteriopathy appears mostly over the age of 40 and after a 10 year history of diabetes (Fig. 6 and 7), but there are earlier cases and after shorter lapses of time [154].

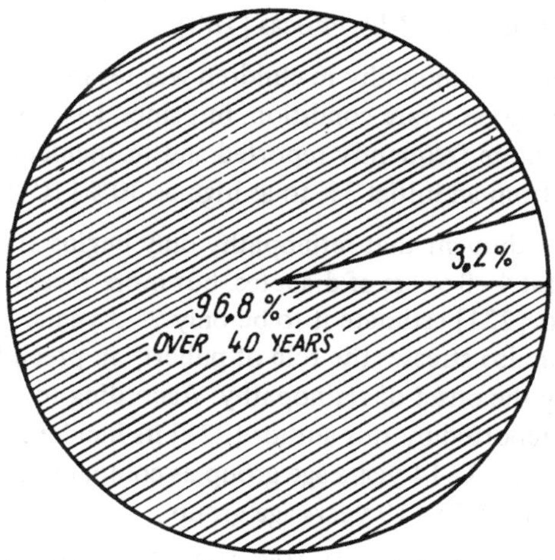

Fig. 6. Percentages of diabetic angiopathy incidence according to age in 3,659 in-patients (1964–1967).

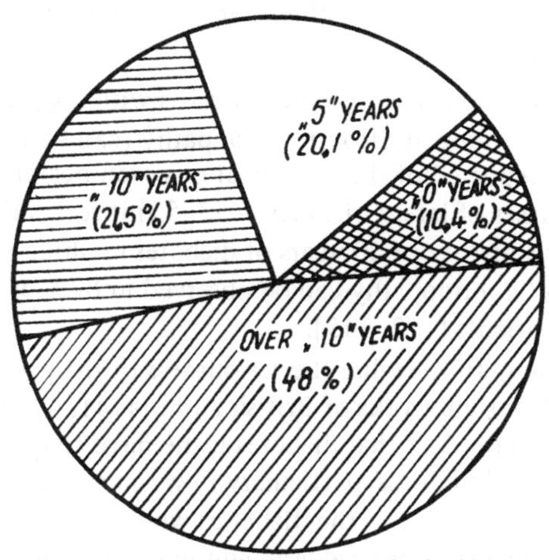

Fig. 7. Percentages of diabetic angiopathy incidence according to the duration of diabetes mellitus in 3,659 in-patients (1964–1967).

B. Diabetic Microangiopathy

The prevalence of diabetic microangiopathy has been investigated especially with regard to its two chief clinical patterns: diabetic retinopathy and diabetic nephropathy.

It has been claimed that 1/3 to 1/2 of all diabetic patients suffer from diabetic retinopathy [178]. Janert et al. found it in 28.8% of a group of 3,000 diabetic out-patients (109) and in 33% of 2,600 hospitalized diabetics [108]. Similar figures have been reported by others, such as 30% by Morisiani [163] and 46.5% by Phocas [180].

Diabetic retinopathy in children was regarded 30 years ago as a rare condition, but since 1947 it has been more frequently reported and its incidence rose from an initial 3% to as high as 30% [104].

It was thought that retinopathy only begins after at least 4–8 years of diabetes, but more recent works [221] estimate it to be only 2–3 years. Unger also stresses the role of puberty in precipitating the onset of retinopathy. According to data reported by this author [221] its incidence is 4% in the 9–14 years age group as compared to 14% in the 15–19 years age group.

Numerous authors [79, 108, 109, 171, 180] maintain that diabetic retinopathy is predominant in females, while many others deny this [104, 124, 125, 145].

If controversial information persists with regard to the beginning of diabetic retinopathy (cases have been reported of the complications even beginning in phases of latent diabetes – 53, 52) it seems that after a history of 20 years of diabetes mellitus diabetic retinopathy can be observed in 82% of the patients [112, 145].

One may fully realise the seriousness of the problem from the works of British authors [41, 42, 43] who established that diabetes is the most frequent cause of blindness, particulary in women. It was found that most of the diabetics who became blind were adults or elderly and in this context diabetic retinopathy is the most important complication leading to blindness.

As for diabetic nephropathy, the other more thoroughly investigated diabetic microangiopathy, most of the clinical and pathological studies have found its incidence rose with the duration of the diabetes [215]. The onset of the renal complication is, however, difficult to date, especially since the electronmicroscopic studies indicate it as almost simultaneous with the apparent onset of the diabetes itself. (See Chap. IV, p. 105.)

It is more difficult to estimate the most frequent age of onset of diabetic nephropathy than that of diabetic retinopathy, because renal investigations are less informative in the early stage. It might, however, be postulated that ageing accelerates the evolution of nodular lesions in this late complication of diabetes mellitus.

Just as with diabetic retinopathy, a sex-linked differentiation has not yet been demonstrated [171]. Many authors stress the prevalance of the complication in females [215].

Finally, there are data favouring the hypothesis that diabetic nephropathy is associated with poor control of diabetes [215].

The coexistence of diabetic retinopathy with diabetic nephropathy and other aspects of diabetic angiopathy must be ascertained for both theoretical and practical reasons. It has long been thought that diabetic retinopathy is a sequel of the long-lasting renal disorder in the diabetic patient, as in Kimmelstiel-Wilson's disease [135]. More recent work suggests that diabetic retinopathy and diabetic nephropathy are found simultaneously in the same patient, but neither can be regarded as secondary to the other [108, 109]. Petrides [178] states less categorically that the above association only occurs in special circumstances, as for instance during the last three months of pregnancy. Other authors continue to question the coexistence of these two microangiopathic localizations in diabetes mellitus [165].

Investigating this correlation in post-mortem material, Ashton found diabetic retinopathy in 64.7% of the diabetic subjects explored, but only in 36.9% of these did he also find diabetic nephropathy. Diabetic retinopathy alone was found in 45% of the subjects [135].

Lieb [135] claimed that the incidence of the association between diabetic retinopathy and diabetic nephropathy increases with the severity of the former, that is, when it reaches more advanced stages. Fischer [79] reached similar conclusions having compared a group of 40 diabetic subjects with proliferative diabetic retinopathy, in which nephropathy was found in only two cases, with another group of 40 patients with plain diabetic retinopathy, 17 of whom had no signs of nephropathy.

According to Otto et al. [171] minimal retinopathy is associated with diabetic nephropathy in 33% of the cases, while for more severe forms, including proliferative retinopathy, the incidence rises to 78%. The author found a 91% overall percentage of diabetic retinopathy in patients suffering from diabetic nephropathy. This suggests that the glomerular nodule of diabetic nephropathy is a much more advanced capillary lesion than the first signs of ocular microangiopathy. If so, the presence in some subjects of diabetic nephropathy without concomitant retinopathy becomes more difficult to explain.

Various modalities of diabetic angiopathy have also been found in association with diabetic neuropathy [77, 208].

Feudell [77] reported in 1964 that there is a statistically significant correlation between diabetic neuropathy and diabetic angiopathy. The fact that clinical diagnosis usually favours one of the forms of diabetic angiopathy – the arteriopathic or microangiopathic type – localized in a given area of the organism, seems to be an important peculiarity of these late vascular complications, namely that their fairly ubiquitous character goes hand in hand with a tendency to preponderance in one particular area. This local preponderance against a generalized pathological background may depend on various secondary

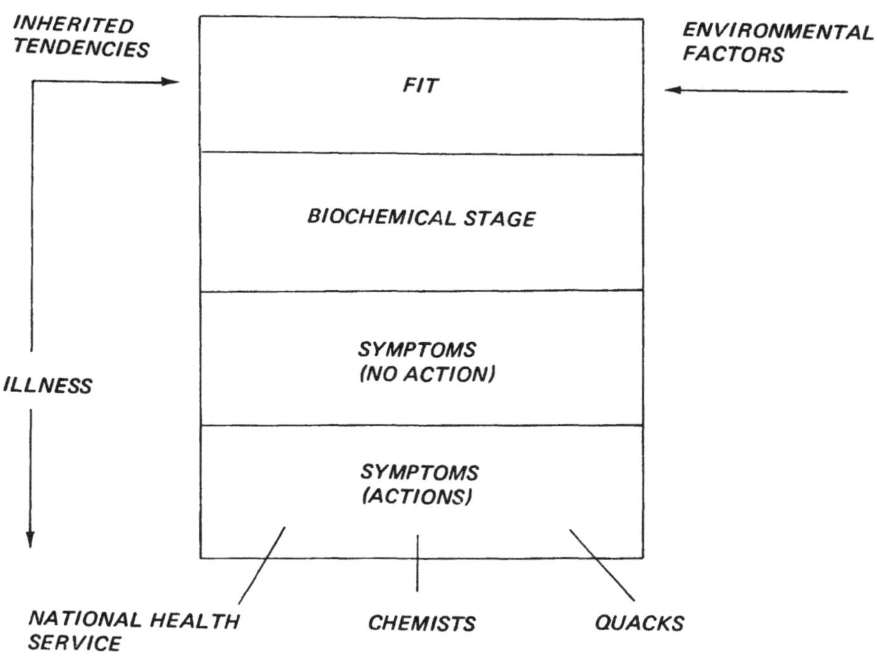

Fig. 8. Manifestation of diabetic angiopathy and patient's solicitation for adequate treatment (Butterfield).

causes, which may be inherited or acquired. Hence, the order of onset and importance of symptoms, will indicate to the physician the particular course taken by diabetic angiopathy in every single case.

As for the subsequent course of the complication, prophylactic and curative management acquires an outstanding importance, and largely depends on whether the patient calls a competent physician or is confined to an empirical management of his condition. Butterfield's diagram [32], illustrates the crucial moments on which the evolution of a case depends, taking into account the stage of evolution and the therapy applied, and suggests certain explanations for the wide differences in the course of various cases of diabetic angiopathy (Fig. 8).

We shall close this discussion on the prevalence of diabetic angiopathy by presenting our statistics of the late complications of diabetes mellitus, recorded on 4,875 diabetic subjects admitted between 1961–1967 into the Clinic of Metabolic Diseases and Nutrition in Bucharest. Diabetic angiopathy is considered here in the full sense of the term, including both diabetic arteriopathy (macroangiopathy) and microangiopathy irrespective of the area of their preponderant localization.

The data summarized in Table II pertaints to 2,062 patients with juvenile diabetes, with onset before the age of 25, and to 1,813 patients in which the disease started at an adult age. Figures indicate a preponderance of females and an overall incidence of angiopathic involvment of 44.72%.

Diabetic angiopathy appears in our statistics more frequently associated with adult (59.9%) than with juvenile (34%) diabetes. In all these patients diabetic angiopathy has been proved by clinical signs, laboratory tests (complex functional investigations) or pathological findings with biopsies of the kidney, muscle, skin and liver.

Figures in Table III present the relation between the incidence of diabetic angiopathy and the presumed duration of diabetes mellitus. A graphic representation of the same is shown in Fig. 9.

Table III

Duration of diabetes in years	Incidence of diabetic angiopathy in percent	
	Juvenile diabetes	Adult diabetes
0– 5	26.3	29.9
6– 9	63.6	44.8
11–15	70.4	57.7
16–20	84.2	61.9
21–25	65.6	89.1
26	62.5	100

These figures show the early presence of diabetic angiopathy, during the first five years of the disease, in both types of diabetes and a peak incidence of these complications corresponding to an 18 year history of the disease.

For a comparison with our data, we present in Fig. 10 the average incidence of the late vascular complications found in Sweden, according to the statistics of Grönberg [96]. The curves are of a

Table II

Type of diabetes mellitus	Number of patients	Sex		Patients		Incidence of DA according to type of diabetes	Overall incidence of DA
		F	M	with DA	without DA		
Juvenile	2062	1115	947	955	1107	34 %	
Adult	2813	1495	1318	1225	1588	59.4%	44.72%
Total	4875	2610	2265	2180	2695		

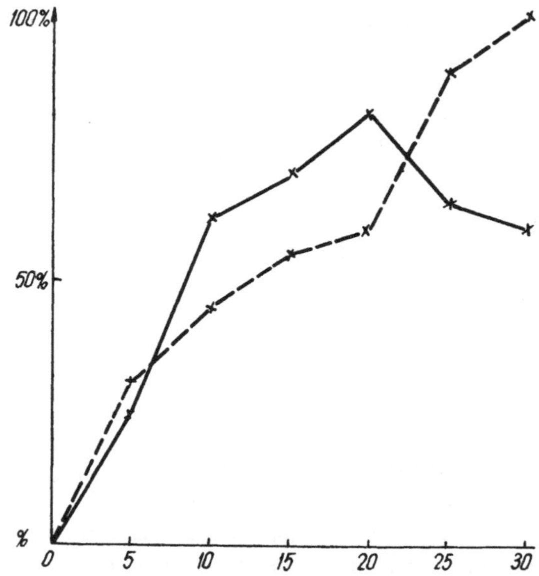

Fig. 9. Incidence of diabetic angiopathy according to the apparent duration of diabetes in juvenile and maturity diabetes (Statistic on 4,875 in-patients).

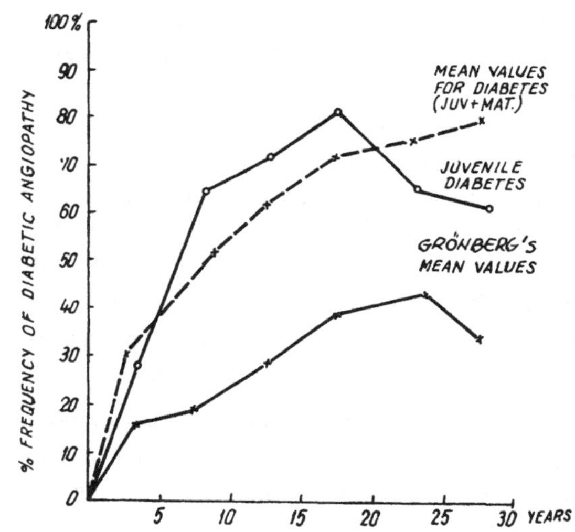

Fig. 10. Diagram for comparison of the diabetic angiopathy according to age in our own and Grönberg's statistics.

quite similar shape (juvenile diabetes is represented in our statistics by a continuous line and in Grönberg's by a broken line). We only compared the two representations of juvenile diabetes

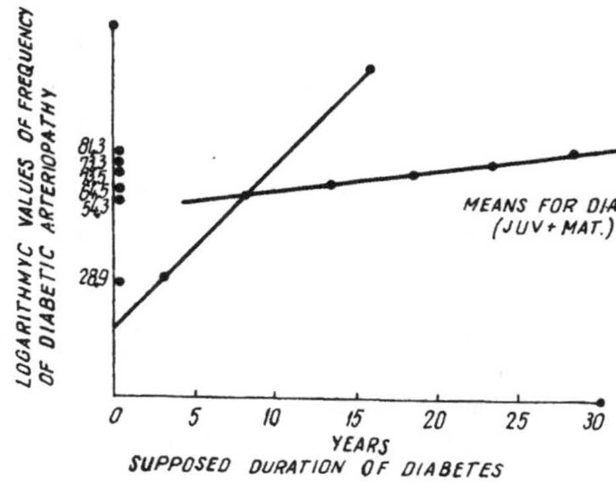

Fig. 11. Semi-logarithmic diagram for the global incidence of diabetic angiopathy, according to the apparent duration of diabetes mellitus.

since Grönberg's statistics only take into account the cases of microangiopathy.

Again Fig. 10, a dotted line represents the average total incidence of both macro- and microangiopathy in our statistics. These data represented on a semi-logarithmic scale (Fig. 11), result in a broken line with two portions of different slope. A first, steeper slope, corresponds to the cases with less than 10 years duration of diabetes and the second portion of milder slope represents the cases that lasted over 10 years. It can be concluded from this that the time interval between the 5th and 10th year after the presumed onset of the disease is a critical one when the incidence of angiopathy suddenly increases. Further increase is gradual and continuous, but occurs at a slower rate.

As regards the possible relation between the incidence of diabetic angiopathy and the type of therapy, the data summarized in Table IV is not sufficient to allow evaluation of the effects – good or bad – of various kinds of therapy [121].

It seems to us that the type of management is less important than whether it resulted in a good, moderate or poor control over the years of therapy.

In this sense, we have been unable to apply the criteria suggested by Keiding [145], much too severe to be applied to large and heterogeneous

Table IV

Diagnosis	Total number of patients		Type of management				
			Insulin 40	IS U. 40	SA	BG	diet only
Juvenile diabetes mellitus	AD	955	440	440	42	33	–
	Without AD	1107	663	430	8	34	2
Diabetes mellitus with maturity onset	AD	1225	346	346	447	84	2
	Without AD	1588	608	354	488	130	8

where: AD = Diabetic Angiopathy

groups of patients. We considered a case to be well-balanced if:

- the general condition was generally good, overweight absent, physical and psychic activities normal,
- clinical signs of diabetes mellitus were absent under therapeutic management,
- hypoglycaemic episodes were avoided,
- glycosuria was reduced to a minimum but not suppressed,
- acetonuria and acidotic episodes were absent,
- diet was maintained under good control [145].

We regarded as moderately balanced a diabetic patient in whom high levels of glycosuria persisted, and blood sugar figures rose over 200 mg% and the history recorded rare acidotic episodes and evidence of wrong therapeutical indications with regard to diet and antidiabetic drug administration.

We included in the group of poor treatment, subjects in which the signs of diabetes did not subside, history was rich in acidotic, precomatous, comatous and even hypoglycaemic episodes, and there were reasons to believe that management had been confused and irregular.

Fig. 12 and 13 represent statistical data on the incidence of diabetic angiopathy in juvenile diabetes mellitus (Fig. 12) und adult diabetes mellitus (Fig. 13), distributed according to the three qualitative forms of long-term management.

With juvenile diabetes, angiopathic involvement is particulary frequent in the "poor treatment" group (Fig. 12). A similar although less marked trend was found amongst maturity onset diabetics (Fig. 13).

In summing up the literature and the personal findings presented above, we feel that a number of correlations of practical importance may be suggested:

a) diabetic angiopathy is a late complication of diabetes mellitus and should be regarded as such once the clinical picture including alterations of the complete vascular system or selected areas has been established. However, its early stages do not always occur in a late period of the disease.

The incidence of this complication reaches a peak at the end of the first decade of the disease.

b) angiopathy prevails in the female, despite the fact that the general incidence of diabetes in the two sexes, indicated in certain statistics is higher in males.

c) a positive correlation seems to exist between the onset and evolution of diabetic angiopathy on the one hand and long-term poor metabolic control of diabetes on the other.

d) no relation could be established between the incidence of diabetic angiopathy and the hypoglycaemic treatment applied.

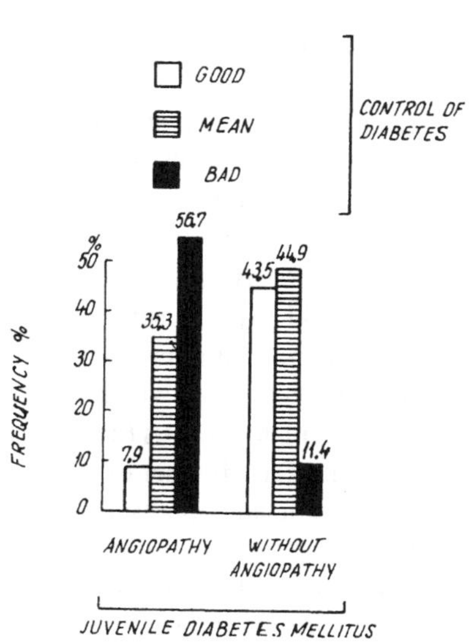

Fig. 12. Correlation between the efficiency of antidiabetic treatment and diabetic angiopathy manifestation in juvenile diabetes mellitus (Statistics on 4,875 in-patients).

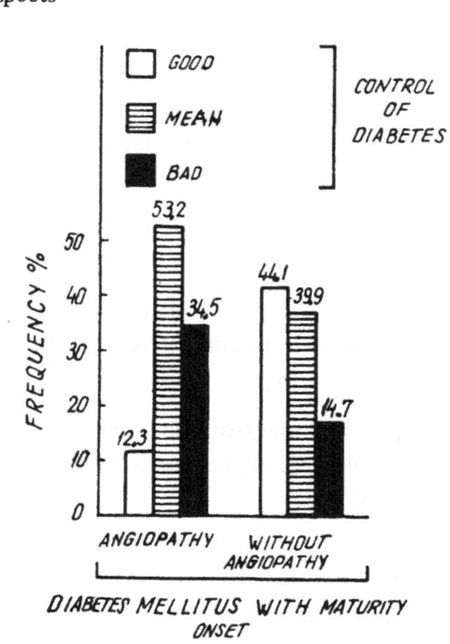

Fig. 13. Correlation between the efficiency of antidiabetic treatment and diabetic angiopathy manifestation in diabetics with maturity onset (Statistics on 4,875 in-patients).

C. Pathological and Electronmicroscopic Studies – characteristic aspects

Regarded as a whole, pathological and electronmicroscopic studies of the blood vessels in diabetes mellitus have revealed certain general characteristics which, while not specific to diabetes only, are grouped in a particular configuration.

Histochemical and microscopic investigations have been performed in almost all organs and more recently electronmicroscopy has brought an outstanding contribution to elucidating ultrastructural aspects. The main aspects described in diabetic angiopathy are presented below.

1. Diabetic Angiopathy of the eye

Diabetic angiopathy of the eye was among the first pathologic patterns to draw attention to the vascular involvement of the disease. Its particular interest lies in the fact that some ocular capillaries – the retinal ones – can be examined "in vivo" and in that the structure of the retinal vessels is intermediate between the structures of the overall systemic and the cerebral ones. Caird et al. [42, 43] describe the retinal vessels as follows: "The retinal arteries have a well-developed median internal elastic lamina, little collagen and no elastic fibres in the media and no nerve fibres. The retinal capillaries resemble those of the brain in having non-fenest rated endothelial cell cytoplasm and their mural cells resemble those found in many other capillaries. They differ from those of other organs in having a thicker basement membrane, both outside the mural cell and outside the endothelial cells at sites where there is no mural cell cytoplasm. The veins are similar to those elsewhere, except that they lack a muscularis. The retina like the brain has no lymph vessels."

The vascular changes found in diabetic retinopathy which will be described in more detail in Chapter III – and those found in the other parts of the eye, can be summed up as follows:

1. microaneurysms of capillaries and veins, sometimes found in the iris, where they make up what is called iritis rubeosa [105];

2. haemorrhage in the deeper retinal layers;

3. presence of the so-called "cytoid bodies" in the nervous tissues, probably subsequent to damage of a capillary area;

4. rubeosis retinae in juvenile diabetes mellitus, due to hypertrophy of the capillaries;

5. vascular proliferation towards the corpus vitrosum, as described in proliferative diabetic retinopathy [135, 136].

From the optic and electronmicroscopic points of view, the pathological aspects appear to consist of [21, 41, 42, 43]:

- thickening of the basement membrane spreading in patches to finally involve the basement membrane as a whole;
- a rise in the number of endothelial cells;
- a fall in the number of mural cells.

In parallel with these aspects a PAS-positive material that cannot be stained with colloidal iron is deposited in the capillary walls [22, 23, 92]. Capillary occlusions are frequent and microaneurysms of the terminal arterial and venous capillaries are fairly characteristic [43].

The extravascular retinal lesions associated with diabetic retinopathy will be dealt with in detail elsewhere. But the above already features some of the general characteristics of diabetic angiopathy, such as the uneven and segmental distribution of the lesions, at least in the early phase and the once more uneven involvement of all the components of the vascular wall.

Besides the retinal lesions, alterations in the bulbar conjunctiva have been described in the children of diabetic mothers as early as 1954 [63]. Recent work of Italian authors [132] confirmed, by light and electronmicroscopic technique, the presence of angiopathy in the conjunctival capillaries. It comprised an uneven thickening of the basement membrane of the conjunctival vessels. The main alterations described here are dilations of the veins, the "sludge" phenomenon, unequal calibre of the veins and microaneurysms ([49, 59, 63, 87, 128, 129] / see Chapter III).

2. Diabetic Angiopathy of the Kidney

The plainest expression of diabetic angiopathy in the kidney – a subject that will be discussed in detail in Chapter IV – is diabetic nephropathy of glomerular origin which was described by Kimmelstiel and Wilson (1936) as eosinophilic nodules in the glomerular area [126]. The subsequent description of a diffuse glomerular sclerosis and of a so-called "exsudative" variety, in which such pathogenical factors as benign sclerosis (common arteriosclerosis) interfere, further extended the importance of diabetic angiopathy and emphasized the interaction and reciprocal potentiating effects of diabetic microangiopathy and macroangiopathy. The concept of nephropathy was gradually widened [61, 62, 205]. A review of the main alterations described in the renal small vessels demonstrates the morphological association of diabetic nephropathy with diabetic microangiopathy in general. They consist of the following:

- a thickening of the basement membrane, regarded by some researchers [21, 56, 151] as the earliest glomerular anomaly, sometimes present even in the stage of inapparent diabetes, but altogether lacking in certain cases of diabetes [21]. The latter fact induced Kimmelstiel in 1966 to deny [119] the specific importance generally attributed to this process.
- a festooned folding of the basement membrane [151] and of the neighbouring endothelial cells, resulting in extensions which seem to penetrate between the respective cells,
- the endothelial cells undergo a sort of swelling and their pores become indistinct here and there, occasionally obliterating some capillary loops [21].
- a proliferation of the mesangial cells, regarded by some authors as the most frequent alteration found in juvenile diabetes [81], and by Kimmelstiel [120] as the primarily involved structure of the diabetic kidney,
- an accumulation of mesangial matrix among the mesangial cells [56],

- the epithelial cells of the glomeruli, podocytes are not extensively altered; although their pedicels may sometimes fuse resulting in coalescence with the basement membrane [151]. This aspect occurs in association with significant proteinuria.
- a thickening of Bowman's membrane [56].

It is obvious that the diabetic alterations of the glomerular vessels widely reproduce those already mentioned in the eye as also those found in other organs. The assimilation of the perithelial cells in the capillary in general, with the mural cells of the retina and the mesangial cells of the kidney offers, according to Kimmelstiel, a specific common denominator to the microvascular pattern of diabetic angiopathy.

Besides these lesions conferring a degree of specificity on the glomerular diabetic angiopathy, aspects have been described similar to those found in collagen diseases in man or rabbit, subsequent to the administration of cortisone (cortisone lesions). These are so-called exsudative phenomena, known as "hyaline fibrinoid" "capsular drops" and "fibrin caps". They consist of PAS-positive material deposits situated (a) between the endothelial cells of the glomerular capillaries and the basement membrane, (b) in the lumen of the capillaries, which acquire a foamy aspect because of their high lipid content, (c) between the "epithelial" parietal cells and the basement membrane of Bowman's capsule. With the electronmicroscope they appear as homogenous, osmiophilic masses, which immunohistochemically, seem to be a sort of fibrinoid-containing gamma globulin and a certain amount of lipids [21].

The alterations in the tubules, mainly comprise:

- partial thickening of the basement membrane, sometimes intruding into the tubular lumen,
- numerous vesicles and vacuoles which have been described in the apical portion of tubular cells, particularly in children and,
- an increased glycogen content found in all renal cells (56).

This brief review of the main alterations noticed in diabetic nephropathy draws attention to the similarity of the renal vascular lesions with microangiopathic findings in other organs. It also contributes, to a certain extent to the understanding of some of the problems of the pathogenesis of diabetic angiopathy.

3. Diabetic Angiopathy in the Muscular System

Diabetic angiopathy in the muscular system has been morphologically investigated especially in the skeletal muscle. Information on muscles in some internal organs, such as for example the heart, is generally grounded on post-mortem observations, since no techniques of obtaining biopsies are yet available.

The light microscopic aspect of small vessels in the skeletal muscles in diabetes mellitus was thoroughly investigated by Goldenberg et al. [92]. They found that lesions involve both the endothelium and the basement membrane of the capillaries. Endothelial alterations range between simple swelling and prominence of the endothelial cells into the lumen and obstruction of the lumen subsequent to proliferation. The latter is more frequent in the small arterioles than in the capillaries themselves.

The most remarkable alterations were again found in the basement membrane. The PAS-positive material deposited there has been described by authors as not staining with colloidal iron according to the Rinehardt-Abu-Hay method.

According to Bloodworth this resistance to staining of the fibrillary network, cannot be regarded as a specific feature of diabetic microangiopathy (21) and hence cannot serve, as Goldenberg et al. advocate, as a specific element for a morphological differential diagnosis of diabetic angiopathy from the common arteriosclerotic lesions.

Similar alterations of the basement membrane have been later described by Zacks [227] in 5 patients. The author stated that he was unable to correlate the light and electronmicroscopic findings with the degree of metabolic control of the diabetes. The thickening of the basement membrane was confirmed by this author and later by Bencosme et al. [15]. The latter did not find narrowing of the lumen in the medium and small arterioles. The basement membrane in the capillaries, described as composed of very thin concentric lamellae, grows to a thickness of 25,000 Å while in the normal subject it ranges between 1,000–6,000 Å. The fibrillary structure itself is accentuated in the basement membrane of diabetic subjects, which was explained by Bencosme as subsequent to the swelling of the basement membrane. Bencosme et al. described in the areas where this swelling occurs, the presence of heaps consisting of a variable number of compact masses of osmiophilic material, probably lipidic. Their size reaches 400 Å to 1 microne diameter and over.

Our own electronmicroscopic investigations on puncture biopsy specimens obtained from leg muscles or from surgical interventions as well as on post-mortem examinations, generally confirm the above data. (See Chapter VI, p. 184)

- an uneven and segmentary distribution of the alterations. This is very obvious for instance in Fig. 14 and 15, illustrating specimens where aspects from the muscles of the thigh and the abdomen of subjects in whom amputation was performed (because of peripheral ischaemic syndromes).
- the fact that all the layers of the small vessel walls are involved, but in an uneven manner, changing from vessel to vessel and in the same patient. This refers both to the thickening of the basement membrane, estimated by us on electronmicroscope pictures (Figs. 16, 17, 18) according to the procedure recommended by Siperstein [206], and to the endothelial altera-alterations. In vessels with a perimeter of the basement membrane of 14.8–15.2 microns, we have been able to observe an average thickness of 2,000 to 2,500 Å (figs. 16, 17, 18) as compared to a thickness of 980–1,050 Å found in normal subjects in the same perimeter range.

A comparison of the alterations found in the basement membrane of capillaries from the leg muscles and from the kidney of the same patient (diabetic) by simultaneous biopsy of muscle and right kidney demonstrated the uneven involvement of the vessels of the two organs compare Figs. 18 and 19.

- the same unevenness and variability from vessel to vessel and from organ to organ has been observed in the capillary endothelium. We compared the electronmicroscopic aspects of endothelia in the vessels of the leg muscles and liver sinusoids in specimens obtained by simultaneous punctures of these organs in the same subject [46]. We regard the results of this study as important since diabetic angiopathy has been investigated in the liver almost exclusively in the small ramifications of the hepatic artery, but not at the level of the hepatic sinusoids, which are the typical capillaries of that organ. It will be shown below in this section that the existence of endothelial proliferation and hypertrophy in the hepatic sinusoid is different from the process that occurs in the same subject in the muscular capillaries.

This difference might be illustrated by comparing Figs. 20 and 21, both belonging to a controlled diabetic subject, with a 10 year history of the disease.

Unlike the capillaries of skeletal muscles, those of the human heart have only been investigated in diabetes mellitus by light microscopy on post-mortem specimens. As regards the small arterioles and the coronaries, many data confirm the presence of alterations of an arteriosclerotic type and the fact that the evolution of the diabetes mellitus enhances the development of this kind of lesion.

In our researches we also resorted to post-mortem material from diabetic subjects and we systematically found deposits of PAS-positive material on the walls of the myocardial arterioles and capillaries (Fig. 22).

There are no electronmicroscopic investigations of the diabetic human myocardium [56], but in experimental diabetes Orth and Morgan in 1962 [169] reported indirect evidence of a deficit in the myocardic microcirculation, describing a picture

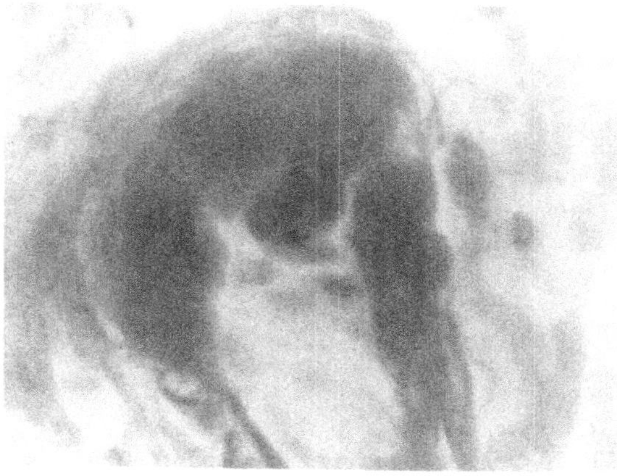

Fig. 14. M. A. Thigh muscle capillary in a diabetic woman with diabetic angiopathy. Great subendothelial accumulation of PAS-positive material.

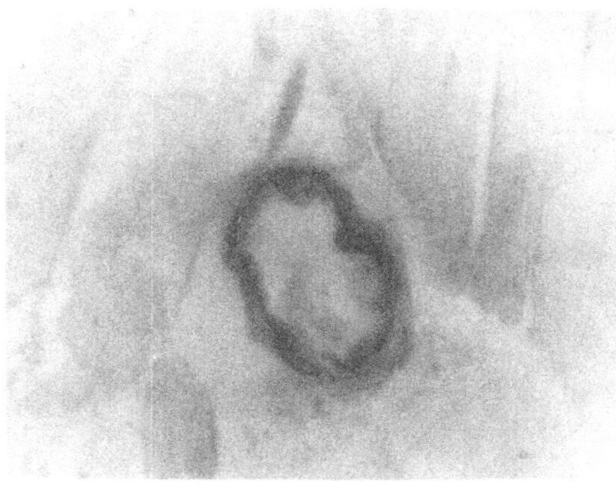

Fig. 15. M. A. Same patient as in fig. 14. Small vessel from the abdominal muscles. Accumulation of PAS-positive material in the walls with prominence of the larger endothelial cell in the vascular lumen.

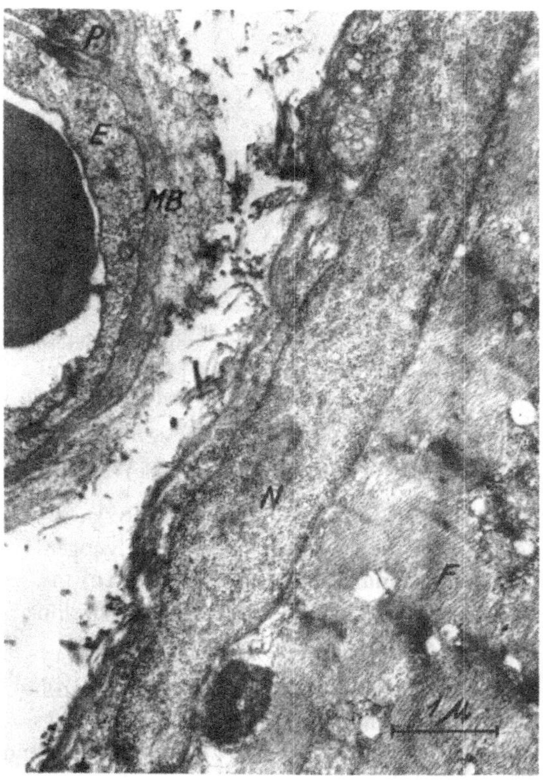

Fig. 16. L. I. Healthy individual. Capillary from shank muscle. MB = normal basement membrane; E = normal endothelial cell; P = pericyte; N = nucleus in muscle cell; F = striated muscle fibres (20,000 x).

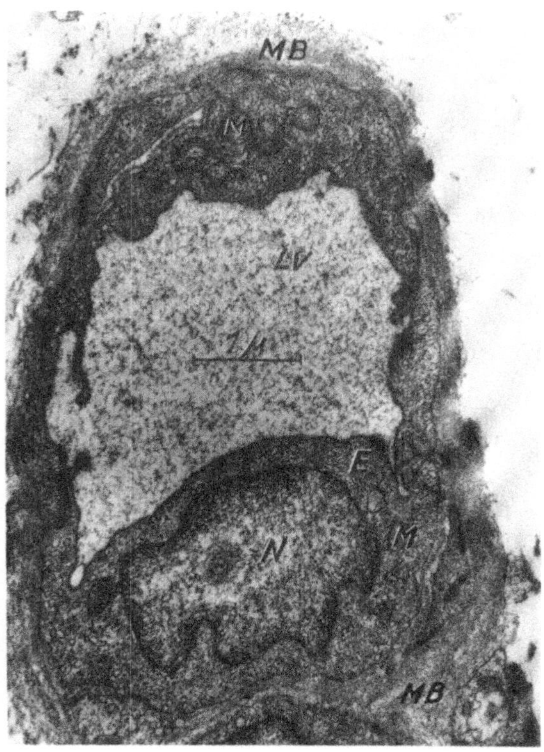

Fig. 17. S. F. Shank muscle capillary in a diabetic subject without apparent symptoms of diabetic angiopathy. MB = fibrillar and slightly thickened basement membrane; E = hypertrophic endothelial cell; N = nucleus in the E; M = mitochondria in the E; LV = vascular lumen (20,000 x).

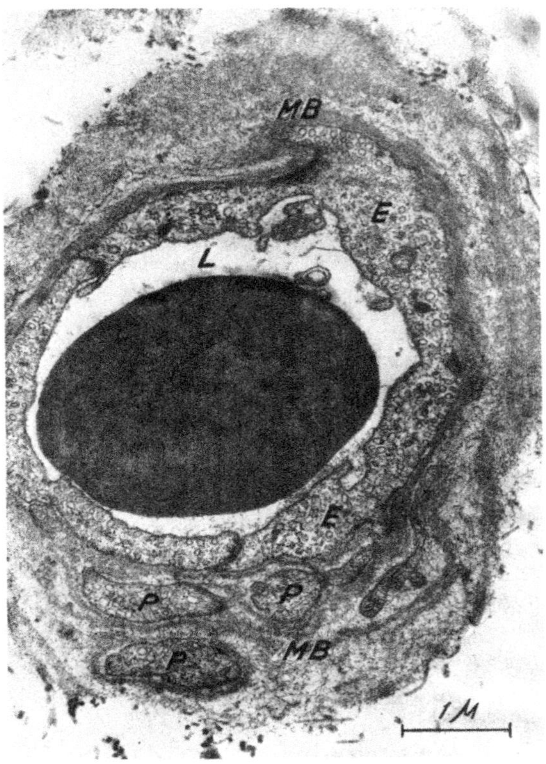

Fig. 18. D. C. Shank muscle capillary in mis-treated diabetes mellitus with diabetic angiopathy. MB = thickened basement membrane including pericytes (PC); E = hypertrophic endothelial cell; L = vessel lumen; H = erythrocyte (20,000 x).

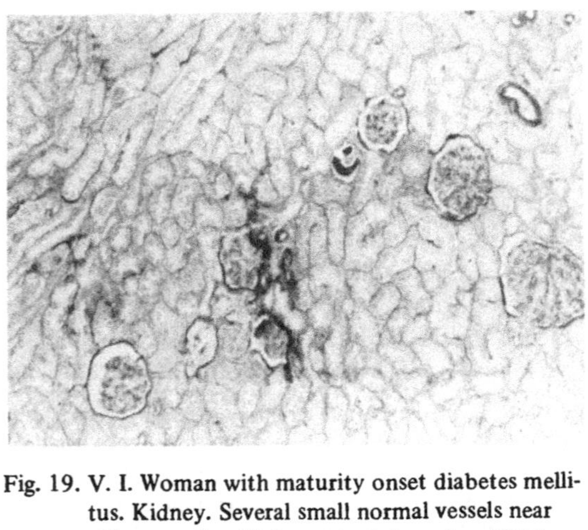

Fig. 19. V. I. Woman with maturity onset diabetes mellitus. Kidney. Several small normal vessels near other vessels with important deposits of PAS-positive material.

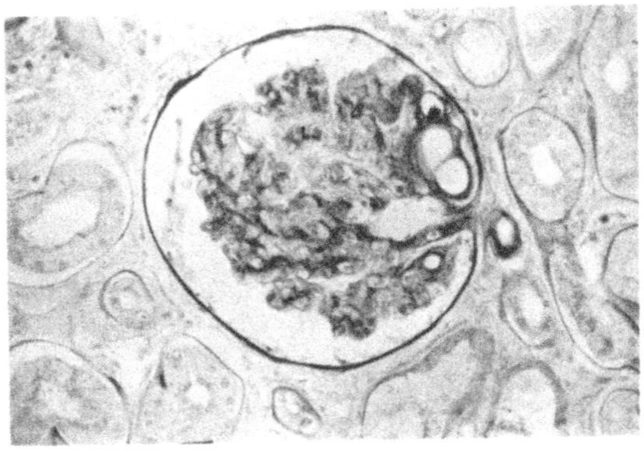

Fig. 20. Same person as in fig. 19. Deposits of PAS-positive material in the renal glomerulae.

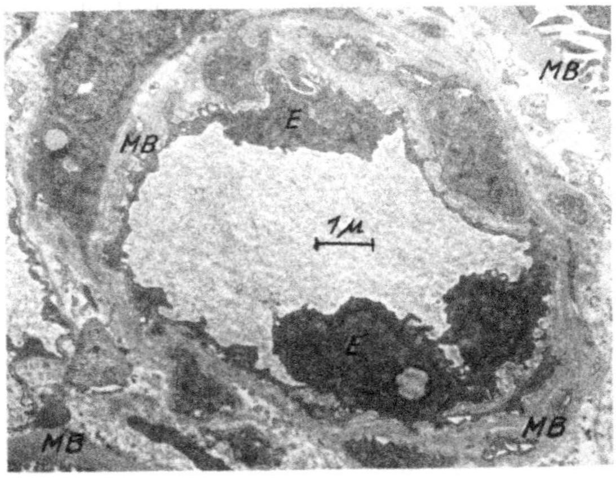

Fig. 21. I. A. Bioptic material from kidney. Diabetes mellitus. MB = thickened basement membrane of a small intraglomerular vessel. Endothelial hyperplasia (E) (8,000 x).

similar to that found in myocardial anoxia. It consisted of the disappearance of the glycogen-containing granules, increased hydration of the sarcoplasma and an early mitochondrial swelling with accumulation of osmiophilic bodies.

All these light microscopical alterations, corroborated with certain electrocardiographic findings, reviewed in detail in Chapter V, show the existence of macro- and microangiopathy in the human myocardium in diabetes mellitus. Its ultrastructural picture may be similar to that described in the animal treated with alloxan, a fact which remains to be demonstrated in the future.

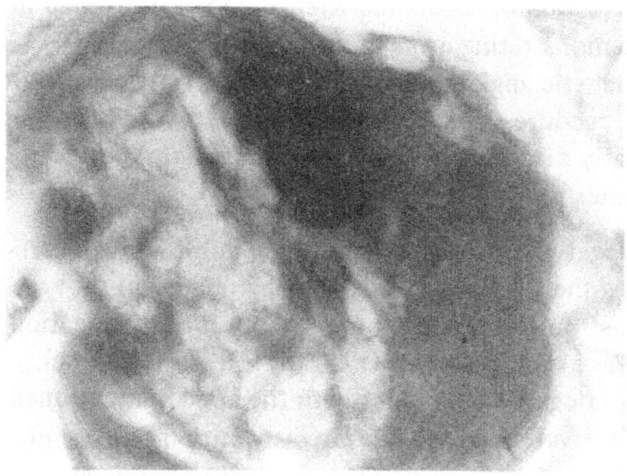

Fig. 22. V. A. Woman with diabetic coma. Necroptic material from the heart. Thickened walls of coronaries with abnormal deposits of PAS-positive material.

4. Diabetic Angiopathy in the Digestive Tract

Only in recent years has diabetic angiopathy in the digestive tract been more thoroughly investigated [4, 5]. Most of the available data rely on postmortem examinations and less on specimens obtained by biopsy or during surgery [5]. More recently biopsy specimens have been obtained by new procedures from the oral, gastric, intestinal and rectal mucous membranes [25, 159].

In the majority of these cases concomitant diabetic nephropathy and retinopathy and often also diabetic neuropathy were found.

In the oral mucous membrane Angerval [4, 5] found the same thickening aspect of the vascular walls, with accumulation of PAS-positive material and reduction of the vascular lumen, eventually producing total obstruction. Worth mentioning is his observation of the patchy distribution of the process, almost normal areas alternating with others of obvious diabetic angiopathy. At the same time, although the presence of a true endothelial proliferation cannot be demonstrated, a high number and prominence of the endothelial cells was often observed.

Similar lesions have been described all along the digestive tract, although post-mortem alterations sometimes rendered their interpretation difficult. Diabetic angiopathy was usually present in other organs as well. In a number of patients from the Clinic of Metabolics Disease and Nutrition in Bucharest, light microscopy after PAS-staining showed the same aspects, namely thickening of the walls of the small vessels by deposits of PAS-positive material, patchy distribution and uneven involvement of the vascular walls (Figs. 23, 24, 25, 26).

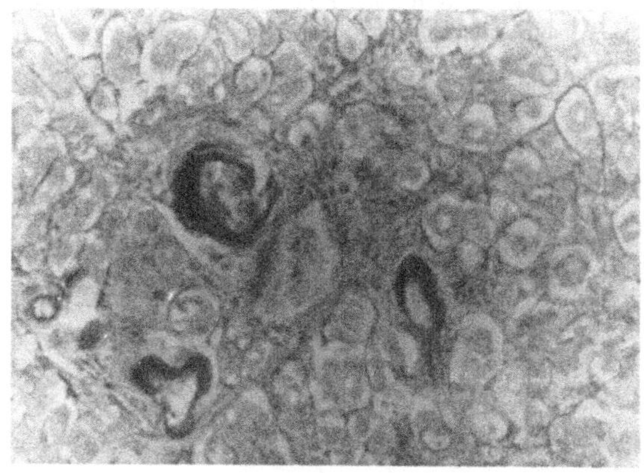

Fig. 23. I. P. Diabetes mellitus with peripheral angiopathy Necroptic material. Pancreas. Thickened walls of arterioles with accumulation of PAS-positive material.

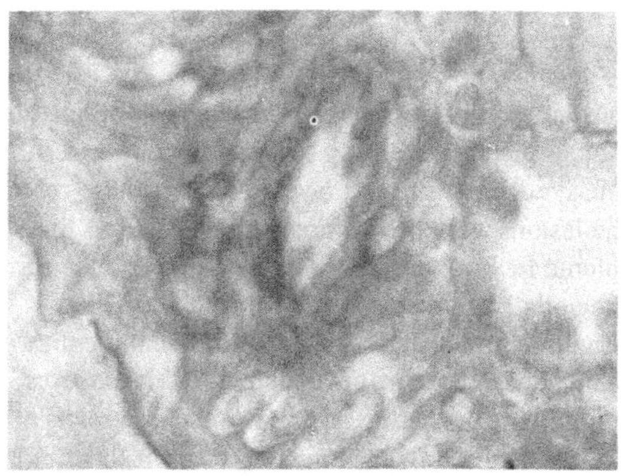

Fig. 24. I. P. Light microscopic aspect of intestinal wall. Arteriolae rich in PAS-positvie material.

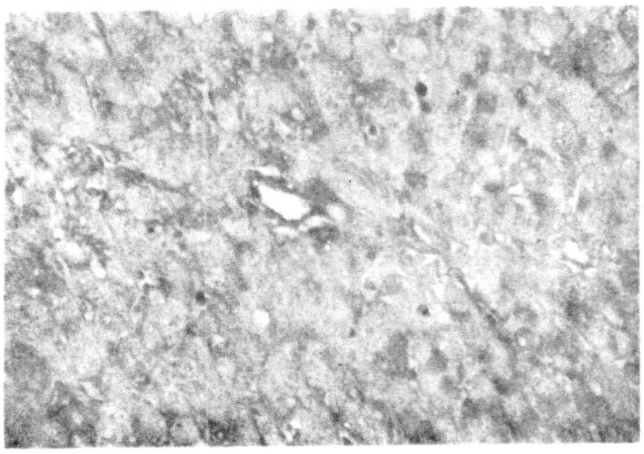

Fig. 25. Light microscopic aspect of the liver in necroptic material. Arteriolae rich in PAS-positive material deposited in their walls.

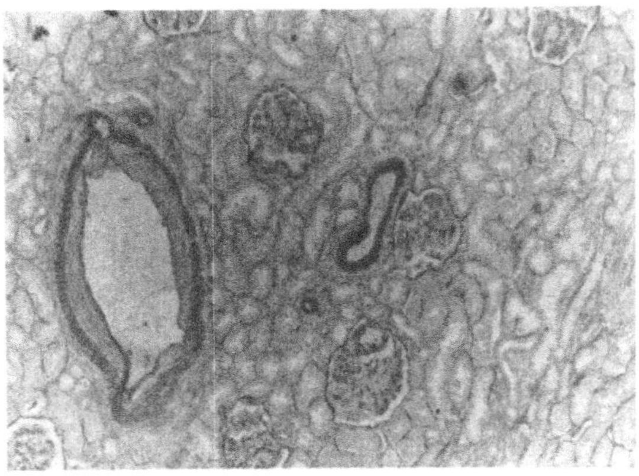

Fig. 26. Light microscopic aspect of the kidney in necroptic material. Kidney arteriolae with large deposits of PAS-positive material in the walls.

Particularly interesting data have been obtained in biopsy specimens during surgery in vascular ischaemic syndromes of the bowel [142]. In these cases, the lesions were predominantly localized at the splenic flexure, a point of critical importance in the collateral vascularization of the bowel [95]. It will be noted that a transient ischaemic colitis seems to be more often associated with diabetes, subsequent to the involvement of small vessels in the bowel. Pathological investigation in this field was limited to standard staining techniques for routine light microscopy.

In 1968, Missmahl and Rieman [159] succeeded in demonstrating on rectal biopsies the presence of diabetic angiopathy at that level and advanced the procedure as a harmless and useful method for the early diagnosis of this late complication of diabetes mellitus.

Negative reports have also been published concerning the presence of diabetic angiopathy in the gastrointestinal tract, even where the complication was identified in other organs [16, 25, 28]. Such findings are consistent with the already mentioned observation of the uneven distribution of disseminated diabetic angiopathy in the various organs of the body.

Of the organs associated with the gastrointestinal tract, the liver has been most studied, as it has been easier to biopsy. However, as we have already stated, these studies were almost exclusively focussed on the small branches of the hepatic artery [56, 229], and therefore they only dealt with type A capillaries. Thus, the alterations of the type B capillaries have been ignored, perhaps because the thickening of the basement membrane has been regarded as the most important element of the process. Moreover, many authors considered that in the picture of diabetic angiopathy, the role of the endothelial cells is of little importance [1, 159] or even totally irrelevant [88]. Nevertheless, the hepatic sinusoids represent a model of the type B capillaries which, because of the particular structure of the liver and the absence of a basement membrane, permits a detailed examination of the endothelial cell and of the Kupfer cell, probably derived from the former.

To this end we performed biopsies in 28 diabetic and 2 normal subjects. The diabetics (19 females and 9 male) had diabetic histories of from 1 to 7 years duration, were under insulin therapy and on an adequate diet. Eight subjects suffered from juvenile diabetes mellitus – one of them with lipoatrophic diabetes mellitus. The other 20 had diabetes mellitus with maturity onset. Previous examination with the light microscope elminated from this group the subjects in which microscopic evidence of any other hepatic condition was found (chronic hepatitis). Consequently, in 17 of our subjects, we were justified in regarding any alteration as exclusively related to the presence of diabetes mellitus [46]. On clinical examination and standard laboratory investigation of the liver, all our diabetic patients seemed to be in the normal range. Muscle biopsies were also performed on the two healthy subjects and 4 of the diabetic subjects, for electronmicroscopic examination. We found the following:

a) In the skeletal muscles a thickening of the basement membrane and a remarkable proliferation of the endothelial cells overlapping each other. The large number of cell organelles, the particular aspect of the nuclei and the abundant and sometimes giant microvilli were proof of the participation of the endothelial cells in the general metabolic abnormality of diabetes mellitus. The monstrous hypertrophy of these cells sometimes almost completely obstructed the vascular lumen. These aspects were in contrast to those found in normal subjects (Fig. 27).

b) In all our diabetic patients, the hepatic sinusoids showed simple swelling of isolated endothelial cells and exuberant growth of long sinous microvilli leading to the total obstruction of the sinusoidal lumen (Fig. 28, 29, 30). The presence was noted in all these cells of gigantic nuclei with corrugated membranes, filling most of the cell. The cytoplasm was comparatively rich in mitochondria, dense bodies and electrondense inclusions. The smooth endoplasmic reticulum was often found to be very wide while the pinocytotic vesicules were rarer than in healthy subjects (Figs. 28, 29, 30, 31, 32).

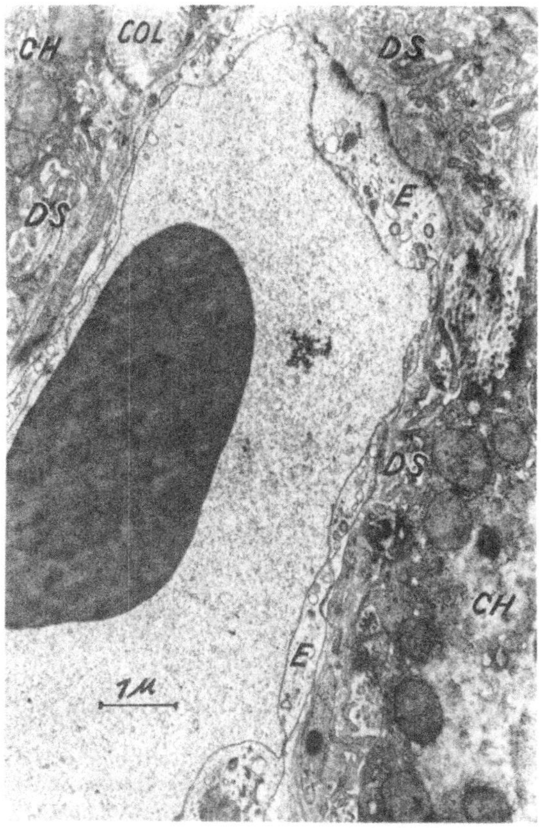

Fig. 28. Liver biopsy in a normal subject. Liver sinusoidal capillaries with unistratificated endothelial cells (E). DS = Disse's space; CH = hepatocytes; COL = collagen fibres in Disse's space.

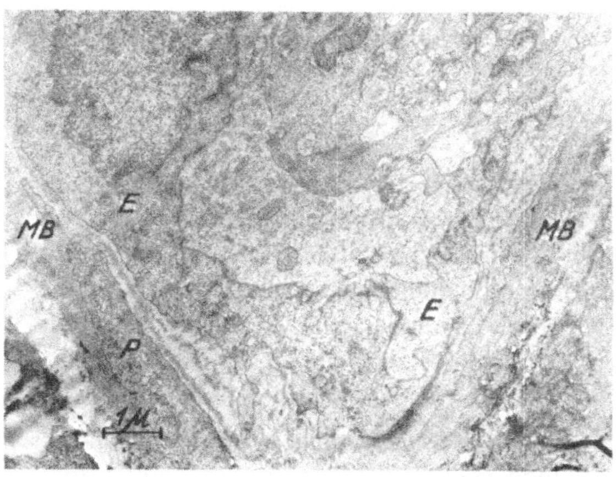

Fig. 27. M. N. Diabetes mellitus with angiopathy. Muscular biopsy of the shank. MB = thickened basement membrane including pericytes (P). Hypertrophic endothelial cells (E) with obvious tend to obturate the vessel.

We may sum up the above data as follows:

– the hepatic sinusoidal endothelium participates in the pathological picture of the diabetic angiopathy to almost the same extent as the endothelium of peripheral vessels,

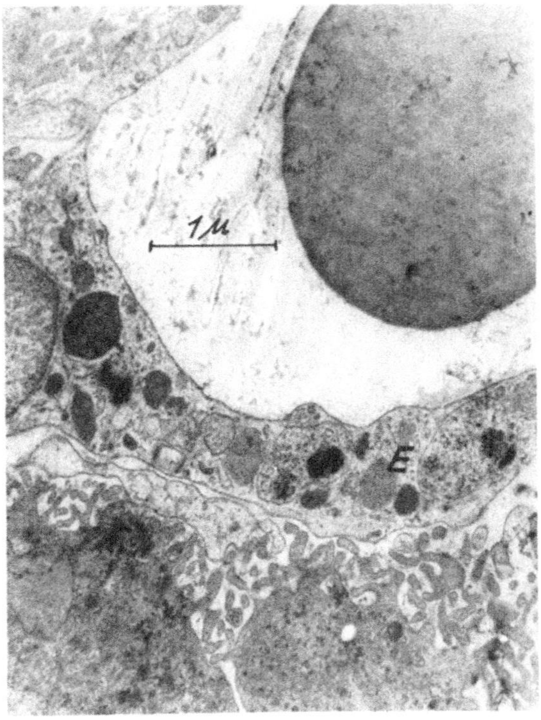

Fig. 29. P. I. Recent diabetes with maturity onset. Liver sinusoidal capillary with unistratificated endothelial cells (E) very similar to those of normal individuals (20,000 x).

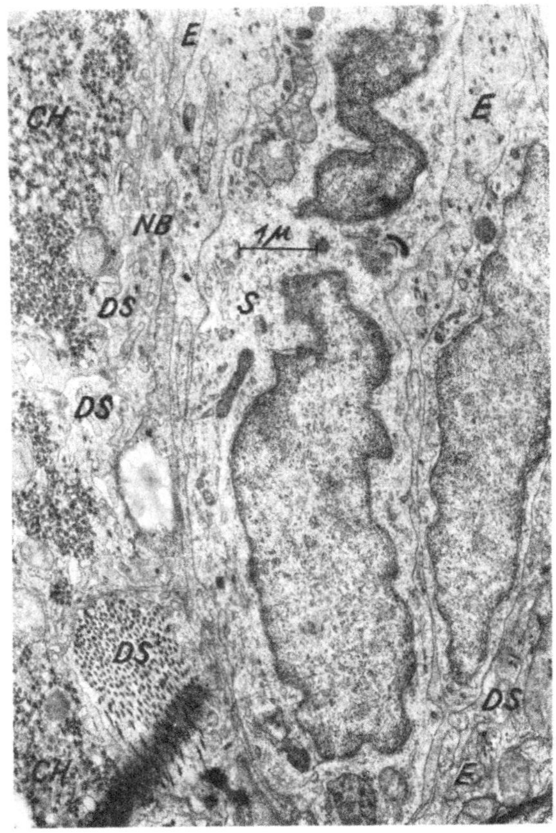

Fig. 30. P. E. Diabetes with maturity onset of long duration. Liver sinusoidal capillary (S) with stratification of endothelial cells (E), rich in cell organites and intracellular inclusions. CH = hepatocytes; DS = Disse's space; NB = diminuation of the microvilli in Disse's space (15,000 x).

– the existence of a hepatic endothelial involvement is significant because it once more confirms the ubiquity of diabetic angiopathy, but it is also significant in itself, as it proves the participation in diabetic angiopathy of the capillaries without the basement membrane, a participation which some authors claimed [22, 23, 92] and others denied [1, 88, 181].

5. Diabetic Angiopathy in the Skin

Diabetic angiopathy in the skin has been less subject to research in spite of the rich clinical picture found at this level.

Light microscopy [1, 25, 66] confirmed the presence of PAS-positive thickening in the capillary walls, especially in the papillae of the dermis and around sweat glands, an aspect we were also able to confirm on skin biopsies (Fig. 33). Special mention should be made of the lesions of dermal lymphatic capillaries, characterized by accumulation of PAS-positive material at the borderline between the capillary and the surrounding tissue.

These lesions have been noticed sooner than those of blood capillaries. This suggests the ubiquitous nature of angiopathy and draws attention to the metabolic disturbances.

A more systematic investigation provided a detailed enumeration of the signs indicating the

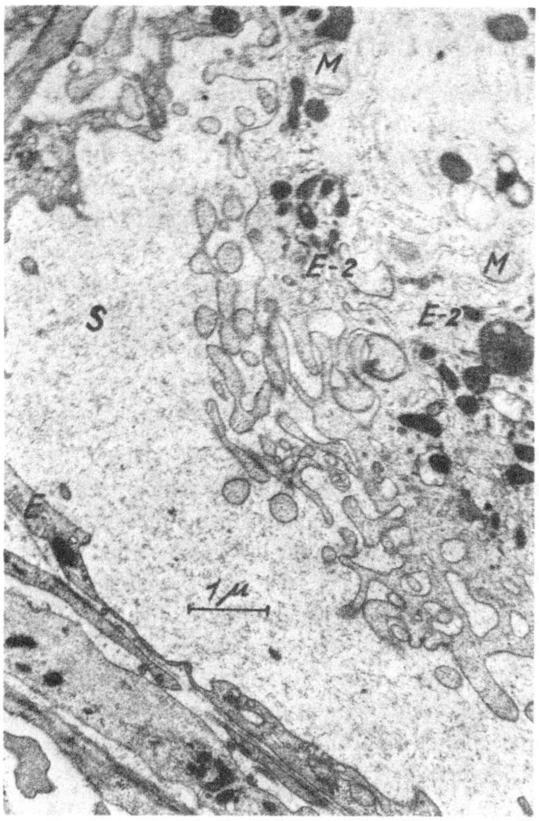

Fig. 31. P. E. Liver biopsy in maturity onset diabetes. Liver sinusoidal capillary with endothelial hyperplasia and hypertrophy (E). Numerous pseudopodes of the endothelial cells. M = mitochondria (15,000 x).

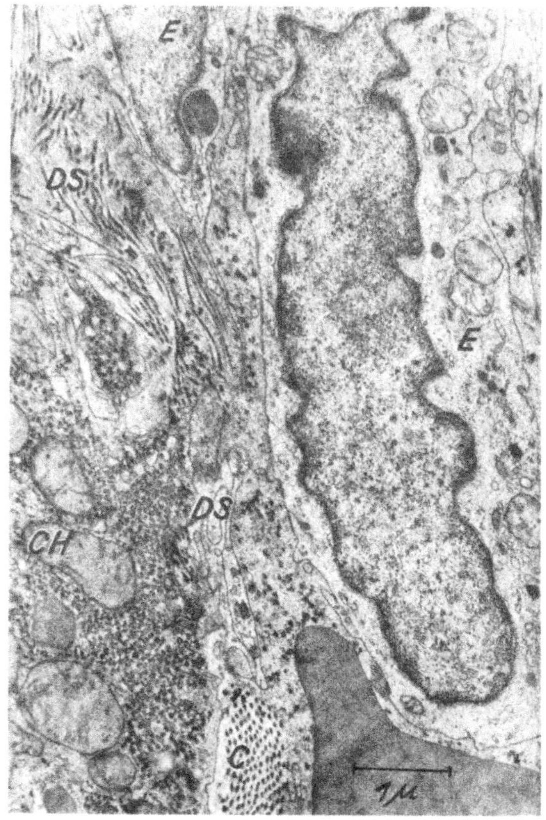

Fig. 32. D. A. Liver biopsy in juvenile diabetes mellitus. Liver sinusoidal capillary with proliferation and hypertrophy of the endothelial cells (E). DS = Disse's space; CH = hepatocytes; C = collagen fibres in Disse's space. Decreased microvilli in Disse's space (16,000 x).

presence of microangiopathy in the skin [181, 193, 194]:

- proliferation of the endothelial cells and subsequent narrowing of the respective vascular lumen,
- thickening of the fibrous adventitia and PAS-positive reaction. Its structure might be (a) dense and homogenous (with a hyaline aspect) or (b) lamellar (with a fibrillary aspect),
- perivascular infiltration with round, mononuclear cells (many mast cells).

The distribution of the skin lesions is uneven in a given patient and even in the same preparation (Fig. 33) one finds normal or almost normal capillaries alongside others with advanced PAS-positive infiltration [194]. In more severe cases, the capillary walls may grow ten times thicker than normal and the process seems to extend along the arterioles and veins. In larger vessels the deviations from the norm are more difficult to percieve.

A classification according to the degree of severity of the anatomical lesions in the skin, as advocated by some authors [130] appears to be useful

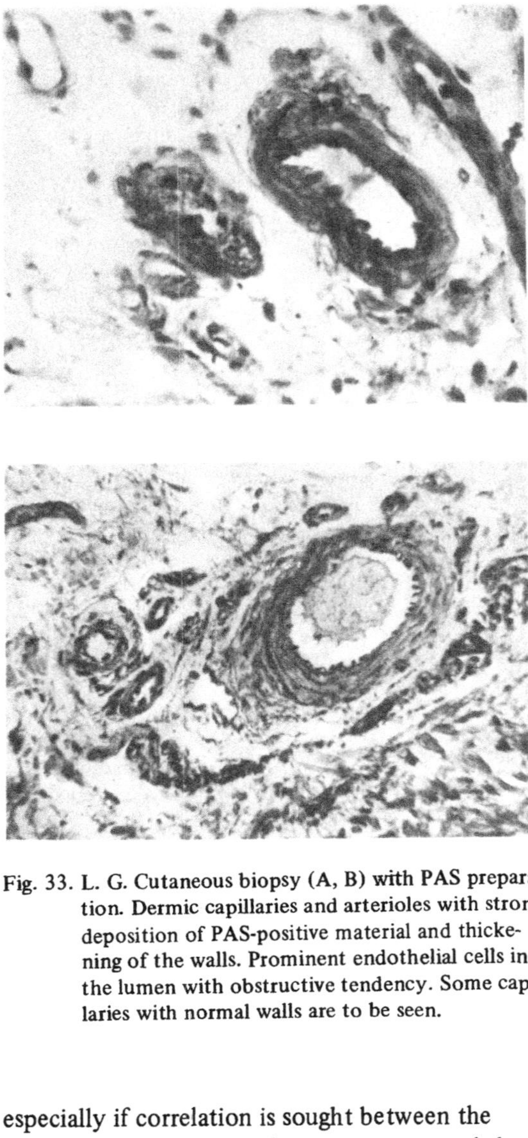

Fig. 33. L. G. Cutaneous biopsy (A, B) with PAS preparation. Dermic capillaries and arterioles with strong deposition of PAS-positive material and thickening of the walls. Prominent endothelial cells in the lumen with obstructive tendency. Some capillaries with normal walls are to be seen.

especially if correlation is sought between the angiopathic alterations of various organs and the duration of the diabetic condition. Such a classification was advanced in 1967 by Larson:

1st degree of skin lesions, also found in healthy individuals, consist of a delicate PAS-positive reaction in vessels mostly in those with thin walls.

2nd degree – in certain small vessels a slight PAS-positive thickening is present.

3rd degree – marked thickening with intense PAS-positive reaction of most of the vessels.

4th degree – extreme thickening of most vessels resulting in total obliteration of vascular lumens.

Statistical evidence in this field is scarce, but there is data indicating that the accumulation of PAS-positive material increases with the duration of the disease. In some cases the PAS-positive depots have a lamellar aspect. The endothelial cells [1] and the number of cells around the altered vessels, were not found to be different from normal ones by all investigators. It should also be mentioned that in the same vessel PAS-positive material accumulation was more obvious on one side of the capillary than on the other.

Immunofluorescent staining [130] enabled the simultaneous ascertaining of the degree of thickening of the capillary wall and of the presence of certain immunoglobulins in the same area. Fluorescent antibody technique provided evidence of the concomitant accumulation of gamma-globulin in various vessels of the dermis [130] and of the PAS-positive thickening of the vascular wall, an important argument in favour of the view, that, pathogenetically, diabetic angiopathy is a phenomenon of self-aggresion.

Electronmicroscopic techniques showed that in most of the skin capillaries of the diabetic subject the walls were thicker than in the normal individual [1]. A material similar in density and structure to that of the basement membrane, accounts for this thickening. It accumulates around the endothelium, incarcerates the pericytes and has sometimes an uneven, lamellar aspect. This latter aspect has also been found in healthy subjects [56, 223], but the overall thickeness of the basement membrane was different.

Some control investigations described a marked polymorphism of the skin capillaries in diabetic and non-diabetic patients, arousing a certain scepticism as regards the possibility of identifying diabetic angiopathy at that level [85].

Earlier works do not mention alterations in the endothelial cells, which however do exist. More recent investigations describe a thickening of the endothelial cells, with occasional proliferation and an increased number of pinocytotic vesicles [164], both more constantly found in patients with a diabetic history of over 10 years. In cases of more recent diabetes (4–10 years) these endothelial changes are less frequent and they are altogether missing in cases where the disease is less than 2 years [164, 173] old.

Recently, Romani et al. [193] described the same alterations of the small vessels of the skin in obesity, finding that in diabetes they are more frequent (in 80.7% of diabetic patients as compared to 59.6% of the obese) and more severe.

We may conclude that the most frequent alteration is a thickening of the basement membrane. It seems to have an early start, even in latent diabetes, since it was found in so many obese patients, and to advance with the duration of the disease. Changes in the capillary endothelium have been less extensively investigated and their participation in the cutaneous processes of diabetic angiopathy requires further study.

A great number of circulatory disorders of diabetes mellitus, both of the arteriopathic and microangiopathic type, have macroscopic expression in the skin. Such is the cutaneous expression of the diabetic arteriopathy in the lower limbs and the so-called necrobiosis lipoidica diabeticorum [113] in which light microscopy revealed the already mentioned alterations of the small vessels. The degree of necrobiosis differs with the distance between the vessel and the necrobiotic focus (4th degree in the focus, 3rd degree at its periphery, 2nd and 1st degrees at a distance [113]). These observations also illustrate the uneven and segmentary distribution of the pathological alterations in diabetic angiopathy.

6. Diabetic Angiopathy in Diabetic Neuropathy

It is still controversial whether diabetic neuropathy should be regarded as a form of diabetic angiopathy. Researchers during the 1930's and 1940's sought for a solution by investigating the nerves and the nervōus system. But Muri demonstrated as early as 1949 [166] that microscopic findings in the nervous system do not offer a satisfactory explanation of the clinical symptomatology of diabetic neuropathy. The following facts suggest that neuropathy is to be associated with angiopathy:

1. the higher incidence of diabetic neuropathy over the age of 40;

2. the frequent association of diabetic angiopathy and diabetic neuropathy, to a statistically significant degree [77].

Such facts induced Fagerberg [73] in 1956 to explain the neurological signs of diabetic neuropathy as due to the involvement of the small vessels of the peripheral nerves.

Subsequently Dreyfus claimed in 1957 [64], on the ground of a detailed study of the oculomotor nerve, that the findings reported by him and his co-workers might very well correspond to a moderate ischaemia of the nerve.

In 1959 Ellenberg and Krainer [68] admitted the possible vascular origin of the neuropathic symptoms found by them in the detailed examination of a patient. They did not observe vascular occlusion phenomena. The extremely varied picture found in the peripheral nerves, where very severe lesions of the nerve fibres alternate with well conserved areas, suggests a vascular origin similar to that of the neuropathies found in periarteritis nodosa.

In three cases of diabetes mellitus with peripheral neuropathy, Reske-Nielsen and Lundabaek [189] described, in 1963, vascular lesions very similar to those considered as typical for diabetic angiopathy.

In 1965, Fagerberg [73] contributed once more to the problem by reporting biopsy findings in 151 crural nerves from diabetic patients. He aimed at demonstrating that the most frequent abnormal finding in patients suffering from diabetic neuropathy is a non-inflammatory, patchy degeneration of the medullary sheath. Wall thickening, PAS-positive deposit and lumen narrowing were found in the intraneural vessels, histochemically equivalent to the alterations described in the retina and the kidney. The vascular alterations were actually found in association with nerve lesions.

This point of view was further supported by subsequent research with new observations on the histological aspects of vascular sclerosis in the peripheral nerves and the coeliac plexus in diabetic neuropathy [93].

The alteration of Schwann's cells in diabetic neuropathy consists, at electronmicroscopic level, of a thickening of the basement membrane and accumulation of phospholipids in the cytoplasm. The former is also found in diabetic angiopathy and particularly in diabetic nephropathy [20].

The similarity between diabetic neuropathy and diabetic angiopathy is also suggested by reports on alterations found in the internal ear [110] and in diabetic amyotrophy [94]. After examining the internal ear of 32 diabetic subjects, Jorgensen reported an uneven involvement of the capillaries in various segments of this organ. PAS-positive thickening of the capillary walls was found in the vascular striae and in the stapedius and tensor tympani muscles, but not in the capillary network of the spiral ligament in the vestibular portion of the labyrinth. It was suggested that the process is equivalent to a diabetic angiopathy of the labyrinth vessels [60, 110].

In patients with diabetic amyotrophy, electronmicroscopic investigation showed a degree of microangiopathic involvement quite similar to that found in diabetics without this complication. The vascular factor might interfere in the determination of this condition if it is associated with other metabolic disorders [99].

The following main objections have been raised according to Ellenberg [68, 69] against the identification of diabetic neuropathy with diabetic angiopathy:

- the comparative rarity of neuropathic symptoms in non-diabetic patients with signs of advanced arteritis obliterans,
- the acute onset
- the marked improvement found with many patients,
- the frequent involvement of the autonomic nervous system,
- the presence of diabetic neuropathy in patients free from other signs of vascular complications [208] and
- the high incidence of cases of diabetic neuropathy having an asymmetrical picture, which rules out a general vascular condition [182].

These objections raise the problem whether diabetic neuropathy is the consequence of an ischaemic process or/and of the dysmetabolic state specific to diabetes mellitus.

Some of the main objections to the theory that angiopathy causes neuropathy, enumerated above, are removed if one accepts that diabetic microangiopathic changes cannot be confused with arteriosclerosis. These angiopathic changes are characterised by uneven segmentary distribution, so, regardless of its anatomical ubiquity, it is usually present only in certain areas.

On the other hand, some of the works which deny that diabetic angiopathy brings about diabetic neuropathy, appear to be inconclusive, either because they rely on unique biopsies, or because they disregard the general histological picture of diabetic angiopathy. Midtgaard et al. [152], for instance, eliminated angiopathy as a pathogenic factor of visceral diabetic neuropathy on the ground of a single jejunal biopsy performed at 95 cm distance from the teeth and in one of the illustrations published with the article (Fig. 1), the interpretation of the electronmicroscopic picture mentions neither the thickening of the basement membrane, nor an endothelial hypertrophy almost completely obstructing the lumen of the capillary.

It is no less true that the alteration of nerve metabolism is also to be taken into account when considering the factors which determine and precipitate the onset of a diabetic neuropathy. Certain researches performed in experimental diabetes will be reviewed in Chapter VII, substantiating the role of these disorders.

Undoubtedly at our present stage no exclusive conclusion can be drawn on this matter. The presence of diabetic angiopathy in diabetic neuropathy is a fact that cannot be denied, but it is the same with the metabolic disorder of diabetes mellitus, which ultimately is among the factors determining diabetic angiopathy itself [89]. An eclectric standpoint, linking together metabolic disorders and irrigation defects caused by diabetic angiopathy, appears to be the best, for the moment.

Summing up these studies of microscopic and ultrastructural morphology in diabetic angiopathy several general conclusions can be formulated which seem to characterize the whole picture of this late complication of diabetes mellitus:

- diabetic angiopathy, with its modalities of macro- and microangiopathy, has an ubiquitous nature and a comparatively early onset in the course of diabetes mellitus.
- in spite of its disseminated character, areas of large pathological alteration generating clinical symptomatology have an uneven and segmentary distribution [1, 130],
- all the components of the vascular wall participate in the picture of diabetic angiopathy, but not to the same extent. Alterations in the basement membrane, of the endothelium or plain arteriosclerotic lesions may in turn be predominant,
- the degree of angiopathic involvement of various organs is uneven, so that in spite of the disseminated character of the complication, there are in each diabetic regions or organs whose involvement dominates the clinical pattern,
- certain statistical data suggest a parallelism between diabetic angiopathy as a whole and the duration of the diabetic condition, but such a correlation is not obvious in all the studies on this subject. It is most likely that the structural stage of diabetic angiopathy is preceded by a functional stage.

D. Investigations on the Functional Stage of Diabetic Angiopathy

The onset of the well-known lesions of the small and medium vessels in diabetes mellitus seems to be preceded by a long functional stage. This stage has an early start and a changing picture and may be reversed by adequate management. Its presence can be demonstrated by investigations of the structure of the small vessels and their behaviour in particular circumstances.

As regards morphology, MacKenzie described as early as 1892 the varicose aneurysm-like aspect of certain capillaries in the diabetic, and Krauss in 1912 reported an "active dilation" of the capillaries resulting in a decreased pressure in the capillary bed. Klingmüller showed that blood flow is very slow in the capillaries of the diabetic subject. Subsequently, Gänslen and Bock suggested that these phenomena are transient and are to be regarded as consecutive to the metabolic disorders that occur in diabetes mellitus [191].

Similar conclusions have been more recently reached by Jutte [114], who ascribed the functional venous dilations in diabetes to an inconstant state of hypoxia, brought about by the typical metabolic disorders of this disease and their reversibility to the therapeutical correction of these disorders.

Ditzel in 1968 [63] reviewed data in favour of the existence of a "functional microangiopathy" and quoted retinal, skin, conjunctival and renal aspects already reported by other authors. In the kidney, for instance, investigations with radioactive cyanocobalamine showed a significant increase in the glomerular filtration rate, which seems to be reversible [8]. This might explain the low blood creatinine values found in diabetes without other signs of diabetic nephropathy [9]. These renal aspects will be detailed in Chapter IV.

Functional disorders in the capillaries of the diabetic are present and can be demonstrated by testing the capillary permeability [44, 191]. Low permeability is found for water and protein, as well as for bilirubin. The functional character of this alteration is suggested by the fact that if the capillary permeability varies for different investigated substances, this rules out the hypothesis of a simple thickening of membranes that should equally hinder all transcapillary migrations. For

Table V. Average values of the capillary permeability in diabetic and non-diabetic patients

Diagnosis	Nr. of cases	Blood protein in mg %	pHy ml %	p. Prot. mg %	Pr. f. gm %	p. Bil. gm %	Bil. f. mg %
Normal subjects	20	7.45	14	0.7	5	0.21	2.74
Diabetic subjects	20	7.58	9.32	0	0	0.21	2.73

pHy – transcapillary hydric loss by filtration
p. Prot. – loss in circulating proteins by transcapillary filtration
Pr. f. – Proteins in glomerular filtration (gm %)
Bil. f. – Bile pigments in glomerular filtration (mg %)
p. Bil. – loss in circulating bile pigments by transcapillary filtration. (Values obtained with a modified Landis' test.) [44, 45]

instance, in alloxan-induced diabetic rats, bromophenol blue leaves the circulation as easily as a macromolecular dextran solution [200]. In fact, capillary permeability in the diabetic deviates greatly from normal for the hydric compound, while bile pigment permeability is only slightly changed [44] (Table V).

It is worth mentioning here that variations in the concentration of certain components of the internal enviroment were found to induce changes in the capillary permeability. An increase in NEFA – whose importance in the pathogenesis of diabetic angiopathy has been emphasized in several recent works [186, 187] when occurring within a short interval, hinders the penetration of glucose in tissues [12].

The same permeability disorder, which consists of an increase of the filtration threshold, might possibly participate in the modification of the clearance of circulating insulin, as found in the researches of Butterfield et al. [30, 31, 32, 33, 34, 35, 36, 37, 38, 39, 40].

The procedure of these authors consists of investigating individuals resting in bed after an overnight fast. Plastic catheters are inserted in the brachial artery and the antecubital vein which drains the deep muscular compartment of the forearm (Fig. 34).

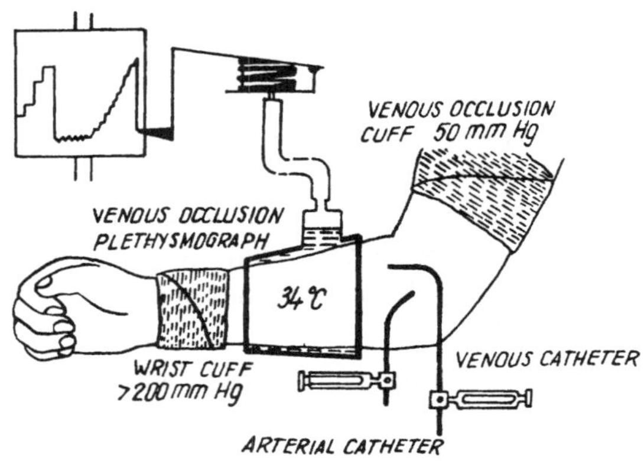

Fig. 34. Diagram of the arrangement for studying the vascular tissue exchanges in the human forearm. Position of venous and arterial catheters, of the plethysmograph and cuffs at the wrist and forearm to ensure the venous occlusion (Butterfield).

The location of the venous catheter is carefully adjusted so as to obtain venous (dark) blood, that should further darken if slight muscular exercise is performed in the forearm. This procedure shows whether the catheterized vein is draining blood mainly from the muscular system. It thus becomes possible to obtain arterial and venous blood samples simultaneously and at one minute intervals. According to the requirements of the experiment, exchanges of glucose, pyruvate, NEFA, insulin labelled with radioactive iodine Evans Blue, etc. in the forearm tissue and muscles in particular may be investigated. Before taking any blood sample, circulation to the hand is arrested in order to prevent the contamination of the blood samples with arterial blood from the arterio-venous (AV) shunts in the finger pulps and the palm.

In order to estimate the exchange of glucose and other substances, blood flow in the forearm is measured with a water plethysmograph at 34°C using a venous collecting pressure of 40–60 mm Hg. The calculated blood flow should be multiplied by the corresponding arteriovenous difference. Certain corrections are required in order to estimate the exchange between blood and the extracellular fluid (ECF) before calculating the cellular uptake of glucose.

This procedure has been used for the study of insulin uptake in the brain, the experimental set-up being completed for that experiment by the insertion, under X-ray control, of a radioopaque catheter into the superior jugular bulb, by subclaviar route. A small catheter inserted into a foot-vein served for the infusion of glucose and insulin.

The permeability of all catheters was maintained with heparinized saline (2 units per ml). Cerebral blood flow was estimated according to the procedure of Malle and Veal with Xe^{133} [37] (Fig. 35].

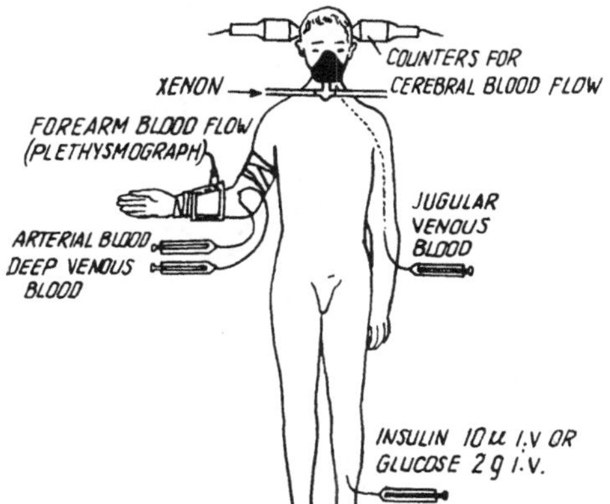

Fig. 35. Device for studying the peripheral and cerebral tissue metabolism (Butterfield).

Various studies of pathophysiology in diabetes and obesity have been performed with the above procedure, particularly with regard to the exchange of hormones and the circulation of metabolisable substances across the vascular wall.

1. During an oGTT, glucose uptake estimates were performed at 15 minute intervals, for 2–2½ hours from the start of the test.

In these experiments, the administration of 50 gm glucose resulted, in control subjects, in values of 0.85 mg/100 ml per minute glucose in the fore-arm samples, as compared to 0.35 mg/100 ml per minute in adult diabetics and 0.08 mg/100 ml per minute in the samples from patients with juvenile diabetes. As expected, individuals in the last group showed no sign of glucose uptake, indicating the absence of any effect of endogenous insulin release following the administration of glucose. It was also found that among the tissue of the controls glucose uptake was greater in lean subjects than in fat ones. All these results become more significant if the calculations are performed assuming a muscular mass of 30 kg. Of the total amount administered, muscular uptake becomes 46 gm in the lean subjects, as compared to 16 gm in the fat and 12 gm in adult diabetics. These findings and especially those in the obese, are consistent with the idea of a functional vascular disorder in the early phases of diabetes, as well as with the morphological findings recently reported by Romani et al. on microangiopathic alterations in the obese [193].

It was found that in the passage of glucose from the blood into the tissues there exists a true threshold, differing in the normal individual as compared to the diabetic (Fig. 36A, B), and that administration of insulin results in a shift of this threshold towards the normal. This is another phenomenon expressing the functional character of some vascular disorders of the diabetic, preceding what might be called a structural angiopathy. Several questions arose, subsequent to these studies. Does the abnormal uptake of glucose in the diabetic pertain to the presence of insulin antagonists in the blood stream? Is it due to a low clear-

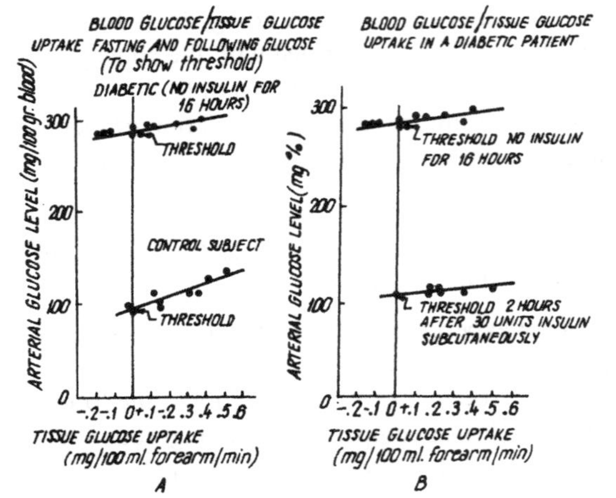

Fig. 36. A. Glucose uptake in normal and diabetic subjects. The existence of a vascular threshold which regulates the quantity of glucose leaving the vessel is demonstrated. B.-Effect of insulin on the vascular threshold for glucose (Butterfield).

ence of insulin from the blood stream into the muscular tissue? And if the clearance of insulin is normal, is it a disturbed metabolic response of the cells to the administered insulin?

2. In order to answer these questions, lightly iodine labelled (I^{131}) insulin was injected into the brachial artery with a measured amount of Evans blue for plasma determinations. Insulin and Evans blue content were checked in muscle venous blood. This enabled the calculation of the clearance of circulating insulin and the subsequent response to glucose. It was thus demonstrated that insulin clearance in the non-diabetic depends directly on the concentration and that for each molecule of insulin that leaves the blood stream, some 2×10^6 molecules of dextrose enter the muscle. It was found that, in the diabetic, insulin clearance is reduced by approximately one half, but that the insulin-dextrose ratio remains unchanged, that is $1 : 2 \times 10^6$. It was then concluded that in the diabetic there is an inability to filtrate insulin from the blood stream into surrounding tissues. This phenomenon was also found in the non-diabetic obese and it is proportional to the degree of obesity.

It is important to mention that investigation of the brain resulted in absolutely identical findings.

This is one more example of the vascular involvement in diabetes mellitus. The changes in the glucose threshold, the influence of insulin and the passage of insulin from the blood stream into the cerebral extravascular space, are displayed in Figs. 37 and 38.

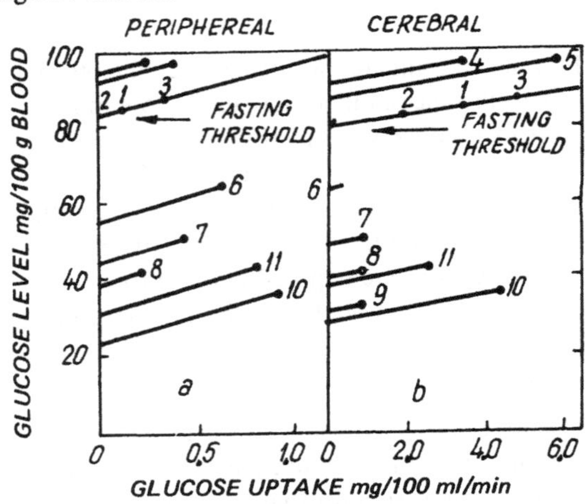

Fig. 37. Fasting threshold for glucose and its subsequent modification in (a) peripheral tissues and (b) cerebral tissues. The 1–5 noted points are before insulin administrations and 6–11 after insulin (Butterfield).

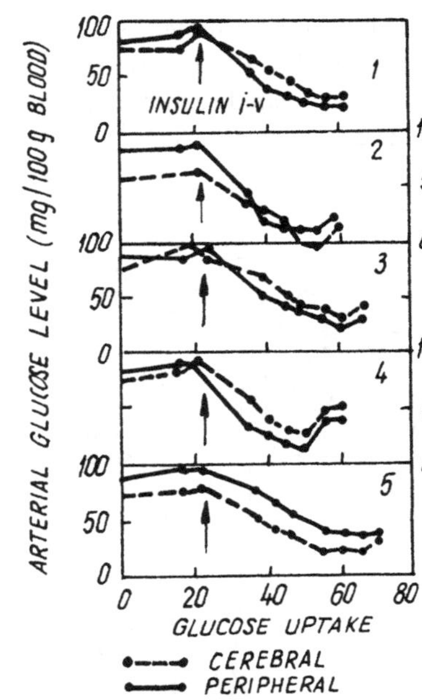

Fig. 38. The peripheral and cerebral thresholds for glucose in 5 volunteers and their modification after intravenous administration of insulin (Butterfield).

Other functional changes preceding any symptomatology have been described. Feinberg et al. [76] (1967) found in 73% of 907 children suffering from diabetes mellitus, abnormal tracings of the digital arterial pulse, without dicrotic waves, in no apparent relation to the severity of the diabetic condition. This is probably related to changes in the tonicity and elasticity of the walls of the small arterioles, a functional manifestation which is present much earlier than true diabetic angiopathy.

Plethysmographic investigations, performed in order to determine the reactivity of the vessels to epinephrine, also revealed differences between diabetic and normal subjects. It was noted that secondary increase in the blood flow reached 2.6 ± 1.31 ml per minute per 100 mg tissue in diabetics as compared to 5.4 ± 1.51 ml in the normal [15].

In 1916, Weiss described the typical aspect of the capillaries in the diabetic. His findings were confirmed [191] since the phenomenon was described again in 1967 by Terry et al. [214]. These authors failed to establish any relation between the aspect they called nodular apical elongation and the severity of the diabetic condition or the presence of some complication.

All this indicates that the onset of diabetic angiopathy follows a long period of early, variable and reversible processes occurring in the circulation in the small vessels. They represent a true functional diabetic angiopathy, which has no manifest clinical and pathological symptoms, but can be identified by special tests of the functioning of small vessels in all the areas of the body.

E. Pathophysiological Problems of Diabetic Angiopathy. Pathogenetical Theories

It is our aim, and a very hard one at that, to give a satisfactory answer to a number of problems raised by this complication of diabetes mellitus. Some of them have already been formulated in the preceding subsections. Here they are in brief:

a) the preferential involvement of the small vessels.

b) the disseminated, ubiquitous character of the disease

c) against the background of this disseminated character, the trend of the complication to become manifest and preponderant in an organ or a group of organs

d) the mechanism of the functional disorders that precede and accompany diabetic angiopathy

e) the pathogenetic relation between diabetic macro- and microangiopathy

f) the relationship between the duration of diabetic history and a given angiopathic picture

g) the relation between the degree of metabolic control of diabetes and diabetic angiopathy.

The current theories advanced as an explanation of some or all of these peculiarities of diabetic angiopathy, can be grouped under two headings:

1. one which regards diabetic angiopathy as an independent disorder, having a course parallel to that of diabetes, but not as a complication of the latter. According to this view, there is no correlation with the duration of diabetes and with the state of metabolic balance, diabetic angiopathy being an independent disorder similar to arteriosclerosis, with an independent course.

2. a second regards diabetic angiopathy, and especially microangiopathy, as a direct consequence of diabetes mellitus.

The tendency to regard *diabetic angiopathy as a condition independent of diabetes mellitus* is based on the hypothesis that no causal relationship exists between the metabolic disorder underlying diabetes mellitus and the alterations of the small vessels. This was suggested mainly by the many reports of alterations of the small vessels in various organs, consisting of thickening of the basement membrane, found in patients with latent diabetes mellitus or even during the so-called prediabetic states [1, 62, 63, 193], as well as by the

observation of vascular alterations regarded as typical of diabetes in patients free from any metabolic disorder [43, 69].
The onset of diabetic angiopathy is related by the supporters of this theory to factors other than diabetes itself, for instance to genetical and pathoimmunological factors. As regards genetics, it was suggested that the same gene might determine the alterations of carbohydrate metabolism and vascular disorders [58].

Several facts speak against this genetical outlook:

a) the investigations which led to the formulation of the genetical theory have rarely been performed on non-diabetic subjects [43].

b) the genetical outlook cannot explain those cases in which diabetes develops subsequent to a pancreatic condition (pancreatitis, pancreatectomy), or a hepatopancreatic condition (haemochromatosis) [58], or endocrine disease [43]. If accepted as an absolute truth, this outlook would imply in all these particular situations a hardly acceptable coincidence between a condition acquired more or less at random (diabetes mellitus) and pre-existing genetical alteration. The only possible but not demonstrated explanation would be that diabetes mellitus, once started, releases hidden genetical potentialities.

c) a similar argument is raised by the presence of angiopathy in experimental diabetes. This includes the retinopathy of alloxan-induced diabetes, found in the monkey, the dog and the rat, in the diabetes following pancreatectomy in the rat, and finally in the experimental hormonal diabetes induced either by the administration of growth hormone alone, or by associating it with cortisone, in the dog, the Chinese hamster and the rat [43].

d) investigations performed in the early stages of diabetes mellitus do not always find evidence of thickening of the basement membrane [120, 170]. The term "early" is emphasized because the apparent onset of diabetes mellitus, comparatively easy to diagnose, is often confused with the real onset of the condition, difficult to ascertain in most cases.

e) in most reports, the estimation of the process of thickenining is empirical. Recent researches carried out by Siperstein et al. [206], show that such a thickening cannot be ascertained by a simple estimation, even of a photograph taken under the electronmicroscope. A precise and reproducible technique of measurement is required in order to obtain an objective result. Minute measurements of the basement membrane did not confirm, in all the cases of recent juvenile diabetes mellitus, the presence of the thickening in the basement membrane [43], in spite of the remarkably high incidence of this alteration in the muscle capillaries [206].

In conclusion, it is most likely that the idea of a special genetic factor determining diabetic angiopathy does not correspond to reality. It is contradicted by numerous observations in the diabetic population and in experimental diabetes. Similar conclusions seem to result from the long-term statistics of the ACB, if one takes into account for each year the incidence of diabetes mellitus with diabetic heredity (see Fig. 1) and the percentage this group represents in the total number of patients. Fig. 39 shows particularly well that the percentage of patients with diabetic heredity factors remained almost constant alongside the continuous increase in the number of patients, while the incidence of the late complications of diabetes increased proportionally with the number of patients, with the average duration of the diabetes and with the applied therapy (see the subchapter on the conditions of the onset of the diabetic angiopathy) Chap. II p. 18.
During the last decade, an alternative explanation based on pathoimmunological arguments, has been suggested, of diabetic angiopathy as having an independent course from that of diabetes mellitus. However, the respective experimental data, interpreted by some authors as in favour of the independence of diabetic angiopathy, might just as well be brought into agreement with the opposite viewpoint according to which diabetic angiopathy depends on the duration of diabetes and the degree of metabolic control achieved by management.

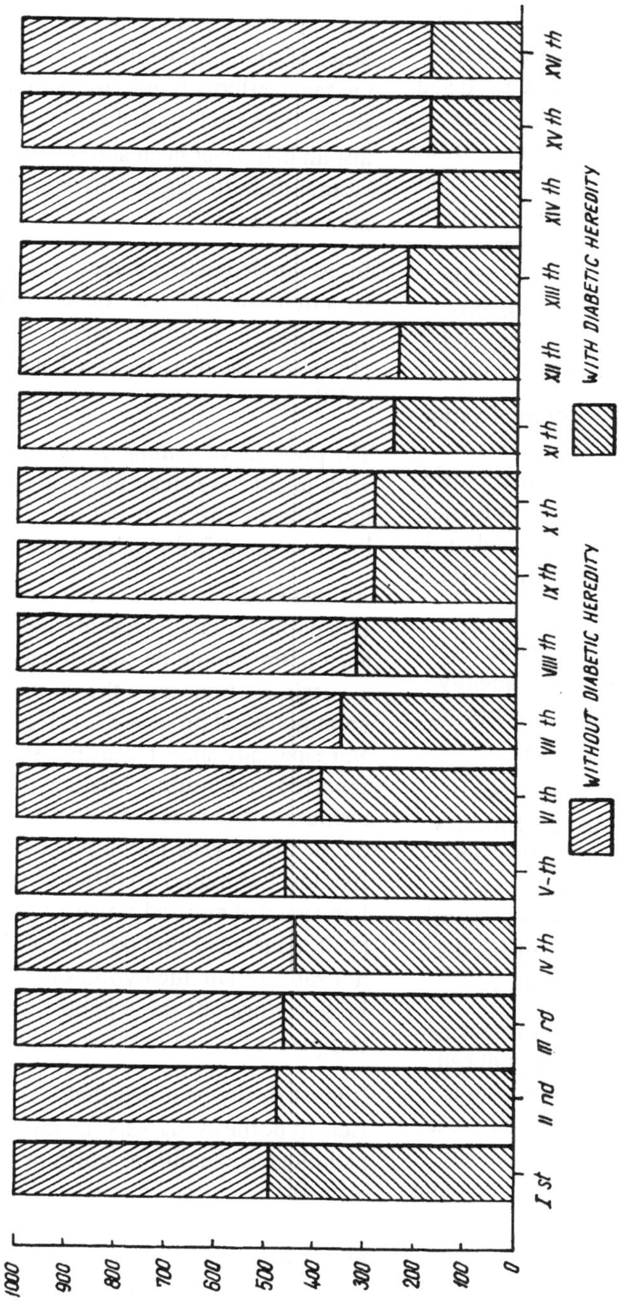

Fig. 39. Registered diagram in the A.C.B., showing the frequency of diabetic heredity.

Fluorescent antibody techniques brought about important progress in this field [130]. As early as 1958, Taft et al. [130] using this procedure, found evidence of the presence of gamma-globulin in the glomerular basement membrane of the diabetic. The fact was subsequently confirmed in 1960 and 1962 by Freedman et al., who found the same gamma-globulin in the basement membrane of the other renal blood vessels [130]. Another outstanding fact was observed on that occasion, namely the lack of specificity of the immunofluorescent picture obtained in diabetes mellitus. The same appearances are found in non-diabetic patients suffering from chronic glomerulonephritis (and from systemic lupus erythematosus [22, 130].

The immunohistochemical investigation of various organs indicated that, of the blood proteins, gamma-globulins are found in the basement membrane of the retinal vessels, of Langerhans islands, of the placenta, of the amputated limbs and in skin biopsies. No other protein fraction of the blood is so widespread in diabetes mellitus.

The binding ability of insulin at the site of the diabetic renal vascular lesions was subsequently studied in post-mortem specimens, using bovine insulin conjugated with fluorescein [18].

Insulin binding was found in 95 of the cases of glomerulosclerosis, in the PAS-positive fibrillary network of the vessels with "proliferative" endothelial lesions, as well as in the basement membrane of the tubular cells or of Bowman's capsule. Insulin uptake was also noted in 13% of the diabetic kidneys free from glomerular lesions.

The above researches as well as studies performed on other tissues from diabetic patients, induced some authors [18, 23] to suggest that insulin is bound in the tissues by an antigen-antibody reaction. This would be in keeping with the already mentioned finding of gamma globulin in the same areas in which binding of insulin occurs. Nevertheless, insulin binding exceeds by far the amounts of gamma-globulin found at the binding site.

On the other hand, Blumenthal et al. [23], by immunizing rabbits with insulin, succeeded in obtaining proliferative vascular alterations, nodular glomerulosclerosis and retinal aneurysms. Insulin binding in the basement membrane was found in these cases in the absence of any disorder of cabohydrate metabolism [58]. Since the same authors found insulin binding to occur also in the vessels of diabetic patients to whom insulin had never been administrated,they suggested that diabetic angiopathy might be an autoimmune disease.

In insulin-dependent diabetics, the level of vascular auto-antibodies was found to be higher than in healthy subjects which suggests that their process of vascular ageing is advanced almost 20 years [230].

The presence of gamma-globulins in the vascular walls might have an aetiological significance [130], the releasing antigen being either exogenous insulin, or a "modified" endogenous insulin.

All these arguments in favour of the hypothesis of a pathoimmunological mechanism of diabetic angiopathy should be considered, however, with a certain caution, since the interpretation of immunological processes is still problematical [58] and especially since recent investigations [130] reported that insulin "binding" in the basement membrane and in any other cells largely depends on the histological techniques used. With some fixation techniques no differences could be found between diabetic and non-diabetic subjects. Larson [130] concluded that our present knowledge does not substantiate the hypothesis that insulin would be the antigen of the supposed antigen-antibody complexes located in the small vessels.

It must finally be noted that while the immunological hypothesis suggests the idea of a separate pathological condition, which might undergo a different evolution from that of diabetes, the same hypothesis also applies to a view based on close relationship, from cause to effect, between diabetic angiopathy and diabetes mellitus. Taking into account all the limitations imposed by our present knowledge, the relations of diabetes mellitus, of its metabolic disorders and of diabetic

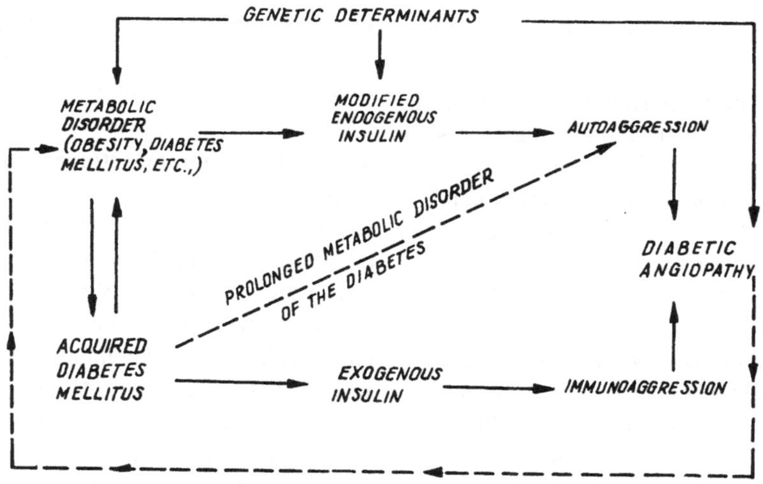

Fig. 40. Possible correlations between genetic and immunologic factors in determining diabetic angiopathy.

vasculopathy, with the genetic factors on the one hand and the phenomenon of antigenic binding of insulin, on the other hand, might be understood as they are figured in Fig. 40.

Genetic determinants		
Metabolic disorders (including trend to obesity, diabetes)	Modified endogenous insulin	Self-aggression
Acquired diabetes mellitus	exogenous insulin	Immunoaggression

The theories regarding the pathogenesis of diabetic angiopathy as a complication of diabetes mellitus assume a dysmetabolic and/or endocrine mechanism dependent on, or concomitant with, the diabetic condition.

The hypothesis grounded on dysmetabolic disorders aims at giving a satisfactory explanation of the functional phase of diabetic angiopathy, of the disorders of permeability associated with it and some of the morphological elements of this late complication of diabetes, such as the thickening of the basement membrane of the capillaries, the endothelial proliferation and the microocclusions, especially in the retina, with or without venous aneurysms.

The chemical structure of the thickened basement membrane was the starting point of numerous metabolic speculations. For a long time it was thought that the mucopolysaccharides are the main constituents of the basement membranes, since they are fixed in a network of protein fibres. More recent works demonstrated, however, that the dry substance of the renal basement membrane contains 28.8% collagen (as tropho-collagen) and 39.6% non-collagen proteins. Lipoid content was found to represent 16.9% (35% as phosphotides). The acid mucopolysaccharides, supposed to predominate on the endothelial side of the renal basement membrane, represent a much smaller part of the membrane constituents than it was originally thought [223].

Particular attention was first paid to all phenomena indicating the presence of disorders in the *metabolism of glycoproteins*, subsequent to the observation of PAS-positive material in the basement membrane of small vessels in diabetics. This material consists, according to Angervall [4, 5] of neutral mucopolysaccharides. The mucopolysaccharides are supposed to penetrate more easily into the vascular wall, because of their small molecules [114].

It was found that the proportion of glycoproteins, which migrate during electrophoresis together with the alpha$_1$- and alpha$_2$-globulins, is normal or slightly above the normal range in cases, of controlled diabetes [52, 90, 117, 156, 157], but increases significantly if angiopathy is present [156], especially with regard to alpha$_2$-glycoproteins [80]. Hence, new hypotheses as regards pathogenesis, such as the very clearly formulated outlook of Lubetzky [141], according to which, glucose, either absorbed or synthesised in the organism, may take one of the following three metabolic pathways:

- glycolysis, with possible deviation to liposynthesis
- glycogen formation
- integration into molecules of glycoprotein.

In diabetes, decreased glycolysis due to the absolute or relative insulin deficit results in an excess of non-metabolised glucose. It may be partially or totally discharged in the urine, or directed towards glycoprotein formation, since this process does not require the presence of insulin [67, 209]. In the latter alternative storage of glycoproteins in the vascular walls and thickening of the basement membranes results.

This view is also supported by reports of disorders in the metabolism of mucopolysaccharides in diabetics [58] in that the half-life of mucopolysaccharides is three times longer than normal [130]. There is also some evidence that the hyaline matter found in the glomeruli in diabetic nephropathy is identical with that absorbed in the capillary walls of the retina in diabetic retinopathy and is, as recently demonstrated, a glycoprotein [84].

Although the mucopolysaccharides, which predominate in the tissues, are less stable than glycoproteins circulating in the serum, arguments like those quoted above remain attractive. The rise in alpha$_2$-globulins, frequently found in the diabetic, is often regarded as an indirect indication of an increase in the circulating glycoproteins and consequently an alarming sign or indication of the presence of diabetic angiopathy [115, 183]. A concomitant increase in alpha$_2$-glycoproteins has been demonstrated in most of these cases [113, 115].

As regards glycoprotein storage in the vascular walls, or their possible synthesis at that level, this seems to occur independently from the storage of fat, another process thought to play an important role in the pathogenesis of the degenerative vascular lesions [84]. This point may be crucial in differentiating biochemical common arteriosclerosis from diabetic angiopathy. Metabolic disorder in the former may occur predominantly in fat storage, while in the latter, it may occur initially in the glycoprotein area, in spite of some arteriosclerotic features associated with the disease in its more advanced or macroangiopathic stages.

Once deposited in the basement membrane, glycoproteins become metabolically inert and undergo a very slow degradation in the organism [43]. This might explain why therapy applied after the formation of these depots fails to improve the damaged vessels. In such cases one can only hope to prevent further depositing in the vascular walls. Some recent works [206] based on objective investigations of the thickening of the capillary walls seem to contradict this optimistic outlook. These authors claim that the deposition of glycoproteins occurs very early in the course of diabetes, initially in the muscular capillaries and later in the kidney and the retina, the latter phenomenon depending on the duration of diabetes and the degree of therapeutical control. In some of our patients with chemical diabetes (Fig. 41), we found the same sequence of events, in that we found no clinical or paraclinical signs, either of diabetic angiopathy or of manifest diabetes mellitus, while thickening of the basement membrane in the muscular capillaries was already evident. This has been already mentioned in this work and also reported by other authors [193]. The early trend to store glycoprotein in the muscular capillaries once more illustrates a main feature of diabetic angiopathy. The disorder is generalized to the whole organism, but becomes manifest at a given moment in given organs.

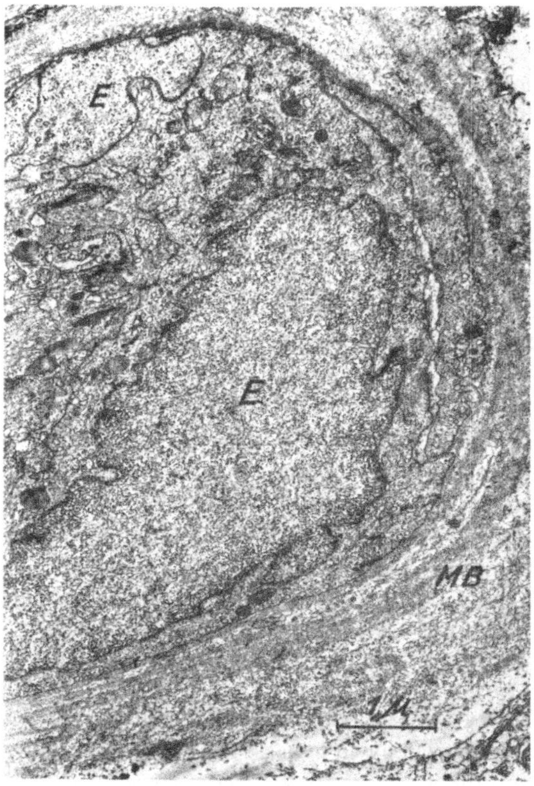

Fig. 41. S. Fl. Muscular biopsy in an obese woman with early alteration of glycoregulation. There is a trend to thickening of the basement membrane (MB). Alteration of the endothelial cells (E) (20,000 x).

Many observations performed on normal, prediabetic and diabetic subjects as well as on animals with experimental diabetes [206] emphasize the lack of correlation between the degree of glycoprotein storage in the basement membrane of the small vessels and the blood sugar level. This finding served as a starting point for criticism of the advocates of a causal relationship between the state of metabolic control of diabetes and the onset of diabetic angiopathy. But in fact the observation demonstrates no more than that the disorder affects a different level of carbohydrate metabolism, as suggested by Lubetzky [141].

Further criticism of the viewpoint that the disorders of glycoprotein metabolism result in diabetic angiopathy relies on the following observations [43]

- that the PAS-reaction, on which the hypothesis is grounded does not necessarily imply, when positive, the presence of polysaccharides.
- that there is no conclusive evidence that a rise in the level of circulating glycoproteins always precedes the onset of diabetic angiopathy [206], and some researchers failed to find a significant correlation between glycoprotein blood level and the development of vascular complications in diabetes mellitus. Quantitative variations in serum glycoproteins have also been described in many non-diabetic subjects, for instance in cases of high blood pressure and non-diabetic vasculopathies [118].
- that the analysis of the composition of the basement membrane indicated as its main carbohydrate compound a glucose-galactose disaccharide, while the circulating glycoproteins contain glucosamine.
- that it has not been possible to demonstrate that an insulin deficit is associated with an increase in glycoprotein synthesis.

Therefore, the hypothesis based on the role of glycoproteins in the onset of diabetic angiopathy cannot yet be regarded as substantiated, in spite of the fact that it answers a number of questions raised by this complication. It does not appear to be the unique mode of pathogenesis of the process. Further investigations may possibly concentrate on the qualitative aspects of glycoproteins in diabetes mellitus, rather than on the quantitive ones, as is the case at present.

The role of lipids in the development of diabetic angiopathy is suggested by a number of facts reported in the literature. Histochemical examination of the glomerular alterations found in diabetic nephropathy have revealed that besides mucopolysaccharides, neutral lipids and cholesterin are present in the basement membrane. Wilens et al. [226] claimed in 1951 that accumulation of fat in the glomeruli is essential at the onset of glomerulosclerosis, and the so-called fibrinoid nodules of diabetic nephropathy have a similar histochemical behaviour to that of the alterations observed in arteriosclerosis.

Hartcroft [101] subsequently described the presence of fat emboli in the renal capillaries and considered them as the cause of diabetic nephropathy. Cook obtained an experimental retinopathy with microaneurysms by injecting fat and Chester [51] believes that lipaemia associated with some local anomaly of the capillary or arteriolar wall may result in the formation of local lipid thrombi.

The intervention of fat in the development of diabetic angiopathy seems most likely in the cases of lipoatrophic diabetes. We followed such a patient for eight years and observed the gradual and parallel onset of a macroangiopathy and diffuse diabetic microangiopathy [177]. The intervention of lipids in the genesis of the late complications of diabetes mellitus is also supported by a negative finding, namely the low incidence of diabetic angiopathy in patients with mucoviscidosis and diabetes mellitus. One of the features of this condition is a low blood cholesterol level [184].

Some disorder of fat metabolism is undoubtedly associated with diabetes mellitus. Diabetic hyperlipaemia is regarded by some authors as exclusively due to mobilization [228], by others as being induced by the intake of fat [10, 11, 19]. Both mechanisms are likely and to be concomitant, successive or alternative. Experimental research on diabetes in the rat demonstrated, for instance, that hyperlipaemia in the acute stage is of the former type – of mobilization – while in the chronic stage of experimentally induced diabetes, when the ketosis subsides, hyperlipaemia depends on fat intake [196]. That both mechanisms interfere in human diabetes is suggested by the evolution of dyslipaemic states in patients with lipotrophic diabetes mellitus. The important hyperlipaemia due to mobilization was found here to depend to a certain extent on the level of fat intake, since changes in the fat content of the diet bring about systematic changes in the blood fat level [91, 177].

Qualitatively speaking, diabetic hyperlipaemia is characterized by an increase in the low-density lipoproteins (see Table VI), and a subsequent increase in NEFA [48, 98, 176, 187].

Table VI

Density Class	Value	Lipoproteine fraction	mμ Molecular diameter	Lipid content	Total Protein content	Predominant amino-acids	Tg	Phospholipids	Cholesterol	Nefa
High	> 1063	Lipoalbumin α_1-Lipoprotein	0.0038	40 %	40–60 %	Asparaginate	–	–	–	++++ +++
	1063–1019	β_1-Lipoprotein	0.02			Serine	+	+++	++++ +++	±
Low	1019–1006	α_2-Lipoprotein	0.03	40 %	40–60 %	Arginine glutamate	+++	+++ ++	+++	± –
	< 1006	β_2-Lipoprotein	0.04 0.07			Threonine	+++++	++	++	
	Chylomicrons		0.5– 1.5 mμ	90 %	2 %		++++++ +	+	+ –	++

The triglycerides rise at the same time. It will be noted that the range of these variations of the circulating lipids is wider in diabetic than in normal subjects. NEFA and plasma glycerol rise in these patients after physical effort, indicating a process of excessive fat mobilization [48] and an inability of the haemostatic mechanisms to maintain certain blood components at a constant level.

The connection between these variations and diabetic angiopathy is still obscure. There are however certain facts worth mentioning. The acute increase in NEFA in certain experimental conditions, for instance, inhibits the movement of glucose in the tissues as well as the stimulating effect of insulin on this process. This rise of the glucose threshold and fall of insulin clearance has been regarded as playing a role in the determination of diabetic angiopathy [12]. But these phenomena may equally occur in an inverted sequence, the rise of NEFA being the consequence of a pathological modification in the filtration threshold of glucose and in the clearance of insulin [74].

A more likely correlation between hyperlipaemia in diabetes mellitus and the vascular disorders complicating this condition is represented by diabetic macroangiopathy, a process very similar to common arteriosclerosis both in morphology and clinical picture. It is difficult to correlate lipaemic disorders with diabetic microangiopathy, because the study of variations of total lipaemia or of certain lipidic compounds does not permit conclusions in individual cases. As a matter of fact the common content of all fractions in fatty acids (see Table VI), and the insolubility of the fatty acids in the watery biological enviroment brings about three consequences:

- the changes in all the lipid fractions usually occur in the same direction,
- all lipids have a common transport mechanism and
- comparative investigations are difficult owing to the wide dispersion of the normal values [131, 212, 219].

The interest of all these investigations depends on whether one admits that the disorder of fat metabolism precedes the pathological vascular alterations, This is becoming increasingly important as data from epidemiological research shows that the significance of hyperlipaemia lies in an inversely proportional ratio with age: the younger the patient, the greater the risk of vascular disease. There is a directly proportional ratio between the risk of a vascular lesion and the level of lipaemia [17]. But there are studies which start from the exactly opposite standpoint, regarding hyperlipaemia as secondary to the diabetic vascular condition and not as its cause [198]. According to this view, the casual link consists of a "circulation deficit" in the pancreas or in other organs [69].

In analogy with the results of the study of arteriosclerosis, *hypercholesterolaemia* has been considered one of the causal factors of diabetic angiopathy by many authors.

Most of the blood cholesterol is of the non-esterified type [184] and predominantly transported by beta-lipoproteins (see Table VI) [188]. The rise of cholesterol in diabetes mellitus is most likely due to a reduction in the rate of its metabolism [141].

The fact that high blood cholesterol levels are associated with a low fibrinolytic activity of the serum and a parallel increase in plasma fibrinogen, served as an argument to those who believe that cholesterol is implicated in the pathogenesis of diabetic microgiopathy [213].

Triglycerides have also been supposed to play a role in the pathogenesis of diabetic angiopathy, although some authors [106] believe that high blood levels may occur for long periods, in diabetic patients, in no relation with the presence or absence of vascular complications. Other authors [11] even consider that a high triglyceride level is often the consequence of chronic renal failure, without being the cause of diabetes or of the vascular complication itself. The only element suggesting a possible role of triglycerides in the onset of the late complications of diabetes mellitus is the fact that their blood level depends to some extent on the state of metabolic balance of diabetes [146], while diabetic angiopathy is known to occur more frequently in the absence of an adequate management of the disease. But this proof is too indirect to be of great significance in the discussion of the pathogenesis of diabetic angiopathy and of microangiopathy in particular [2].

It has been suggested that a deficit in lipaemia "clearing-factor" might also interfere in the process. Many authors consider this factor identical to lipoprotein lipase, in spite of the fact that its rate of clearing, its reversibility by protamine and its dependence on the amount of available heparin argue against its similarity to an enzyme [228].

In normal circumstances, an increase in chylomicronaemia cannot bring about the release of sufficient heparin-like substances to rapidly influence a process of clearing. This inability might be even more marked in the diabetic and result in persistent dyslipaemic states. The so-called lipoprotein lipase activity has therefore been investigated with a view to a possible correlation with the onset and evolution of diabetic angiopathy. The research performed by Jones in 1966 did not succeed in demonstrating any differences in the activity of the clearing-factor in various categories of diabetic patients, insulin dependent or insulin independent, with and without hyperlipaemia, with hyperlipaemia and ketoacidosis or in patients with recurrent hypoglycaemic states. This pathogenetical hypothesis of diabetic angiopathy was accordingly discredited [176].

Free fatty acids are the most labile lipid fraction, with a half-life of only a few minutes. But the speculations regarding the pathogenesis based on their responses to any change of energy metabolism are still far from convincing, because it is very difficult to grasp the unceasing variations and adjustments which occur between the synthesis of fatty acids in the tissues and their formation by splitting up of the plasma glycerides [228]. No correlation was obtained between the rise in NEFA and the duration of diabetes, the age of onset, the severity of the condition and requirments of insulin [80], although there is some evidence of their influence on insulin activity [153, 186] and insulin release [169].

In chromatographic studies of the fatty acids in diabetic subjects with and without diabetic angiopathy, Schrade et al. in 1960 and 1963 [201, 202] and Tuna et al. in 1968 [217], found no decrease in the concentration of any circulating fatty acid, including the non-saturated ones. At the same time, none of the major complications of diabetes mellitus could be associated with some specific pattern of circulating NEFA Changes in NEFA have only been reported in relation to the state of metabolic balance or unbalance of the condition. A transient large release of fat from depots probably occurs during uncontrolled episodes, resulting also in changes in the blood concentration of NEFA.

The fact must also be borne in mind that the storage of fat, such as occurs in diabetic retinopathy and other forms of diabetic microangiopathy, is in no way an outstanding event, except for the hard exsudates found in the late stages of diabetic retinopathy.

The microaneurysms found in diabetic retinopathy, attributed by Chester [51] to fat thrombi, also occur in other pathological conditions with an entirely different metabolic background. The hypothesis of a specific disorder of fat metabolism, associated with diabetes mellitus and alone responsible for diabetic angiopathy, therefore remains doubtful and unlikely. Hyperlipaemia, with or without the intervention of fat thrombi, is just one auxiliary factor in an insufficiently understood complex mechanism.

An *alteration in the metabolism of protein* may also play a role in bringing about diabetic angiopathy. Balo [90] suggested that a change in the capillary permeability might permit blood proteins to penetrate into the vascular walls and contribute to their thickening and to the onset of the fibrinoid necrosis found in diabetic macroangiopathy. This process was partly confirmed in elderly non-diabetics and in arteriosclerotic subjects by investigations of differential capillary permeability [6, 7, 44] and implies that the proportion of globulins

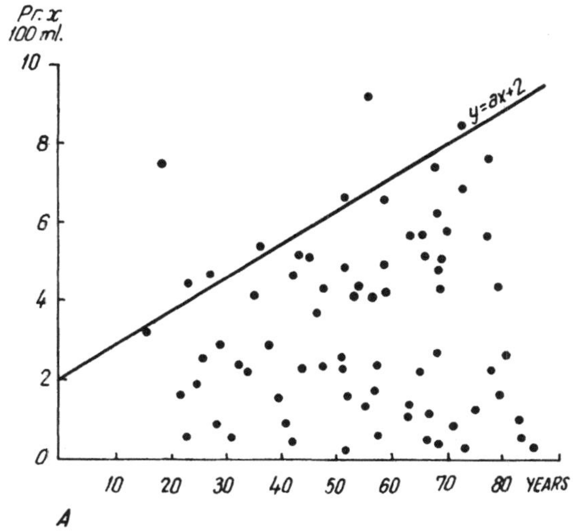

Fig. 42

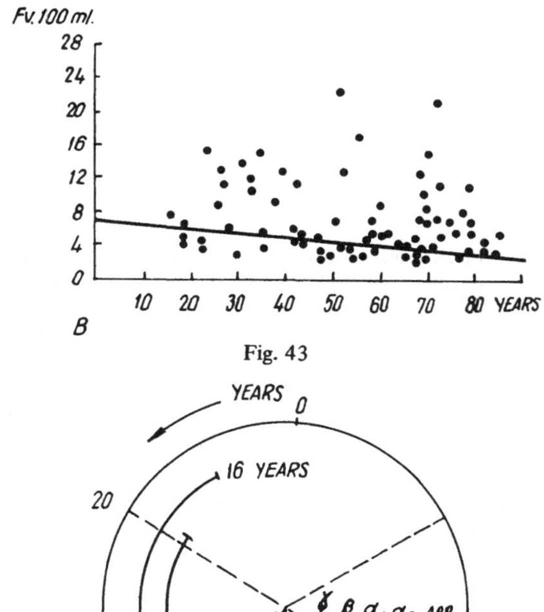

Fig. 43

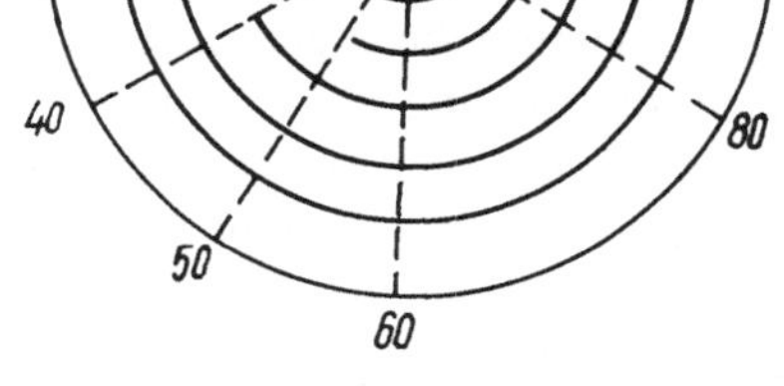

Fig. 44

Fig. 42, 43, 44. Correlation among liquid transcapillary filtration (fig. 42), protein transcapillary filtration (fig. 43) and electrophoretic fractions filtration according to the age (fig. 44).

with large molecules passing through the capillary wall increases with the age of the subject (Fig. 42, 43, 44). The process was not found, however, in young diabetics, in spite of the fact that they are not exempt from this late complication of diabetes.

The mechanism suggested by Balo might operate to a certain extent in cases of diabetes in aged subjects, but cannot be extended to all cases of diabetic angiopathy. Nevertheless, the interference in the course of diabetes of some disorders of protein metabolism-most probably an alteration of protein synthesis-can hardly be excluded. This was suggested to us by recent research in which we observed a specific appearance suggesting dysfunction of the rough endoplasmic reticulum in the diabetic [155]. We examined 262 hepatic biopsy specimens by light microscopy and isolated 25 diabetic patients in whom no signs of hepatic involvement were found, apart from the dysmetabolic picture typical of the condition. In this group we subsequently performed an electronmicroscopical study and found, besides the typical disposition of nuclear and cytoplasmic gycogen, certain remarkable aspects which have received little attention in the literature.

Modifications at the hepatic pole of the hepatocytes were found, consisting of a diminished number of microvilli and enlarged Disse's spaces, filled with an amorphous, slightly osmiophilic matter, probably a protein (Fig. 45, 46, 47). These alterations co-exist with almost normal tissue in other cell areas in the same individual.

In many cases a particular disposition of the mitochondria was noticed, either around the nucleus (see Fig. 48) or around the biliary canaliculi (see Fig. 49), separated by wide cytoplasmic areas poor in organites (Fig. 48, 49, 50, 51, 55). These appearances were frequently associated with a breaking up of the mitochondrial crista into fragments, changes in their disposition (Fig. 56) and homogenity of the mitochondrial content (Figs. 48, 49).

We also found in most of the cases examined by electronmicroscopy a preponderance of the smooth

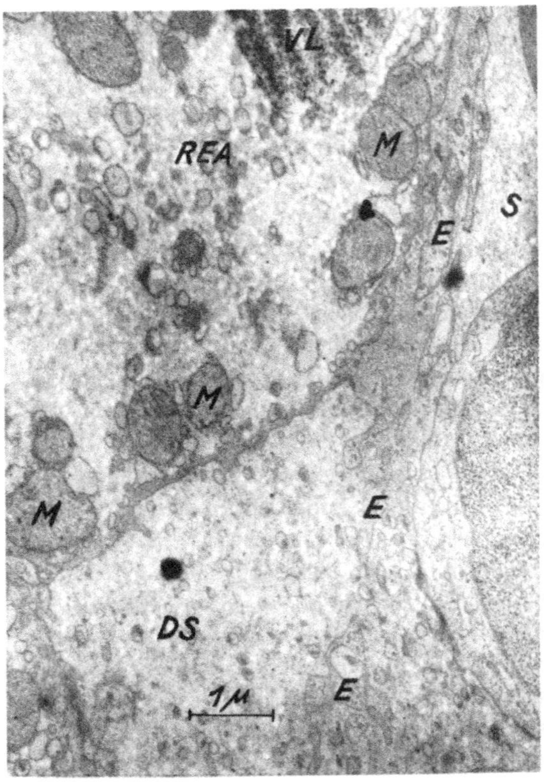

Fig. 45. P. I. Liver biopsy in a young diabetic. Decreased number of microvilli in Disse's space (DS). Mitochondria (M) situated in the peripheric area of the hepatocyte. Hyperplasia of the smooth endoplasmic reticulum (REA) with tendency to sacular dilation. Lipidic vacuolae (VL). Sinusoidal capillary (S). Endothelial cells(E). (16,000 x).

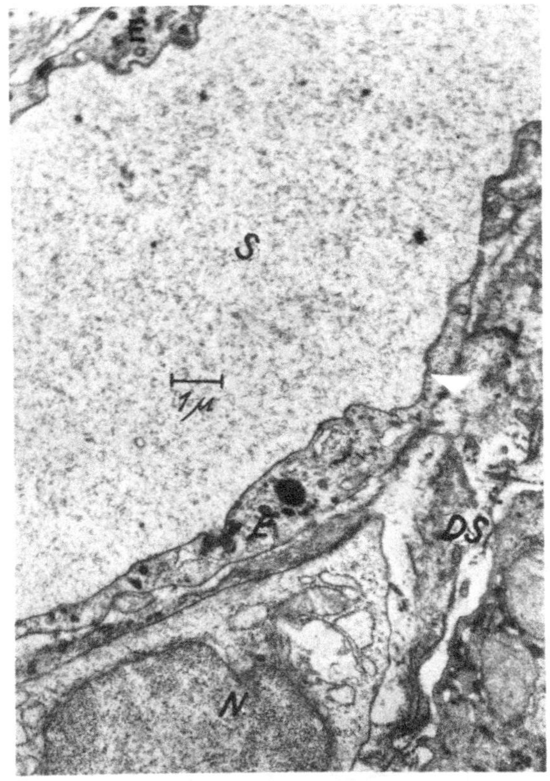

Fig. 46. P. A. Liver biopsy in a woman with maturity onset diabetes mellitus. Decreased number of microvilli in Disse's space (DS) which is slightly enlarged. E = endothelial cell. S = liver sinusoidal capillary (10,000 x).

endoplasmic reticulum (Figs. 50, 51, 52, 53, 54), variable from patient to patient and even among hepatocytes in the same patient. This fact has not been particulary emphasized up to now in the descriptions of the ultrastructure of hepatocytes in the diabetic, although the important role played by the smooth endoplasmic reticulum in the metabolism of glycogen is generally admitted.

We frequently found in our patients another alteration not yet described in diabetes. The endoplasmic rough reticulum is poor and disposed around the mitochondria of the hepatocytes. This appearance is very obvious in Fig. 54, but can also be observed in specimens from other patients (Figs. 45, 50, 51, 52, 53, 55). A particularly obvious perimitochondrial disposition was also found in an endothelial cell from a diabetic child (Fig. 47). This last finding is especially important because it illustrates the general character of disorder which underlies the alteration and because the presence of this pattern in this endothelial cell suggests that the same process occurs in other endothelial cells as well. This implies the involvement of the small vessels and the possible role of this alteration in the pathogenesis of diabetic angiopathy.

The intracytoplasmic alterations found in diabetes mellitus suggest the existence of a dysmeta-

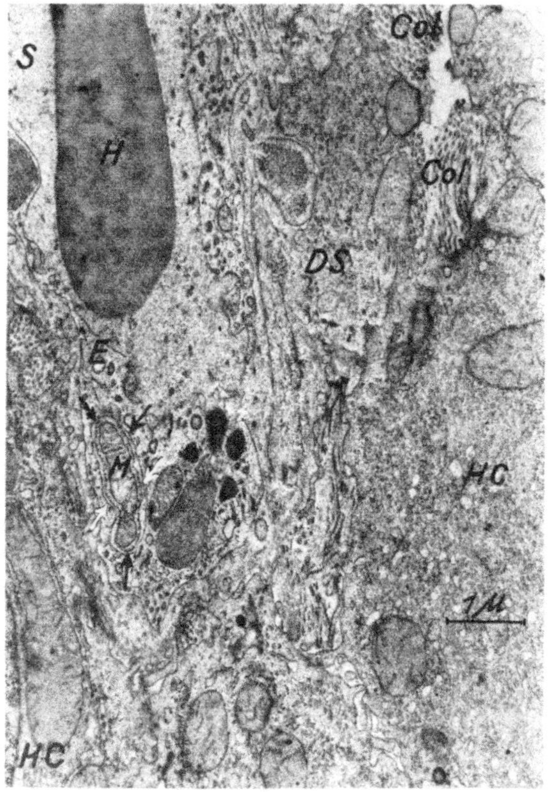

Fig. 47. D. A. Liver biopsy from a child with juvenile diabetes mellitus. Enlarged Disse's spaces (DS) with decreased number of microvilli. Inside an endothelial cell (E) there are mitochondria (M) with crown disposed rough endoplasmic reticulum (arrows). Col = sectioned collagen fibres. S = liver sinusoidal capillary with erythrocyte inside (H). HC = hepatocytes (8,000 x)

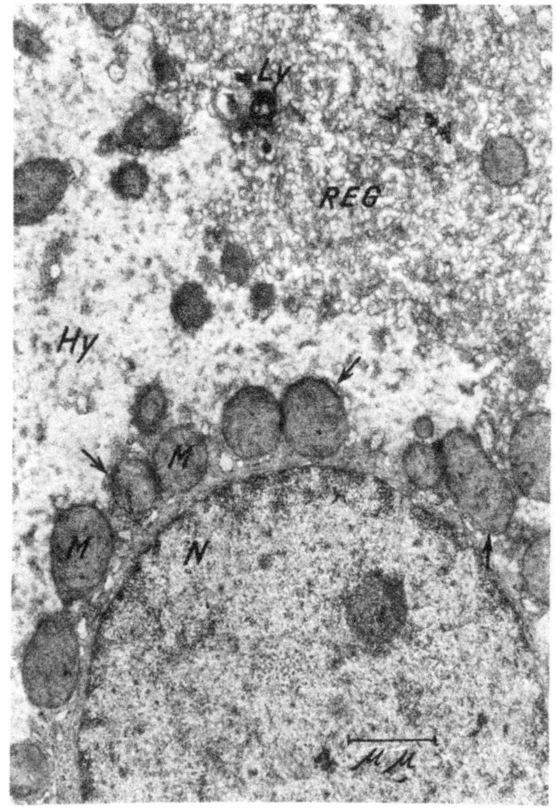

Fig. 48. S. M. Liver biopsy in a child with infantile diabetes mellitus. Crown arrangement of mitochondria (M) around the nucleus (N). Large areas of cytoplasm (Hy) without cellular organites. Rough endoplasmic reticulum (REG) irregularly distributed in the cell. Ly = lysosome (16,000 x).

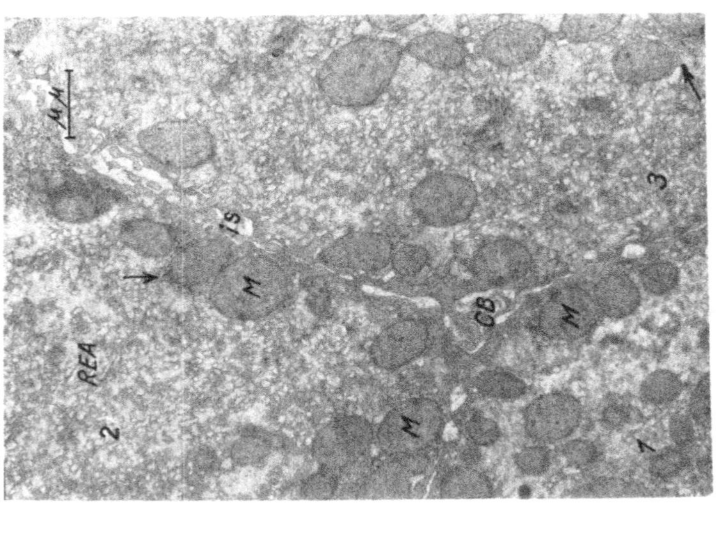

Fig. 49. Same patient as in fig. 48. Arrangement of the mitochondria (M) pericanalicular (CB = biliary canaliculus) and around the intercellular spaces (IS). Typical perimitochondrial location of the rough endoplasmic reticulum (arrows). Numbers 1, 2, 3, indicate the three hepatocytes. REA = smooth endoplasmic reticulum (8,500 x).

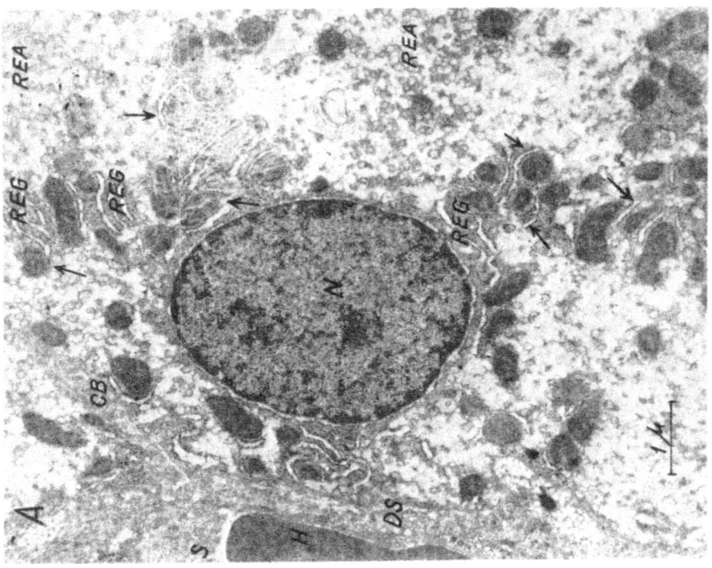

Fig. 50. D. A. Juvenile diabetes mellitus. General view of hepatocyte. N = nucleus; REA = smooth endoplasmic reticulum; REG = rough endoplasmic reticulum with predominantly perimitochondrial arrangement (arrows). Liver sinusoidal capillary (S) with an erythrocyte in side (H); CB = biliary canaliculus; DS = Disse's space (8,500 x).

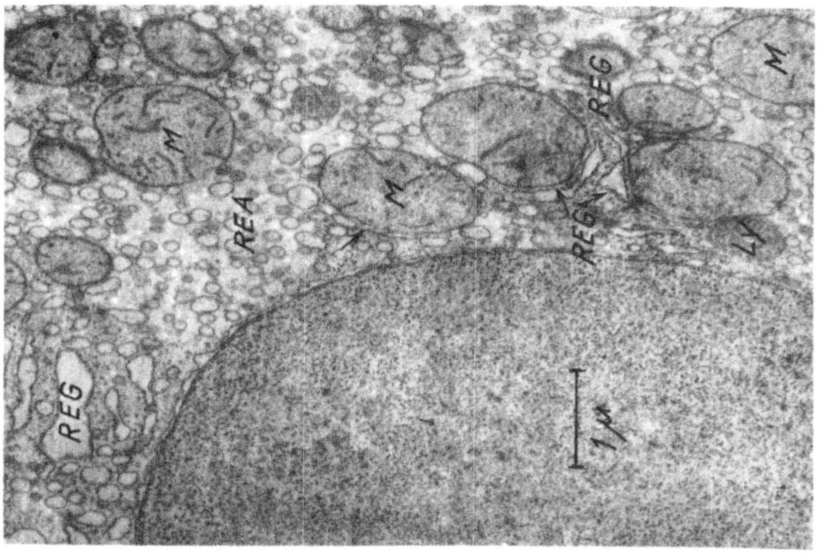

Fig. 52. P. B. Liver from patient with maturity onset diabetes. Smooth endoplasmic reticulum proliferation (REA). Perimitochondrial location of remains of the rough endoplasmic reticulum (REG). M = mitochondria Ly = lysosome (20,000 x).

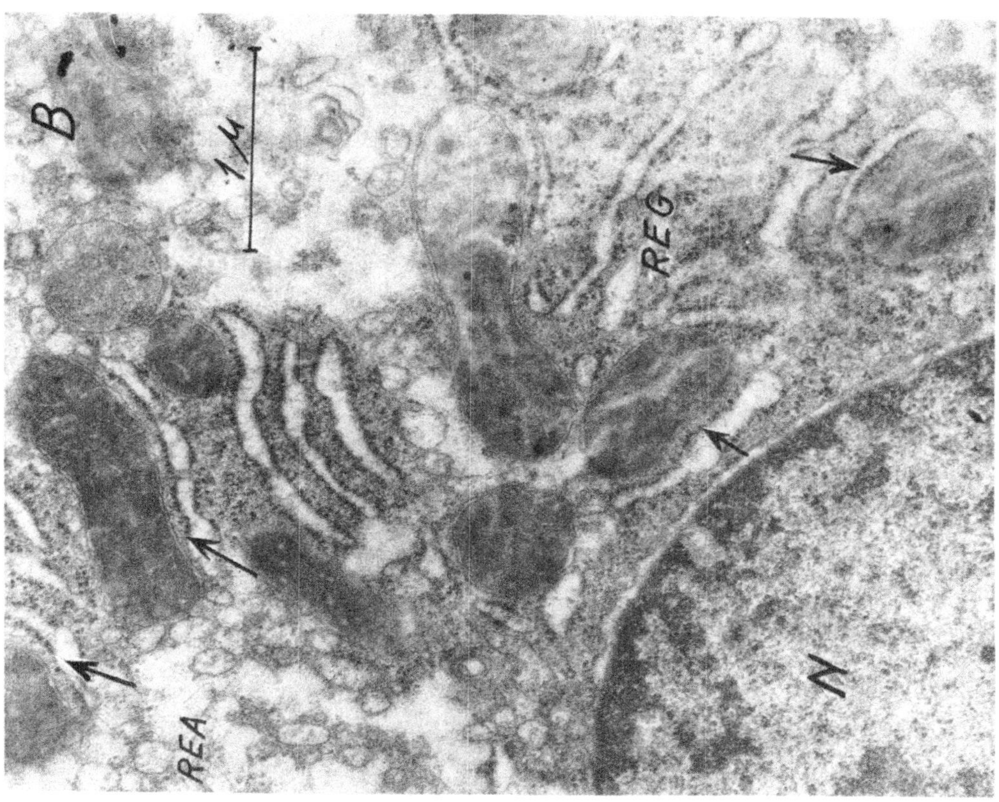

Fig. 51. Detail from fig. 50. Perimitochondrial location of the rough endoplasmic retuculum (REG, arrows). REA = smooth endoplasmic reticulum (20,000 x).

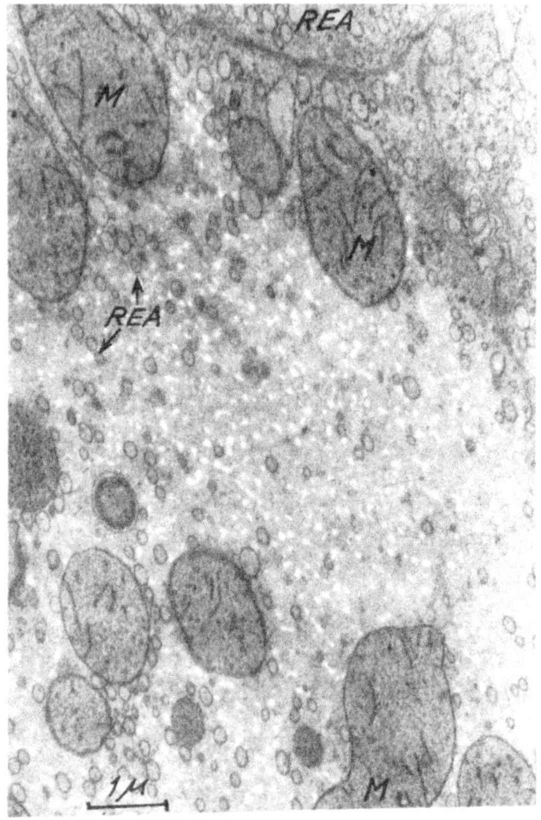

Fig. 53. M. C. Biopsy of the liver in juvenile diabetes mellitus. Decrease of the smooth (REA) and rough endoplasmic reticulum. Large areas of cytoplasm without organites. Modification in the state and size of mitochondria (M) (16,000 x).

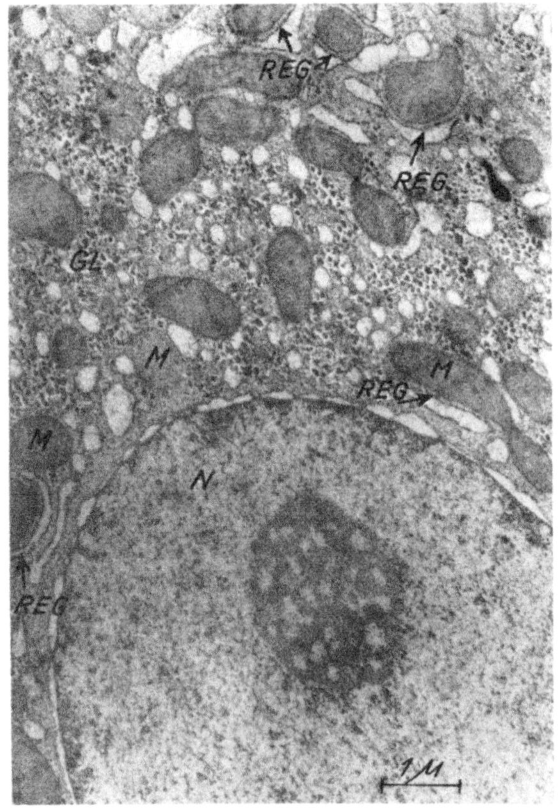

Fig. 54. Diabetes mellitus with maturity onset. Intense accumulation with glycogen of the hepatocytes (GL). Perinuclear location of mitochondria (M) and perimitochondrial arrangement of the rough endoplasmic reticulum (REG, arrows). Modification of the nuclear (N) membrane (8,500 x).

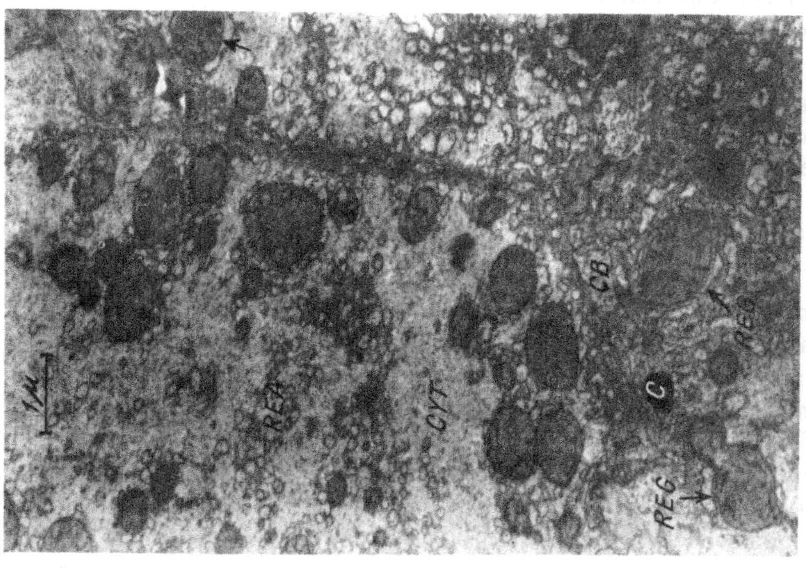

Fig. 55. L. G. Bioptic section of the liver in juvenile lipoatrophic diabetes. Smooth endoplasmic reticulum proliferation (REA) with perimitochondrial location of rest of rough endoplasmic reticulum (REG, arrows). CYF = cytoplasm without organites; C = cytosomes (8,500 x).

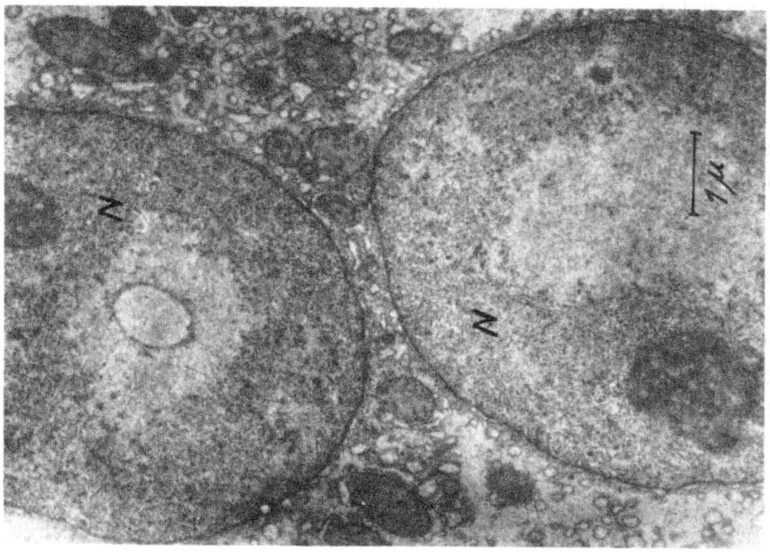

Fig. 56. L. G. Lipoatrophic diabetes. Same aspect of liver cytoplasm as in fig. 55. Hepatic intranuclear (N) accumulation of glycogen (14,000 x).

bolic state that involves the lipid and carbohydrate compartments to the same extent as the protein one. The proliferation of the smooth endoplasmic reticulum may be evidence of some kind of effort to perform glycogenesis or maybe to store glycogen in the cytoplasm.

The reduction and perimitochondrial disposition of the rough endoplasmic reticulum occurs in animals after prolonged fasting and its presence in diabetes indicates either that some factor acts as a toxin on the liver or, more likely, indicates the existence of a state of altered metabolism. We advance this hypothesis bearing in mind the role played by the rough endoplasmic reticulum through its ribosomes containing RNA, in the synthesis and uptake of amino-acids in the proteins. The perimitochondrial disposition of the remainder of the rough reticulum in diabetes mellitus, observed in starvation when feeding is resumed, might be the expression of an effort by the hepatocytes to compensate for a protein metabolic disorder.

The disposition of the ribosomes in heaps situated far from the endoplasmic reticulum may be interpreted in the same way.

A number of recent investigations have demonstrated that in diabetes the capacity of hepatic ribosomes to synthesize proteins is altered at the level of information transcription. Under the same circumstances, in muscle ribosomes the translation of information is altered [216].

An alteration in the cycle of mitochondrial "pulsation" in the course of acute experimental diabetes in the rabbit [157] has been described. It might be related to such findings as the perimitochrondrial disposition of the stripes of rough endoplasmic granular reticulum and the coronary disposition of the often distorted mitochondria around the nucleus or around the biliary canalicule, leaving large areas of cell hyaloplasm without organelles. The presence of a large number of morphologically abnormal mitochondria may have the same significance, indicating a multiple metabolic disorder, including that of protein metabolism.

Finally, the relatively frequently found reduction in the number of microvilli of Disse's spaces, usually wide and full of a slightly osmiophilic substance, is similar to a process found both experimentally and in man, in states of prolonged starvation [56] suggesting the probable inability to incorporate metabolisable substances, due to a relative deficiency of the hepatic cell.

It was recently reported (1968) that an insulin deficit diminishes the rate of lipoprotein formation. This might be significant with regard to the relationship between the disorders of fat and protein metabolism and diabetic angiopathy, because it might bring about a reduction in the rate of discharge of the triglycerides as very low density lipoproteins [1020 Sf.]. The process was demonstrated experimentally in the perfused liver [225].

In Fig. 57 we tried to schematize the vicious circle which can be deduced from the ensemble of all the metabolic disorders described in diabetes mellitus, their effects upon the vessels and the possible relationships with the pathogenesis of diabetic angiopathy. In this multifactorial determination the latter appears to us to depend on the degree of metabolic control of the diabetes and the duration of the diabetic condition. Comparing this diagram with that of Fig. 40, one obtains a picture of the multiple determination of the onset and evolution of diabetic angiopathy in man, the pathogenesis of which is not yet completely elucidated. Numerous other findings related to the influence of endocrine glands and their disorders in diabetic angiopathy, its onset, its pattern of evolution and its connection with diabetes in general, are also to be taken into account. We shall briefly review, in the following, the main implications of the various endocrine glands in the pathogenesis of diabetic angiopathy, their theoretical background and therapeutical consequence.

The role of the anterior pituitary in the development of diabetic angiopathy is still being investigated by many authors. It was suggested both by the diabetogenic effect of some pituitary hormones [133, 142, 179] and by the evidence of the influence of the pituitary gland on the course of

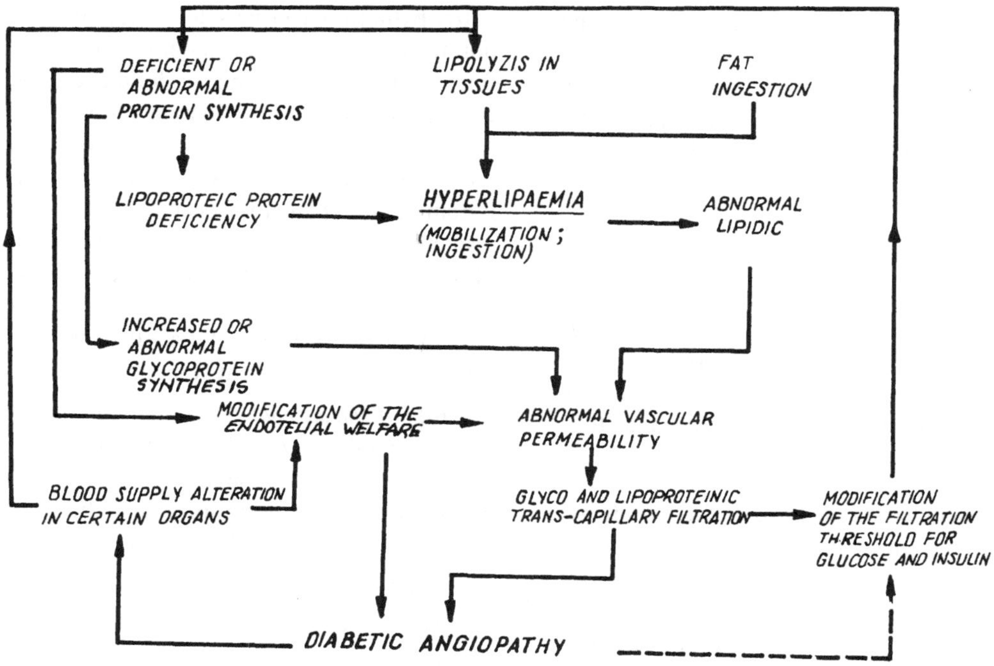

Fig. 57. Metabolic interactions in determining the diabetic angiopathy.

some kinds of diabetic angiopathy. Poulsen's observation is famous in this respect, reporting a case of diabetic retinopathy in a woman, who underwent a spontaneous inprovement following an episode of acute post-partum failure of the anterior pituitary gland (Sheehan's syndrome). Fifteen years later the subject was found at post-mortem examination to have a total and selective necrosis of the anterior lobe [100]. The observation aroused much controversy Caird et al. [42, 43] expressed their opinion that in this case an acute episode of diabetic retinopathy was arrested after delivery. The report stimulated the management of diabetic retinopathy by hypophysectomy, and an almost equal number of successes and failures have since been reported [43, 44, 142, 148, 150].

A few reports of diabetes mellitus subsiding after acute panhypopituitarism [27] also attest the role played by the pituitary gland in the course of certain varieties of diabetes mellitus and maybe in diabetic angiopathy as well.

As for the diabetogenic effect of certain pituitary hormones, Luft [142] considers it unlikely to be due to ACTH, TSH or to gonadotrophic hormones, but reports numerous data that suggest a diabetogenic and ketogenic efect of HGH. The hypothesis relies upon the following observations:

- daily administration of an amount of HGH to a normal non-diabetic subject, results after 1–2 days in an alteration of glucose tolerance that may reach diabetic levels,
- given as above to non-diabetic, hypophysectomized subjects, HGH brings about, besides the above effects, hyperglycaemia, glycosuria, polyuria and sometimes ketonuria and even nitrogen retention,
- in cases of hypophysectomy performed in subjects with juvenile diabetes, the administration of small doses of HGH results in a deterioration of the diabetic condition and acidosis. This reaction occurs neither in the adult nor in juvenile diabetes, if the pituitary gland has not been removed,

- in prediabetic states, the intravenous administration of sulphonylureas results in significantly increased levels of circulating HGH at the end of the test, indicating a hyperresponsiveness of the releasing mechanisms of HGH [24].

The observation reported by Young [53] is also noteworthy. He claimed that HGH becomes diabetogenic only when the hormone cannot exert its effect on its normal effector tissue, cartilage. That is why pituitary gigantism is generally not associated with diabetes mellitus, unlike acromegaly, in which cartilage no longer responds to HGH.

It was concluded on the basis of these findings that insulin protects the organism against the diabetogenic effect of HGH. This is corroborated by the observation that the administration of HGH to normal subjects results in an increased release of insulin [140] in spite of the concomitant reduction in glucose tolerance. The same finding was noted in hypophysectomized, non-diabetic subjects and in patients with acromegaly [142].

A further step, after the demonstration of the diabetogenic effect of HGH, consisted in experiments which proved that the administration of HGH to the dog may result in microangiopathy [70, 102].

Pfeifer's investigations [179] on prediabetic subjects confirmed the role of HGH, but also proved that the overactivity of the hormone cannot wholly explain the biochemical alterations and the obesity often occurring in these patients. He argues in favour of the interference of a second factor, that he believes to be ACTH or an ACTH-like substance, responsible for the excessive lipolysis found in prediabetes.

ACTH was also postulated as promoting diabetic angiopathy and maintaining a state of metabolic unbalance, by its suprarenal effects. Thus, at least two pituitary hormones appear to play a role in the process we are studying. The final result probably depends on the dominating hormone in the pituitary secretion. Another example of alternative pathological effects depending on the main hormonal secretion of the anterior pituitary is found in the bones. If, in an older diabetic patient, the pituitary secretion is dominated by ACTH, signs of chronic hypercorticism such as osteoporosis will develop gradually. On the contrary, if HGH is dominant, hyperostosis occurs [26]. The response of the vessels to various circumstances of pituitary dominance cannot be anticipated, but the great variation in the results of hypophysectomy in the management of diabetic retinopathy already indicates different responses.

The role of the adrenal glands in maintaining a metabolic imbalance in the diabetic and in bringing about diabetic angiopathy remains controversial. As for the anterior pituitary, the attention was drawn to the adrenals by several facts such as:

- the indubitable existence of a diabetogenic effect of the adrenal hormones and,
- reports on improvement in the course of diabetic angiopathy subsequent to adrenalectomy [133, 137].

The diabetogenic effects exerted by the medullo-suprarenal gland are proved by the reports that phaeochromocytoma is frequently associated with an inhibition of insulin secretion, [86, 133, 224], with hyperglycaemia rising to diabetic levels [162] and with alterations of the fundus and the electrocardiogram suggesting the involvement of the small vessels [153].

The effects exerted by the medullo-suprarenal gland form another example illustrating the concept of differentiated responses depending on stimulations at various levels. Epinephrine and norepinephrine, potassium ions, glucagon. ACTH, TSH, LH, all exert an effect on adenyl cyclase, catalysing the intracellular formation of cyclic 3′5′-AMP(cAMP). It is known that cAMP is a second messenger stimulating the discharge of insulin (Fig. 58). Therefore epinephrine, by stimulating the accumulation of cAMP in some tissues, would be expected to stimulate insulin discharge. But, it actually inhibits it. In an attempt to explain this seemingly paradoxical behaviour, some researchers have concluded that receptors of the pancreatic cells result in various effects on the synthesis and consequently on the amount of cAMP present in the insulin-secreting cell. Epinephrine activates both adenyl cyclase and the alpha receptors, so that the insulin releasing effect is counteracted [140, 218].

The fact that the stimulating effects of glucagon, ACTH and STH upon insulin discharge are enhanced in the presence of glucose suggests that there is a relation between the activation of the adenyl cyclase system, cAMP and the metabolism of glucose in the beta cell itself. The possible common denominator is the concept of differentiated responses of the various organs to the same stimuli, at different moments. The presence of glucose is the main stimulus for insulin secretion and the hormones which act upon adenyl cyclase or those which concomitantly activate the beta and alpha cells at different moments will determine different metabolic responses to the same stimuli, both in the normal and in the diabetic subject. It may then be concluded that any therapy based on a hypothesis that regards diabetic angiopathy as determined by the disorder of a single gland or hormone, disregards the concept stated above. This could explain the therapeutic successes and failures which have obscured the pathogenesis of diabetic angiopathy. In any case the medullo-adrenal hormones do not play an important role in this condition, excepting phaeochromocytoma, where increased glycaemia is associated with other pathogenetic alterations.

The possible role of the adrenocortical hormones in maintaining metabolic imbalance in the diabetic subject in spite of therapy, or in specifically bringing about diabetic angiopathy, is suggested by the existence of a syndrome, the Cushingoid hypercorticism of obesity [3] as well as by the existence of diabetes of the type called "cortisone" type [179] or the secondary extra-pancreatic diabetes following excessive cortisol production [153]. These are usually benign diabetic conditions in which the most advanced angiopathic complications consist of the presence of retinal microaneurysms [148], but not in a true diabetic retinopathy.

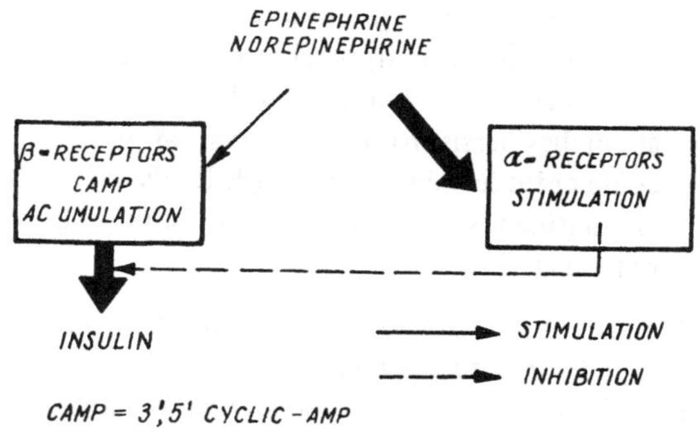

Fig. 58. Epinephrine and norepinephrine action on α- and β-pancreatic receptors.

Uncertainty has lately increased with regard to the effects of the adrenocortical hormones on diabetic angiopathy because adrenalectomies performed in diabetic retinopathy did not yield encouraging results and because an association between diabetes mellitus and Addison's disease has been described during the last decades [137, 174]: Diabetes mellitus was found some time after adrenal failure.

The role of the thyroid hormones. The thyroid hyperfunction in Graves-Basedow disease may be associated with a mild diabetic syndrome, or may aggravate the course of a pre-existing or associated pancreatic diabetes. In this latter case, taking into account the relationship between the state of compensation of diabetes and diabetic angiopathy, one might suppose that the thyroid hyperfunction plays an auxiliary role in precipitating an angiopathic complication. A direct intervention of the thyroid hormones on the small vessels has not yet been described.

Thyrotropin, which also stimulates the discharge of insulin in the presence of glucose and the activation of cAMP, has no known effect on the small vessels [140].

Controversy persists over *the possible role of insulin* in the pathogenesis of diabetic angiopathy, and over whether insulin therapy can cause the onset and progression of diabetic angiopathy [176]. In favour of its role are a number of findings in angiopathic patients, especially of the macroangiopathic type such as:

- many subjects with premature coronary artery disease suffer from hyperglycaemia or give abnormal glucose tolerance tests. These anomalies persist for long intervals after an acute episode. Abnormally high levels of circulating insulin have also been found in these patients [231].

One cannot state for sure whether these high levels are due to an actual rise in the threshold of filtration of insulin from the blood stream to the extravascular space, as suggested by Butterfield et al. [31], or a variety of inactive insulin, subsequent to a molecular modification or to some insulin antagonists [222]. There is a similarity between the behaviour of these patients and the obese subjects, and the presence of a vascular lesion makes the hypothesis of the pathogenetic role of a primarily increased insulin level very attractive.

- abnormally high insulin responses to oral glucose were found in elderly patients suffering from myocardial ischaemia or cerebral angiopathy [72, 107, 198, 212, 219].
- in 73% of the coronary patients a rise in the insulin-antagonist synalbumin was found, compared with an incidence of 23% found in normal controls [222].
- there is indirect experimental evidence that rabbits made insulin-dependent with alloxan and subsequently put on an atherogenic diet, proved to be more resistant to the onset of arteriosclerosis than normal rabbits. The administration of insulin reversed this effect and the regression of the arteriosclerotic lesions was also delayed after discontinuation of the atherogenic diet. Similarly the delaying action of oestrogen on atherochia formation is antagonised by insulin.

According to Stochs et al. insulin has an indirect role, by creating a state of insensitivity to its own action. As a result, the diabetes is difficult to control and, therefore, the trend of vascular complications is created. This interpretation is supported by the results of Elkeles et al. who found a greater incidence of diabetic angiopathy in patients slightly responsive to insulin therapy [210].

Statistical investigations performed in the Antidiabetic Centre in Bucharest on 16,000 outpatients and 4,875 diabetics admitted to hospital, showed (Table IV) that the incidence of insulin-requiring patients was higher in the group of subjects without diabetic angiopathy. On the other hand, Figs. 13 and 14 show that an inadequate metabolic control of diabetes, usually due to a relative or absolute insufficiency of insulin dosage, stimulates the onset of diabetic angiopathy. Therefore, it seems more likely that insulin protects against diabetic angiopathy than that it promotes the complication.

The roles of glucagon and LH in the pathogenesis of diabetic angiopathy appear to be entirely insignificant in spite of the fact that they stimulate adenyl cyclase and increase the amount of cAMP in most of the tissues. They would be expected to activate the secretion of insulin, but it seems that much higher concentrations of cAMP than the physiological ones are required to effect this. Therefore, other effects of these hormones prevail over that of insulin stimulation [140]. But even if we admit that they exert an insulin-stimulating activity, a deleterious effect of insulin remains to be proved.

The idiopathic or primary hypothyroidism associated with diabetes mellitus has for a long time been regarded as a rare event [112]. Its accepted incidence was 0.03 %. The investigations of Baron in 1955 [13] in England, based on determinations of basal metabolism, revealed an incidence of 0.07%. Modern methods for the diagnosis of hypothyroidism, indicated an incidence of 1.7%. It would need to be much more frequent to invoke its role in the pathogenesis of diabetic angiopathy [153].

This short review of the possible effects of the main hormones on the onset of diabetic angiopathy shows that some of them might be regarded as factors that could accelerate the course of a diabetic angiopathy, but none appears to determine it.

The various therapeutical interventions performed either by blocking the activity of some hormones supposed to interfere with the onset of diabetic angiopathy, or by removing the respective endocrine glands, did not result in evidence of a direct and favourable effect on the large or small vessels. – Their effects consisted only in removing a possible accelerating effect, by the improvement of a general dysmetabolic state.

The intervention of endocrine factors in diabetic angiopathy, by speeding up the course of the condition, partly explains why the degree of small vessel involvement increases with the metabolic imbalance and the duration of diabetes. However, no standard interval can be named after which angiopathy is present in all cases of diabetes. The various combinations of endocrine dysfunction described in pathology confirm the concept of differentiated responses and explain why in apparently similar circumstances two patients may behave quite differently.

The ubiquitous character of diabetic angiopathy is also consistent with the humoral mechanism of this complication, but the preponderant involvement of the vessels in a given organ cannot be explained substantially by endocrine interventions.

The unified vascular hypothesis relies on some findings suggesting that the etiological factor of the various vascular lesions may be a disorder in the blood supply of the vascular walls by the vasa vasorum.

Findings in Bürger's disease, "pulseless disease", mediocalcinosis, etc. and in experimental arteriosclerosis [196] seem to support this outlook. Recently Levy reported facts suggesting that ATS phenomena originate in an obliterating arteritis bringing about the obstruction of the vasa vasorum. According to this hypothesis, there is no arteritis or arteriosclerosis specific to diabetes mellitus, and the reaction to colloidal iron, suggested as a test for differentiating common ATS from diabetic angiopathy [92] cannot he significant, since many other related conditions have a common positive PAS reaction. Hence, diabetes mellitus might only be an element precipitating or speeding up the process.

This view is, however, unable to explain the fact that in common arteriosclerosis, large vessel involvement may be as advanced as to cause gross symptomatology, while microangiopathy is seldom present.

The reverse statement also appears to contain some truth. In cases of diabetes mellitus with generalized microangiopathy, we do not always find generalized diabetic macroangiopathy. It is therefore more likely that if vasa vasorum do play a role in bringing about diabetic angiopathy, they are not the unique determining factor.

It may be concluded that none of the above factors can be assigned the role of main determining factor, a plural causality appears more likely. In the pathogenesis of angiopathy, the principle of differentiated responses may operate, in the sense that different pathogenetic factors result in different responses, depending on many metabolic, genetic, exogenous, etc. peculiarities are permanently at work in the organism.

Chapter III Ocular Microangiopathy

Ocular microangiopathy is of particular practical and theoretical interest because (a) its incidence has steadily increased since the discovery of insulin therapy, (b) the prognosis has failed to improve, therapeutic results are poor and controversial, owing to the fact that (c) the present knowledge of the pathophysiology of the conditions is still incomplete, in spite of its apparent accessibility for clinical investigation.

According to certain authors [60], ocular microangiopathic complications occur in all patients after a 15–25 year history of diabetes. Romani et al. [129] found ocular angiopathy in 49 out of 57 diabetics investigated (86 %), while Whittington [153, 154] reported retinopathy in 2/3 of the patients with a diabetic history longer than 20 years. According to the same author, at the moment when the diabetic condition was diagnosed, which did not always correspond to the onset of the disease, retinopathy, was already present in 6% of patients younger than 60 years and in 11% of those over that age.

The different incidences to be found by various authors and in various periods of time can be assigned to several factors among which:

- the very concept of ocular involvement in the diabetic differs from author to author and from one period to another;
- the incidence found at a given moment depends on the development of the diagnostic procedures at the respective moment;
- earlier statistics do not correlate the prevalence of the late complications of diabetes, including the ocular ones, with age, duration of diabetes and sex (Grönberg) [71]. The therapeutic

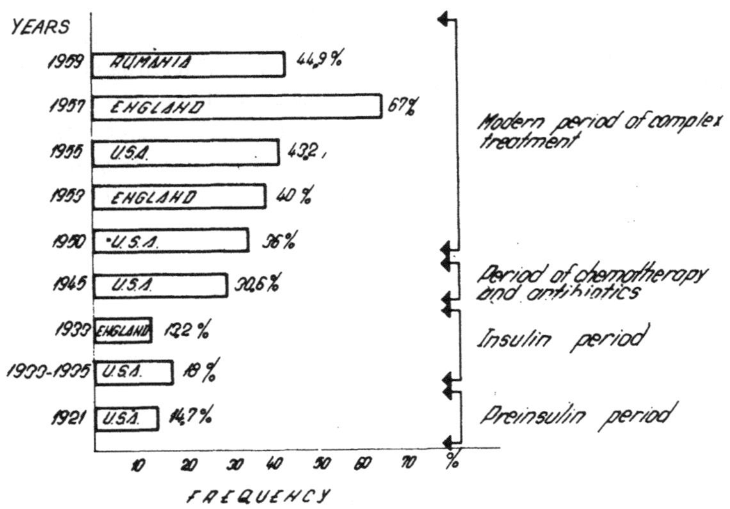

Fig. 1. The incidence of diabetic retinopathy between 1921 and 1959 in terms of different treatment periods.

period during which the respective statistical investigation was performed, is of particular importance. For instance, the incidence of diabetic retinopathy was remarkably low during the preinsulin period (Fig. 1), the real incidence being probably hidden by the high death rate. It is noteworthy however that statistical data published in various countries at various times show that there was no substantial rise in the incidence of retinopathy after the introduction of insulin therapy. A greater increase was recorded following the advent of chemical and antibiotic antiinfectious therapy, when the incidence of ocular complications was doubled over a short time. Subsequently, during the period of complex management of the disease, and as the average life span of the diabetic patients was markedly increased, incidence figures rose further and became very high (Fig. 1).

Statistics in most of the largest countries recorded incidences between 40 and 60% for ocular complications. Rumania stands at the level of 44.9 %, nearest to figures published for the United States, Britain, Sweden [71] and even for south-east Europe [123].

Prognosis is rather poor in ocular complications in general and in retinopathy in particular, as illustrated by the fact that diabetes has become one of the main causes of acquired blindness in the adult, accounting for 8 to 15% of the cases. Diabetic retinopathy results in a sudden or gradual fall in visual acuity leading to blindness in 15–90 % of the cases. Caird et al. [24, 25, 27] give the same prognosis, finding that 5 years from the first ophthalmic symptoms, diabetic retinopathy leads to blindness in 15–50% of cases, while among patients in whom haemorrhage in the vitreous occurs, after only 4 years sight is preserved in 1/3, affected in 1/3 and lost in 1/3.

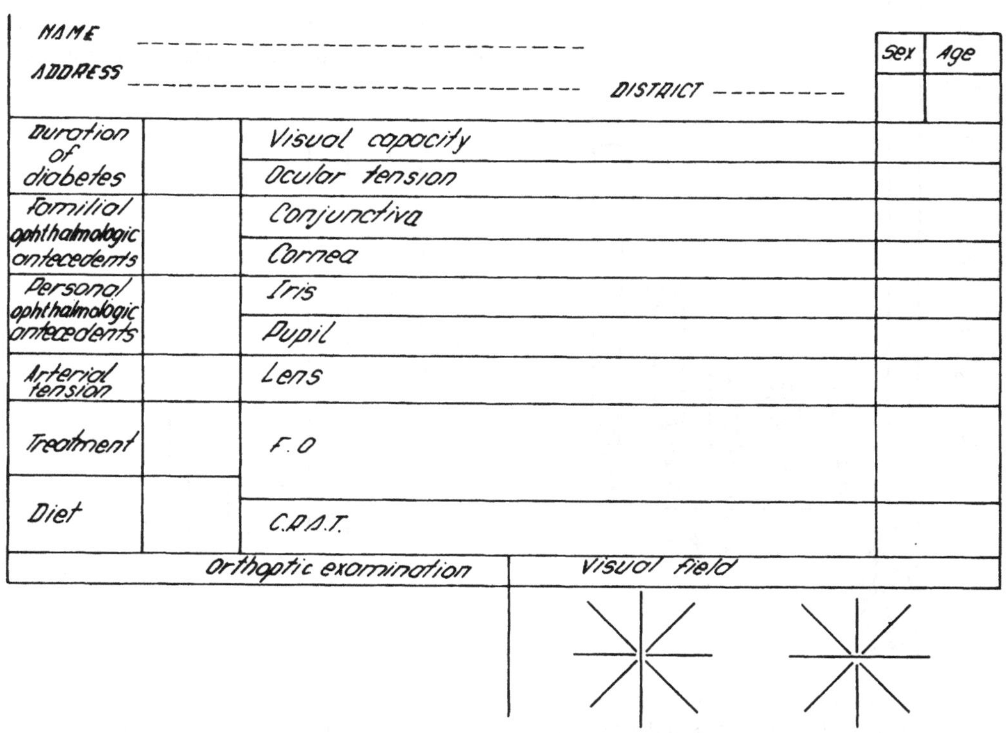

Fig. 2. Record card for ocular angiopathy registration used in the Antidiabetic Centre in Bucharest.

A study by Beetham [13] on 109 cases of proliferative retinopathy showed adequate sight in only 39 out of 65 young subjects after 5 years, and in only 15 out of 44 cases of mature diabetes, after 3½ years.

According to Azerad [10] prognosis does not depend on sex or the duration of the disease, but appears to be worse in patients over the age of 35. Some 10% of the diabetics die during the first 5 years of retinopathy and 40% of them die after ten years.

It appears that the numerous problems raised by diabetic ocular microangiopathy can only be answered by investigating the various aspects of the complication on large groups of patients over long periods. It is to this end that the ACB, has adopted the system of recording on a special card all the ophthalmological data of the patients, collected by a small group of specialists familiar with the ocular problems of the diabetic (Fig. 2). Besides some general data, every examination concerning the anterior and posterior poles, the visual field, etc. is recorded (Fig. 2/III). Such examinations have been performed in 920 diabetic patients selected at random, that is in the order of their registration at the centre, in order to avoid bias.

52 % of the patients were over the age of 60. As no significant difference was recorded in the distribution according to sex, only total figures have been considered in the diagram (Fig. 3/III).

The distribution according to the duration of the diabetes showed 11.6% patients with a history of less than 1 year, 34% between 1–5 years, 28.3% between 5–10 years, 19.7% between 10–20 years, and a small percentage of diabetics with a history exceeding 20 years (Fig. 4/III).

Four categories of treatment have been established: plain diet, insulin management, oral treatment

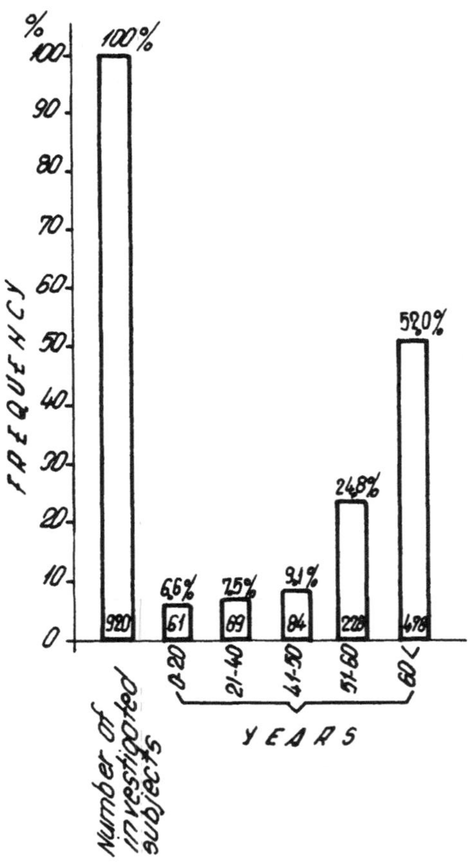

Fig. 3. Age distribution of ocular diabetic microangiopathy in 920 registered diabetics in the Antidiabetic Centre in Bucharest.

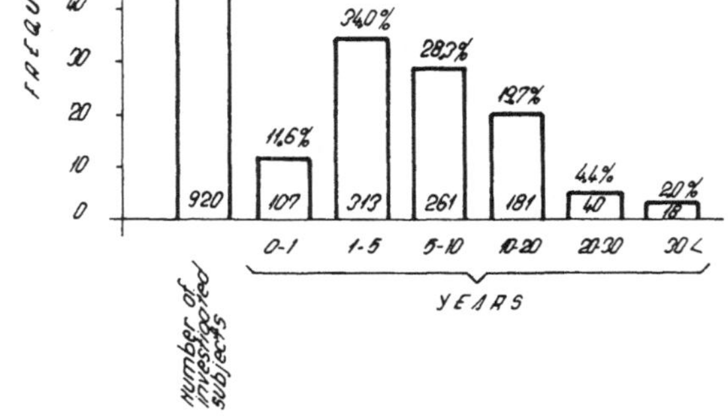

Fig. 4. Duration of diabetic disease and incidence of ocular microangiopathy in 920 registered diabetics in the Antidiabetic Centre in Bucharest.

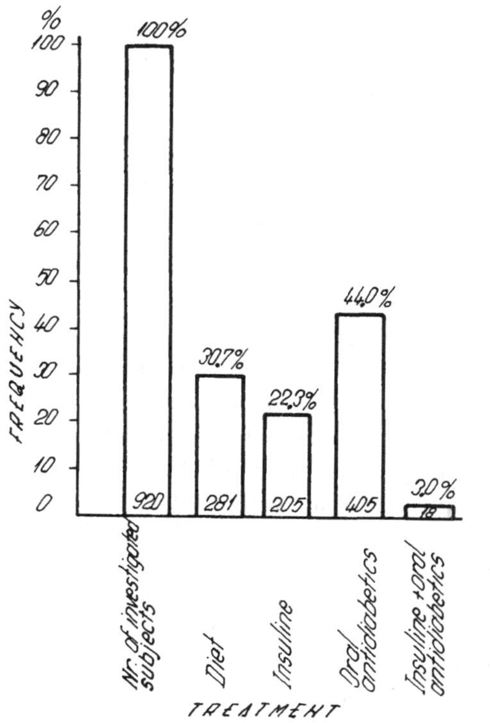

Fig. 5. Treatment of diabetes and occurrence of ocular angiopathy in 920 recorded patients in the Antidiabetic Centre in Bucharest.

and combined insulin and oral treatment. All kinds of drug management were associated with special diets 30.7 % of the patients have been controlled by plain diet therapy, 22.3 % by insulin, 44 % by oral management (hypoglycaemic sulphonamides, biguanides or both) and 3 % by insulin and oral therapy (Fig. 5/III).

Ophthalmological investigations were concentrated on the changes in the anterior pole (conjunctiva, iris and lens) and in the posterior pole (fundus oculi).

Conjunctival alterations were found in 49.5%, of the cases, iridal alterations in 28.8%, crystalline (lens) alterations in 49.4%, and retinal (by fundus oculi examination) in 44.9% (Fig. 6/III), [113, 114].

The following subsections will deal with the problems of prevalence and incidence, clinical features, prophylaxis and therapy of the main patterns of ocular diabetic microangiopathy by resorting to data from the literature and from the ACB between 1942 and 1969.

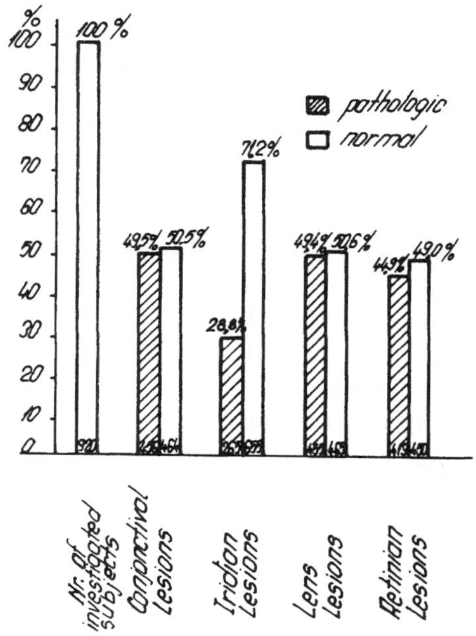

Fig. 6. Incidence of main ocular complications in 920 diabetics recorded by the Antidiabetic Centre in Bucharest.

A. Alterations of the Anterior Ocular Pole

1. Diabetic Alterations of the Conjunctiva

The conjunctiva is among the eye structures with the richest blood supply. The blood vessels originating in arteries which penetrate the eye at the internal and external ocular angles form the two vascular arches (arcus tarseus and arcus externus) whose further ramifications pass through various local glandular elements and develop into a rich capillary network under the conjunctival epithelium [125].

Biomicroscopical and microphotographic examinations systematically performed in diabetic subjects often show vascular alterations such as conjuncti-cal aneurysms, venular dilation with a consecutive change in the venule/arteriole ratio. These appearances are seen at the various stages of diabetic angiopathy but are also found sometimes in non-diabetic subjects. The problem consists of deciding whether they might be attributed to the diabetes. Chazan et al. [31] give the following classification of vascular conjunctival abnormalities in diabetes mellitus:

1. *Collateral veins:*
   a) the modification of the venule/arteriole ratio
   b) uniform venular dilation
   c) uneven venular dilation
   d) micropools
   e) sludging of the blood
2. *Postcapillary venules*
   a) tortuosities
   b) congestions
   c) sludging
3. *Capillaries*
   a) ischaemia (sometimes)
   b) terminal or diffuse narrowing
   c) micropools
   d) sludging
4. *Branching arterioles*
   diameter modifications
5. *Terminal arterioles*
   a) narrowing
   b) sludging

The general arteriolar-venular anastomoses are notable in capillary ischaemia.

Ditzel et al. [42, 44, 45] used the biomicroscopic method to investigate the alterations in the terminal conjunctival blood vessels in diabetes mellitus. They found a preponderance of capillary enlargement, with a high venule/arteriole ratio and a saccular or fusiform enlargement of the venules. Venular dilation was associated with microscopic oedema.

According to Whittington [134, 135] the only significant aneurysms for the diagnosis of diabetes mellitus are those of the spherical berry-like type. Such aneurysms have been found in about 40.3% of diabetics. The fusiform aneurysms seem to relate to arterial hypertension and the saccular ones to arteriosclerosis. It should, however, be noted that 15% of normal adults may have such aneurysmal dilations. The same author reported that the venule-arteriole ratio is modified in 10–15 % of the non-diabetic subjects.

The observations of Ditzel [42, 44], who reported venular dilations in 47 % of 70 diabetic children, are highly significant however, because they refer to a group of subjects under adult age.

On the other hand, more recent electron microscopic investigation [94] of the conjunctival vessels in biopsy specimens from diabetic subjects showed various degrees of thickening of the vascular basement membrane, proliferation of the endothelial cells and hyperplasia of the arteriolar muscular layer, together with an obvious reduction in the membranous elastic structures. These changes are similar to those found in investigations of other organs and regions of the body in diabetic subjects (see Chapter II).

A systematical biomicroscopic examination has been performed in the conjunctival vessels of the 920 diabetic patients under study at the ACB
The following were recorded as being a significant irregularity of arterioles and venules, aneurysmal alteration, high venule/ arteriole ratio, spontaneous conjunctival ecchymosis, conjunctival oedema, and circumscribed avascular hyaline infiltration of the conjunctiva [117] (Fig. 14–19).

Pathological alterations of the conjunctiva were found in 49.5% of these patients (Fig. 6/III). Fig. 7, 8, 9, 10, 11, 12 and 13/III and Tables I and II show the distribution of these angiopathic findings according to age, duration of diabetes and the treatment applied [113, 114] (see p. 249).

It should be noted that the incidence is close to that reported by Ditzel, who reported it in 47% of the investigated children [49, 113, 114].

The high percentage of conjunctival vascular alteration found in diabetes mellitus reveals the great importance of the systematic examination of the anterior pole of the eye and of the conjunctiva in

Table I. Conjunctival lesions. Distribution according to sex, age and duration of diabetes

Present age (yrs)		Duration of diabetes 0–1 yrs	1–5 yrs	5–10 yrs	10–20 yrs	20–30 yrs	> 30 yrs	Total	Overall total	%
0–20	M	2	2	–	1	–	–	5	11	2.4
	W	1	2	3	–	–	–	6		
21–40	M	1	4	5	2	5	–	17	26	5.7
	W	1	–	3	5	–	–	9		
41–50	M	3	11	4	1	–	–	19	39	8.5
	W	1	4	7	8	–	–	20		
51–60	M	14	21	14	7	1	–	57	115	25.2
	W	9	20	18	8	2	1	58		
>60	M	11	33	39	35	14	6	138	265	58.2
	W	14	52	45	14	1	1	127		
Total		57	149	138	81	23	8	456	456	–
%		12.5	32.66	30.2	17.8	5.04	1.8	–	–	–

M = MEN; W = WOMEN;

Table II. Conjunctival lesions. Distribution according to the duration of diabetes and the management applied

Management	Duration of diabetes 0–1 yrs	1–5 yrs	5–10 yrs	10–20 yrs	20–30 yrs	>30 yrs	Total	%
Diet alone	28	56	48	15	2	2	151	33.1
Diet + Insulin	6	23	20	19	10	3	81	17.8
Diet + Oral antidiabetic drugs	22	67	66	40	11	3	209	45.9
Diet + Insulin + Oral drugs	1	3	4	7	–	–	15	3.2
Total	57	149	138	81	23	8	456	–
%	12.5	32.66	30.2	17.8	5.04	1.8	–	–

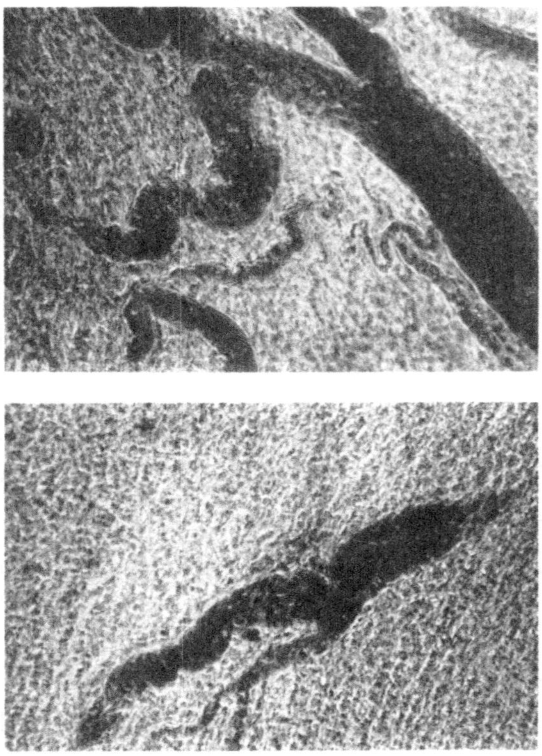

Fig. 14. R. M., 33 years old woman. Juvenile diabetes mellitus Appreciated duration of the disease about 7 years. A.-Conjunctival biopsy: vessels of different diameter with venular tortuosities. The small ones overflow in a bigger, enlarged venule. Modification of the arteriole/venule ratio in favour of the venule. B.-Narrowing of the blood flow, possibly resulting in an aneurismal enlargement.

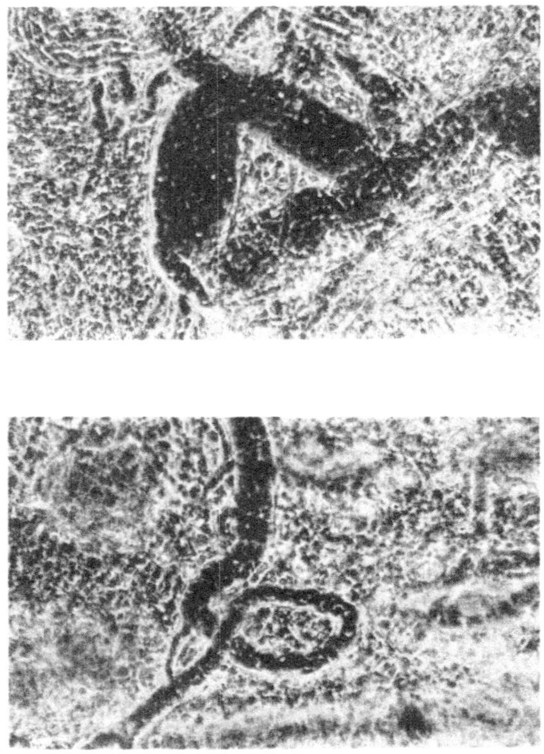

Fig. 15. Conjunctival ocular biopsies from a 50 year old diabetic patient. Treatment with oral hypoglycaemics and diet. Probable duration of the disease 6 years

A. Enlarged venule with variable diameter. Sludging of blood erythrocytes.

B. very enlarged venule with irregularities of its diameter, surrounded by numerous small tortuous venules.

particular. This examination is important since the lesions occur at early stages of the disease and are preceded by a reversible functional stage [48], easy to diagnose. While some authors regard these stages as preceding the onset of retinal microangiopathy, others [113] consider that the changes of permeability and capillary resistance in the conjunctiva are closely related to the retinal alterations without, however, preceding them. There is also a current belief that the two aspects of diabetic microangiopathy are altogether independent [13]. Whatever the relation betwen the microangiopathy of the anterior and posterior poles, (such as precedence, concomitance or independence), it testifies to the particular capillar fragility of the diabetic subject [78].

The incidence of pathological alterations of the anterior pole increases with the age of the subject and to a certain extent with the total number of examined patients. This might suggest that the lesions are non-specific, since they have also been

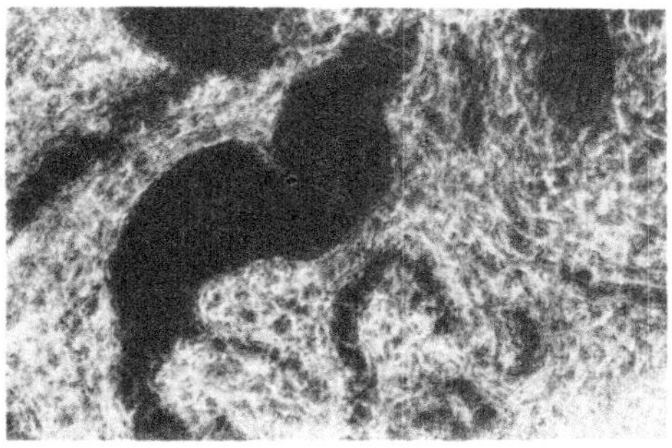

Fig. 16. C. P. 59 year old man with diabetes. Duration of diabetes 9 years.
Pseudo-aneurysmal enlargement of the principal venule. Sinuosities and tortuousity with sludging of the neighbouring vessels.

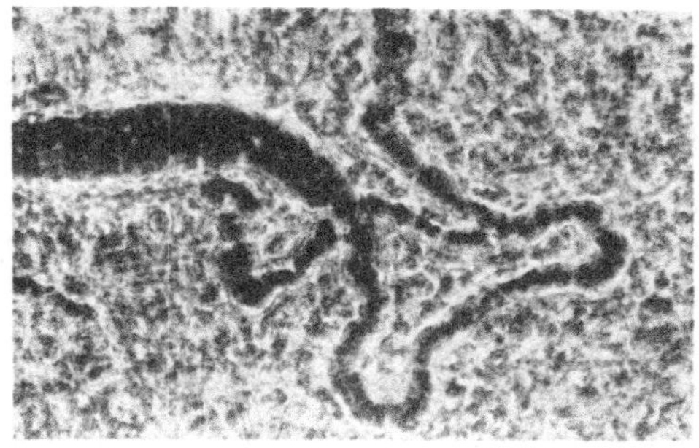

Fig. 18. S. D. 65 year old diabetic. Duration of diabetes about 16 years.
Inequality in the diameter of a sinuous venule with sludging.

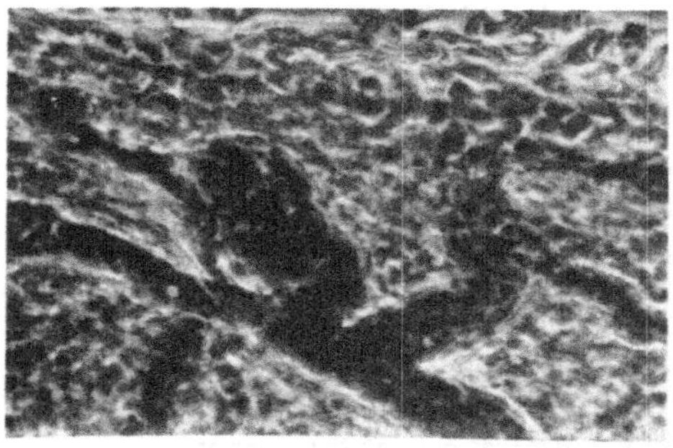

Fig. 17. P. V. 46 year old man with maturity onset diabetes. Duration of diabetes 2 years. Tolbutamide.
Sacciforme dilation of a venule with variable diameter. Sludge.

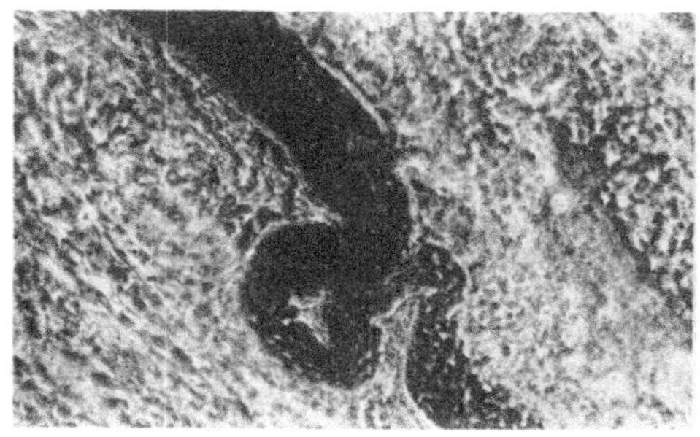

Fig. 19. N. A. 59 year old woman with maturity onset diabetes. Duration of diabetes about 23 years.
Sinuous venule with inequality of diameter and sludging.

found in aged non-diabetic subjects. However, the diabetic condition aggravates their character, increases their incidence and precipitates their onset at earlier ages.

The distribution of lesions according to the duration of the disease yields much higher percentages for the shorter duration (see Table I and Fig. 20 and 21/III). This might be partly due to the small number of patients with longer duration of the diabetes, but also to the fact that certain vascular conjunctival alterations are of a functional character, reversible by adequate management.

Poor control of the diabetes seems to be one of the factors favouring and precipitating the onset of the conjunctival vascular alterations. Diabetes appears to accelerate the normal vascular ageing

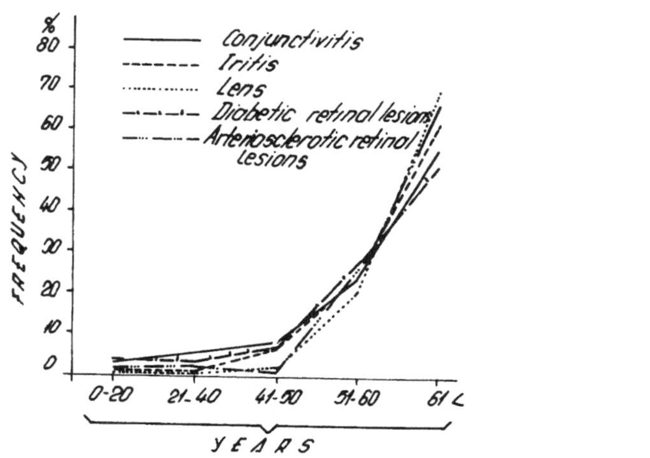

Fig. 20. Age distribution of various ocular complications of diabetes in the statistics of the Antidiabetic Centre in Bucharest.

of the conjunctival vessels and its effect is even more obvious in cases incorrectly treated. [12, 18, 27, 37, 46, 81, 91, 95, 115, 141].

In our research, conjunctival complications are more frequent in diabetics treated by oral therapy (45.8%) than in those managed by insulin (17.8%) (Table II, Fig. 21/III and 22/III). This treatment difference suggests either that the oral predisposes to a greater extent to conjunctival vascular complications, or that the benign character of the

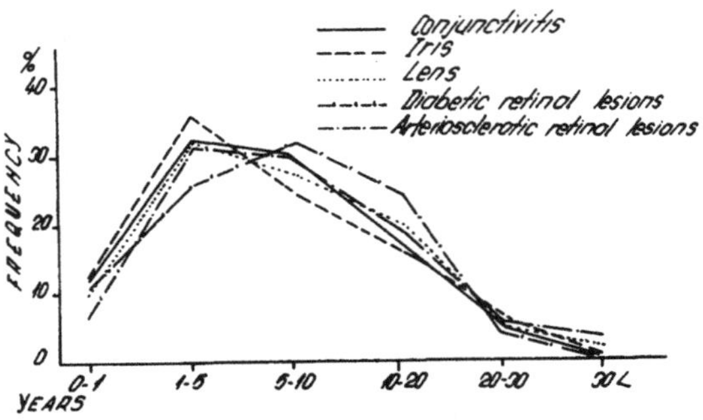

Fig. 21. Distribution of the various diabetic ocular complications according to the possible duration of the disease. Statistics of the Antidiabetic Centre in Bucharest.

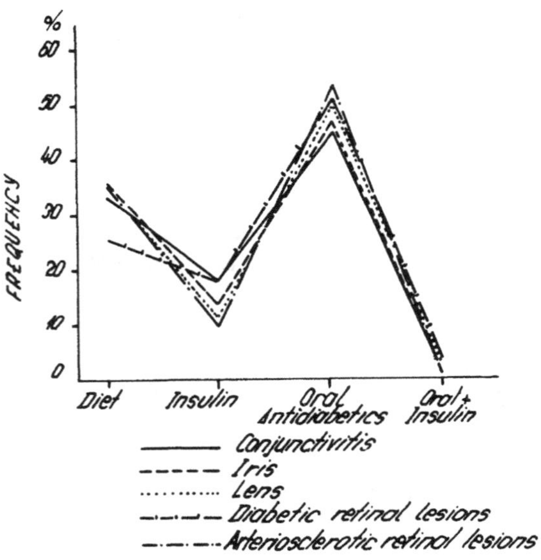

Fig. 22. Percentual distribution of the various ocular diabetic complications according to the applied antidiabetic treatment. Statistics of the Antidiabetic Centre in Bucharest (A.C.B).

disease in these patients keeps them metabolically unbalanced for a longer period. Another possible conclusion from these statistics is that the administration of insulin may be necessary in cases insufficiently balanced by oral therapy or if they have incipient vascular conjunctival alterations.

In summary one has to emphasize the practical importance of the examination of the bulbar conjunctiva and if necessary of biopsy specimens, which permit an early diagnosis of microangiopathy. Although the specificity of the lesions of small vessels in the area is not definite, their high incidence in the diabetic raises important problems with regard to pathogenesis, therapy and prognosis. Mention should also be made of the high frequency of cunjunctival vascular alterations in diabetics treated with oral hypoglycaemic drugs, compared to patients treated with insulin. This probably indicates the importance of adequate control of the diabetes.

2. Diabetic Alterations of the cornea

The alterations of the cornea in diabetes have not been investigated so thoroughly, because they are much less frequent than the other ocular lesions and also because it is much more difficult to determine whether they are specifically of diabetic origin. Authorities still consider that besides the late corneal lesions complicating certain alterations of the iris (rubeosis iridis), no other alterations may be regarded as specific to diabetes [40]. Nevertheless, more recent contributions throw new light on the corneal changes during diabetes [36, 81].

In a classification of the corneal lesions in the diabetic, Collier [151] described:

Keratopathies associated with diabetic coma, featured by ocular hypertension and folding of the cornea.

Keratitis associated with other diabetic ocular complications, particularly with iridic alterations. Diabetic iridis, is for instance, frequently complicated by a deep keratitis which may take the shape of a central parenchymatous keratitis, of the punctata or striate variety. The rubeosis iridis found in diabetic subjects is often complicated by ocular hypertension with subsequent bullous or oedematous corneal alterations.

A corneal endothelial melanosis has also been described which occurs during the degeneration of the iridic pigment sheet, often found in diabetics.

Other keratopathies, in the diabetic. These affect the anterior third of the cornea, and often last only for short intervals, which explains why they are rarely described and only if a careful and systematic examination of the cornea has been performed. Among this group, the diabetic epithelial keratodystrophia punctata seems to be a pathognomonic condition. It consists of epithelial dystrophic fluoresceine-retaining sites with a centrally situated loss of substance circumscribed by an epithelial halo of microvesicles slightly prominent on the corneal surface. These lesions are situated on the lower half of the cornea, in paralimbic position, and show no trend to run together. Their course is short and benign.

A recurrent corneal ulcer has also been described in diabetes, associated with subconjunctival haemorrhage and nodular keratitis, consisting of small, grey, round, opaque areas in the anterior corneal parenchyma. A long course sometimes results in nodular corneal scars.

Corneal degenerations in diabetics. Central or marginal, these consist of folds of Bowman's membrane or of Descemet's membrane. The specificity of these lesions is controversial. Corneal dystrophies and pigmentation of the cornea have also been reported in diabetics. Corneal epithelial melanosis, nodular keratopathy and folding of Descemet's membrane are regarded as important features of diabetic corneal lesions.

The incidence of corneal lesions in diabetic subjects has been reported with a frequency of 8–30 % [81].

The systematic examination of the group of 920 diabetics in the ACB revealed corneal lesions in only 17 patients (1.8 %). Lesions were mostly dystrophic or degenerative, and more frequent in patients over the age of 40.

Duration of diabetes ranged in these patients between 1 and 20 years.

As regards therapy, of 17 patients found with corneal lesions 10 were on oral antidiabetic therapy, 5 on diet alone and 2 on insulin [113, 114].

It should be noted that those authors who investigated corneal lesions in diabetes mellitus failed to correlate their incidence with the age, or the duration and severity of the diabetic condition.

3. Diabetic Alterations of the Iris

Iridic alterations in diabetes mellitus have been reported as occurring comparatively rarely. Thus, the incidence of rubeosis iridis varies from less than 1% to 5% [27]. It is usually described as bilateral and often results in irreversible blindness.

Diabetic iritis is also rarely reported, with an incidence around 1.3%. This figure approximately equals that found for iritis in non-diabetics, an argument in favour of its unspecific character [27]. Whittington [154], who regards diabetic iritis as a specific complication, reported even lower incidences and considers it a rare pathologic condition.

Pigment depositing on the anterior face of the iris and on the posterior face of the cornea is reported in higher percentages, in about 10%, of cases while deposit in the lens may occur in some 3%.

Comparing these data with those found by the ACB, certain differences can be found, probably accounted for by the fact that the group of ophthalmologists who performed the observations were particularly interested in discovering the earliest modifications occurring in the anterior pole of the eye during diabetes mellitus.

The iridic changes found in the group of patients investigated by the ACB were only of pigmentary and vascular character and occurred in 265 patients, 28.8% of the total (Fig. 6/III).

The distribution of the iridic lesions according to the age of the patients indicates a higher incidence with increasing age, 25.3 % in the 51–60 years group and 65.6 % in the group over 60. This suggests a probable relation between degenerative lesions and biological age, irrespective of the presence of diabetes (Fig. 20/III, Table III), especially since there is no parallelism between the incidence of the lesion and diabetes duration throughout the distribution. The iridic lesions are more frequent in the groups of a 1–5 and 5–10 years history of diabetes (35.8 and 24.9 % respectively). As a matter of fact, most of the patients belong to these categories (Fig. 21/III, Table III).

The correlation between the iridic lesions and the type of management shows a higher incidence among patients treated with oral drugs (47.2 %) or diet alone (35.4 %), and less in patients treated with insulin (13.5 %), (Table IV, Fig. 22/III). That means that more than 80% of the patients with iridic lesions were treated with oral drugs or by diet. These data suggest either that there is a lack of parallelism between these complications and the severity of the diabetic condition, or that a possible protective role is exerted by insulin, resulting in a better metabolic balance. The study of iridic lesions of the diabetic has led to the following conclusions:

- iridic alterations were found in almost 30% of the investigated subjects (Fig. 23–26);
- pigmentary and vascular alterations are predominant;

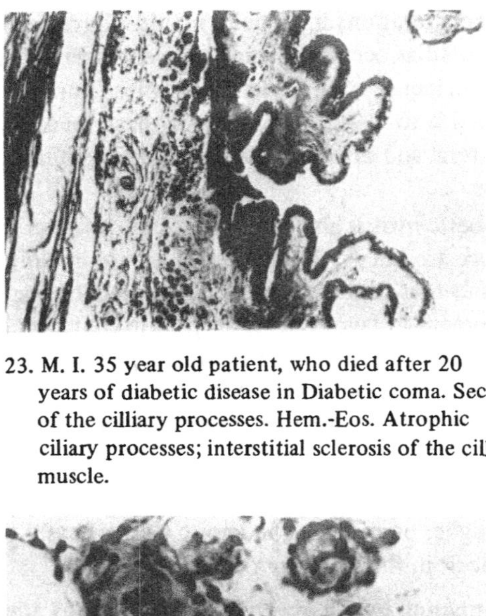

Fig. 23. M. I. 35 year old patient, who died after 20 years of diabetic disease in Diabetic coma. Section of the cilliary processes. Hem.-Eos. Atrophic ciliary processes; interstitial sclerosis of the cilliar muscle.

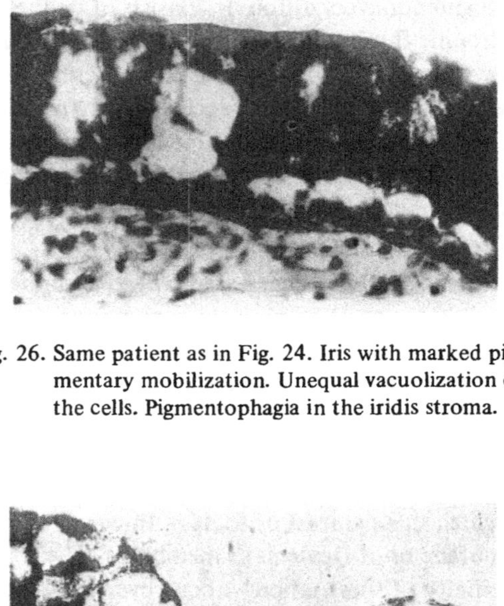

Fig. 26. Same patient as in Fig. 24. Iris with marked pigmentary mobilization. Unequal vacuolization of the cells. Pigmentophagia in the iridis stroma.

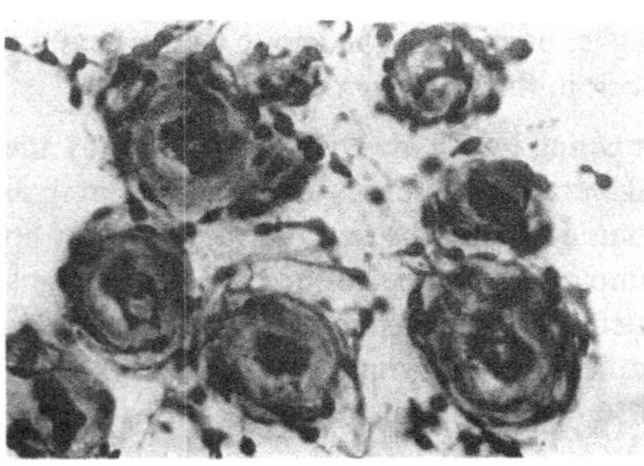

Fig. 24. D. M. 16 year old boy, died with Coma diabetica. Iridian vessels (Hem.Eos). Endothelial proliferation completely obturating the vascular lumen. Thickening of the vascular walls. Oedema.

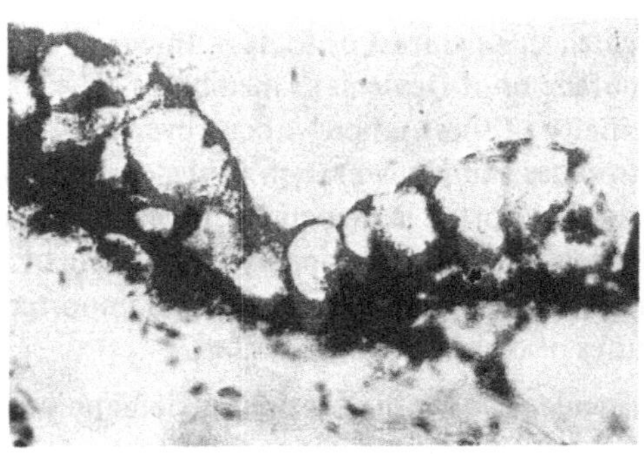

Fig. 25. Same patient as in Fig. 24. Iridian epithelium dystrophy with unequal vacuolazition.

Table III. Lesion of the iris. Distribution according to sex, age and duration of diabetes

Present age (yrs)	Sex	Duration of diabetes						Total	Overall total	%
		0–1 yrs	1–5 yrs	5–10 yrs	10–20 yrs	20–30 yrs	> 30 yrs			
0–20	M	–	–	–	–	–	–	–	3	1.1
	W	1	2	–	–	–	–	3		
21–40	M	1	–	–	–	1	–	2	2	0.7
	W	–	–	–	–	–	–	–		
41–50	M	1	5	1	–	–	–	7	19	7.2
	W	–	3	4	5	–	–	12		
51–60	M	4	13	8	5	2	–	32	67	25.3
	W	8	11	10	6	–	–	35		
> 60	M	7	23	13	20	13	3	79	174	65.7
	W	11	38	30	9	4	3	95		
Total		33	95	66	45	20	6	265	265	–
%		12.4	35.9	24.9	17.0	7.5	2.3	–	–	–

M = MEN; W = WOMEN;

Table IV. Lesions of the iris. Distribution according to the duration of diabetes

Management	Duration of diabetes						Total	%
	0–1 yrs	1–5 yrs	5–10 yrs	10–20 yrs	20–30 yrs	> 30 yrs		
Diet alone	20	39	26	6	2	1	94	35.5
Diet + Insulin	2	8	8	11	4	3	36	13.5
Diet + Oral antidiabetic drugs	10	45	32	23	13	2	125	47.2
Diet + Insulin + Oral drugs	1	3	–	5	1	–	10	3.8
Total	33	95	66	45	20	6	265	–
%	12.4	35.9	24.9	17.0	7.5	2.3	–	–

– incidence is significantly higher in patients treated by oral drugs or diet alone than in those treated with insulin.

Intraocular nutrition depends on blood supply and on the aqueous humour discharged by the ciliary epithelium. Alteration in any of these elements might underlie the ocular complications of diabetes mellitus, namely of retinopathy, glaucoma, cataracta, iridopathy and even of the corneal complications. In diabetics besides the common vascular alterations of the microangiopathic process [157], a remarkable thickening of the basement membrane of the ciliary bodies was found. This might offer a consistent explanation for the pathogenesis of the alterations of the iris, lens and other ocular structures, even if it does not cover all the clinical findings and their evolution [12, 157].

Blumenthal et al. [17] performed investigations with fluorescent insulin, which was retained in the glomerular nodules in diabetic nephropathy. Similar findings have been reported in other diabetic microangiopathic lesions. Outstanding among these is the report of Coleman et al. [31] who described the process in the thickened basement membrane of the ciliary epithelium. These observations might substantiate a summing up of the present knowledge on the pathogenesis of diabetic microangiopathy in general (see Chapter II) and of the iridic alterations in particular. It has also been suggested that vascular neoformation both in the retina and the iris might be stimulated by the presence of a metabolic by-product, reaching the iris through the aqueous and vitreous bodies [27].

Experimental work on animals shows that ischaemia in the area of the ciliary arteries plays an important role in vascular neoformation. No such process was demonstrated in man.

Iridic alterations may be due to pigmentary, vascular or inflammatory disorders.

a) The main pigmentary alteration is cystic degeneration of the pigmentary epithelium, resulting in depigmented areas and the formation of vacuoles on the anterior surface of the iris. The discharged pigment is stored in the neighbouring tissues.

Light microscopic examinations demonstrate the Presence of vacuoles filled with PAS-positive material. Such glycogen infiltrations are not specific to diabetes mellitus and represent a phase that precedes the degeneration of the pigment cell [27] which undergoes swelling, lengthening and proliferation and final disintegration. Its possible adherence to the capsule of the lens brings about the storage of the discharged pigment in the latter.

The picture is that of "diabetic iridopathy" and has an obvious degenerative character.

The sclerosis of the iridic vessels, as well as the atrophy and depigmentation of the iris confer on that organ the appearance of a strip of rigid connective tissue which accounts for the diminished photomotor reflex activity.

b) Among the iridic vascular alterations in diabetes, rubeosis iridis has been the most thoroughly investigated. It consists of a non-inflammatory vascular proliferation in the upper layers of the iridal stroma, which develops into a particulary severe secondary glaucoma. The delicate network of newly formed capillaries gives the iris a reddish tint. These neogenetic vessels appear to consist only of an endothelium and to be very poor in connective tissue, hence their easy bleeding [27]. The biomicroscopical examination shows that the neogenetic capillaries originate from the pigmentary collar, which they never invade, and spread in a radial direction, giving rise to a rich anastomatic system. They reach the deep layers of the iridic tissue and occasionally group together into prominent vascular agglomerations. An associated inflammatory process, as well as the iridic atrophy subsequently promote ectropion uvae and finally result in the formation of a pupillary membrans [27].

The radial and peripheral extension of the neogenetic vessels results in an increase in intraocular pressure which leads to the onset of a painful, incurable, haemorrhagic glaucoma [12]. In certain cases, however, the neogenetic vessels may spontaneously subside together with the increased intraocular pressure [27]. Rubeosis iridis is regarded as specific to diabetes mellitus only when it is bilateral. In most cases, the process of new vessel formation is asymmetrical, predominating in one eye.

Some authors distinguish between true diabetic rubeosis and posthaemorrhagic rubeosis [46]. True diabetic rubeosis is bilateral and starts at the level of the pigmentary collar of the pupilla in irregular vascular agglomerations. It only begins after many years of diabetes, and in the absence of haemorrhage, while posthaemorrhagic rubeosis follows several months after a thrombosis of the central vein or a hyphema, both subsequent to glaucoma. True rubeosis generally precedes glaucoma, while posthaemorrhagic glaucoma follows it. According to most authors, rubeosis iridis precedes and is always associated with diabetic retinopathy featured by severe preretinal haemorrhage [66], finally resulting in the glaucoma of diabetes mellitus [153, 154].

c) Diabetic inflammatory alterations of the iris include the very rare and much contested diabetic iriditis. According to various investigators, the true nature of diabetic iriditis is an infectious iridocyclitis which occurs on a particular metabolically altered substratum. The diabetic condition appears to confer to this inflammatory complication a particular pattern consisting of a marked pericorneal vasculopathy with conjunctival chemosis, very dilated veins and a thick albuminous exudate which fills the anterior chamber and rapidly subsides under antidiabetic management.

Other authors [134, 135] do not share this opinion and consider that the process is specific to diabetes and characterized by an extreme vascularization of the pericorneal tissues, marked oedema of the conjunctiva, sinuous veins filled with blood near the limbus, by the presence of an exudate looking like the uncooked white of an egg and by new vessel formation similar to that found in rubeosis. In the early stages, ocular pressure is low and the symptoms subside in some 3 weeks with effective antidiabetic management.

4. Diabetic Alterations of the Lens

The lesions of the lens have been long known but controversy persists as to whether these lesions result from or are only associated with diabetes mellitus. General agreement exists upon the presence of the alterations of the lens in young diabetic subjects and the specific form of the diabetic cataract in young diabetes.

The lesions of the lens in diabetes are regarded today as subsequent to the hyperglycaemic state, which results in an excessive accumulation of sorbitol [26, 27]. Glucose is the main nutritive element of the lens and its filtration into the lens does not depend on the presence of insulin, but the fact that the hormone controls glycaemia accounts for the correlation between the metabolic imbalance and the incidence of lens alterations in diabetes mellitus.

In fact, the lens is an isolated organ [27] deprived of blood vessels and nerves and suspended on the ciliary body. Its nutrition occurs only by imbibitition from the environment, hence an alteration cannot be regarded as a pure expression of diabetic microangiopathy.

In spite of the above remarks, we shall briefly review the data reported in the literature and the experience of the ACB on the prevalence of lens alterations. The literature suggests that there is a significant relation between the duration of the diabetic condition and the incidence of the alteration. On the other hand, the complication appears to be preponderant in females. Caird [25], Whittington [135], Burditt and Caird [21] found that after a 10 year diabetic history, 5–11 % of the patients show some degree of lens involvement, and its incidence rises to 23–32 % after 20 years. As regard lens opacity in juvenile diabetes, the figures reported by various authors range between 2 and 56% [21, 25].

In the ACB lens alterations were found in 455 of the examined patients, that is in almost 50 % (Fig. 6/III). Considering the various alterations of the lens (opacity, condensation) apart from the deve-

Table V. Lesions of the lens. Distribution according to sex, age and duration of diabetes

Present age (yrs)	Sex	Duration of diabetes						Total	Overall total	%
		0–1 yrs	1–5 yrs	5–10 yrs	10–20 yrs	20–30 yrs	> 30 yrs			
0–20	M	–	–	–	–	–	–	–	2	0.4
	W	–	–	2	–	–	–	2		
21–40	M	–	–	–	–	–	–	–	4	0.9
	W	1	1	1	1	–	–	4		
41–50	M	1	3	1	–	–	–	5	13	2.9
	W		2	4	2	–	–	8		
51–60	M	7	16	9	7	–	–	39	100	22.0
	W	9	27	15	8	1	1	61		
> 60	M	13	41	37	51	22	8	172	336	73.8
	W	15	55	58	27	4	5	164		
Total		46	145	127	96	27	14	455	455	–
%		10.1	31.8	28.0	21.0	5.9	3.2	–	–	–

M = MEN; W = WOMEN;

Table VI. Lesions of the lens. Distribution according to the duration of diabetes and to the type of antidiabetic management

Management	Duration of diabetes						Total	%
	0–1 yrs	1–5 yrs	5–10 yrs	10–20 yrs	20–30 yrs	> 30 yrs		
Diet alone	26	63	45	20	1	6	161	35.4
Diet + Insulin	3	10	13	14	7	3	50	11.0
Diet + Oral antidiabetic drugs	17	70	64	54	18	5	228	50.1
Diet + Insulin + Oral drugs	–	2	5	8	1		16	3.5
Total	46	145	127	96	27	14	455	–
%	10.1	31.8	28.0	21.0	5.9	3.2	–	–

loped cataract, the former were found in 421 patients (45.7 %) and the latter in 34 (3.7 %). The first figure is very near to that found in the literature (40 %), while for cataract higher figures have been reported (5–7 %).

The distribution of lens alterations according to the age of the patients shows that the incidence of the complication increases with age: 2.9 % for the 41–50 years interval, 22% between 51–60 years and 73.8% over 60 years of age (Fig. 20/III, Table V). It should be noted that no case of constituted cataract was under the age of 40, and that 26 out of the 34 patients with cataract were over 60. These data suggest that biological ageing in the diabetic enhances the disorders of the lens in general and cataract in particular.

In our statistics, the incidence of lens alterations is higher in the cases with a short diabetic history (1–10 years). This is either due to the late onset of diabetes in older individuals, or the early disorders may be, to a certain extent, reversed by therapy (Fig. 21/III, Table V).

The method of treatment appears to be particularly significant. It was found that 85% of the lens alterations occur in patients treated with oral antidiabetic drugs (50.1 %) and by diet alone (35.4 %), while among the patients treated with insulin the incidence was only 11 % (Fig. 22/III, Table VI).

The incidence of opacity of the lens, and of subcapsular vacuoles, alterations which are to a certain extent reversible is therefore fairly high in young diabetic subjects.

Diabetic cataract in the young is characterized by: early onset (mostly under the age of 25), rapid course to maturation into a soft intumescent cataract and bilaterality of the lesions. The process obviously proceeds at a much slower rate if the diabetic condition is under adequate control. The biomicroscopical aspect of diabetic cataract in the young is “shaggy” or “snowstorm-like”. Early opacities are subcapsular, and the cortex acquires an ice-like aspect as the vacuoles dissociate the fibres. The chronic cataract in which diabetes is incriminated is posterior subcapsular.

Senile cataract in the diabetic is in no way different from the picture of common senile cataract. According to Dolfus’ statistics (quoted by 40), there is no significant difference between the incidence of cataract in diabetic and non-diabetic subjects over the age of 40.

It might be concluded from the above that the disorders of the lens are only indirectly the consequence of a microangiopathy in so far as the microangiopathic process, involving the intraocular vascular network, brings about conditions promoting the onset of such disorders in that isolated organ.

It should however be noted that alterations of the lens are particularly frequent in the diabetic (50%), and that age and therapy are in a significant correlation with the onset of the process. The fact is also worth remembering that in our statistics the incidence of lens alterations is much lower (11%) in patients treated with insulin than in those treated by diet only or with oral antidiabetic drugs.

B. Alterations of the Posterior Ocular Pole

1. Diabetic Retinopathy

Since the retinal alterations may be readily observed by ophthalmoscopic examination and photographic recording, they are among the most important clinical signs of diabetic microangiopathy and one of the earliest positive indications of the presence of this degenerative complication in diabetes mellitus.

The retinal lesions consist of a variable association of seven elements: microaneurysms, anomalies of the retinal veins, haemorrhage, exudates, new vessel formation, glial proliferation and vitreous detachment [25, 27]. A classification of the various patterns of evolution of diabetic retinopathy is required both for establishing clinical criteria to estimate the severity of the complication and for statistical investigation. Various stages have been defined by grouping the symptoms of diabetic retinopathy, although actual cases seldom fit the respective classification [25, 40].

The classification adopted at the ACB for the investigation of the prevalence of the condition and for clinical purposes divides diabetic retinopathy into 4 stages R_1, R_2, R_3 and R_4, taking into account the lesions found in the more severely involved eye. There is also a fifth group in the tables-R_5, for patients in whom some other type of retinopathy has been diagnosed (hypertensive, arteriosclerotic, etc) [122], on the ground of modifications in vascular calibre (arteriolar spasticity), shape (sunous arterioles and veins), the crossing sign (Salus Gunn), etc.

The following four stages were considered as significant for statistical studies on the incidence and prevalence of diabetic retinopathy.

Stage I (R-1) – segmental perimacular venous enlargements, primitive or associated with retinal xanthosis.

Stage II (R-2) – microaneurysms and punctiform exudates.

Stage III (R_3) – haemorrhage, confluent exudates, pigment alteration and lesions of the major veins.

Stage IV (R-4) – vascular proliferation with preretinal haemorrhage (proliferative retinitis), retinal degeneration and eventually secondary glaucoma.

Investigations at the ACB, on the prevalence of microangiopathic disorders found in the posterior pole of the eye, in 1,920 diabetic patients selected at random from cases recorded during the 1968–1969 interval, resulted in the following observations:

Retinal lesions were found in 44.9% of the cases, a figure fairly near to that recorded for cunjunctival lesions (49.5%) and for alterations of the lens (49.4%) (Fig. 6, 113, 114/III).

The distribution of diabetic retinopathy according to sex yielded results much too insignificant to be reported in detail. The higher number of women with diabetic retinopathy is accounted for by the fact that diabetes itself is more frequent in females [27, 135, 136, 154].

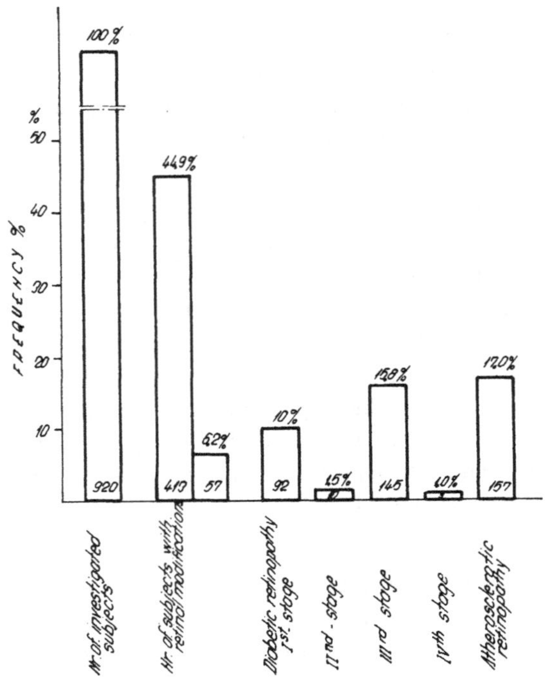

Fig. 27. Incidence of the various stages of diabetic retinopathy (stages I, II, III and IV) as well as of the arteriosclerotic retinopathy in 920 patients of the A.C.B.

As regards the distribution according to the stage of the alterations, 11% were found to be in stages I and II (R_1 and R_2), 16.7% in stages III and IV (R_3 and R_4) while the other 17 % were arteriosclerotic, with no specific diabetic character (Fig. 27/III, Table VII–XII). As compared to the total number of retinal lesions, retinopathy in stages I and II represents 25%, that in stages III and IV 37 % and arteriosclerotic retinopathy 37 %. It should be noted that fundus examination failed in 57 patients (6.2%), because of lens alterations which prevented a conclusive fundus examination. It might be assumed that retinopathy was to be found in most of these patients.

The figure found for the incidence of the lesions in stages I and II (11%) is similar to that reported by Walker [130] and Hardin [66]. Swelling and congestion of the retinal veins is the most important symptom in the early stages of diabetes while

Table VII. Diabetic retinopathy. Distribution of the lesions in stages I and II ($R_1 + R_2$) according to sex, age and duration of diabetes

Present age (yrs)	Sex	Duration of diabetes						Total	Overall total	%
		0–1 yrs	1–5 yrs	5–10 yrs	10–20 yrs	20–30 yrs	> 30 yrs			
0–20	M	–	1	–	–	–	–	1	7	6.9
	W	–	4	1	1	–	–	6		
21–40	M	1	–	–	–	1	–	2	3	2.9
	W	–	1	–	–	–	–	1		
41–50	M	–	3	3	–	–	–	6	8	7.9
	W	–	1	1	–	–	–	2		
51–60	M	1	3	5	4	–	–	13	24	23.5
	W	3	2	5	1	–	–	11		
> 60	M	3	8	5	5	1	2	24	60	58.8
	W	7	14	8	6	1	–	36		
Total		15	37	28	17	3	2	102	102	–
%		14.7	36.3	27.5	16.7	2.9	1.9	–	–	–

M = MEN; W = WOMEN;

the other alterations of the retina, such as microaneurysms and haemorrhage, begin later. These early changes of diabetes (clinical or preclinical) are reversible under an adequate management of the disease. On the other hand, tendency to develop thrombosis, intravitreous haemorrhage and proliferative retinopathy is retained [87, 114]. The distribution of the lesions in stage I (R_1) according to age, yielded for the 0–20 years age group an incidence of 7.6%, the highest percentage of retinal lesions for that age group (Fig. 28/III). The highest figures were recorded in the older age groups, probably due to the higher number of cases or to the fact reported by other authors [134, 135] that the older the subjects, the earlier retinopathy begins. Severe forms of diabetic retinopathy are more frequent during juvenile diabetes although Levin has shown that a mature diabetes can also lead to a severe form in case of pancreatic beta cell deficiency.

The distribution of the lesions in stage I according to the duration of the diabetes confirms the presence of the complication in recent diabetes, since the highest percentage (35.8%) was recorded in the 1–5 year duration group (Fig. 28/III). Among the cases of diabetes with a history of less then 5 years, 52% were found with retinal alterations in stage I, while the incidence for other stages in the same age group was lower.

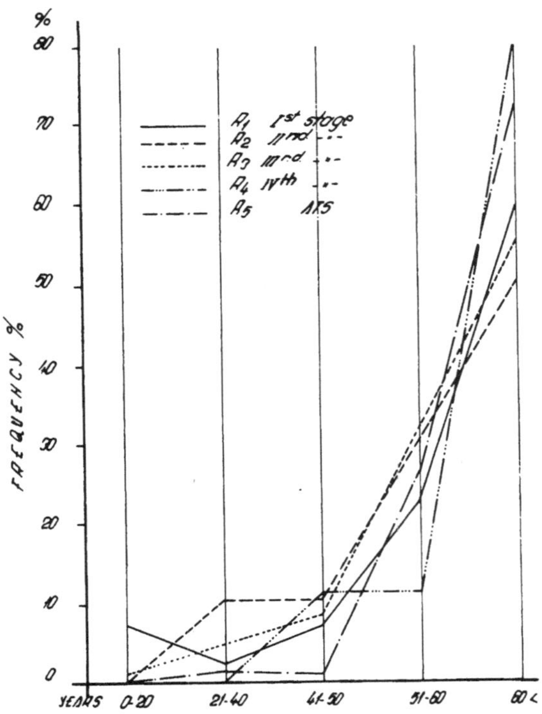

Fig. 28. Age distribution of the various stages (I, II, III, IV) of diabetic retinopathy and arteriosclerotic retinopathy in diabetics. Statistics of the A.C.B.

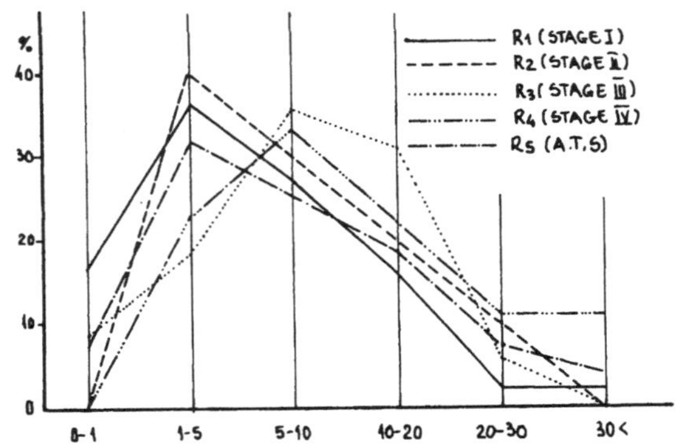

Fig. 29. Percentual distribution of the various stages (I, II, III, and IV) of diabetic retinopathy and of arterio-sclerotic retinopathy in diabetics according to the supposed duration of the diabetic disease. Statistics of the A.C.B.

The highest incidence of cases with lesions in stage II (R_2) was found in recent diabetes (1–5 years duration) (Fig. 29/III).

It is known that the key lesion of stage II (R_2), capillary microaneurysm, while particularly frequent with diabetes mellitus, is not absolutely specific to it and may be brought about by various factors found in several pathological conditions [4, 120]. Investigations using fluorescent techniques and electroretinograms have also confirmed the presence of retinal alteration in the early stages of diabetes [55, 80, 137, 139].

Correlations between antidiabetic therapy and retinal involvement will be dealt with in a general discussion concerning retinal lesions, since they all seem to depend on the type of therapy (Fig. 30/III). Table VIII.

The distribution of the retinal alterations in stages III and IV according to age shows their predominance in older patients (54.5% of stage III lesions and 78% of stage IV lesions were found in patients over the age of 60). Only 0.7% of the alterations in stage IV (R_4) was recorded in patients under 40 years of age (Fig. 28/III).

Considering prevalence in relation to the duration of diabetic history, most of the lesions in stages III and IV (R_3 and R_4) take longer to appear. While peak figures for stages I and II fall in the 1–5 years duration group, the percentage of stage III and IV lesions was at its highest in patients with a 5–10 year history of the disease, and was also high in others with a 10–20 year diabetic history (Gig. 29/III, Table IX).

The small percentage of cases having advanced retinal alterations found with long duration diabetes may be due to the small number of such patients in the investigated group, or to the fact that only diabetics with milder arterial lesions survive for longer intervals.

The unspecific lesions grouped under the heading R_5, such as hypertensive and arteriosclerotic retinopathy, occurred in 17 % of all the patients examined and 37% of the cases in which some retinal in-

Table VIII. Diabetic retinopathy. Distribution of the lesions in stage I and II ($R_1 + R_2$) according to the duration of diabetes and to type of management

Management	Duration of diabetes						Total	%
	0–1 yrs	1–5 yrs	5–10 yrs	10–20 yrs	20–30 yrs	> 30 yrs		
Diet alone	9	9	6	1	–	–	25	24.5
Diet + Insulin	1	8	4	3	1	–	17	16.7
Diet + Oral antidiabetic drugs	5	18	17	12	2	2	56	54.9
Diet + Insulin + Oral drugs	–	2	1	1	–	–	4	3.9
Total	15	37	28	17	3	2	102	–
%	14.7	36.3	27.5	16.7	2.9	1.9	–	–

Table IX. Diabetic retinopathy. Distribution of the lesions in stages III and IV ($R_3 + R_4$) according to sex, age and duration of the diabetes

Present age yrs		Duration of diabetes						Total	Overall total	%
		0–1 yrs	1–5 yrs	5–10 yrs	10–20 yrs	20–30 yrs	> 30 yrs			
0–20	M	–	–	–	–	–	–	–	1	0.6
	W	–	–	–	1	–	–	1		
21–40	M	–	1	–	1	–	–	2	7	4.5
	W	–	–	3	2	–	–	5		
41–50	M	1	1	1	1	–	–	4	13	8.5
	W	–	1	6	2	–	–	9		
51–60	M	5	5	8	6	2	–	26	47	30.5
	W	4	3	5	7	2	–	21		
> 60	M	1	6	16	18	5	–	46	86	55.9
	W	1	12	16	9	1	1	40		
Total		12	29	55	47	10	1	154	154	–
%		7.8	18.8	35.8	30.5	6.5	0.6	–	–	–

M = MEN; W = WOMEN;

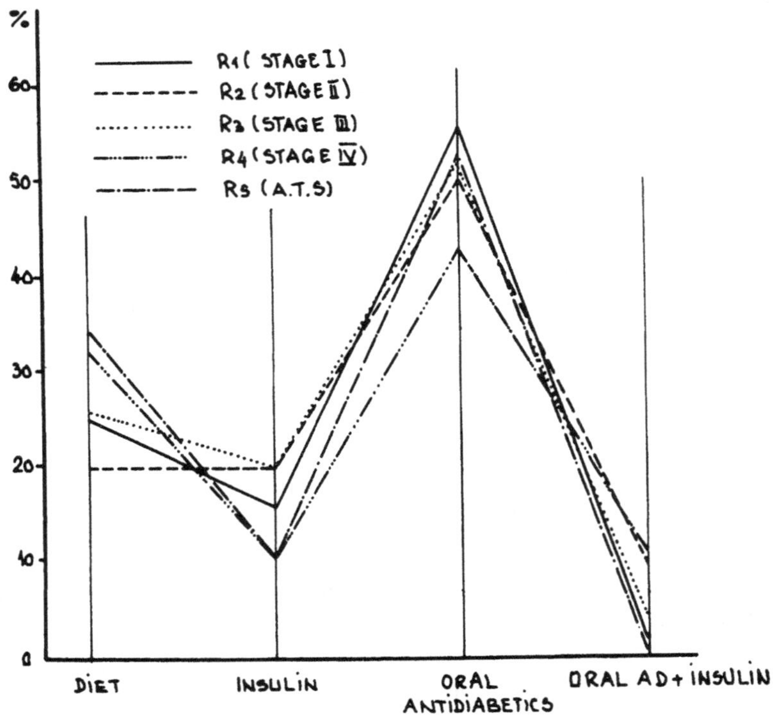

Fig. 30. Percentual distribution of the various evolutive stages (I, II, III and IV) of diabetic retinopathy and of arteriosclerotic retinopathy in diabetics (stage V) according to the kind of treatment applied. Statistics of the A.C.B.

volvement was found. Most of the subjects belong to the older age groups: 70.7 % were over 60 and the complication was virtually absent under the age of 50. This particular distribution favours the specificity of the retinopathy described in diabetes and its differentiation from the arteriosclerotic and hypertensive vascular lesions found in the eye (Table XI/III, Fig. 20/III and 28/III).

Mention has already been made of a group of 57 subjects (6.2%) in which alterations of the lens prevented fundus examination (Fig. 27/III). Retinopathy was probably present in most of these patients and its diagnosis would have increased the overall incidence of retinopathy. Taking into account that 44 of these patients (77%) were over the age of 60, cataract should be regarded as a highly probable occurrence.

The distribution of retinopathy according to the kind of antidiabetic management suggested important pathogenetic and therapeutic implications. In the following, all stages of retinopathic alteration will be dealt with as a whole, since their distributions are very similar. It was found that retinopathy, like all the other ocular alterations in diabetes, is most frequently found (over 50%) in the group of patients controlled by oral therapy, and is at its lowest in patients treated with insulin (16.6% for stages I and II, 18.8% for stages III and IV), (Fig. 22/III and 30/III, Tables VIII, X and XII).

The group of patients treated with insulin associated with oral drugs is too small to permit analysis.

It results that more than 75% of the cases with retinal involvement were treated with oral drugs, by diet alone and fewer than a quarter (1/5) with insulin.

Table X. Diabetic retinopathy. Distribution of the lesions in stages III and IV ($R_3 + R_4$) according to the duration of the diabetes and to the type of antidiabetic management

Management		Duration of diabetes					Total	%
	0–1 yrs	1–5 yrs	5–10 yrs	10–20 yrs	20–30 yrs	> 30 yrs		
Diet alone	5	7	23	6	–	–	41	26.5
Diet + Insulin	1	3	8	13	3	1	29	18.8
Diet + Oral antidiabetic drugs	6	19	24	22	6	–	77	50.2
Diet + Insulin + Oral drugs	–	–	–	6	1	–	7	4.5
Total	12	29	55	47	10	1	154	–
%	7.8	18.8	35.8	30.5	6.5	0.6	–	–

Table XI. Retinopathy in the diabetic. Distribution of the alterations of atherosclerotic type (R_5) according to the duration of diabetes

Present age yrs	Sex	Duration of diabetes						Total	Overall total	%
		0–1 yrs	1–5 yrs	5–10 yrs	10–20 yrs	20–30 yrs	> 30 yrs			
0–20	M	–	1	–	–	–	–	1	1	0.6
	W	–	–	–	–	–	–	–		
21–40	M	–	–	–	1	–	–	1	2	1.3
	W	–	–	1	–	–	–	1		
41–50	M	–	–	–	–	–	–	–	2	1.3
	W	–	–	1	1	–	–	2		
51–60	M	3	6	5	4	·	–	18	41	26.1
	W	2	10	7	4	–	–	23		
> 60	M	2	16	9	15	10	4	56	111	70.7
	W	4	17	24	6	1	3	55		
Total		11	50	47	31	11	7	157	157	–
%		7.0	31.9	29.9	19.8	7.0	4.4	–	–	–

M = MEN; W = WOMEN;

These findings once more suggest that insulin exerts a protective role in ocular microangiopathy or, at least, that it affords a better control of the diabetic condition. The data permit an even wider conjecture (apparently benign diabetes resulting in more severe complications, the noxious role of sulphonamide therapy, etc).

It cannot be decided for certain, however, whether the low incidence of retinopathy with insulin therapy is directly due to insulin, or to a better control of the disease.

As far as visual ability of the patients with retinal complications is concerned, it depends on the extent of the alterations of the fundus and on their location on the retina. This accounts for the high number [135] of diabetic patients in which sight is only mildly affected, in spite of haemorrhage and exudate. According to British statistics [25], the risk of blindness does not exceed 7%, even after 30 years of diabetic history.

It should also be noted that in the USA incidence of diabetes among the blind is 8.4 %, which

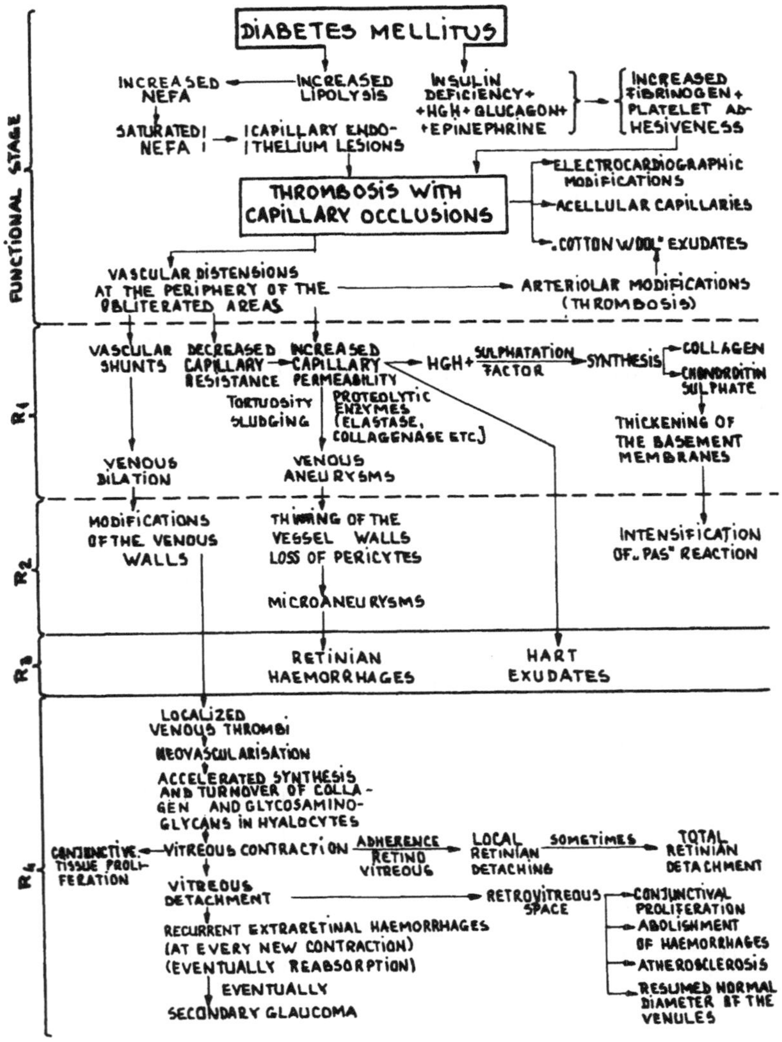

Fig. 31. Diagram of the stages of development of diabetic retinopathy.

Table XII. Retinopathy in the diabetic. Distribution of the lesions of atherosclerotic type (R_5) according to the duration of diabetes and type of management

Management	Duration of diabetes						Total	%
	0–1 yrs	1–5 yrs	5–10 yrs	10–20 yrs	20–30 yrs	> 30 yrs		
Diet alone	6	25	16	5	–	4	56	35.7
Diet + Insulin	–	3	4	6	2	1	16	10.2
Diet + Oral antidiabetic drugs	5	21	26	20	9	2	83	52.8
Diet + Insulin + Oral drugs	–	1	1	–	–	–	2	1.3
Total	11	50	47	31	11	7	157	–
%	7.0	31.9	29.9	19.8	7.0	4.4	–	–

amounts to 1% of the total number of known diabetics [64]. In accordance with recent statistics in Wales, diabetic retinopathy accounts for 7% of the blind, a figure very near to that found in the USA. The overall incidence of blindness in all diabetics was 2.7 % and that of blindness due to retinopathy 1.9 % [25]. The overall incidence of blindness by retinopathy in all age groups in the population is 0.6 %, a figure 11–29 times higher than that of blindness due to all other causes [22, 23]. There are no similar statistics for Rumania.

With a view to elucidating the importance of age, duration of the disease and the type of management in detecting diabetic ocular complications, these parameters have also been investigated in a group of 156 patients (representing 17 % out of the total of 920 diabetics examined in this study) with a completely normal ophthalmological picture (Tables XIII and XIV).

The incidence of a normal condition obviously decreases with age, from 26.9 % in the 0–20 years group, to 18 % over 50 years (Fig. 32/III).

The percentage of ophthalmologically normal subjects also falls with the duration of the diabetic condition and only 0.6% of the patients with a diabetic history of more than 20 years were free from ocular complications (Fig. 33/III).

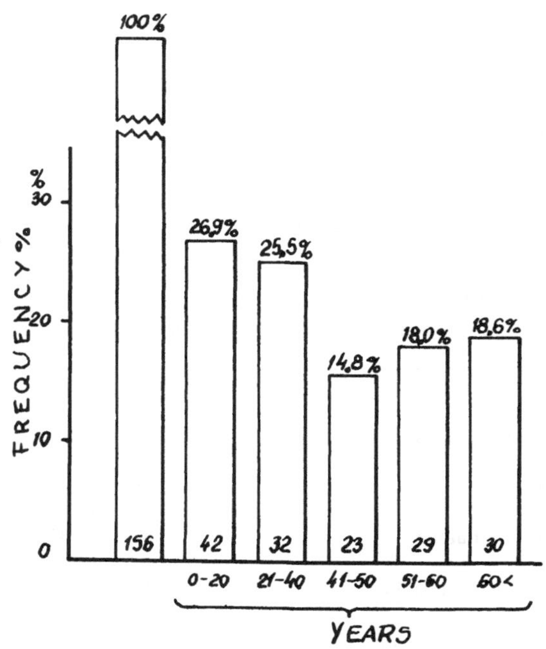

Fig. 32. Diabetics without ocular complications. Age distribution in 156 subjects. Statistics of the A.C.B.

Table XIII. Diabetic patients without ocular complications. Distribution according to sex, age and duration of the diabetic condition

Present age (yrs)	Sex	Duration of diabetes						Total	Overall total	%
		0–1 yrs	1–5 yrs	5–10 yrs	10–20 yrs	20–30 yrs	> 30 yrs			
0–20	M	1	12	6	2	–	–	21	42	26.9
	W	4	9	7	1	–	–	21		
21–40	M	–	6	8	5	–	–	19	32	20.5
	W	–	4	3	6	–	–	13		
41–50	M	5	7	–	2	–	–	14	23	14.7
	W	2	3	3	1	–	–	9		
51–60	M	–	5	4	1	–	–	10	29	18.6
	W	3	12	4	–	–	–	19		
> 60	M	1	6	4	3	–	1	15	30	19.3
	W	3	5	3	3	1	–	15		
Total		19	69	42	24	1	1	156	156	–
%		12.2	44.3	26.9	15.4	0.6	0.6	–	–	–

M = MEN; W = WOMEN;

Table XIV. Diabetic patients without ocular complications. Distribution according to the duration of the diabetic condition and to the type of management

Management	Duration of diabetes						Total	%
	0–1 yrs	1–5 yrs	5–10 yrs	10–20 yrs	20–30 yrs	> 30 yrs		
Diet alone	4	17	11	4	–	1	37	23.8
Diet + Insulin	6	31	22	15	–	–	74	47.3
Diet + Oral antidiabetic drugs	9	19	9	5	1	–	43	27.6
Diet + Insulin + Oral drugs	–	2	–	–	–	–	2	1.3
Total	19	69	42	24	1	1	156	–
%	12.2	44.3	26.9	15.4	0.6	0.6	–	–

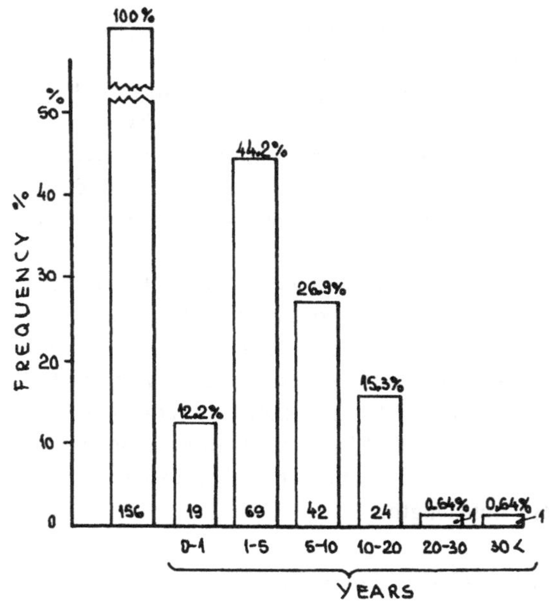

Fig. 33. Diabetics without ocular complications. Distribution according to the supposed duration of the diabetic disease in 156 subjects. Statistics of the A.C.B.

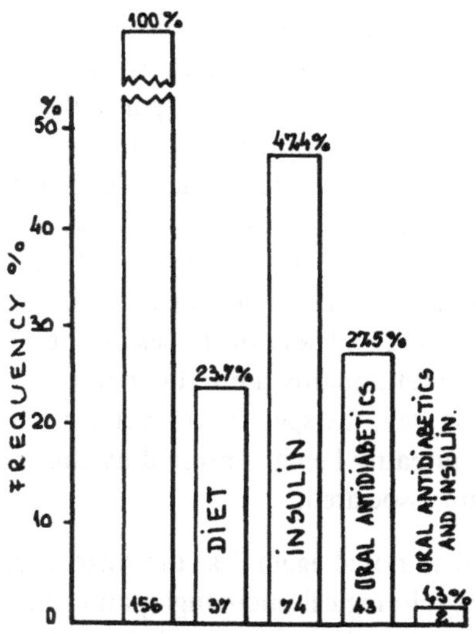

Fig. 34. Diabetics without ocular complications. Distribution according to the kind of treatment applied in 156 subjects (Statistics of the A.C.B.)

As for the distribution of ophthalmologically normal diabetic subjects according to the type of therapy, the figures obtained are consistent with the data presented above, in that 47 % have been treated with insulin, 27.5 % with oral drugs and 23.7% by diet only. This confirms once more that most of the ophthalmologically normal diabetic patients belong to the group receiving insulin (Fig. 34/III).

These investigations on prevalence and incidence may be summarised as follows:

- retinopathy is one of the most frequent ocular complications of diabetes mellitus (44.9%);
- the incidence of the complication rises with age;
- there is a direct correlation between the retinal lesions and the duration of the diabetes in that most of the advanced alterations (stages III and IV) occur in patients with a diabetic history longer than that of the patients with early retinal lesions (stages I and II);
- the incidence of retinal involvement is significantly higher in diabetic subjects treated with oral drugs or only by diet than in patients treated with insulin.

This last conclusion resulting from our data contradicts, to a certain extent, the statements of other authors [64] who maintain that none of the treatments applied at present can improve or retard retinopathy. In our opinion this statement requires a correction, namely that the maintenance of a good metabolic balance in diabetes, irrespective of the type of therapy applied, appears to delay the onset of retinal complications. This also follows from the finding of Adnitt et al. [2] that there is no significant relationship between the progressive tendency of diabetic retinopathy and the average level of glycaemia or the duration of diabetes. It is, however, true that after the onset of retinopathy, one can only aim at slowing down or arresting its advance which is rather difficult with our currently poor therapeutic possiblities. This topic will be discussed in detail in the subsection on therapy.

Pathology. Seven morphological and clinical elements combine, in various proportions, to produce (Fig. 35–44 p. 250) the various stages of the pathomorphological picture of diabetic retinopathy. These are: microaneurysms, vascular anomalies (particularly of the retinal veins), haemorrhage, exudates, new vessel formation, glial proliferation and vitreous detachment [24, 25, 27]. The process as a whole consists of a combination of degenerative, proliferative and exudative alterations of the ocular vessels and parenchyma [16]. Many of the lesions described in diabetic retinopathy are to be met with in other diseases as well, the specific character of diabetic retinopathy being conferred by the way the lesions are associated.

It should be noted again that the stage of established morphological microangiopathic alterations is preceded by a long functional stage. According to recent investigations there is a 10% increase in the average diameter of the retinal veins, as compared to the normal [138, 139, 140]. An increase in the general and especially in the ocular capillary fragility in the diabetic, even in the absence of any obvious angiopathic involvement, might be regarded as another feature of this stage. This last factor plays an unquestionable role in determining the appearance of diabetic retinopathy.

Therefore the view of some authors [78] that the increase of permeability was directly related to the amount of insulin. seems doubtful.

Investigations on general capillary permeability [26] suggest that the changes in permeability depend on the degrees of hepatic, dysmetabolic or inflammatory involvement associated with diabetes mellitus. On the other hand, statistical studies indicate that microangiopathic, ocular complications are more frequent in diabetics who do not receive insulin or in those with a poorer metabolic balance. The hypothesis is more likely therefore, that the increase in capillary fragility and permeability also found in the retina by microangiography with fluoresceine [68] represent a functional stage. The extent of the functional disorder appears to depend on the severity of the metabolic imbalance of diabetes which will, ipso facto, require insulin therapy in order to be corrected [146].

As already mentioned in the previous subsection on prevalence, the clinical course of diabetic retinopathy has been divided into 4 stages. The sequence of the stages may be altered by unusual patterns of combination and the disease may quickly cover a certain stage, be arrested in a more advanced one or regress to an earlier stage.

Stage I (R_1) consists of vascular alterations such as segmentary dilatations of the veins, mostly situated around the macula, and pigment disorders (retinal xanthosis), conferring a yellowish tint to the posterior pole. The venous alterations in this stage are different from the dilation subsequent to thrombosis, in which the vein is expanded along its whole length.

Stage II (R_2) is marked by the onset of aneurysms and punctiform exudates. Aneurysms as such are not specific to diabetes mellitus, but they are distributed in the retina according to a particular pattern in that disease. Their distribution is irregular and involves the posterior pole in particular, reaching the peripheral areas only in later stages. It differs from the distribution found in hypertensive retinitis in that aneurysms in the latter are not isolated but situated at the distal end of a vessel or occur as fusiform dilations of a vessel.

Punctiform exudates in this stage generally appear subsequent to aneurysms, their shape is round, their limits are clear-cut and they occur isolated in the posterior pole area.

Stage III (R_3) is marked by the presence of haemorrhage, confluent exudates, pigment alterations and lesions of the large vessels. It should be noted that among all varieties of retinitis the diabetic one shows the strongest disposition to haemorrhage.

- The microaneurysms bring about small spherical haemorrhages located in the deep layers of the retina. With the advance of the disease, they might multiply and exceed the perimacular area.
- The old punctiform exudates might increase during this stage, multiply and become con-

fluent. An important differential diagnostic feature is the unaffected macula (Fig. 37–39).

- The late pigmentary alterations are bilateral and consist of hypo- and hyperpigmentary patches located in the macular area.
- Alterations to the large vessels during this stage consist of irregularities in the size of the veins. Dilations may be saccular or moniliform, and result in haemorrhage and perivenous oedema. The latter, invaded by connective tissue, brings about the bending of the venous segment to fixed loops.

Stage IV (R_4) is marked by vascular proliferation, preretinal haemorrhage, proliferative retinitis, degeneration of the retina, detachment of the retina and secondary glaucoma.

This division into stages gives a somewhat schematic picture of the course of diabetic retinopathy. It may nevertheless, be useful in summing up a given state in a patient and comparing it with previous pathological pictures in the same subject or with other patients, by permanently referring to the therapy applied in each case. It is also true that an objective estimate of the evolution of a case depends on the accurate definition of the respective lesions. All the seven elements which build up the picture of diabetic retinopathy will therefore be reviewed in detail in the following.

Microaneurysms are small red patches described by some authors as "blood patches", located either along the large vessels of the retina, or, more often, far from the latter. These formations are not specific to diabetes mellitus [27]. Bloodworth [6] discovered four different types:

a) thin-walled, saccular or spherical microaneurysms with a diameter of 30–150 microns. They are associated with capillary dilations reaching a size 2–3 times the normal capillary diameter (varicous dilations), or with U-shaped capillary loops [16–107].

b) in a later stage, the well of the aneurysm undergoes mucopolysaccharide impregnation and endothelial proliferation. Both processes result in a thickening of the respective microaneurysm and eventually in its obstruction, what Bloodworth called hyalinized or thrombotic aneurysm.

c) another type of microaneurysm, either resulting from the former, or developing simultaneously, is characterized by a thick basement membrane in several layers, poor in pericytes [16, 107].

d) microaneurysms have also been described in which the proliferation of the basement membrane, the infiltration with red cells and the marked decrease of the vascular parietal cells finally results in the disappearance of the aneurysm itself [33, 34] (Fig. 16).

According to certain authors [6, 7, 8, 9, 151, 152] the increase in the number of intervascular mesodermic strands in diabetic retinopathy is at the origin of retinal aneurysms. These strands are inserted on the walls of the small retinal vessels and are produced by the mechanical effect exerted by the existing turgor of the retina in diabetes mellitus.

Vascular anomalies particularly of the retinal vessels, are a second element of diabetic retinopathy [24, 25, 26, 27]. They consist of capillary, arterial and vascular dilations produced either by the already mentioned functional disorders, or by the anatomical processes described in Chapter II (Pathomorphology of diabetic microangiopathy), namely the thickening of the basement membrane and endothelial cell proliferation.

The capillary diameter is mostly irregular in diabetes mellitus [16], with significant narrowings at intervals of 100 to 1000 microns, which can hinder the normal blood flow.

The dilations of the venules, [102, 153], are spindleshaped in the beginning but subsequently grow along the vein and appear like small sausages. They occur mostly around the papilla and, by growing, may reach the periphery of the retina Such winding, varicoid veins, occasionally penetrate the vitreous body (Fig. 43 p. 250).

Haemorrhages [16] are a result of the alterations in the capillary walls. They occur in the deep plexiform layers of the retina and, being isolated and disseminated, have been called punctiform haemorrhages [107]. Their location is characteristic of diabetic retinopathy, namely among the temporal branches of the arteria centralis retinae, next to the macula and the papilla [16, 154] (Fig. 40 and 44).

The size of the haemorrhage may subsequently increase, resulting in ruptures into the vitreous.

Proliferative retinopathy may bring about important haemorrhage in the deepest retinal layers, with severe disorders of sight (Fig. 42–43).

Exudates or what is described under that denomination in diabetic retinopathy, may be divided into two categories:

a) waxy exudates, of a fan-like shape, with digits, located in the outer plexiform layer. They are of a white or yellowish colour, isolated in the early stages and subsequently joining into irregular islands with clear-cut limits around the macula [153]. In association with the small haemorrhagic points they build up the picture called "diabetic retinitis punctata" (Fig. 35, 36). These exudates are made up of hyaline and lipid material and may also contain red cells. Their origin is still obscure, but they may be made up of blood serum [14] and/or breakdown products of the retina itself, as suggested by the presence of areas of retinal degeneration in their proximity [16]. No direct communication has been found between such an exudate and any ruptured blood vessel;

b) exudates shaped as cotton-wool plaques are collections of degenerate nerve fibres, cells and glial fibres as well as the PAS-positive spherical formations called "cytoid bodies". These exudates are most probably of ischaemic origin and occur in the retinal layers composed of nerve fibres, ganglion cells and glial cells. They readily penetrate into the vitreous and contain a small amount of lipid. The average persistence of cotton-wool exudates depends on the patient's age. Their half life duration is 8.1 months under 40 and 17.2 months after 40. They are preceded by capillary anomalies and conditioned by arteriolar occlusions, while capillary ischaemia continues even after their disappearance [99, 97].

They are similar to those in arterial hypertension, being differentiated only by associated vascular anomalies. Capillary anomalies precede the emergence of vascular occlusions which are necessary for the appearance of cotton-wool exudates (see Fig. 41) [96, 97]. Retinal degeneration may occur not only in circumscribed areas, but also as a diffuse and irregular loss of ganglion and nerve cells in both granular layers: degenerative alterations of the cones, and swelling and breaking up of numerous nerve fibres in the plexiform layers [14].

New vessel formation represents, in a certain sense, a reaction, an attempt to replace the areas of haemorrhage and exudate by healthy tissue. This process results in the stellated appearance centered around the macula (Fig. 41). Such areas may cover a surface of 200–300 microns and are surrounded by a fine vascular proliferative reaction. New vessel formation may occur in any stage of diabetic retinopathy and usually starts at the periphery of the papilla. In subsequent stages, vessels from the papilla and the surrounding retinal area penetrate into the vitreous [107].

New vessel formation starts by the spontaneous generation of bundles of intra- and preretinal new capillaries, usually originating in venules and only exceptionally in arterioles.

New vessel formation occurs in three stages (acc. 72):

1. A first stage, lasting for 6 to 18 months, is marked by vascular loops and anastomoses. The new vessels are deprived of perivascular connective tissue support, excepting some fine connective fibres. Accordingly, this stage was called that of the "naked vessels". Small retinal haemorrhages may occur at the end of the stage.

2. The following stage, lasting for 1 to 2 years, comprises an increase in the number of new vessels and the gradual condensation of connective

tissue around them. An outstanding feature of this stage is the marked trend to subhyaloid and vitreous haemorrhage, originating in the fine capillary vessels.

3. The third stage, that of healing, is featured by a considerable fall in the number of new vessels and the marked growth of the surrounding connective tissue. Haemorrhage occurs less often during this stage. In spite of these apparently favourable changes, sight often deteriorates consequent to the mechanical occlusion caused by the fibrous strands and to detachement of the retina under the traction of the same fibres. Blindness may finally occur either through the above process, or by secondary glaucoma [72]. Diabetic retinopathy is generally bilateral, but important differences may be found between the two eyes, in the extent and severity of the alterations [109] (Fig. 44).

The relation between diabetic retinopathy and other microangiopathic involvements, especially the renal ones, have been subject to much controversy. It has already been stated that in spite of its ubiquity in diabetes mellitus at a given moment, the microangiopathic process tends to be preponderant in a certain area of the organism. Furthermore certain microangiopathic locations are easier to explore in the earlier stages.

It has long been claimed, for instance, that there is no parallelism between the course of diabetic retinopathy and diabetic nephropathy. The practice of renal biopsy has provided rich evidence that the ocular microangiopathic alterations set in at the same time as the characteristic nodules of diabetic nephropathy [4, 21, 64, 68, 92, 93, 100, 134]. The previously presumed lack of parallelism was due to the fact that the clinical investigation of the eye reveals microangiopathic involvement earlier than do renal tests (see Chapter IV). This is also true for other parts of the organism and maybe for the diabetic macroangiopathy whose early coronary involvements will be discussed in Chapter V of the present work.

Symptomatology and Prognosis. There is no strict relationship between the alterations in diabetic retinopathy and visual acuity. The ophthalmoscopical findings are not always consistent with the clinical and functional ones. This discrepancy relates to (a) the variable location of the microangiopathic lesions on the retina, i. e. if the lesions are superficial, they affect the perceptive neurons and (b) to the type and extent of the respective lesions. Taking into account that the fovea, site of maximal visual acuity, is a practically avascular area [15] and that a more or less similar situation exists in the deep layers of the retina which are important in visual perception [154], it means that only secondary degenerative processes may bring about a fall or loss of visual acuity in these areas of the eye. The fact that the vessels involved by microangiopathy are situated only on the internal layer, that of the nerve fibres, suggests that the reduction of visual acuity occurs by some other means.

Considering the position of the vessels with regard to the area where proper visual perception occurs, it may be concluded that retinopathic alterations interfere with sight in the following situations:

a) Large retinal or preretinal haemorrhages, eventually associated with loss of transparency of the vitreous. The sudden changes in visual acuity reported by some diabetic patients should be related to such retinal and preretinal haemorrhages.

b) degenerative alterations consisting of large exudates involving the macula and the fovea itself. They result in a gradual loss of sight, associated with scotomate and reductions in the visual field;

c) in the presence of glial proliferation involving the macula [27], or of detachment of the retina, or if a secondary glaucoma occurs, sight is usually irreversibly lost. According to Whittington [154], deterioration of the transparency of the vitreous due to haemorrhage or glial proliferation is the main cause of blindness in juvenile diabetes mellitus. Blindness in these cases is usually total and occurs after a diabetic history of 10 to 16 years.

In the case of mature and senile diabetes, loss of sight usually occurs subsequent to large exudates and is not always total, a certain degree of visual ability being preserved. Unlike juvenile diabetes mellitus, the deterioration of sight occurs much sooner, sometimes even before diabetes mellitus has been diagnosed. Out of the seven elements of the complex picture of diabetic retinopathy, only microaneurysms and the anomalies of the retinal veins do not result in disorders of vision. The risk of blindness increases as the other elements, grow and tend to involve the macula, as in fact most often happens. It would be most important both from symptomatic and prognostic points of view to ascertain the reversibility of the lesions. In fact, microaneurysms, small haemorrhages and punctiform exudates are reversible to a certain, though unpredictable, extent. A few reports have been published on the reversibility of certain more severe aspects of microangiopathy, in which the retinal tissue itself was not affected. The cotton-wool exudates are essentially degenerative processes and their effect on visual acuity is usually irreversible. Similarly, no clinical remission can be practically expected in retinal detachment, glaucoma, haemorrhagic diabetic glaucoma, often associated with proliferative diabetic retinopathy, or other diabetic angiopathic manifestations [82]. It follows from the above that from the point of view of the risk of blindness, the various aspects of diabetic retinopathy can be divided into benign and malignant. The benign aspects of diabetic retinopathy include:

a) the functional stages of diabetic retinopathy;
b) the presence of microaneurysms;
c) the presence of venous anomalies;
d) the punctiform haemorrhages
e) mixed aspects consisting of some or all of the above elements (from a to d)

The malignant aspects of diabetic retinopathy include:

a) vascular proliferation
b) glial proliferation
c) extensive degenerative processes in the macula: cotton-wool plaque exudates
d) haemorrhages in the vitreous
e) secondary detachment of the retina and
f) secondary glaucoma.

The process which consists of vascular proliferation, consecutive haemorrhage in the vitreous and subsequent connective tissue invasion was called proliferation diabetic retinopathy or "retinitis proliferans". In fact, this aspect should be named according to Whittington [131, 135] *a venous proliferative angiopathy,* since this points to the predominantly venous origin of the new vessel formation in diabetic retinopathy. The clinical investigation of diabetic retinopathy, implies the use of the following methods:

1. The classical methods of ophthalmoscopy and determination of the visual field which generally yield sufficient data to enable the practitioner to diagnose the condition and estimate its severity. Photographs of the fundus should be taken in order to follow the course of the disease and avoid bias in the estimate of the lesions found at a given moment.

2. Special methods of investigation such as fluorescein angiography, electroretinography, electro-oculography and scotometry. Fluorescein angiography gives a very clear picture of the microaneurysms and the general state of the retinal circulation, but the procedure is still too sophisticated to be applied routinely. Electroretinography is mainly used for estimating the state of the fundus where an opaque lens prevents ophthalmological examination. Results with this method are still uncertain and the same can be said of electro-oculography, a method that can, theroetically, yield some information on the electric potentials associated with the chemical processes involved in retinal metabolism. Scotometry is, on the contrary, a most valuable method of ascertaining sight disorders of which the patient is sometimes unaware, thus enabling the taking of therapeutical and prophylactic measures aiming at slowing down or arresting the evolution of the process [27].

3. Additional data can be obtained by clinical laboratory tests revealing the presence of a dysmetabolic process which might exert some influence on the course of diabetic retinopathy.

a) Just as with other aspects of diabetic angiopathy (see Chapter II), the ocular complications are associated with a marked increase of the alpha-2 globulin fraction. The extent of tissue damage is proportional to the rise of this electrophoretic fraction [83] and ipso facto there is a correlation between its blood level and the extent of the lesions of diabetic retinopathy. Nevertheless the test is not specific to this complication nor to diabetic microangiopathy in general, since similar rises are found with any destructive process in the organism (malignant disease, postoperative disease, chronic suppurative diseases, etc [74];

b) the determination of serum lipids is more relevant to the degree of control of diabetes mellitus than to the presence of an ocular complication. Hypercholesterolaemia, hypertriglyceridaemia, and an increase in NEFA, yield significant information concerning the risk of any microangiopathic complication, including diabetic retinopathy. Repeated determinations, may serve for checking the effectiveness of the general therapeutic control of diabetes mellitus and as indicators for diet adjustment;

c) some endocrine indexes have been granted a diagnostic significance, such as;

- the determination of urinary 17-hydroxycorticoids, in the presumption of a suprarenal hyperactivity in diabetic retinopathy;
- the data obtained from the determination of the growth hormone, supposed to be concerned in the pathogenesis of retinopathy. Since pituitary suppresion has been used to treat the complication, results have been inconclusive and the method has not been adopted as a routine test.

Pathophysiological problems of diabetic retinopathy: As far as pathogenetic hypotheses significant for therapy are concerned, the considerations stated in Chapter II on general pathophysiology of microangiopathy are also valid in the case of diabetic retinopathy. The pathogenetic evolution of diabetic retinopathy is shown in the diagram below (according to Sevin) (Fig. 31) [135, 136]. Some special problems raised by the ocular complication, however, deserve special discussion.

1. Is there an inborn predisposition to diabetic retinopathy, since not all diabetic subjects experience this complication and since even in cases of diabetes of the same duration the degree of ocular involvement differs from patient to patient? Fischer's investigations [63, 64, 65] attempted to demonstrate the role of a genetic factor, but the facts suggest rather that the degree of metabolic compensation all along the course of the diabetes, the type of management, the age at which the diabetes commenced, the duration of the disease and the possibility of its existence before diagnosis, are elements which, considered as a whole, could well account for the differences observed in the course and extent of the retinal complications.

2. Does the therapeutical intervention and the degree of compensation of diabetes interfere with the course of an already existing diabetic retinopathy, or is the progress of the latter independent of these factors? For the moment, the answer to this question is ambiguous. On the one hand, it is admitted that the formation of deposits of glycoproteins in the vascular walls in diabetic microangiopathy is an irreversible phenomenon, on the other hand, remissions have been described in certain stages of diabetic retinopathy. While the latter alternative cannot be denied, and should stimulate an active standpoint in the management of the ocular complications, the former does not imply that therapy is hopeless. On the contrary, if a return to normal is out of the question, therapy should aim at arresting the advance of the respective pathological process.

3. Is insulin therapy useful or harmful in retinal complications?

It has already been mentioned that a deficiency in insulin at the cellular level results in an alteration in the functional integrity of the small vessels (venules, arterioles, capillaries). Tonicity is lost and permeability rises in excess. This first stage is, to a certain extent, reversible, as indicated in our research by the lack of advanced retinal alterations (stage IV) in recent onset diabetes. If the process is not arrested in that stage of functional microangiopathy the exudate resulting from vasodilation and increased permeability infiltrates the basement membrane with plasmatic compounds which stimulate the endothelial cells to discharge acid mucopolysaccharides. A first consequence of the prolonged dilation and stasis is the onset of capillary microaneurysms [6, 155]. In fluorescence angiography, microaneurysms with a rich cellular wall are perfused without losing the fluorescein, unlike those with a partially hyalinized wall. The wholly acellular capillaries are not perfused [97]. The exudates provoke damage to the basement membrane function resulting in a hyaline change which consequently enhances the pericyte degeneration [119].

The gradual thickening of the walls of arterioles and venules brings about the obstruction of the respective vessels with subsequent stasis and anoxia of the retinal tissues. The normal metabolic exchanges are disturbed, abnormal metabolites accumulate and stimulate the formation of new vessels [84].

The initial functional alterations become associated with irreversible degenerative lesions aggravating the prognosis of the disease (degenerative microangiopathy).

It has been claimed that the retina has a high capacity for glucose metabolism, even in the absence of insulin. Nevertheless, the absence of the hormone at the cellular level brings about an increase in the catabolism of fat and a consecutive rise in circulating fatty acids [154]. The latter are partly oxidized and partly incorporated and esterified in the fatty tissues. This process may also occur in the intima of the blood vessels. The disorder in the metabolism of fatty acids may involve the retinal vessels too and result in excessive depositing of glycoproteins on the thickened basement membrane.

The important role played by insulin in the prophylaxis of the ocular complications of diabetes is also suggested by the fact reported by some authors and also found by us in some isolated cases that retinal complications are rare in diabetic patients with a history of repeated episodes of hypoglycaemia [102].

Data from the literature and personal experience entitle the authors to answer the above questions on special and general pathophysiology in diabetic microangiopathy by the following considerations:

- diabetic retinopathy is part of the ubiquitous diabetic microangiopathy and one of the major locations of that complication;
- there is a correlation between the duration of diabetes, the degree of metabolic control and the type and extent of diabetic retinopathy;
- there is a relationship between the age at which diabetes begins and the type of retinopathy eventually associated with it. The risk of blindness differs accordingly;
- certain metabolic disorders associated with diabetic mellitus (e. g. the dyslipaemic states) interfere with the rate of evolution of the ocular complication.

These conclusions suggest that the therapy of the ocular complications of diabetes in general and of retinopathy in particular should be an active one, in spite of the fact that its results are still inconclusive, as shown in the following.

2. The Therapy of Diabetic Retinopathy

Many therapeutical measures have been recommended in the management of diabetic retinopathy, but their effectiveness is uncertain. They are based on several elements supposed to interfere with its pathogenesis. These are:

a) The general metabolic balance and metabolic disorders in particular areas.

b) The alterations of capillary permeability and

c) Hormonal balance.

a) Therapeutic Measures Concerning Metabolic Balance

1. The maintenance of diabetes in a state of metabolic balance [18] is a matter of caution [95], even if the influence of metabolic imbalance on the

course of diabetic retinopathy is still controversial. This is especially true in cases of a possible reversibility of some lesions of diabetic retinopathy in patients in whom the only previous management had consisted of strictly controlled diet [53, 54, 55]. Another argument in favour of a complex therapy is the fact that a thorough control of the metabolic balance of diabetes mellitus tends to reestablish the normal level of serum triglycerides [111], supposed to play a significant role in the pathogenesis of this vascular complication of diabetes.

In the statistics of the Clinic of Metabolic and Nutritional Diseases in Bucharest, as well as in other series reported in the literature, the lowest incidence of retinal alterations was found in the groups of patients in whom a good metabolic balance had been obtained by diet restrictions and insulin therapy. Incidence figures in these groups were in sharp contrast to those of retinal complications found in diabetic patients poorly controlled by diet alone or associated with antidiabetic sulphonamides. Further analysis of the statistics of the ACB showed that patients in the latter group either refused to submit to a necessary insulin therapy or overlooked dietary restrictions in the hope that the effect of the modern oral therapy would keep their "mild" diabetes under control.

The above facts suggest that the maintenance of metabolic balance in a case of diabetes mellitus should be regarded at least as a method of preventing too rapid an advance of a process inevitably associated with the disease, if not as a possibly effective prophylaxis of the complication [37, 38, 39, 58, 74, 86, 87, 90, 91, 110, 112, 141].

2. It has also been claimed that the *reduction of the serum levels of cholesterol and triglycerides* to normal values has some therapeutical worth since some authors have assumed that there is a correlation between the fat content of the hard exudates in diabetic retinopathy and general disorders in fat metabolism. Various measures have been recommended with this aim in view:

a) It has been reported [56, 94] that hard exudates in diabetic retinopathy recede under a low fat diet containing a certain proportion of corn oil. Unfortunately, while exudates in the fundus actually disappear more rapidly, the deteriorated visual acuity does not improve accordingly. Some authors prescribe a daily diet containing some 20 gm of animal fat supplemented by some 60 gm unsaturated vegetable fat in order to obtain a normal spectrum of serum lipids [94]. Others restrict total fat intake even further (to 17–19 gm daily according to body weight) but concomitantly allow free intake of protein [57, 121, 150].

It should be noted that such dietary restrictions are meant to be associated with cholesterol and blood sugar lowering drug therapy, as detailed below, in order to potentiate their effect. Insulin requirements have also been found to be lower under these therapeutic conditions [57].

Table I/V (p. 145) may serve as a guide for diet prescriptions in disorders in the lipid fractions.

Hyperlipoproteinaemia of Types I and III is expected to improve under fat intake restrictions associated with the carbohydrate restrictions which are compulsory in diabetes mellitus, while hyperlipoproteinemia of type V requires a diet, low in total calories.

b) The administration of drugs inducing hypocholesterolaemia and hypolipaemia appears to be efficient in cases of hyperlipoproteinaemia of types II and IV (s. Table I/V).

The exudates in diabetic retinopathy often recede following the administration of a combination of clofibrate (ethyl-chlorophenoxy isobutarate) and androsterone, but clofibrate alone, without androsterone may be just as effective [77, 79, 120]. In both cases, however, sight does not improve with the resorption of the exudates [77], either because degenerative alterations (called cytoid degeneration) persist at the site of the resorbed exudates [16], or because of a neuronal degeneration that may precede the formation of the [77] exudates [16, 157, 152]. The two processes may be associated.

Favourable results have been reported but not confirmed following the administration over several months of an antihaemorrhagic drug associated with heparin and alphachymotrypsin [40].

It is admitted that if any of these therapies result in a fall in serum cholesterol levels of more than 10–15%, the alterations of the fundus are found to be improved in 73–81.5% of treated subjects [41, 77, 79]. The drugs appear to be more efficient in female patients [71].

The use of certain biguanides, such as phenformine, appears to be indicated as frequently as clofibrate. Even if the latter exerts a more important hypolipaemic effect [104, 116, 117], the biguanides also improve the metabolic balance of diabetes mellitus and induce weight loss [116, 119], thus interfering with three elements which, according to our present knowledge, contribute to the onset, maintenance and determination of diabetic retinopathy.

Jensen and Lundbaeck (quoted by 118) reported that in 4 patients treated with PAS for several months, the exudates subsided. The authors assigned the resorption of the retinal exudates to the hypocholesterolaemic effect of PAS.

b) Therapy Controlling Capillary Permeability. Haemorrhages and Vascular Proliferations

a) General therapy consists of the administration of drugs having an effect on the vascular wall, such as vitamins P and K [145] with or without vitamin C. Calcium-containing drugs favouring blood coagulability as well as haemostatic drugs (Clauden, Adrenoxil. Presomen, Dicynone, etc.) [145] are also advisable. According to Sèvin, calcium dobesylate is superior to calcium etymsylate; both of them, however, normalize the capillary resistance and permeability while they are being administered [136]. Their greatest efficiency is recorded in the early periods of diabetic retinopathy.

b) *Local therapy:*

- Radiotherapy. It has been claimed that 3–5 months of radiotherapy result in a decrease in the calibre of small and medium vessels, without undue side effects on glial tissue, retinal haemorrhage and exudates. Subsequent comparative investigations failed to confirm these results [27, 118].
- Photocoagulation or laser beam therapy [14] may serve to destroy the preretinal new vessels, but not the intravitreous ones or those around the optic disc. The procedure implies the risk of retinal detachment, but seems logical, unlike radiotherapy, particularly in the early stages of proliferative diabetic retinopathy, or if possible, shortly before its appearance [136]. The best results have been recorded in patients aged between 40 and 50. In young patients photocoagulation has a rather pernicious effect [135].

c) Hormonal Therapy

1. Adrenalectomy has been suggested as a means of affecting the course of diabetic retinopathy, but it proved completely ineffective. Moreover, before such a surgical intervention was recommended, some authors have claimed that the administration of cortisone and of ACTH were favourable to the same ocular complication [60].

2. Hypophysectomy appears to have yielded favourable results in certain circumstances. This therapeutic intervention has been recommended during the last 15 years, considering both the very severe prognosis of the proliferative diabetic retinitis, leading to blindness in 50% of the cases in 5 years [13, 25] and the poor results obtained with other procedures. Removal or destruction of the pituitary must be as complete as possible to obtain satisfactory results [59] and prevent new vessel formation in the retina [80, 81, 118].

The following surgical procedures have been recommended for hypophysectomy:

- transfrontal approach
- oro-naso-transsphenoidal approach [75, 76]
- section of the pituitary stalk [43, 62, 132]

Other procedures for the destruction of the pituitary gland are:

- transsphenoidal destruction by application of cold or heat [1, 156] or the implantation of $Ytrium_{90}$ [88, 89].

– external irradiation by supervoltage X-rays [42], or heavy particles [102], or cobalt therapy [144]. These procedures are indicated in cases which cannot be treated by surgery. Their common drawback is variable, partial and progressive destruction.

Hypophysectomy is indicated in the cases of proliferative retinopathy with preretinal haemorrhage in the vitreous without affecting the macula [30, 88, 89, 127]. It should not be performed in cases of retinopathy with microaneurysms and retinal haemorrhage which do not seriously impede visual ability, or in cases in which the final fibrous proliferation has already occurred. Hypophysectomy rarely interferes with the hard retinal exudates [88]. However Ytrium$_{90}$ implantation reduced the half-life of cotton-wool exudates to 2–3 months, on average [96].

Most of the authors consider that the patient should be observed during a preliminary period of 1 to 6 months of strictly correct management of the diabetes, in order to ascertain whether the process of ocular microangiopathy is progressive. Hypophysectomy should be ruled out in cases of extensive renal damage, in hypertensive patients with coronary disease and in diabetic patients with some other symptoms of evolutive macro-angiopathic involvement. The surgical intervention should also be withheld in the presence of chronic infection and in advanced diabetic neuropathy, particularly if associated with postural hypotension in older subjects.

In estimating the results of the surgical intervention one should remember the trend to spontaneous remission of microaneurysms, retinal haemorrhages and punctiform exudates, as found in some 30% of the younger patients [22, 23]. Even proliferative retinopathy may spontaneously arrest its evolution, irrespective of pituitary surgery [13, 20, 53, 54, 55]. Operative deathrate through surgical procedures has been estimated at about 4% as against the 10% death rate through irradiation procedures [135, 136].

It has been claimed that if the above indications are observed, the surgical intervention improves or arrests the evolution of the retinopathy in over 50% of the patients [20]. Unfortunately the reported series are not conclusive, lacking adequate control.

Joplin [89] reported that Ytrium$_{90}$ implantations in a small series of patients improved retinal haemorrhage in 50 % of the cases, inhibited new vessel formation in 30 % and venous dilatation in 20 %, as compared to a control group.

According to Rucker [132], sight was preserved in one third of the operated patients while all the controls became blind. It is not known whether hypophysectomy, or the destruction of the pituitary also improves diabetic microangiopathy or macroangiopathy [62].

It has been reported, however, by many authors, that in certain patients, in spite of this heroic therapy, diabetic retinopathy inexorably pursues its fatal course [135].

It has also been argued that the reported improvements might be due to better control of the diabetes. The argument does not stand since the improvement, if any, begins in the first days after the operation. The effect was also assigned to a possible resorption of the retinal oedema and clearing up of the vitreous, as well as to a fall in the level of circulating growth hormone

The risks of interfering with the pituitary can be summed up as follows:

– operative death, reported in 8.8 %–11.2 of the cases, depending on the surgical technique.

– secondary meningitis

– renal failure, which accounts for some 40% of the deaths. Hypophysectomy seems to worsen preexisting renal conditions, as the lack of somatotrophic hormone decreases glomerular activity.

– endocrine disorders like persistent diabetes insipidus (25–50% of cases) and total hypopituitarism [30] require close supervision and adequate substitutive treatment. The administration of cortisone should be started during the

operation, that of thyroxine 2–3 months later, together with androgens and oestrogens.
If diabetes insipidus occurs, pitresine should be given [30].

- the effects of hypophysectomy on diabetes are absolutely noteworthy. The requirements for insulin fall after the intervention by 30 to 100%, sensitivity to insulin rises and great oscillations can be recorded in the course of the basic disease, which may end in a fatal hypoglycaemic episode.

According to Lundbeack [109], one third of the operated patients show an improvement of the visual capacity which can sometimes be only transient. It has also been noticed that hypophysectomy does not affect the average life span of the diabetic.

3. Other hormonal therapies have been suggested, such as the administration of anabolic steroids, alone or in association with antidiabetic biguanides. The results are not encouraging, however.

Chapter IV Renal Diabetic Angiopathy

A. Pathomorphology of the Renal Diabetic Angiopathy

Renal angiopathy, one of the severest late complications of diabetes, may become manifest as diabetic microangiopathy and/or diabetic macroangiopathy.

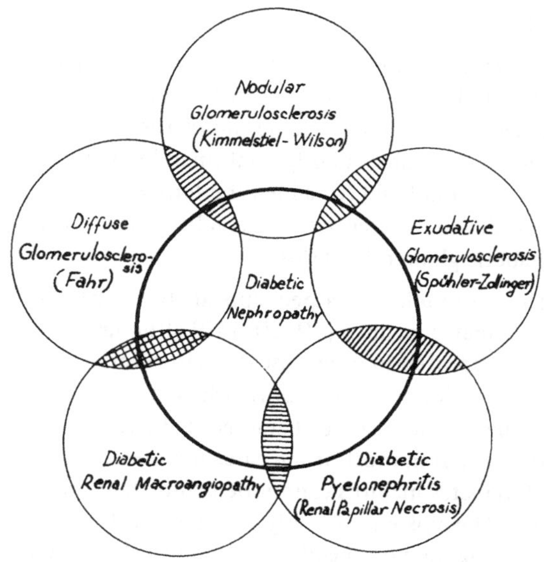

Fig. 99. The concept of "Diabetic nephropathy" and its correlation with the various kidney troubles during diabetes mellitus.

1. Microangiopathy essentially involves the glomerules as nodular, diffuse or exudative glomerulosclerosis. Any of these types may be found alone or associated, conferring a characteristic polymorphism to the picture. The association of nodular glomerulosclerosis and diffuse glomerulosclerosis is particularly common [79, 80].

2. The macroangiopathic involvement or the renal arteriosclerosis in the diabetic, morphologically and clinically overlaps common arteriosclerosis, but the dysmetabolic background of the underlying diabetes mellitus confers a specific pattern on this complication.

The several varieties of diabetic microangiopathy and the macroangiopathic alterations of the kidney may be found separately or together, or associated with pyelonephritis. All these complications contribute to the wider pathological entity called by Aschoff diabetic nephropathy [40] (see Fig. 99).

There is a great variety of possible associations among the various types of microangiopathy as well as of the latter with renal macroangiopathy. This might account partially for the peculiarities found in the evolution of this late complication of diabetes and it explains the intricate character of the renal pathological process in most diabetic patients (Fig. 99). It should be noted that microangiopathy is much more frequently encountered in a diabetic patient with renal involvement/than arteriolosclerosis or diabetic pyelonephritis. Although certain authors [18] postulate that the association between renal papillary necrosis and diabetic glomerulosclerosis is so rare that the two complications might be regarded as excluding each other, more recent data invalidate this statement [136].

The present section will concentrate upon diabetic microangiopathy and macroangiopathy, in spite of the fact that in the clinical description, one cannot disregard the other components of diabetic nephropathy and is compelled to present the clinical picture as a whole. In fact, although the Kimmelstiel-Wilson syndrome corresponds to a specific alteration of diabetes mellitus, it actually refers to the picture of diabetic nephropathy as a whole.

1. Renal Diabetic Microangiopathy

Renal diabetic microangiopathy, a complication involving the renal glomerular vessels, may be found in three separate pathomorphological varieties.

1. The nodular glomerulosclerosis was described in 1946 by Kimmelstiel and Wilson [79, 80] and called "intercapillary glomerulosclerosis". The finding was subsequently confirmed by many authors and Bell [10] added the term *nodular*, in order to differentiate the condition from diffuse diabetic glomerulosclerosis.

This morphological aspect appears to be specific to diabetes mellitus [79, 80, 140] although it has been reported in other diseases. However, a closer examination of those reports which appear to challenge the specific character of the lesion, shows that in most of the cases the presence of diabetes mellitus cannot be completely ruled out. The existence of only very few works claiming the non-specific character of the nodular lesion is a confirmation of its diabetic specificity [37, 40, 56, 147], especially since nodular glomerulosclerosis is often asymptomatic and consequently ignored [1].

Morphologically, the nodular lesion consists of accumulations of hyaline material, staining intensively with PAS but not with Alcyan blue. The nodules are disposed in a particular pattern, at the periphery of the glomerular tuft [89, 90]. They are spherical, ovoid or cone-shaped [147] with a diameter of between 20 and 200 millimicrons.

The central portion of the nodule is mostly homogeneous and its periphery contains several picnotic nuclei incorporated into the hyaline mass. Several glomerular capillaries can be found on its surface [90]. The glomeruli involved in the process may be larger than the normal average [1] or rarely, smaller. Bowman's space looks normal [147]

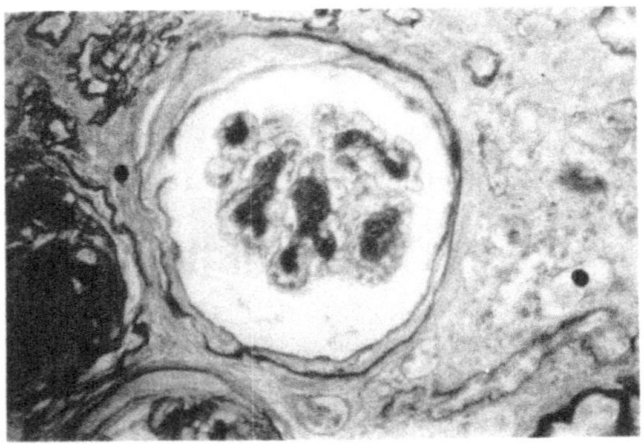

Fig. 100. Nodular glomerulosclerosis in juvenile diabetes mellitus. Diabetes duration about 10 years.

(Fig. 100, 101). In most cases, the basement membrane and Bowman's membrane do not look thickened.

These findings suggest that the main alteration in nodular diabetic glomerulosclerosis does not occur in the capillary wall itself, but most probably in the intercapillary space of the mesangium.

The nodules described by Kimmelstiel and Wilson appear to be composed of a glycoprotein [49, 89] different from the mucopolysaccharides of the basement membrane. This contradicts the hypothesis that the process is related to an excessive production of mucopolysaccharide of this type [89] (see the subsection on the histochemistry of diabetic nephropathy, p. 117).

The nodular changes may involve either a few or most of the glomeruli. One or several nodules may be found in the same glomerulus [49, 147]. They may be small or may fill most of the glomerulus [97]. PAS-positive material is often found between the nodules as well as in nodule-free glomeruli [97]. If a nodule lies close to a small and dilated capillary, it tends to diminish its lumen [2].

2. Diffuse diabetic glomerulosclerosis was the most controversial of the renal complications of diabetes mellitus. It was described in the same year (1942) by Fahr [44] and Bell [10,11] as a non-specific renal alteration, morphologically different from the nodular glomerulosclerosis of Kimmel-

stiel and Wilson and consisting of the accumulation of PAS-positive material in the walls of the glomerular capillaries [1, 2] which consequently thicken. At an early stage, the PAS-positive material accumulates in the central part of the glomerulus. Subsequently it spreads, thickening the capillary walls.

Various authors [10, 79, 80] have expressed different views regarding the role of the basement membrane in the glomerular tuft. More recent research [17, 32], confirmed by electronmicroscopy has concluded that the main change in diffuse diabetic glomerulosclerosis is the thickening of the basement membrane (Fig. 101).

Several morphological changes differentiate diffuse diabetic glomerulosclerosis from other pathological conditions:

- the alterations are located axially and begin at the periphery of the glomerulus, as in the normal subject, and in direct ratio with age [147];

- in the kidneys of subjects with diffuse diabetic glomerulosclerosis, the glomeruli retain their normal diameter or grow even larger. This feature is common in this pathological condition and is also found in ageing, membranous glomerulonephritis and extramembranous glomerulonephritis [4]. The association of arteriolar alterations confers a particular picture quite specific to diabetes mellitus at this stage [147]. It should be noted that various glomerular alterations can occur simultaneously in the same subject, hypertrophy in some glomeruli and hyaline transformation in others [45];

- the proliferation of endothelial cells [14, 16] also occurs in disseminated lupus erythematosus, but not in ageing, arterial hypertension and non-diabetic bilateral glomerulonephritis. No confusion is possible with disseminated lupus erythematosus because of the features mentioned above [116];

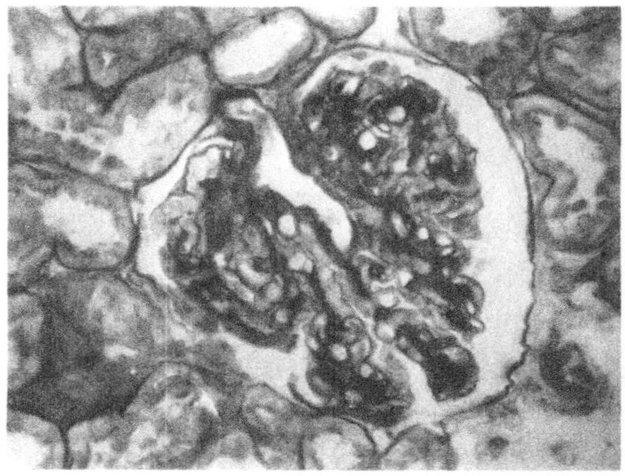

Fig. 101. Diffuse glomerulosclerosis in juvenile diabetes mellitus. Presumed duration of diabetes about 11–12 years. (PAS).

3. The exudative glomerulosclerosis in diabetes mellitus is characterised by the shapes usually called "fibrin cap" and "capsular drop". They were first reported in diabetes by Spühler and Zollinger in 1943 under the name of "fibrinoide kappen" [143]. The term "fibrin cap" was first used in 1952 by Barrie et al. [5]. In 1954 Anderson [1] suggested that the process is the expression of an exudative glomerulosclerosis.

The "fibrin cap" is a crescent-shaped body, displaying eosinophilic but not argentophilic staining and is located at the external convex edge of a glomerular capillary. The term "fibrinoid" is due to its staining blue with Mallory. Unlike fibrin, it does not contain fibres.

A similar accumulation of fibrinoid material occurring in Bowman's capsule, takes the shape of a spindle or of a "falling" drop, hence its name of "capsular drop" (Fig. 102, 103).

The subsequent development of these formations is still not completely elucidated. According to some authors, the fibrin cap is never invaded by fibroblast cells [147] while others claim [5] that the capsular drop is rapidly invaded by fibroblasts thus becoming connective tissue (Fig. 104).

The fibrin deposits are not specific to diabetes mellitus. They have also been reported in the

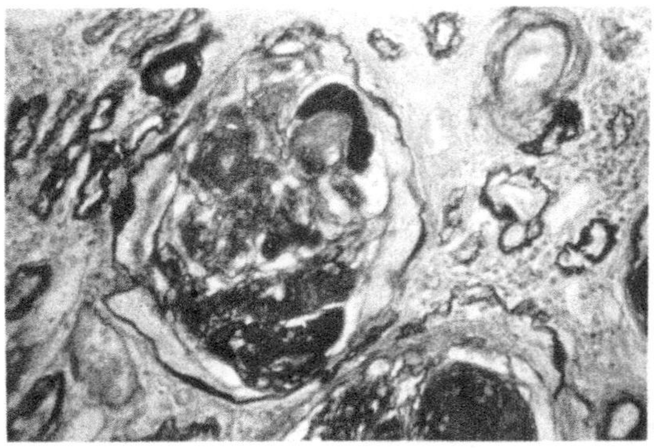

Fig. 102. Exudative diabetic glomerulosclerosis in the kidney of a woman with juvenile diabetes mellitus. Fibrin cap. (PAS).

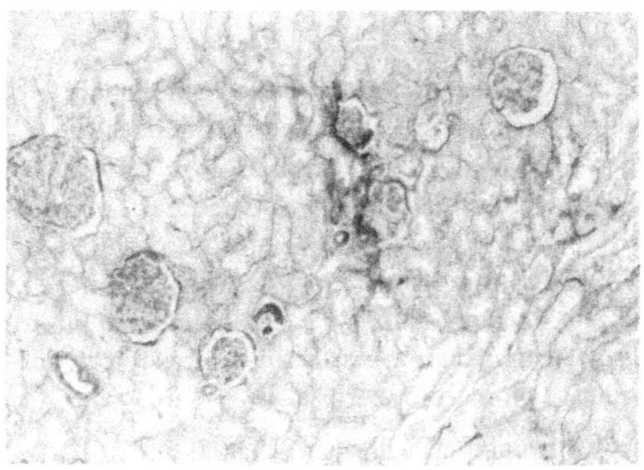

Fig. 103.

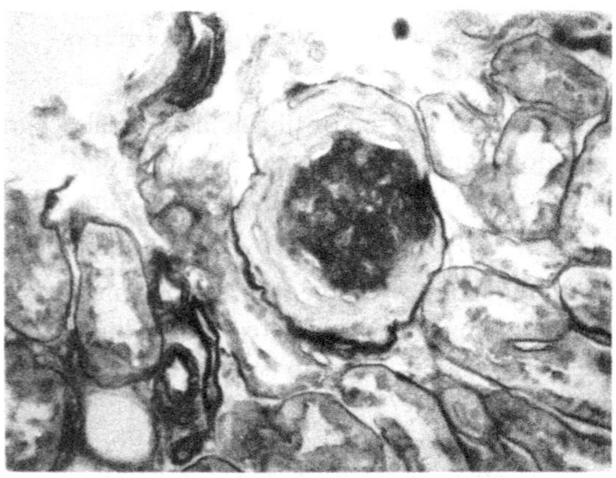

Fig. 104. Terminal stage of a diabetic nephropathy (PAS) in juvenile diabetes (estimated duration of the disease: 17 years).

atherosclerotic kidney as well as in non-diabetic chronic glomerulonephritis. The tendency rather is to confer some diabetic specificity on the capsular drop [5, 147].

2. Renal Macroangiopathy in the Diabetic

This condition involves the afferent and efferent arterioles of the glomerulus and the small nutritive vessels of the kidney.

The specific morphological feature is the proliferation of endothelial cells. According to Blumenthal et al. [16] this is to a certain extent common to all vascular alterations in the diabetic. Their possible immuno-aggressive origin was mentioned in Section II (p. 48). In diabetic microangiopathy, this feature also occurs in all the small vessels without basement membrane even the B type capillary vessels [20, 33].

Deposits of PAS-positive material in the arteriolar walls have also been described. The initial deposit resembles a fibrillar structure, subsequently undergoing a process of hyalinization, the so-called renal hyalinosis [107]. This confers on the vessels an aspect typical of arteriosclerosis. The thickening of the basement membrane adds to the picture which includes elements of diabetic microangiopathy and arteriosclerosis.

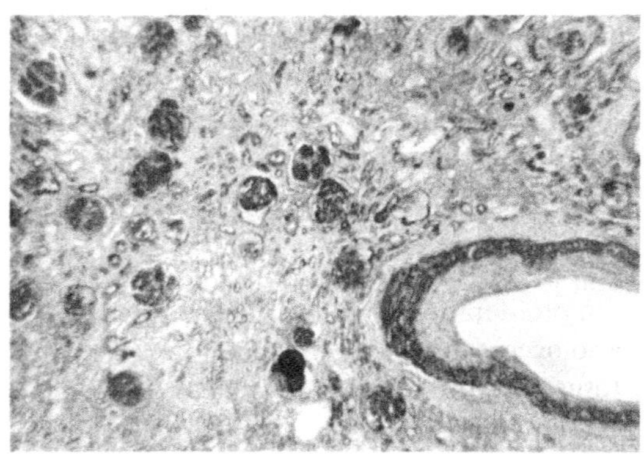

Fig. 105. Diabetic macroangiopathy of the extraglomerular vessels in maturity onset diabetes mellitus. Estimated duration of the disease: 9 years. IPAS).

Renal vascular hyalinosis occurs in almost every elderly diabetic, its progress paralleling widespread glomerular damage. The process involves the small renal arteries, the arterioles and the arterioles of the glomerular pediculus, but sparing the afferent arterioles in most cases [107].

The lesions are rare in the small interlobar and interlobular vessels of the renal parenchyma [16]. They generally occur in the renal hilum (Fig. 105).

3. Ultrastructure of the Renal Diabetic Vascular Lesions

Renal diabetic microangiopathy is highly interesting for ultrastructural studies since the renal glomerulus is one of the most common locations of diabetic angiopathy.

The following ultrastructural aspects have been described by electronmicroscopic investigation, some of them occurring pre-eminently in diabetes mellitus.

According to Kimmelstiel [79, 80], the renal structures initially affected in diabetus mellitus are the *glomerular lobules and their axial area.* These

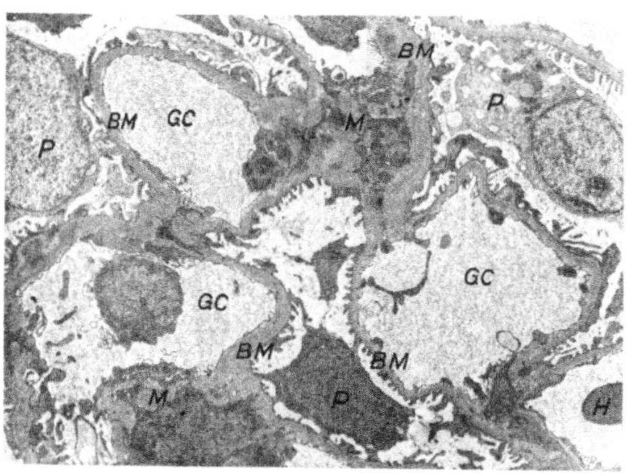

Fig. 106. F. I., boy, 13 years, recently discovered diabetes mellitus. Kidney biopsy. Widening of the strands of mesangial matrix (M) with increased density and quantity of the mesangial matrix. Here and there, presence of thickening of the basement membrane (BM). Foldings in the mesangial area. Glomerular loops (GC) with normal lumen. P = podocytes (glomerular epithelial cells). (6,000 ×).

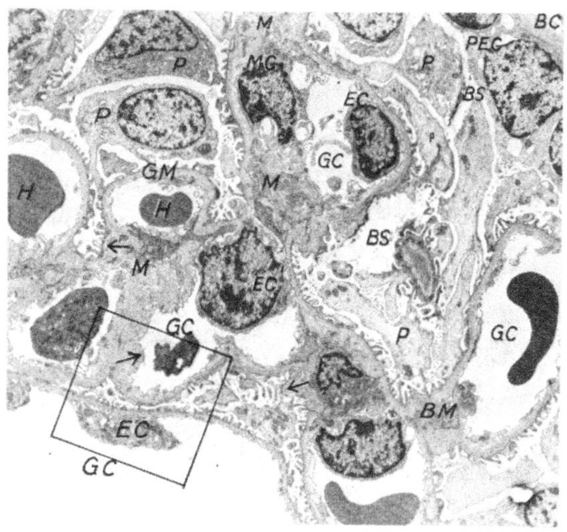

Fig. 107 A. U. D., 6 year old girl, with juvenile diabetes mellitus. GC = glomerular capillary, partially obtured by the intense mesangial matrix (M) proliferation. Basement membrane (BM) thickening. EC = endothelial cell. MC = mesangial cell. H = erythrocyte. BC = Bowman's capsule. BS = Bowman's space. PEC = capsular epithelial cell. P = glomerular epithelial cell (Podocyte). (6,000 ×).

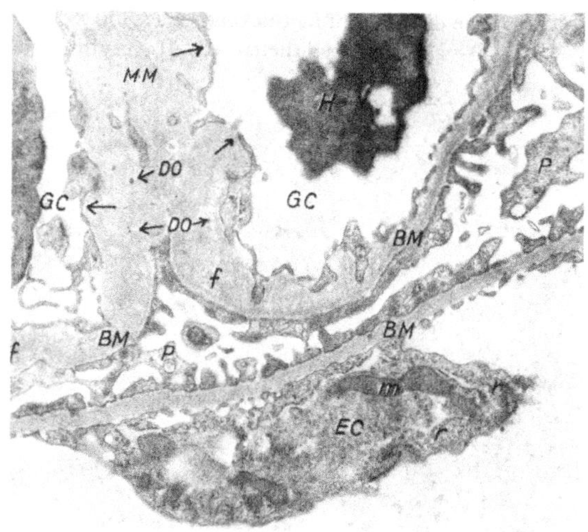

Fig. 107 B. Partial enlargement of Fig. 107 A. MM = thickened mesangial matrix. Arrows = direction of formation of the basement membrane (BM) deposits. Exaggerated fibrillarity (f) and deposits of granular and electrondense material (DO) in the basement membrane; m = mitochondria; r = ribosomes and polyribosomes in the endothelial cell; P = glomerular epithelial cells (24,000 ×).

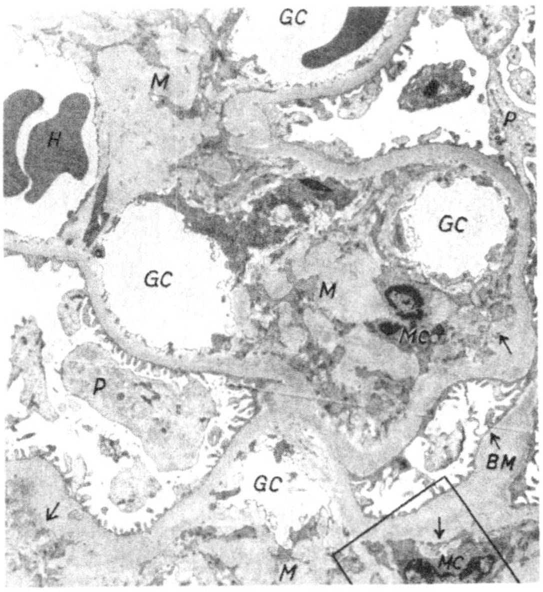

Fig. 108 A. D. L., young woman of 19. Juvenile diabetes mellitus, discovered 13 years ago. M = nodular mesangial proliferation in the axial area of the glomerulus. GC = glomerular capillaries, sometimes quite obturated. MC = mesangial cells; BM = basement membrane (the arrows indicate the direction of its thickening). (6,000 ×). P = glomerular epithelial cells; H = erythrocyte.

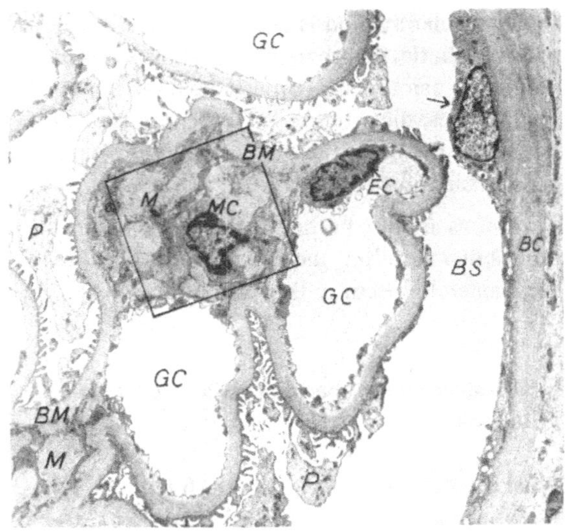

Fig. 109 A. Same patients as in Fig. 108 A & B. Axial nodular diabetic glomerulosclerosis. M = non-homogenous mesangial matrix; MC = mesangial cell; EC = endothelial cell; GC = glomerular capillary; P = glomerular epithelial cell; BM = Bowman's space; BC = Bowman's capsule; moderately thickened; arrow: capsular epithelial cell. (6,000 ×).

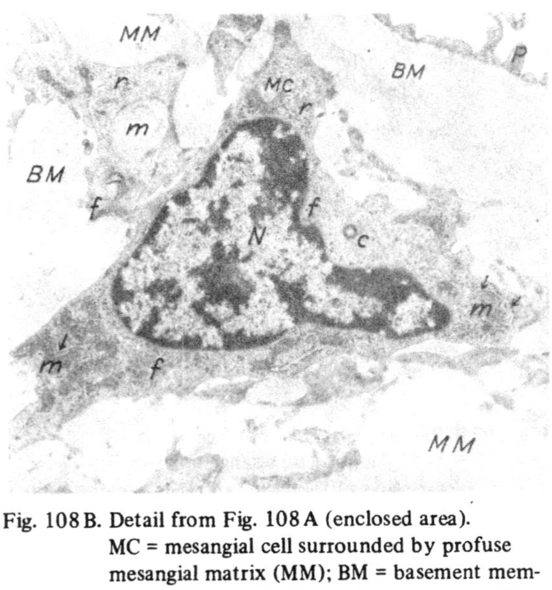

Fig. 108 B. Detail from Fig. 108 A (enclosed area). MC = mesangial cell surrounded by profuse mesangial matrix (MM); BM = basement membrane (thickened); C = centrosome; m = mitochondria, some of them modified; r = free ribosomes; arrows = perimitochondrial disposition of the rough reticulum; f = fibrillar modification of the cytoplasms; P = glomerular epithelial cells. N = nucleus (24,000 ×).

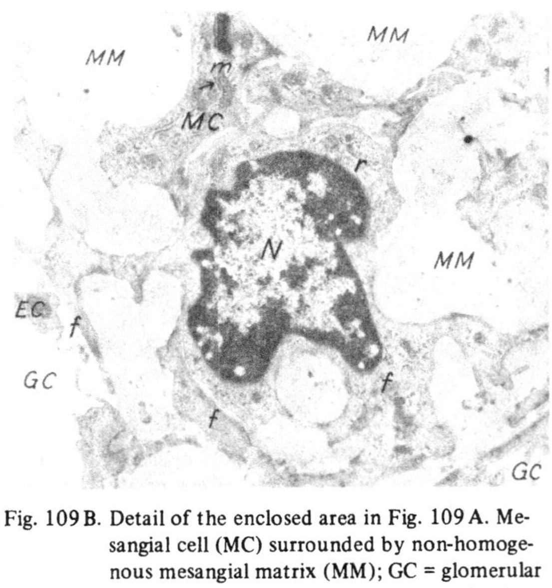

Fig. 109 B. Detail of the enclosed area in Fig. 109 A. Mesangial cell (MC) surrounded by non-homogenous mesangial matrix (MM); GC = glomerular capillary; EC = endothelial cell; m = mitochondria; r = free ribosomes; arrow = perimitochondrial disposition of the rough endoplasmatic reticulum; f = fibrillar modification of the mesangial cytoplasm; N = mesangial cell nucleus. (24,000 ×).

lobules, normally made up of two or several, often clover-shaped, glomerular capillaries, circumscribe an axial intercapillary space, the mesangium [73, 104]. It is here that the most characteristic alterations of diabetic nephropathy occur.

A widening of the strands of mesangial matrix occurs first (Fig. 106), associated with a variable increase in density which approaches or even exceeds the basement membrane density (Fig. 107 A) A remarkable increase in the quantity of mesangial matrix takes place concurrently. This will lead to the formation of the typical nodular lesions of diabetic glomerulosclerosis (Figs. 107 A and B, 108 A and B, 109 A and B).

Fibril-like formations can sometimes be noticed within the mesangial matrix.

The mesangial cells are also involved in this process. Farquhar [46, 47, 48] considers they are characterized by a decrease in the number of cytoplasmic organelles. Besides this relative scarcity, which is not always evident, our pictures often show pathological alterations of these organelles. For instance alterations in the shape of mitochondria are frequent (Fig. 108 B). Quite often, intracytoplasmic, fibril-like formations are seen (Figs. 108 and 109 B), although equally often, the cytoplasm looks normal.

Free ribosomes are very numerous (Figs. 108, 109 B, 110, 115, 121). They are frequently associated with the endoplasmic reticulum, tending to a perimitochondrial grouping (Figs. 108 B, 109 B, 110, 119). Suzuki described them as electron-dense material [146].

Electron-dense droplets in the cytoplasm were also described as being of lipidic nature (Fig. 121).

Alterations in the shape of nuclei are also frequent (Figs. 107 A, 108 A and B, 109 A and B, 110, 111, 112).

In some mesangial cells active centrioles can be noticed (Figs. 108, 110).

The alterations of the glomerular capillary basement membrane are the most precocious and frequent in diabetes. They consist of thickening and

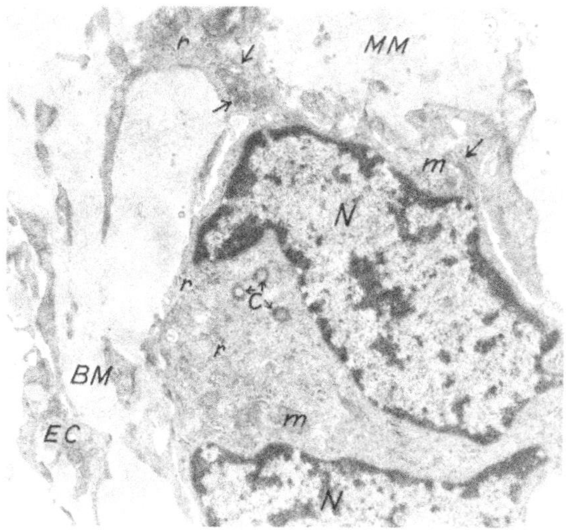

Fig. 110. Diabetic glomerulosclerosis. Mesangial cell with particular shape of the nucleus (N); c = centrioles; MM = mesangial matrix; r = ribosomes; BM = basement membrane; EC = endothelial cell; arrows = perimitochondrial disposition of the rough endoplasmic reticulum (24,000 ×).

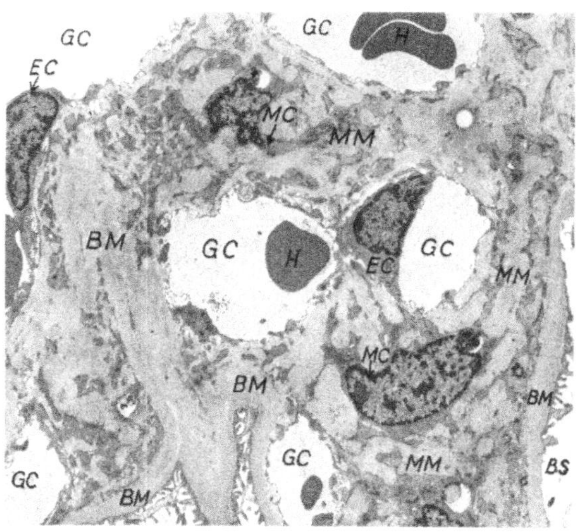

Fig. 111. Glomerulosclerosis diabetica. GC = glomerular capillaries partially obturated by the mesangial matrix (MM) proliferation. Thickening and folding of the basement membrane (BM). EC = endothelial cell; MC = mesangial cell. (Young girl with diabetes mellitus) (6,000 ×).

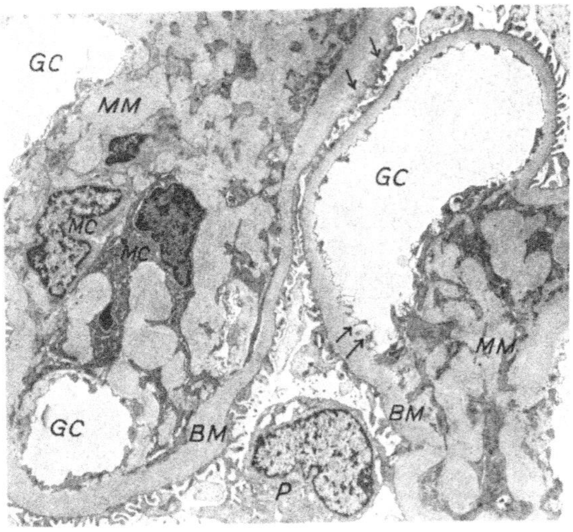

Fig. 112. Young girl glomerulosclerosis diabetica. Mesangial matrix (MM) proliferation including mesangial cells (MC). GC: glomerular capillaries during the obturating process. Arrows = directioı of the thickening process of the basement membrane (BM). P = glomerular epithelial cell. (6,000 X).

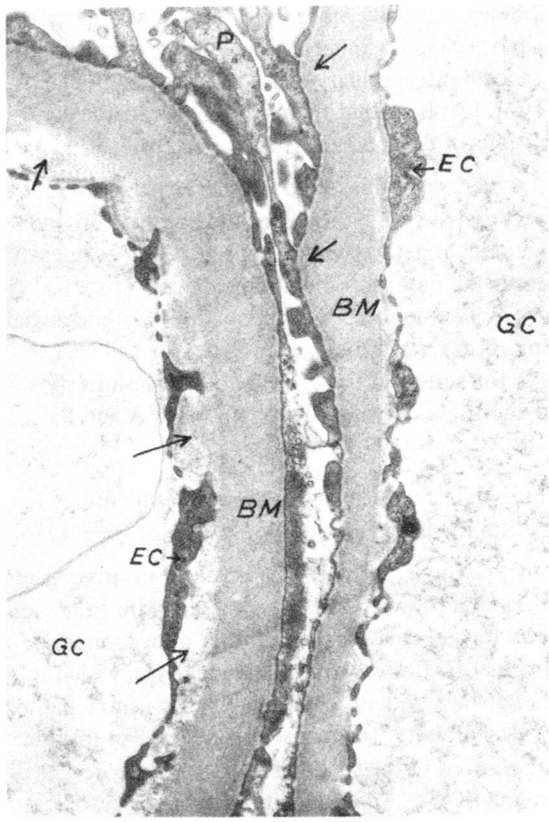

Fig. 113 B. Glomerulosclerosis diabetica. Basement membrane (BM) during the pathologic thickening process (arrows). The process develops either to the glomerular capillary's lumen or towards the Bowman's space. EC = endothelial cell; P = glomerular epithelial cell. (16,000 X).

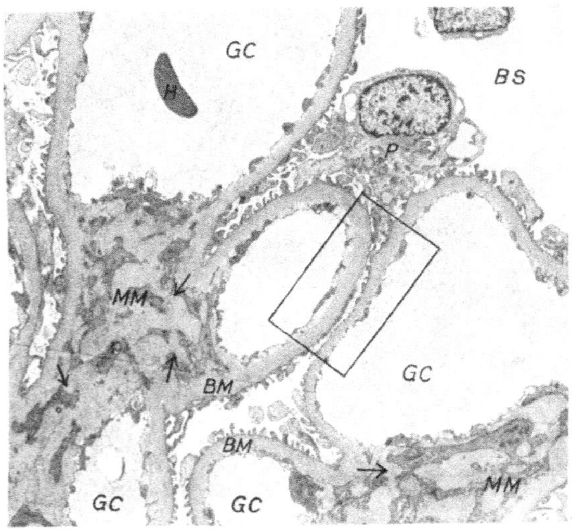

Fig. 113 A. Diabetic glomerulosclerosis. Nodular proliferation of the mesangial matrix (MM). Thickening of the basement membrane (BM). (the arrows indicate the direction of the thickening progress). GC = glomerular capillaries (some are in course of obturation). BS = Bowman's space. H = erythrocyte. (6,000 X).

folding of the basement membrane with exaggerated fibrillarity and deposits of granular material [12] leading to folding and fusion of capillary loops [73] (Figs. 106, 107 A and B, 108 A, 109 A) up to their complete obliteration (Fig. 107 A, 108 A, 111, 112, 113 A). Mesangial proliferation participates equally in the obliteration of capillaries, sometimes appearing as the main determining factor (Fig. 106, 108 A, 112).

The thickening of the basement membranes is the result of deposits accumulating towards:

a) the glomerular capillary lumen (Figs. 107 B, 112, 113 B, 114, 117, 120, 126);

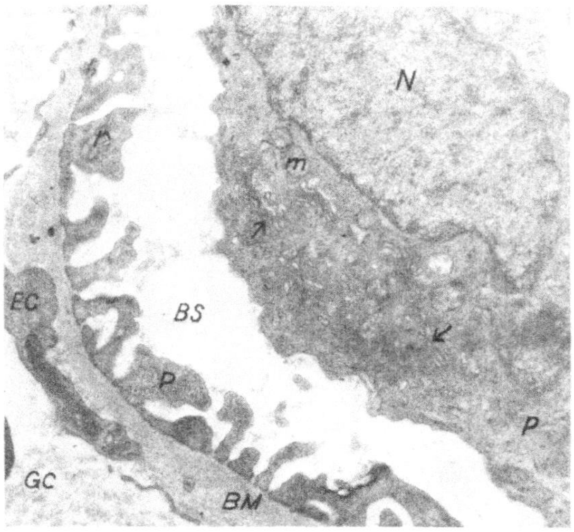

Fig. 114. Thickening of the basement membrane (BM) with clear deplacement of the endothelial cells (EC) towards the lumen of the glomerular capillary (GC). BS = Bowman's space with a great glomerular epithelial cell (P). Arrows indicate some tubular structures in its cytoplasm. m = mitochondria; r = free ribosomes (24,000 ×).

b) the axial area of the glomerular lobule (Figs. 108A, 113A, 115, 116, 117);

c) Bowman's space, under the glomerular epithelial cells (Figs. 112, 113B, 116, 117, 121), sometimes resulting in the fusion of two neighbouring basement membranes (Fig. 107B).

d) Bowman's space and glomerular capillary lumen simultaneously (Fig. 107B, 108A, 112, 113B).

During the process of basement membrane thickening, accumulations of electron-dense granular material occur on both the capsular and capillary side (Figs. 114, 115, 116, 117) and the middle area of the basement membrane. Thus some authors [46, 47, 48] supposed it to be an exudative lesion, different from the fibrinoid deposits occurring during LED, eclampsia and various types of glomerulonephritis [12, 48, 30].

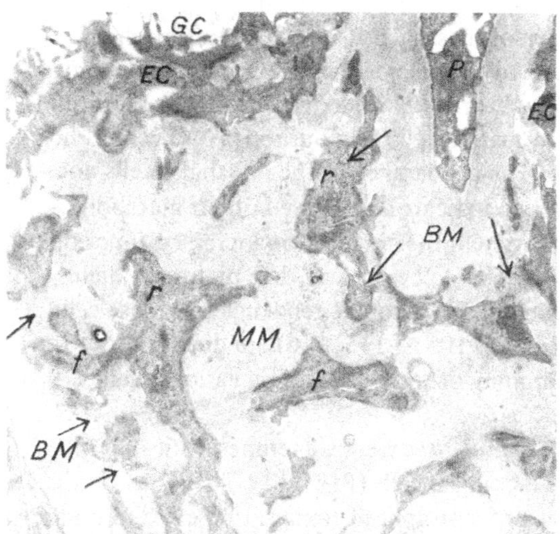

Fig. 115. Nodular diabetic glomerulosclerosis. Detail from a nodular lesion. MM = mesangial matrix with non-homogenous appearance; BM = basement membrane; thickening develops towards the axial area indicated by the arrows. P = glomerular epithelial cells with free ribosomes (r) and fibrillar formations (f). EC = endothelial cell; GC = glomerular capillary. (24,000 ×).

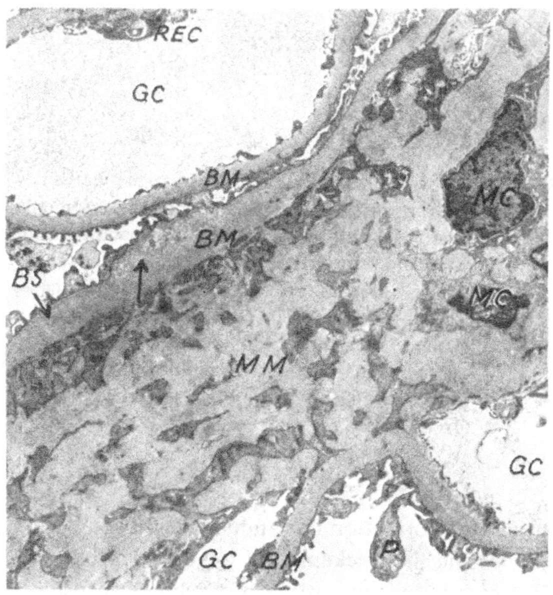

Fig. 116. Nodular diabetic glomerulosclerosis. Thickening of the basement membrane (BM) directed towards the capsular space (BS) as indicated by the arrows. Mesangial matrix (MM) whose strong proliferation includes many mesangial cells (MC). Glomerular capillaries (GC) sometimes with apparently normal basement membrane. EC = endothelial cells. P = glomerular epithelial cells (6,000 ×).

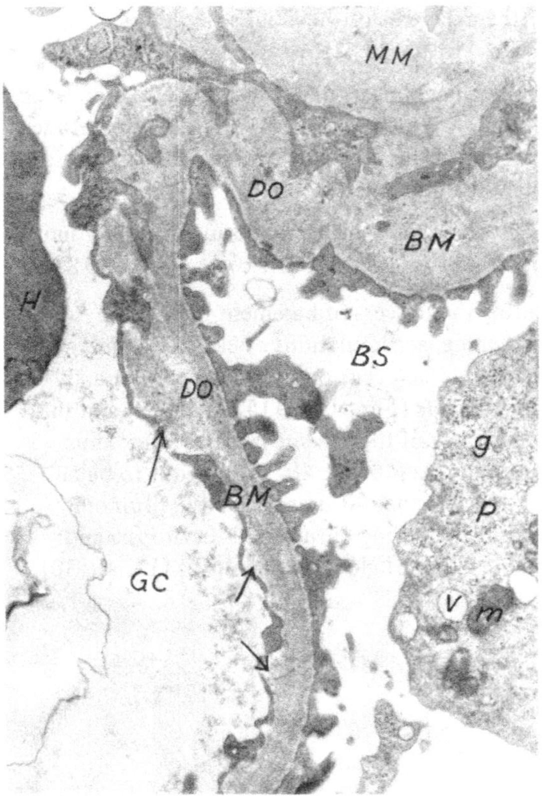

Fig. 117. Diabetic glomerulosclerosis. Mesangial matrix (MM) proliferation. Thickening of the basement membrane (BM) with some dense opacities inside (DO) and prominence into the glomerular capillary (GC) lumen (arrows). BS = capsular space with an epithelial cell (P). V = vacuoles in this glomerular epithelial cell, and g = electron-dense granular material disseminated in the cytoplasm; m = mitochondria; H = erythrocytes (16,000 ×).

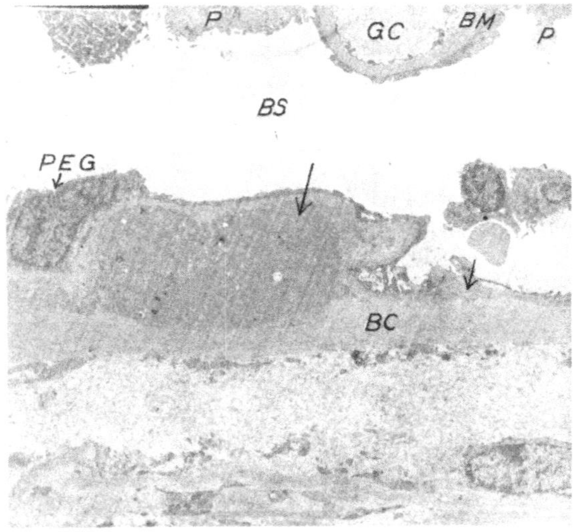

Fig. 118. Diabetic glomerulosclerosis. Accumulation of non-homogenous material into Bowman's capsule (BC) (arrows) PEC = capsular epithelial cells; BS = Bowman's space; GC = glomerular capillary with basement membrane (BM); P = glomerular epithelial cell. (6,000 ×).

Besides the formation of Kimmelstiel-Wilson nodules and the thickening of the capillary basement membrane, alterations of Bowman's capsule are frequently noticed in the form of electron-dense deposits on the glomerular sides of the capsule. This might account for the formation of the so-called *"capsular drops"* in diabetic glomerulosclerosis (Figs. 118, 127).

Although there are a great number of hypotheses to account for the formation of these deposits, none has yet been confirmed. The accumulation of mesangial matrix was, for instance, ascribed to a decrease in the activity of mesangial cells which could no longer discard the accumulated material [73]. In our series of pictures, however, the appearance of the mesangial cells does not seem to indicate a decrease in their metabolic activity. On the contrary an increased functional level seems to be present. The pictures which might suggest atrophic tendencies in these cells (Fig. 106, 108A, 115, 116) are due rather to the sectioning of the cell body on various planes.

Myelinic figures were sometimes noticed within the mesangial cells (Fig. 119). They may be the result of a prolonged toxic action exerted on the cell. The existence of such an action is compatible with a supposed increase in metabolic activity, and a diversion from normal pathways. This phenomenon could also be related to the accumulation of basement membrane-like material [73].

Relative hypertrophy of the glomerular endothelium has been frequently noticed (Fig. 111, 120,

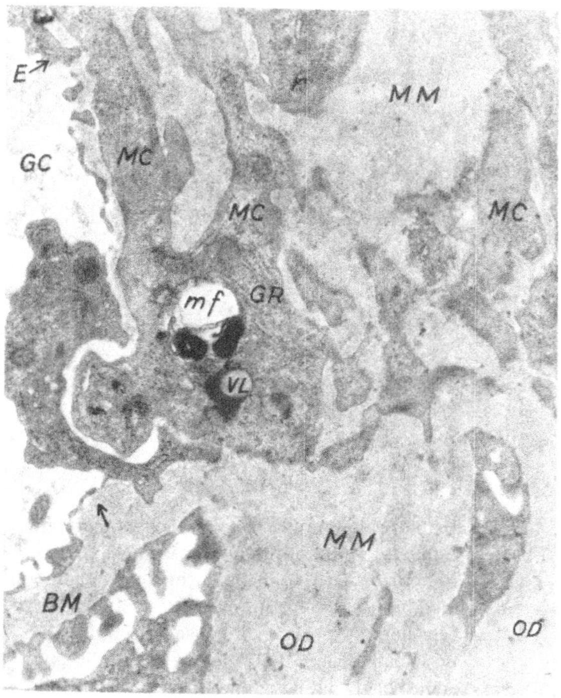

Fig. 119. Diabetic glomerulosclerosis. Intense proliferation of the mesangial matrix (MM) with frequent dense opacities in side (OD). Thickening basement membrane (BM) especially towards the glomerular capillary (GC) lumen (arrow). MC = mesangial cell, rich in rough endoplasmic reticulum (GR), containing myelenic figures (mf), vacuoles (V) probably with lipidic material and free ribosomes (r).
E = endothelial layer (16,000 X).

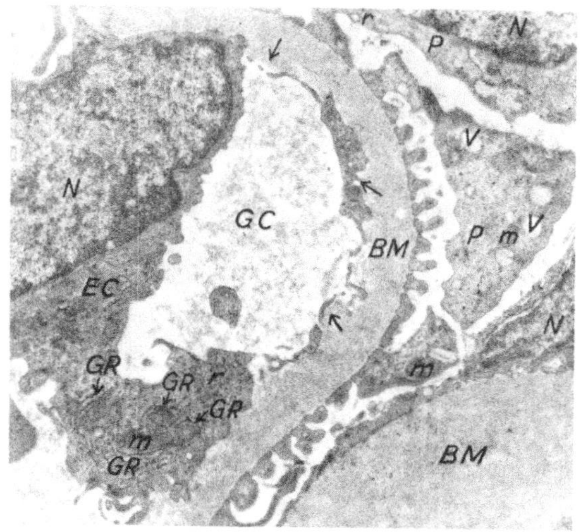

Fig. 120. Diabetic glomerulosclerosis. EC = endothelial cell and P = epithelial cell in the capsular space. Thickening of the basement membrane (BM) especially in the direction of the glomerular capillary (GC) lumen, protruding the endothelial layer (arrows). N = nucleus. GR = rough endothelial reticulum, sometimes with perimitochondrial arrangement; m = mitochondria; V = vacuole; r = free ribosomes. (16,000 X).

122). Unlike mesangial cells, however, whose relative scarcity of cytoplasmic organelles could be postulated, the endothelial cells seem to preserve them unaltered. Numerous free and polyribosomes could be observed (Fig. 107B, 120, 121). In a number of cases, a perimitochondrial disposition of the rough endoplasmic reticulum was observed (Fig. 120). This appearance is very similar to the endothelial cells of hepatic sinusoides (Fig. 48).

The nucleus of the glomerular endothelial cells is rather festooned (Fig. 121), although, quite often, its appearance is not different from that of normal endothelial cells (Figs. 107A, 120, 122).

We also noticed a tendency of endothelial cells to detach themselves from their basement membrane (Figs. 107B, 113B).

The swelling and vacuolization of glomerular endothelial cells was mostly described in those cases where a severe nephrotic syndrome was also present [12].

The alterations of glomerular epithelial cells were studied to a lesser degree. They are not spared by diabetic metabolic disturbances. The following aspects could be described:

- Their tendency to expand on very wide areas of the glomerular interlobular spaces by gripping at several glomerular lobules at the same time (Figs. 107A, 122).
- The cytoplasm has a remarkable vacuolar aspect (Figs. 107A, 108A, 109A, 112, 113A, 114, 117, 120, 122, 123, 124, 125, 126) which it

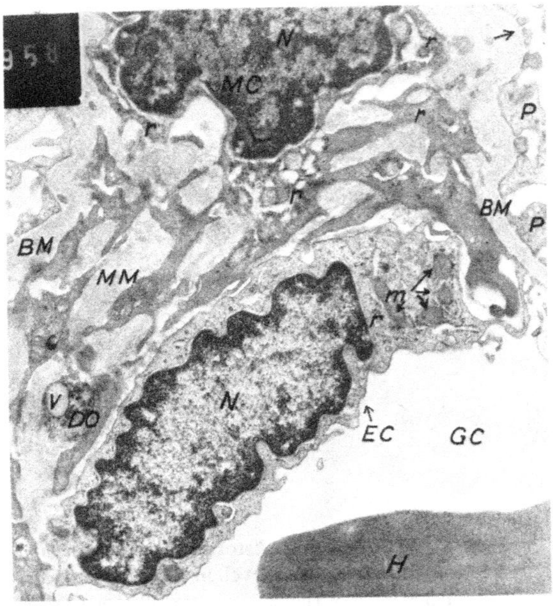

Fig. 121. Diabetic glomerulosclerosis. Endothelial cell (EC) and mesangial cell (MC) with very irregularly shaped nucleus (N). Mesangial matrix (MM) proliferation including some vacuoles (V) as well as electrondense opacities (DO). Thickened and folded basement membrane (BM). P = glomerular epithelial cells; r = free ribosomes; GC = glomerular capillary; H = erythrocyte (10,000 ×).

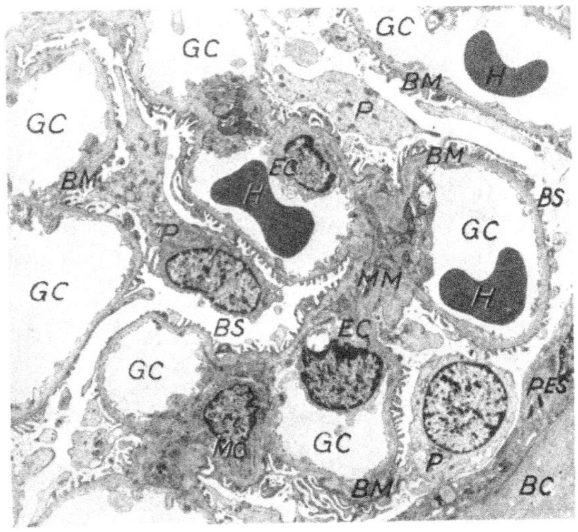

Fig. 122. Diabetic glomerulosclerosis. GC = glomerular capillary; MM = proliferated mesangial matrix; BM = irregularly folded and thickened basement membrane; H = erythrocyte; BC = Bowman's capsule. PEC = capsular epithelial cell; BS = Bowman's space; MC = mesangial cell; EC = endothelial cell; P = glomerular epithelial cell (Podocyte) (6,000 ×).

shares with the epithelial cells on the inner side of Bowman's capsule (Fig. 127).

These vacuoles are sometimes electron-transparent and seem to be formed by dilations of the ergastoplasmic reticulum. At other times, they are made up of amorphous, electrosemiopaque material (Fig. 123).

- The Golgi membranes are sometimes well developed (Figs. 123, 124). A marked development of the Golgi membranes in glomerular epithelial cells is very often seen in animals with a physiological protein loss in the urine [33].
- The increase of intracytoplasmic fibrils sometimes covering the entire cytoplasm (Fig. 123, 125, 126).
- In numerous glomerular epithelial cells, electron-dense granulations are spread all over the cytoplasm, sometimes grouped as polyribosomes (Figs. 123, 124, 125, 126).
- Occasionally, the pedicles merge into one another (Figs. 125, 126).

Thus diabetic renal microangiopathy may affect all the components of the glomerulus. Without being specific alterations, as a whole they build up the pattern of diabetic glomerulosclerosis and partially account for the clinical manifestations of this complication. One further remark is necessary to round off the ultrastructural histologic pattern: the thickening of the basement membrane also occurs in the renal tubules (Fig. 128, 131) when diabetic nephropathy is in an advanced stage.

Renal diabetic macroangiopathy. The alterations of the arterioles in the kidney are not different from those in other organs of the diabetic (see also section II p. 28), but their extension is often remarkable. These alterations, which under light microscopic investigation are very similar to those

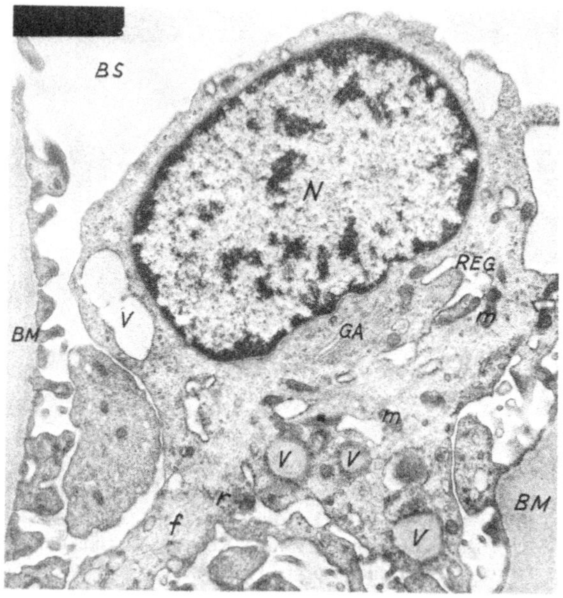

Fig. 123. Diabetic glomerulosclerosis. Glomerular epithelial cell with numerous vacuoles (V) possibly formed from the dilated rough endoplasmatic reticulum (REG). Golgi apparatus (GA); m = mitochondria; BM = thickened basement membrane; f = fibrilles inside the cytoplasm. (24,000 X). N = nucleus.

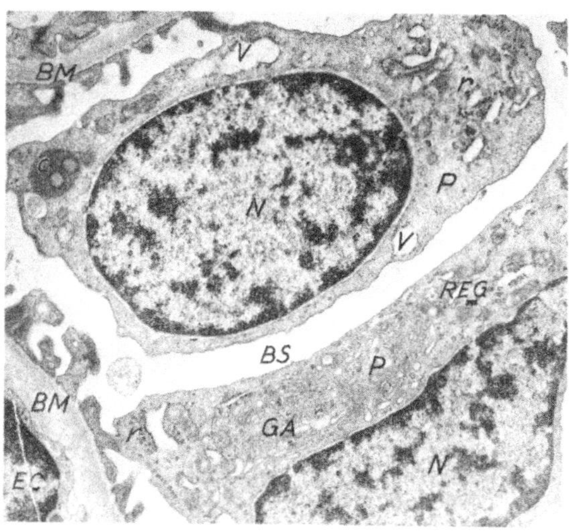

Fig. 124. Diabetic glomerulosclerosis. Two glomerular epithelial cells (P); N = nucleus; GA = Golgi apparatus; REG = rough endoplasmatic reticulum, saccular shape and sometimes dilated as to manage true vacuoles (V); r = free ribosomes m = mitochondria; c = centrosomes; BS = Bowman's space; EC = endothelial cell (24,000 X).

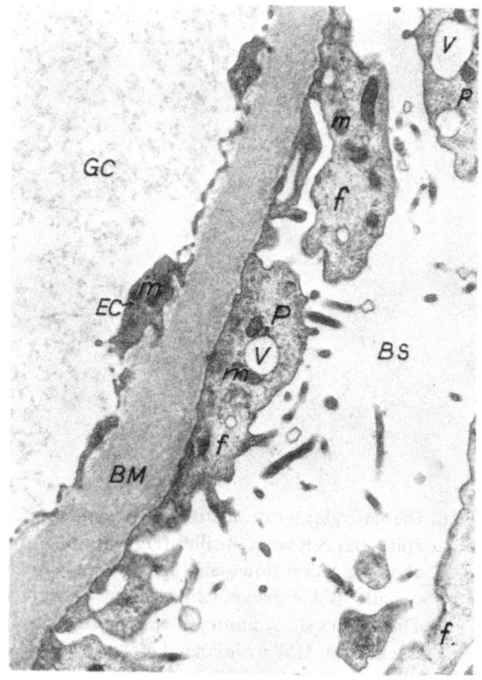

Fig. 125. Diabetic glomerulosclerosis. Glomerular epithelial cells (P) with numerous vacuoles (V) probably managed by the dilation of the rough endoplasmic reticulum; f = fibrilles m = mitochondria; BS = Bowman's space; EC = endothelial layer in the glomerular capillary (GC); BM = basement membrane (notice its fibrillar aspect) (10,000 X).

in other vessels of the body, look very much like aspects in the renal glomerulus, particularly Bowman's capsule with the electron microscope material, denser than the basement membrane itself, can be noticed. They lie under the latter, penetrating between the layers of arteriolar walls (Fig. 128, 129 A and B, 130). The resulting wall-thickening may contribute to a decrease in the vascular lumen and to modifications of local haemodynamics.

4. Histochemistry of the Renal Alterations in Diabetes Mellitus

The data pertaining to the histochemistry of the lesions in diabetic nephropathy is still comparatively poor and inconclusive. Hypotheses have

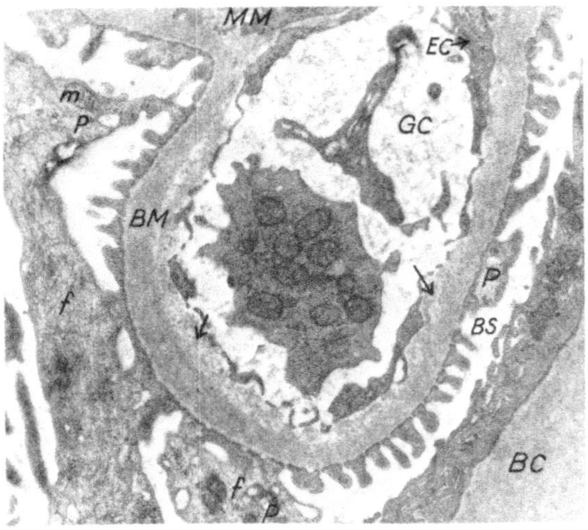

Fig. 126. Diabetic glomerulosclerosis. P = glomerular epithelial cell with fibrilles (f) inside; M = mitochondria; BS = Bowman's space; BC = Bowman's capsule; BM = thickened basement membrane. The arrows show points of subendothelial (EC) thickening; MM = mesangial matrix; GC = glomerular capillary (16,000 X).

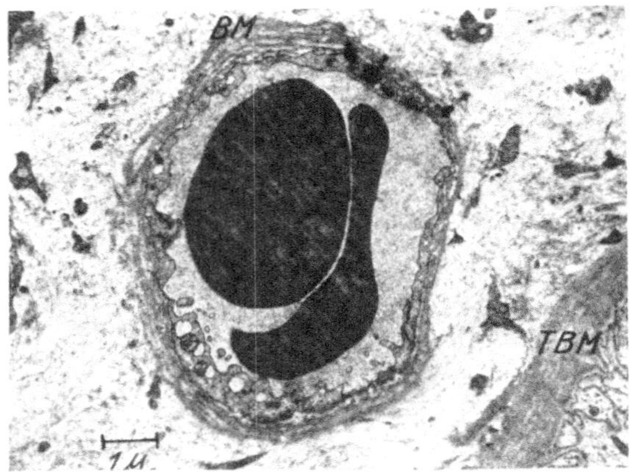

Fig. 128. Diabetic glomerulosclerosis. Small intrarenal, extraglomerular vessel. Thickened basement membrane (BM) at one of its poles. TBM = tubular basement membrane. Remarkable thickening with fibrillar aspects. (6,000 X).

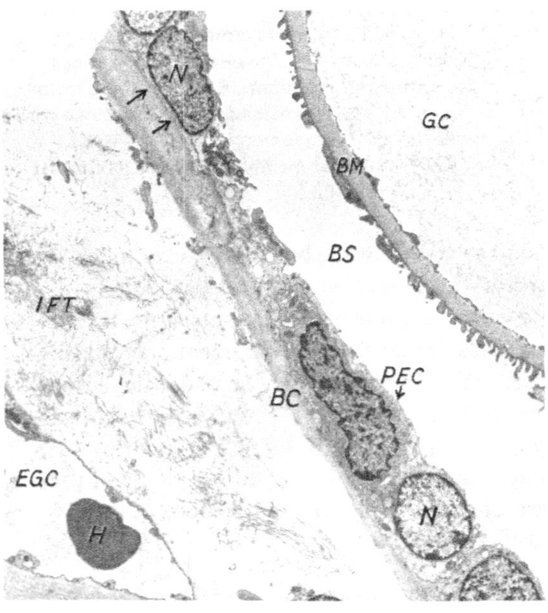

Fig. 127. Diabetic glomerulosclerosis. Bowman's capsule (BC) partially thickened (arrows). Epithelial capsular layer (PEC); BS = Bowman's space; GC = glomerular capillary with its basement membrane (BM); extraglomerular capillary (EGC) with an erythrocyte (H); IFT = interstitial fibrous tissue. (6,000 X).

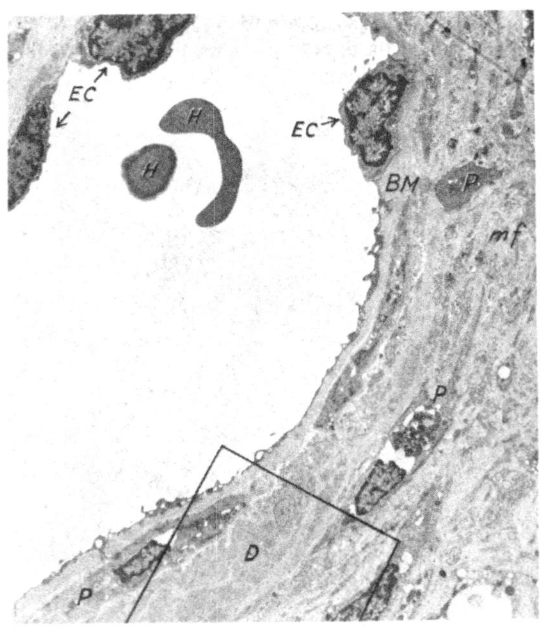

Fig. 129. Renal diabetic macroangiopathy. Highly thickened basement membrane (BM) with big pools of non-homogenous material electronodense (D); P = pericyte; E = endothelial cell; mf = myofibrilles; H = erythrocyte. (6,000 X).

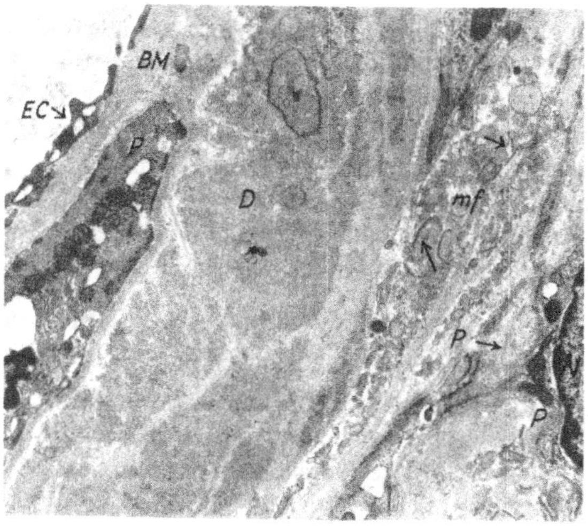

Fig. 129 B. Detail from previous figure (128 A). EC = endothelial cell; BM = thickened basement membrane with big electrondense non-homogenous pools of material inside (D); P = pericyte; Mf = myofibrilles; N = nucleus of a pericyte. (24,000 ×).

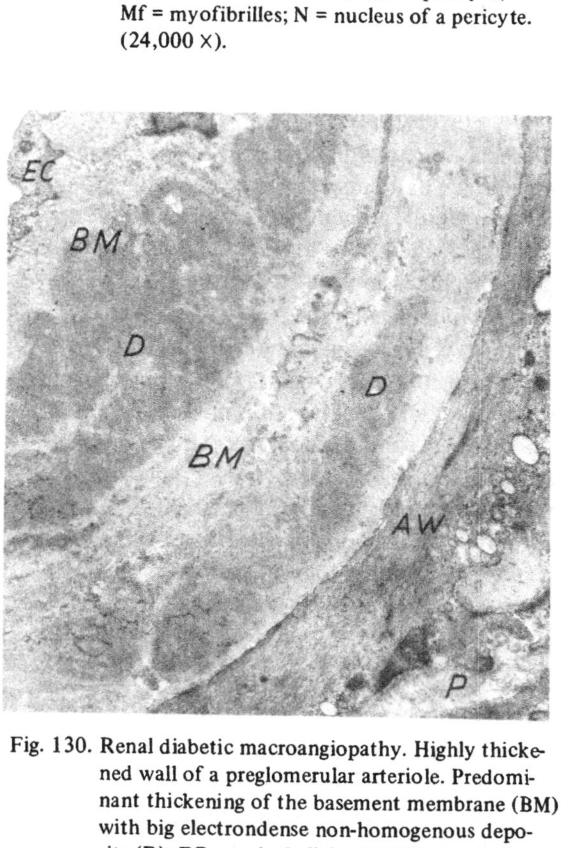

Fig. 130. Renal diabetic macroangiopathy. Highly thickened wall of a preglomerular arteriole. Predominant thickening of the basement membrane (BM) with big electrondense non-homogenous deposits (D); EC = endothelial cell; AW = muscular arteriolar wall; P = pericyte. (24,000 ×).

been advanced, however, with regard to the pathogenesis of this late complication of diabetes mellitus, and therapies recommended, with a view to correcting certain alterations supposed to play a role in the onset of the disease.

This is largely due to the fact that the chemical structure of normal tissues is not yet fully elucidated. On the other hand, experimental research on animals in which the administration of certain substances (such as protamine) [91] resulted in alterations similar to those found in diabetic glomerulosclerosis, cannot be extrapolated to human diabetes mellitus. Therefore, a review of the present state of advances in this field offers a criterion for the estimation of the efficacy, or of the inefficacy of the various treatments applied, and of the natural history of this late complication of diabetes mellitus.

Nodular diabetic glomerulosclerosis, the classical lesion described by Kimmelstiel and Wilson [80], consists, according to many authors [89, 90], of the accumulation of a given substance in the mesangium. The accumulated material originates partly in the bloodstream and is partly synthesized in situ.

A chromatographic analysis of the carbohydrates commonly found in the kidney of the diabetic subject and that of the rat with experimental alloxan diabetes, shows a significant accumulation of glucose (normal 5.00 ± 1.72, diabetic 13.85 ± 11.6 μmol/gm), of sorbitol (normal 3.46 ± 1.22, diabetic 8.92 ± 5.02 μmol/gm) and of fructose (normal 0.20 ± 0.08, diabetic 0.55 ± 0.16 μmol/gm).

The diffuse lesions of the glomerulus or diffuse diabetic glomerulosclerosis is chiefly characterized by a diffuse, uniform or focal [27] thickening of the basement membrane around the capillary vessel [89, 90].

The thickness of the basement membrane varies with age, ranging between 800 and 2,500 Å. In diabetes mellitus it may reach 5,000–8,000 Å and even more [33]. Generally speaking, the basement membrane is nowadays considered [123] as a "copolymer" of a particualr collagen, rich in structural carbohydrates and glycoproteins. It is composed of

85 % protein, 4 % carbohydrates and 11 % fat [2]. The protein contains 7.7 % hydroxyproline, 2.1 % hydroxylysine and a high proportion of glycine (11.2%) [141, 142]. Investigations of the bovine renal cortex questioned the presence of lipids in the basement membrane [142]. According to Spiro, the carbohydrates make up 10 % of the weight of the basement membrane, and are found as glucosylgalactose, mannose, fucose, hexosamine and as sialic acids. Some 50 % of the carbohydrates in the basement membrane are disaccharides, the other half being heterosaccharides. The great number of disaccharide units bound to hydroxylysine are supposed to confer on the basement membrane the chemical properties differentiating it from collagen. The chemical structure of the basement membrane in the glomerular capillaries is very similar to that of the capsule of the lens, suggesting some relationship between renal microangiopathy and certain varieties of loss of transparency of the lens in diabetes mellitus (see Section II p. 27).

It was noted that in the alterations of the histochemical structure occurring in diabetes, the content of carbohydrates, qualitatively similar to those found in the glomerulus of non-diabetic subjects, increases some twenty times. A rise in the proportion of proteins may also occur, but their composition differs from that of the normal individual since they contain some 20 % more hydroxyproline, suggesting an excess of collagen [1, 2].

Some authors also reported increases in the content of mucopolysaccharides, neutral fat, esters of cholesterol and argyrophilic fibres [93]. In diabetes a more intense positive PAS reaction than in normal subjects can be noticed. This is due to the glycoproteins linked to the collagen fibrils. Its greater intensity in the diabetic may be accounted for by [123]:

a) the modification of the normal ratio between collagen and synthesized structural glycoproteins,

b) an abnormal synthesis of macromolecules, or

c) a decrease in the quantity of lysine and the equivalent increase of hydroxylysine and also disaccharide units bound to hydroxylysine [7].

In order to estimate the importance of these qualitative and quantitative chemical modifications, one has to take into account that the basement membrane, which does not contain acid mucopolysaccharides characteristic of the conjunctival fundamental substance, and also phosphatides, glycoproteins and non-collagen proteins, is mainly composed of two particular elements:

- a high proportion of hydroxylysine, a substance found in collagen [118], and
- two types of carbohydrate, a disaccharide, glucosylgalactose, bound hydroxylysine, and a polysaccharide containing hexosamine, galactose, mannose, fucose and sialic acid, most probably bound to asparagine [77].

All these compounds build up the three layers of the basement membrane: where the most important of the thickening of the basement membrane in diabetes is located; and the two "laminae rarae", one internal or subendothelial and the other external or subepithelial.

The spaces among the filaments of the basement membrane, particularly of the lamina densa, are filled by lipids, mucopolysaccharides and non-collagen protein [93]. If there is synthesis of some abnormal macromolecules in diabetic microangiopathy, the molecules may no longer be recognized as "self" by the immunocompetent cells. Thus autoantibodies could result. At present one cannot evaluate this mechanism. However, immunofluorescence studies have demonstrated the presence of antigens situated in the glomerulus in various kinds of glomerulonephritis [70]. Such autoimmune phenomena occurring during diabetic nephropathy are frequent, representing typical reactions to IgG and C'3 antiserums (Fig. 132 A and B).

In summary, it follows that the thickening of the basement membrane occurs in the lamina densa and is associated with an increase in the material contained in that area. The various compounds increase in different proportions, the carbohydrate fractions being the highest. Consequently, the ratio between carbohydrates and proteins, for

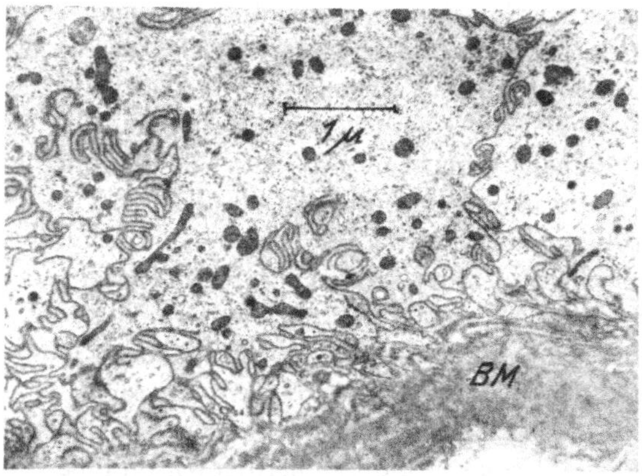

Fig. 131. Diabetic glomerulosclerosis in a young patient. Collecting tubule in the inner zone of medulla. Thickening of the tubular basement membrane (BM) with fibrillar aspect (20,000 ×).

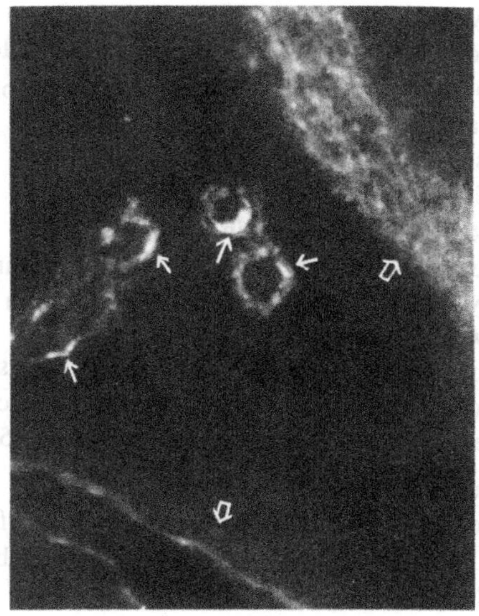

Fig. 132A and B. P. F., 42 year old woman with juvenile diabetes mellitus insulinodependence. Diabetic diffuse glomerulosclerosis in its terminal stage. Fig. A shows (arrows) the area which was explored immunofluorescently in Fig. 130B. Immunofluorescence for IgG and C′3 was found in some periglomerular arterioles (photo Dr. N. Chişu).

instance, which lies around 0.05 in the normal subject, reaches 0.9 in the modified basement membrane of the diabetic and tends towards unity (Fig. 133). At the same time, even if the amount of lipid increases at this level, its share in the total is proportionally changed by the much higher increment in carbohydrates (11%), so that in the diabetic they occupy the third place, representing only 6% of the total content. The association of these quantitative histochemical changes with a qualitative alteration perhaps accounts for the remarkable irreversibility of the entire process.

The nonspecific exudative lesion – "fibrin caps" and "capsular drops" – has often been confused with the nodular glomerulosclerosis described by Kimmelstiel and Wilson. Its histochemical pattern

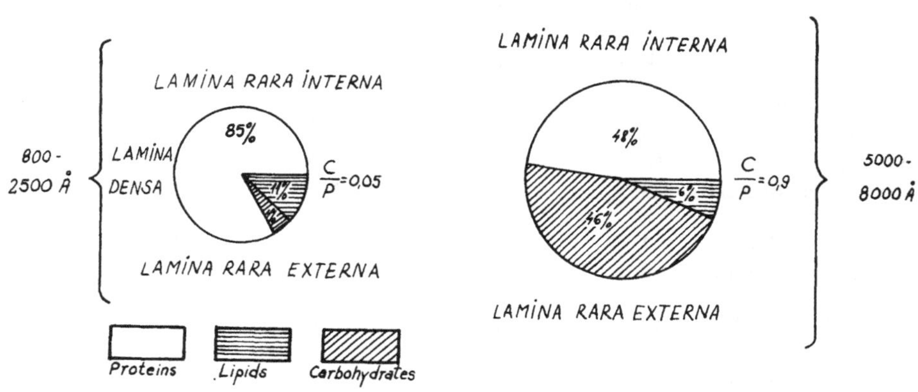

Fig. 133. Histochemical structure of the glomerular basement membrane.

is very similar to that of the alterations found in arteriosclerosis. The fibrin caps contain a protein-carbohydrate-lipid mixture as well as mucopolysaccharides, neutral lipids, cholesterol and its esters and phospholipids [93]. These features usually occur in the capsular space, but may sometimes be found also in the lumen of the glomerular capillaries [89, 90, 93]. The appearance is very similar to that found in animals and in man following the administration of high doses of corticosteroids or ACTH and suggests the existence of a state of corticosuprarenal hyperfunction in the course of diabetes mellitus [90, 151, 152].

The histochemical features of renal diabetic macroangiopathy which overlap with those of diabetic microangiopathy (p. 106) have already been detailed in Section V (p. 143).

B. Prevalence and Incidence

It is interesting to investigate the correlation between the *type of lesion* and its incidence in diabetic subjects since this might help the establishment, for each type, of a clinical equivalent, a pattern of evolution and – as will be subsequently detailed – the life expectation.

Various authors have reported different figures for the incidence of *nodular glomerulosclerosis* in post-mortem specimens, ranging from 10 to 46% of the total number of diabetic subjects examined. A comparison between such figures reported in diabetic and non-diabetic subjects (Table XXI), according to data from the literature and from personal experience has emphasized the specific character of this morphological pattern. Post-mortem examinations in a group of 112 diabetic subjects who died in 1968–1969 were compared with similar examinations in non-diabetic subjects. Nodular lesions of the Kimmelstiel-Wilson type were found in 36 subjects (32.14%) in the former group and only in two subjects (1.7%), in the latter.

As regards the incidence of nodular lesions in renal biopsy specimens various authors have reported figures between 40 and 60 % [29, 90], although some found incidences around 20 % [26] (Table XXI).

In 47 renal biopsies in diabetic subjects, performed in the Clinic of Metabolic Diseases and Nutrition in Bucharest using the Menghini procedure, nodular lesions were found in 14 patients, i.e. in 29.8% of the group (Table XXII). Age, duration of the diabetes and the nature of treatment should

Table XXI: The frequency of nodular glomerulosclerosis (Necropsy material).

Authors (year) of report	Number of patients			Nodular lesions in %	
	Diabetes mellitus absent	Diabetes mellitus present	Total of subjects examined	Non-diabetic	Diabetic
Henderson [68] (1948)	81	313	394	3.6 %	10 %
Zins [152] (1949)	50	50	100	2 %	34 %
Hall [64] (1952)	50	120	170	2 %	38 %
Rogers, Robbins and Heghers [126] (1952)	3	387	?	?	26 %
Bell [10, 11] (1953, 1960)	7	236	?	?	16 %
Lambie and MacFarlane [86] (1955)	2	120	?	?	46 %
Ditscherlein [36] (1964) Clinic of Metabolic Diseases and Nutrition, Bucharest (1968–1969)	112	112	224	1.7 %	32.14 %

Table XXII: The frequency of nodular glomerulosclerosis (Biopsy material).

	Juvenile diabetes mellitus with a duration of 2–8 years	Maturity onset diabetes mellitus with a duration of 2–11 years	Total
Number of renal biopsies	31	16	47
Number of patients with nodular lesions	9	5	14
Incidence (%)	29	51	29.8

undoubtely be taken into account in interpreting this figure. It should be noted that 9 of 14 patients with Kimmelstiel-Wilson lesions had an insulin dependent, juvenile diabetes mellitus, with a duration of 2–8 years. The other 5 patients suffered from diabetes with maturity onset of 2–11 years. Three of the latter had been treated only by a low carbohydrate diet and the other two had been taking antidiabetic sulphonamides for 4 and 6 years respectively. In both groups poor control of the diabetic condition was noted, either due to the instability of the disease (in three of the juvenile cases) or to disregarding therapeutic instructions.

Diffuse glomerulosclerosis is regarded as more frequent than nodular glomerulosclerosis [79]. Incidence figures reported by various authors on biopsy specimens range from 9–59%. This wide variation should probably be assigned to the differences between the investigated groups with regard to age duration of diabetes type of treatment and, possibily, the sex of the subjects.

In post-mortem examinations performed at the Clinic of Metabolic Diseases and Nutrition in Bucharest, this type of renal diabetic complication was found in 25 of 112 diabetic subjects, i.e. in 23% of the post-mortem specimens (Table XXII).

Thomsen [147] found diffuse diabetic glomerulosclerosis in 90% of biopsies from 102 patients. In the 47 diabetics, in whom renal biopsy was performed at the Clinic of Metabolic Diseases and Nutrition in Bucharest, the incidence of diffuse diabetic glomerulosclerosis was higher in patients with maturity onset diabetes than in those with

Table XXIII: The frequency of diffuse glomerulosclerosis (necropsy material).

Authors (year of report)	Total number of patients investigated	Patients with diffuse diabetic glomerulosclerosis	Incidence (%) of glomerulosclerosis in the diabetic subjects
Henderson [68] (1948)	313	31	10 %
Zins [152] (1949)	50	17	34 %
Bell [10, 11] (1953, 1960)	1465	131	9 %
Brun [17] (1953)	24	12	50 %
Darnaud [32] (1956)	60	20	30 %
Hatch [in 147] (1961)	69	41	59 %
Clinic of Metabolic Diseases and Nutrition, Bucharest (1968–1969)	112	25	23 %

Table XXIV: The frequency of diffuse glomerulosclerosis (biopsy material).

	Juvenile diabetes mellitus, duration 2–8 years	Maturity onset diabetes mellitus, duration 2–11 years	Total
Number of renal biopsies	31	16	47
Number of patients with diffuse glomerulosclerosis	6	7	13
Incidence (%)	19	43	27

juvenile diabetes. It should, however, be noted that the duration of the diabetes did not exceed 8–11 years in any of the groups (Table XXIV). Recently, some authors [49] have insisted on the frequent coexistence of nodular and diffuse glomerulosclerosis in diabetics. It has been claimed that the diffuse lesion is always associated with, and even precedes, the nodular lesion [89, 90]. Reubi [120], for instance, has suggested that the nodular lesion, diffuse glomerulosclerosis and exudative glomerulosclerosis (fibrin caps) are different expressions of the same process, which ends in diabetic glomerulosclerosis. This opinion is not shared by all the authors investigating the field, since the nodular lesion may occur with out the distinctive element of diffuse glomerulosclerosis, i. e. thickening of the basement membrane.

Research at the Clinic of Metabolic Diseases and Nutrition in Bucharest has revealed that the two types of lesion coexist in some cases but are found separately in many others. This might explain the differences reported by various authors regarding the incidence of this late complication.

Both in the necropsy and the biopsy specimens the preponderant or exclusively nodular lesions were found to be particularly frequent (Tables XXI and XXIII).

Exudative glomerulosclerosis, characterised by "fibrin cap" and "capsular drops", is of less practical significance than nodular and diffuse glomerulosclerosis. This is particularly important for long-term prognosis, although some authors have suggested that exudative glomerulosclerosis is the earliest stage of nodular glomerulosclerosis [98] or conversely, that the latter is the final stage of the former [90].

More recent detailed descriptions of these alterations have helped to avoid confusion between the exudative and the nodular glomeruloscleroses. In the past, such confusions not only biased statistical conclusions, but also caused certain authors to ignore the specificity of the Kimmelstiel-Wilson nodule in diabetes mellitus.

Alterations similar to those found in diffuse glomerulosclerosis have also been described in arteriosclerosis, in the absence of diabetes mellitus, and in animals given ACTH and/or corticosteroids.

The real incidence of exudative glomerulosclerosis in the diabetic subject has therefore been difficult to estimate. Work published in the same year (1952) suggested percentages ranging from 6–7 % [5] to 47 % [82]. Ditscherlein [37] found this type of lesion in each fifth subject at necropsy and often in association with the diffuse or the nodular types, or both.

In necropsy specimens from 112 diabetic patients at the Clinic of Metabolic Diseases and Nutrition in Bucharest, "fibrin caps" and/or "capsular drops" were found in 9 % of the cases (10 subjects). In the renal biopsy specimens from 47 patients, the incidence was 6.4 % (3 patients). All patients with exudative lesions were adults with a disease duration of 9–11 years.

Renal macroangiopathy or *renal arteriosclerosis* was found in 77% of the cases examined by Ditscherlein [37, 38, 39] and 72% of the cases examined by Franke [51]. It was present in all patients in whom the duration of the diabetes exceeded 10 years.

Statistical analysis of necropsy results has revealed the frequent association between renal arteriosclerosis and diffuse [132] or nodular glomerulosclerosis. This is not surprising, since, experience shows that severe chronic glomerular processes may affect the renal arterioles, by means of a non-specific macroangiopathy, and because macroangiopathy may develop without interfering with the glomerular alteration or in the absence of the latter [139].

The general incidence of renal involvement amounted to 32.8% in 4,975 diabetic patients admitted between 1962 and 1968 to the Clinic of Metabolic Diseases and Nutrition in Bucharest.

A correct estimation of the *relationship between the duration of the diabetic disease and renal diabetic angiopathy* is difficult because:

- there are cases with a long duration of disease in which the presence of a renal diabetic angiopathy is difficult to ascertain [87], and
- it is often difficult to determine the moment of onset of diabetes mellitus, since it does not always coincide with the clinical onset of the condition [40, 132, 139]. Nevertheless, authors today admit that the incidence of the various types of renal involvement in diabetes, particularly the micro- and macroangiopathic types (see) Fig. 99), increases with the duration of the disease [40, 111, 112]. In fact, at the beginning of the century, the mortality due to diabetic nephropathy was estimated at 3% of the total number of diabetic deaths. The figure rose to 10–12% at mid-century and has increased to 57.1% [84] in the last 15 years. It is admitted now that after 11 years of diabetes the presence of a renal microangiopathy is very probable, while it is unlikely to be found in cases lasting less than 5 years [38]. The rise in the incidence of renal vasculopathy in the diabetic has gone, of course, hand in hand with an increase in cardiac and cerebral vascular complications.

The parallelism between the increase in the average life expectation of the diabetic patient, due to the improvement of therapeutic possibilities, and the rise in the incidence of diabetic nephropathy has been so striking that the question arose whether the therapeutic management itself, and insulin therapy in particular, could be held responsible for the renal involvement.

The incidence of diabetic nephropathy in the patient depends on the diagnostic criterion. Utilizing the results of renal biopsy, many authors consider diabetic nephropathy as concomitant with or even preceding the first clinical signs of diabetes mellitus [41, 63, 92]. On the contrary, if the onset of the urinary syndrome and proteinuria in particular, is taken as the criterion, the onset of diabetic nephropathy is regarded as a late event, reaching its peak incidence after 15–24 years of diabetes. Thus, diabetic nephropathy should be regarded as a rare complication in the first ten years of the disease [1, 2], reaching a frequency of 18–30 % after 15 to 20 years. After 20–25 years duration, figures of 25–54 % have been reported for the incidence of renal micro- and macroangiopathy [75].

The hypothesis that the duration of the diabetes plays no important role in determining the incidence of diabetic nephropathy, based on the fact that aspects of glomerulosclerosis may be found in the absence of a manifest diabetes mellitus [41, 132], or in cases diagnosed as prediabetes [34, 107], only shows that the existence of a disorder of carbohydrate metabolism is one of the factors determing the condition, even if the metabolic disorder is a minor one.

Observations at the Clinic of Metabolic Diseases and Nutrition in Bucharest of renal biopsy specimens from 47 patients admitted to hospital and of necropsy specimens from 112 diabetic patients who died in hospital for various reasons, revealed a similar frequency distribution in the two groups (Table XXV). The general shape of the distribution of the types of renal lesion was also found to be similar of course, the subjects in the two groups underwent a certain selection in that they were admitted to hospital or died in hospital, so that the statistical results cannot be regarded as reflecting the general pattern of frequency of renal complications. The investigation is, however, useful because it gives some indication of the proportion between the frequencies of the various types of diabetic microangiopathy and also because it shows the comparatively early onset of this complication in the diabetic patient. In fact, the duration of the diabetic disease ranged between 2–11 years in the 47 patients in which renal biopsy was performed (31 cases of juvenile diabetes and 16 cases of maturity onset diabetes) (see Table XXIV).

In the group of 112 deceased patients the statistical results were less conclusive from this point of view, since the duration of the diabetes ranged from 11/2 to 22 years and the number of cases of maturity onset diabetes largely exceeded those of juvenile diabetes (101 to 11).

After studying *the efficiency of long-term control* of diabetes mellitus in a group of diabetic patients, it was found that the frequency of diabetic nephropathy was higher in patients with poor metabolic control. According to Keiding et al. [78] it was 28 %, compared to 2 % in groups of patients under good metabolic control. In other groups of patients, estimated to be in intermediate degrees of metabolic control, the incidence lay between these extreme figures (17 %). It appears that good metabolic control delays the onset of diabetic nephropathy, just as it does with diabetic retinopathy [77]. Experiments performed on monkeys with alloxan diabetes also suggest that a chronic imbalance in diabetes mellitus promotes the onset of diabetic nephropathy [58, 132].

In the two groups of patients examined by necropsy and by renal biopsy at the Clinic of Metabolic Diseases and Nutrition in Bucharest, the incidence of glomerular lesions was found to be higher in the subjects treated with a low carbohydrate diet and/or oral antidiabetic drugs, than in those treated with an adequate dose of insulin, and by a controlled diet (Table XXVI).

This might be explained, as already suggested in other sections of this work, by the positive role played by a correct metabolic control by insulin, and also by the fact that many of the patients on oral treatment were taking oral antidiabetic drugs, although insulin had been prescribed to them precisely because of the poor results of previous therapy.

Table XXV: The frequency of renal lesions of angiopathic type (necropsy and biopsy material).

Subject group		Patients without renal angiopathic lesions	Renal manifestations of diabetic microangiopathy			The total number of patients with angiopathic renal lesions
			Nodular glomerulosclerosis	Diffuse glomerulosclerosis	Exudative glomerulosclerosis	
47 renal biopsies	Number of patients	17	14	13	3	30
	Frequency %	36.2	29.8	27	6.4	63.8
112 necropsies on diabetic patients	Number of patients	41	36	25	10	71
	Frequency	36.7	32.14	23	9	63.3

Table XXVI: The frequency of glomerular lesions in patients treated with insulin compared to patients treated orally.

Group of subjects	Management	Diabetic nephropathy absent		Diabetic nephropathy present	
		Metabolic control			
		sufficient	poor	sufficient	poor
47 diabetics with renal biopsy	Diet	5	2	2	6
	Oral antidiabetic drugs	3	1	3	9
	Insulin	5	1	4	6
	Total	13	4	9	21
112 diabetics examined by necropsy	Diet	9	2	8	14
	Oral antidiabetic drugs	16	4	11	20
	Insulin	8	2	6	12
	Total	33	8	25	46

The work of Keiding and Marble [78] was among the first to draw attention to the significantly high incidence of diabetic patients with prolonged metabolic inbalance. Subsequently Sherill [135], Engleson [42] and Johnsson [75] reported the same observation, either by comparing groups of patients on controlled or free diets, or by retrospective follow-up of patients on unrestricted diet.

The importance of these observations with regard to the possibility of aprophylaxis of the renal diabetic angiopathy is obvious.

Diabetic nephropathy, under its various aspects, was found in all ages, and *its distribution differences with age group* were considered. In the elderly diabetic the clinical picture is complicated by other pathological conditions, particularly arteriosclerosis, which develop simultaneously with diabetes. The incidence of hypertension is also much higher in elderly patients irrespective of the presence of diabetes.

There are, however, some indications that in cases of equal duration of diabetes, typical diabetic nephropathy is more frequently found in younger than in older diabetics. The same observation was made with regard to diabetic retinopathy [11, 39, 50, 114].

It is difficult to establish a relationship between the prevalence of diabetic nephropathy and the *sex* of the patients, since the results reported by various authors are very different [132]. Such differences may be due to the fact that the statistical investigations performed so far, including those at the Clinic of Metabolic Diseases and Nutrition in Bucharest, rely, according to Danowsky [31], on cross-sectional studies and on long-term observations and checking at pre-established intervals of homogenous groups of patients.

The often-reported comparatively large number of female patients with renal microangiopathy may be due to the generally higher incidence of diabetes mellitus in females (see Section II, Table II, p. 24). There seems to be no difference between the number of sexes if large groups of diabetic patients are compared [38, 39, 114]. One fact should however be noted: glomerulosclerosis associated with proliferation in Bowman's capsule (capsular drop) is more frequent in males [114].

It has been claimed that the clinical picture of diabetic glomerulosclerosis cannot be found in pancreatic diabetes mellitus [2]. This assertion, implying that a supposed genetic factor plays a decisive pathogenetic role, by minimizing the prolonged disorder of the carbohydrate metabolism [95], does not appear to be true. The research of Marble et al. [99] and Becker and Miller [6] demonstrated the presence of diabetic glomerulosclerosis in all types of diabetes mellitus, including the pancreatic type.

It was found that diabetic glomerulosclerosis could be induced experimentally in pancreatectomized or alloxanized dogs [100] and in alloxanized monkeys treated by doses of insulin lower than those required for the daily carbohydrate intake [58]. Such findings rule out the hypothesis that a genetic factor determines the renal localization of diabetic angiopathy. These investigations, and those mentioned in Subsection III (p. 75) emphasize the toxic role played by prolonged metabolic imbalance in diabetes mellitus and deny the specific nephrotoxic effect of particular types of diabetes.

Certain investigators have emphasised the role of *pregnancy* [144] in diabetic women in promoting the development of renal angiopathy. It is more likely that a preexisting renal lesion in a diabetic pregnant woman disturbs the normal course of pregnancy [119].

The *coexistence of diabetic retinopathy and nephropathy* is frequent. Investigations performed by Otto et al. [114] showed that in 86 cases of complicated diabetes, renal and retinal microangiopathy coexisted in 50 patients. In the other 36 cases only one of these organs was predominently involved, namely the retina in 28 and the kidney in 8 cases. The anatomical pattern of the microangiopathy seems to be important since renal microangiopathy is always present if the ophthalmological findings show proliferative diabetic retinopathy [50, 114, 147]. Retinal microaneurysms often coincide with a nodular glomerulosclerosis [3].

Fischer [50] has observed that while the course of proliferative retinopathy is always malignant, that of the associated glomerulosclerosis is not necessarily so.

Kuhlmann et al. [85] consider that the retinal and renal microangiopathic processes undergo a parallel evolution, but for practical reasons the renal alteration is often diagnosed later. This may explain certain reported discrepancies and apparent lack of parallelism. Investigations of experimental diabetes in the dog have confirmed this opinion [115].

The cause of *death in diabetic patients suffering from renal* angiopathy relates to progressive glomerular insufficiency and associated uraemia. However, according to Mohnike [111, 112] a large number of diabetic subjects die from pyelonephritic complications, which belong to the framework of diabetic nephropathy (see Fig. 99, p. 105), but are not of angiopathic nature themselves. Therefore, the effect of renal diabetic angiopathy on the death rate is difficult to estimate.

From the data above, one may attempt a summary of the problems inherent in studies of the prevalence, incidence and mortality of diabetic angiopathy. The conclusions are undoubtedly incomplete and insufficient, since the underlying investigations are not based on long-term observations and the selection of the groups and the methods used are not homogenous.

1. The diabetic microangiopathy which has an ubiquitous character may predominantly involve the kidney, taking a benign or malignant course. Difficult to predict, its development obviously depends on certain factors, among which a good control of the diabetic dysmetabolic state is worth mentioning.

2. There is a correlation between the renal changes in diabetes mellitus and the duration of the

diabetic disease, in that the probability of finding disorders in renal function and microcirculation increases with the duration of the disease.

3. The renal microangiopathy does not appear to be under genetic control and is not related to the sex of patients, but age does seem to be an important factor. Most of the cases, particularly the most severe, occur in the younger patients.

4. Long-term effective treatment of diabetes mellitus, by any therapy, appears to have a positive influence on the course of diabetic nephropathy, delaying or arresting its malignant course.

5. Like most types of diabetic microangiopathy, the renal diabetic microangiopathy begins with a functional stage that precedes, by a long interval, the apparent clinical stage. This may explain why various authors have reported the onset of diabetic nephropathy at different stages, and why certain discrepancies have been found between the pathomorphological and the clinical pictures described in a patient at a given time.

6. The statistics of the Clinic of Metabolic Diseases and Nutrition in Bucharest show that, in 4,875 patients admitted to hospital between 1962 and 1968, diabetic nephropathy of all types was found in 32.8 % of the cases.

C. Clinical Study of the Renal Diabetic Microangiopathies

The correspondence between the pathomorphological pictures resulting from electron and light microscope data, and the clinical symptoms of the renal complications of diabetes mellitus, is still much debated. The situation is further complicated by the fact that not all ultrastructural alterations have a corresponding morphological equivalent in the light microscope picture, and the alterations in renal structure found with both these methods may in their turn have no equivalent in the clinical symptomatology or in kidney function [60, 130].

Disregarding pyelonephritis and necrotic papillitis, inflammatory processes of bacterial origin which may occur in association with any of the anatomical varieties of renal diabetic vasculopathy, one clinical entity remains, the Kimmelstiel-Wilson syndrome. Actually, this clinical syndrome is by no means identical to that described in 1936 by Kimmelstiel and Wilson. These authors described the lesions known today as "nodular glomerulo-clerosis" and the patients studied by them had not only diabetes mellitus, but also oedema, arterial hypertension, proteinuria and renal failure. This collection of symptoms, to which one more facultative symptom should be added, diabetic retinopathy, represents the clinical basis of the so-called Kimmelstiel-Wilson syndrome. Subsequent research has demonstrated that the lesions described by Kimmelstiel and Wilson in the glomerulus of the diabetic subject do not always coincide with the clinical syndrome [57, 59].

There appears to be a much closer relationship between the Kimmelstiel-Wilson syndrome and diffuse glomerulosclerosis [9, 10, 11, 40, 57, 58]. As already mentioned at the beginning of this section (Fig. 99), this morphological alteration is often associated with nodular glomerulosclerosis.

Several explanations of the pathogenesis of the Kimmelstiel-Wilson syndrome have been advanced. It may, for instance be assumed that a restriction of the glomerular filtration rate (GFR) occurs by:

a) the thickening of the basement membrane of the glomerular capillaries, since it is known that the rate of ultrafiltration is inversely proportional to the thickness of the membrane to be crossed:

b) the proliferation of the endothelial cells and the alterations of the mesangium which also affect normal filtration, because of the material accumulated between the internal environment and the space in Bowman's capsule and also because of a possible modification of the selectivity of the cells of the capillary endothelium in general [22, 23];

c) the changes in the glomerular epithelial cells, which fuse together and cover large areas of the external surface of the basement membrane. These modifications are very similar to those described in nephrosis and are probably associated with heavy proteinuria [27]. They may, of course, be a consequence rather than a cause [81].

In fact, none of these alterations can be positively related to the clinical picture of renal diabetic microangiopathy. Further research in the field is needed [81].

1. Clinical Analysis of Kimmelstiel-Wilson Syndrome

The coexistence of renal, vascular, and metabolic features and their association with diabetic retinopathy is highly suggestive, although the correct diagnosis can only be made after renal biopsy [51]. The combination of the symptoms reflecting the ubiquity of the angiopathy with the renal symptomatology may also suggest a diagnosis of diabetic glomerulosclerosis, differentiating it from common nephrosclerosis and the other bilateral renal pathological conditions. A brief analysis of this symptomatology will illustrate the above.

1. The renal symptomatology shows that the target organ of the ubiquitous angiopathic process is the kidney. It includes:

a) proteinuria and eventually other changes in the urinary sediment;

b) oedema, or what has been called the nephrosis of renal diabetic angiopathy, and

c) azotaemia.

2. The vascular alterations in diabetic angiopathy result in arterial hypertension and ultimately heart failure.

3. The metabolic component is represented by one of the most characteristic symptoms of the Kimmelstiel-Wilson syndrome: the insulin requirement gradually falls and in extreme cases glycaemia and glycosuria return to normal.

4. To these three features of the clinical picture of renal diabetic angiopathy, most authors add the highly frequent association of some degree of diabetic retinopathy.

The whole syndrome, undergoes a chronic course, finally resulting in renal failure and death. The course of renal diabetic angiopathy can be roughly divided into several phases:

a) an initial, oligosymptomatic phase consisting of proteinuria and perhaps some symptoms of diabetic retinopathy. This might be regarded as the borderline between the functional and lesional phases, when more information can be obtained from the renal function tests than from the clinical examination of the patient;

b) an intermediate phase in which the clinical picture is of a nephrotic-hypertensive type. Fundus examinations reveal progress towards haemorrhagic or proliferative retinopathy. Progressive reduction in insulin requirements may already be noted;

c) a terminal phase consisting of renal failure, usually associated with proliferative diabetic retinopathy.

Taking into account the duration of the diabetic disease and the age of the patient, Reubi [119, 120] described two general patterns of renal diabetic angiopathy:

1. The typical pattern comprising the whole symptomatology of the disease and mostly found in juvenile diabetics under the age of 40 years;

2. The atypical or oligosymptomatic pattern mostly found with maturity onset diabetes, in older patients. Hypertension and proteinuria are moderate and the deficiency in renal function is minimal.

2. Pathophysiological Symptomatology

Proteinuria is one of the earliest symptoms of renal complication. Intermittent at the beginning, when it corresponds to a moderate renal diabetic microangiopathy [139], it later becomes persistent. It occurs in approximately 2/3 of cases of diabetic nephropathy, i.e. in some 80 % of patients [53, 74] and its incidence and severity increase with the advance of diabetic glomerulosclerosis [139].

Proteinuria is probably the result of an increase in the permeability for protein of the basement membrane of the glomerular capillaries [150], within the general rise in capillary permeability observed in diabetes mellitus [21]. The structural modifications of the endothelial cells and glomerular epithelial cells, as found on electron microscopic examination (see the respective subsection) may perhaps be related to the presence of proteinuria [27].

Proteinuria in diffuse diabetic glomerulosclerosis is often associated with slight haematuria and minor cylindruria. A high urinary white cell count, with heavy haematuria, bacteriuria and pyuria indicates pyelonephritis alone or in association with diabetic glomerulosclerosis. Particular importance has been assigned to the presence in the urine of birefringent bodies, composed of lipids frequently found in diffuse diabetic glomerulosclerosis [57, 59, 122] but which might equally indicate a renal tubular alteration. None of these alternatives-pyelonephritis and associated tubulopathy-imply a typical renal angiopathy, and the presence of the latter becomes unlikely if another unspecific renal alteration of this late complication of diabetes mellitus is positively diagnosed.

The hypoproteinaemia found in the later phases of renal diabetic microangiopathy may be a consequence of this persistent proteinuria, but the possible intervention of some defect in protein metabolism, related to the diabetic disease itself, cannot be ruled out [105]. Electrophoretically, this hypoproteinaemia is characterized by hypoalbuminaemia [71]. According to Thomsen [147], the decrease in serum albumin is inversely related to the degree of proteinuria, but it is obvious that both the disorder in protein synthesis and a low protein intake may play an important role in its mechanism.

Oedema though included in the Kimmelstiel-Wilson syndrome [80], is not always present. Onset of oedema is generally late [112] and does not necessarily imply the existence of a syndrome. Reubi [120] considered that oedema in diabetic subjects under the age of 40 most likely indicates diabetic glomerulosclerosis, but over that age oedema may originate from heart failure, cirrhosis and in renal diseases of another kind. Bell [10, 11] adopts the same standpoint and claims that various degrees of oedema found in diabetic subjects under the age of 30 are due in 90% of cases to diabetic glomerulosclerosis, but the same cause cannot be inferred in subjects over the age of 50. Investigating the relationship between the pathomorphological type of diabetic glomerulosclerosis and the presence of oedema, Gellman [57] found that the latter occurs both in the slight and the severe forms of nodular glomerulosclerosis, but that their incidence, which is not very high [139], rises in direct ratio with the severity of the diffuse glomerulosclerosis [59].

It may be assumed that hypoproteinaemia, i. e. low serum albumin (which may fall below 2.5 gm%) plays a role in the mechanism of oedema in renal angiopathy, but it does not appear to be a determining factor, since in many oedematous patients the albumin level is normal and in many patients with low serum albumin no oedema can be found [147].

Heart failure undoubtedly contributes to oedema in certain cases. Nevertheless, since the nephrotic syndrome is more frequent in young patients, although it was initially described in the older diabetic, this factor may also be regarded as auxiliary and not determining.

The alteration of capillary permeability observed in diabetes [21], in which the endothelial cells of the capillaries in the whole organism lose their controlling function of transcapillary migration, may also play a role in oedema formation.
The alterations in the basement membrane and those found in the ultrastructure of the capillary endothelial cells offer possible morphological evidence of this functional disorder of diabetes [22, 23].

Arterial hypertension, the third symptom of the clinical Kimmelstiel-Wilson syndrome is inconstant, moderate and apparently benign [8]. It appears comparatively late in the course of renal diabetic angiopathy [111, 112]. The relationship between its onset and nodular glomerulosclerosis is doubtful and the symptom seems to originate rather in the process of renal arteriosclerosis [139]. As early as 1942 Fahr [44] claimed that there is no pathogenetical relationship between pure nodular glomerulosclerosis and arterial hypertension. This opinion has been confirmed [24]. Nodular glomerulosclerosis is often associated with a slight rise in diastolic pressure. However, that this increase is not proportional to the severity of the disease [57], [10], cannot be inferred. On the contrary, as well as the influence exerted by renal arteriosclerosis on blood pressure it seems that there is an unquestionable relationship between arterial hypertension and the severity of the diffuse glomerulosclerosis.

Thomsen has shown [147] that the presence of arterial hypertension in diabetic subjects with diabetic microangiopathy depends, to a great extent, on the process of arteriosclerosis, often associated with diffuse glomerulosclerosis, which frequently results in a diminished perfusion of the renal tissue. However the opposite hypothesis is equally possible, i. e. that the presence of arterial hypertension in the Kimmelstiel-Wilson syndrome accelerates the process of arteriosclerosis [124], thus bringing about a true vicious circle. Such a mechanism justifies, to a certain extent, the inclusion of this symptom in the clinical picture of renal diabetic microangiopathy. This might provide an explanation for the fact that arterial hypertension occurs only in 3/4 of the cases of diffuse glomerulosclerosis [84] and why, when present, it reaches very high levels only gradually during the last phases of the renal condition [2, 97].

Azotaemia, which occurs in the late stages of diffuse diabetic glomerulosclerosis is preceded and accompanied by a fall in insulin clearance. The patients tolerate azotaemia well [111, 112] and may live for years with a blood urea of more than 80 mg% [117]. Nevertheless, azotaemia indicates an important reduction of the functional renal tissue and the advance of the disease towards renal failure [150].

It has been estimated that diabetic glomerulosclerosis ends in renal failure in 50–60 % of the diabetic patients suffering from nephropathy [139].

The retention of urea goes hand in hand with an accumulation of the intermediate products of protein breakdown [150], whose toxicity may account for the severity of that stage of the disease. It may be supposed that an accumulation of some of these substances exerts an enzyme inhibiting effect, further aggravating the general dysmetabolic state.

Reduction of insulin requirements. An important differential element in the diagnosis of diabetic glomerulosclerosis is that 20% of the patients [67] suffering from chronic renal insufficiency of non-diabetic origin manifest a low tolerance to glucose and a fasting hyperglycaemia. This may be due to both a diminished secretion of pancreatic insulin and an increased output of glucose by the liver. The latter mechanism is bound to occur since the kidney is known as an important site for insulin degradation. Otherwise, renal failure should always result in an increased blood insulin and therefore, an amelioration of carbohydrate tolerance [145]. This only happens however in diabetic nephropathy, which underlines the specific functional character of this late complication as compared to other nephropathies.

As urea retention increases in diabetic glomerulosclerosis, the insulin requirements often decrease in order to compensate for the preexisting diabetes [25, 254]. This symptom may be found in the hypertensive-oedematous stage.

Several processes have been postulated to account for the diminished glucose tolerance in chronic renal insufficiency of non-diabetic origin, such as:

- a disorder in the synthesis or the discharge of insulin;
- the presence of insulin antagonists in the blood;
- an alteration in the peripheral turnover of glucose;
- an arrest in glycogen formation, causing a fall in the glycogen content of the liver, manifest in the failure of epinephrine and glucagon to induce hyperglycaemia [67].

The explanations advanced for the opposing phenomenon occurring in diffuse diabetic glomerulosclerosis are equally unconvincing. It is very difficult to explain the diminished insulin requirement and the improvement of the diabetic state in this syndrome which, clinically, is quite similar to other bilateral renal diseases, but shows a particular pathomorphological picture. The mechanisms producing the low glucose tolerance in some other renal diseases leading to renal insufficiency, may act in reverse to produce the improved carbohydrate tolerance in diabetic nephropathy i. e.:

- enhanced synthesis and discharge of insulin in the remaining pancreatic tissue;
- blocking of the antiinsulinic effect previously exerted by insulin antagonists;
- improved peripheral utilization of glucose, and
- normalization of the glycogen synthesis in the liver. Several other hypotheses also have been advanced in order to explain the fall in insulin requirements of diabetic patients with angiopathic glomerulosclerosis;
- as uraemic patients are anorexic, the carbohydrate intake [76, 86] or even the general caloric intake [129] may be diminished, with a respective fall in insulin requirements. Other authors are not satisfied with this explanation [66] and in the Clinic of Metabolic Diseases and Nutrition in Bucharest carbohydrate intake could be raised in many such patients to amounts higher than the average carbohydrate intake of the non-diabetic subject;
- delayed breakdown of insulin in the kidney and the liver [121];
- increased penetration of glucose into muscle and fat tissue, as a result of the increased permeability of the capillary wall and cell membrane, as an insulin dependent phenomenon [28];
- metabolic breakdown products are retained in renal insufficiency and exert a hypoglycaemic effect [78]. This hypothesis is refuted by the fact that in other chronic renal insufficiencies under similar circumstances, tolerance to glucose is diminished.

The rise of the renal threshold for circulating glucose, likely to occur in diabetic nephropathy [86], should not be confused with the reduction in insulin requirements [74]. The former phenomenon results in a diminished glycosuria, but comparison with the blood glucose level shows that it does not entail an improvement in the diabetic state, requiring less or no insulin.

In the Clinic of Metabolic Diseases and Nutrition in Bucharest the evaluation of the degree of improvement was investigated in several patients with diabetic glomerulosclerosis. Determined according to the Hagedorn-Jensen method, fasting glucose levels were found to fall gradually. Insulin was reduced, and the carbohydrate intake increased, until a free carbohydrate diet without insulin therapy was reached. In one of these cases, a high concentration of blood urea called for glucose infusions, well tolerated without any insulin correction. The reality of this phenomenon is beyond doubt, but as yet there is no satisfactory explanation.

Anaemia often occurs in diabetic glomerulosclerosis, especially in the stage of chronic renal insufficiency. The blood picture is similar to that found in renal failure of other origins, and generally consists of a hypochromic, or eventually normochromic anaemia. Various statistics have suggested an incidence of 41 to 87.5 %. Singer and Ditscherlein [139] reported an incidence of 66 %.

It seems quite likely that a decreased synthesis of erythropoetin accounts for this anaemia, since no erythropoetin was found in the plasma of uraemic patients with anaemia [150]. However some other factors may also interfere, such as disorders in haemolysis, a haemorrhagic diathesis due to some qualitative defect of the platelets and possibly the hypoproteinaemia associated with chronic renal insufficiency. According to some authors [51] the symptomatic picture should be completed by the late and poor excretion of the contrast substances used for renal radiographs.

3. Renal Function in Diabetic Renal Angiopathy

Various renal function tests may be performed in order: (a) to ascertain the reduction of renal function, (b) to obtain a quantitative estimate of the renal function at a given moment and (c) for the long-term observation of the development of a case of diabetic glomerulosclerosis. It seems that the information obtained by these procedures, considered in isolated figures or in time sequences expressed in diagrams, offers a more objective estimate of the renal function.

Highly important is the determination of the glomerular filtration rate (GFR) using inulin (normal values 114–131 ml/min.), mannitol (normal values 124 ± 19 ml/min.) and/or with endogenous creatine clearances (normal value 137 ml/min.) [15].

Inulin clearance is widely used because it yields better information on the function of the glomerulus (since 95% of inulin is discharged into urine) than for instance, urea clearance (since 40% of the urea is reabsorbed in the renal tubules) [138]. The creatinine clearance, technically simpler to perform, is regarded as more useful for prognosis than for differential diagnosis, and its use is more advisable within complex explorations such as the Romeo test.

It has been reported that the inulin clearance is often diminished in diffuse diabetic glomerulosclerosis, but one should take into account such misleading factors as a possible hypoglycaemia during the test, or the reactions of a very labile autonomic nervous system. It should also be borne in mind that in certain cases of glomerulosclerosis the GFR remains unaffected for a long period. With advanced renal damage, no variations are found with repeated clearances. In nodular diabetic glomerulosclerosis, the figures obtained with this procedure show a great variability and are generally inconclusive [138].

Cases have also been reported with clearance values over or at the upper limit of the normal range. This may occur in very recent diabetes in very young patients, in prediabetes and during pregnancy. In such situations, figures 30–50 % above the normal were found [15]. An increased general capillary permeability, as found in the functional stage of diabetic microangiopathy, might account for such findings [21].

The PAH clearance, at plasma concentrations of 10–13 mg% (normal values 79.5–77 Tm mg/min.), performed to measure TmPAH, i. e. the tubular mass of excretion, is useful for determining whether pyelonephritis is associated with diabetic glomerulosclerosis or not. It is thought that an association of low TmPAH values with high GFR occurs mostly in pyelonephritis [87, 138].

The PAH clearance at plasma concentrations lower than 10 mg% allows the estimation of renal plasma flow (normal value 592–654 ml/min.). Variations in the results of this test in diffuse diabetic glomerulosclerosis are generally parallel to those of the inulin clearance. Hypoglycaemia and pregnancy obviously modify the results.

Regarding the correlation between the results of the renal clearance rate and the main symptoms of renal diabetic angiopathy, it is of interest that:

- persistent proteinuria is often associated with a low inulin clearance, ranging from 60–100 ml/min. Below 50 ml/min. heavy proteinuria is usually found;
- renal oedema often accompanies inulin clearance values lower than 50 ml/min.

As a rule, these methods cannot be used for an early diagnosis of diabetic nephropathy [51]. Morgensen's studies [108, 109, 110] of the "glomerular filtration rate" (GFR) have shown it to be abnormally high in juvenile diabetes of recent onset. The same holds for RPF (renal plasma flow) and TmG (maximum tubular reabsorbtion capacity). Insulin therapy helps in normalizing these abnormalities. Hence, the origin of this disease may be an abnormality of the tone of the afferent and/or efferent vessels of the glomerulus, rather than structural defects in the capillary membrane. The prolonged duration of diabetes mellitus causes a significant decrease of GFR and RPF if proteinuria is simultaneously present. In cases with no proteinuria, this phenomenon is less marked.

It has been agreed that a GFR of less than 30 ml/min. is likely to indicate a fatal prognosis [138].

In the Clinic of Metabolic Diseases and Nutrition in Bucharest the following renal function tests were performed:

1. Creatinine clearance.
2. The complex Romeo test.

Glomerular filtration was investigated by a endogenous creatinine clearance test in 96 diabetic patients aged between 15–75 years. There were 51 male and 45 female subjects and duration of diabetes ranged from 1 to 30 years.

The interpretation of the results took into account the creatinine urinary flow rate, correlated with its plasma concentration [106]. Attention was focussed on the functional glomerular disorders present, their time of onset and their dependence on the duration of the diabetes. Results were expressed as mean values with 95 % confidence intervals, assuming a Gaussion distribution, and using the Students t-test.
Normal values of GFR were found to lie between 100 and 150 ml/min. (with a mean of 137 ml/min.). The patients in the investigated group were then divided into two subgroups:

- those with normal filtration: GFR over 100 ml/min./ 1.73 m^2 – 29 cases, i. e. 30.2 % of the group, and
- those with low filtration: GFR under 100 ml/min./ 1.73 m^2 – 67 cases, i. e. 69.8 % of the group.

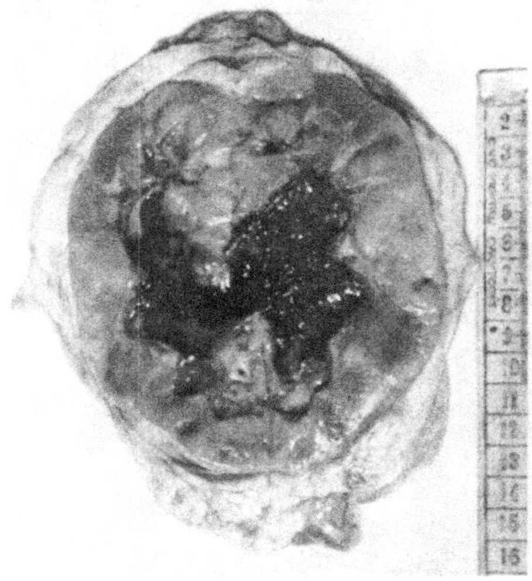

Fig. 134. Renal diabetic papillar necrosis.

Figure 135 compares the obtained distribution with the normal distribution. The C peak represents the distribution of cases in which a GFR higher than 100 ml/min. was found. The C peak almost overlaps the B peak, which represents the normal distribution.

The pathological cases in which the GFR was significantly under the normal value (peak A in figure), show a wide range of values between 13.8 ml/min. and 99.5 ml/min., with an average of 61.8 ± 32 ml/min.

An analysis of this data, taking into account unifactorial criteria, shows the following:

a) The glomerular filtration rate does not appear to depend on the age of the subject (Fig. 136).

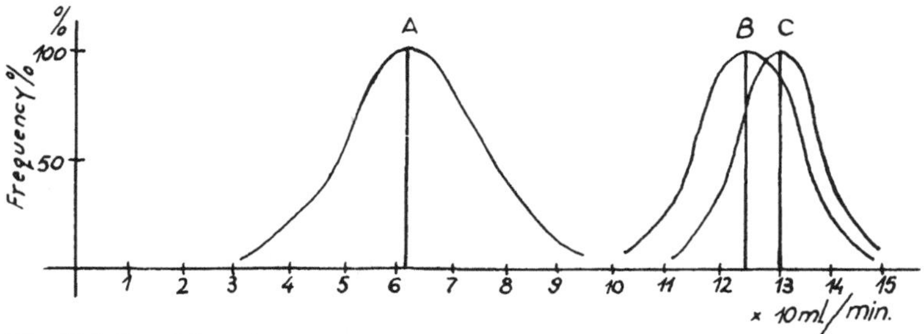

Fig. 135. Renal function testing with clearance of endogenous creatinine. Distribution of the cases in which the diabetic renal disturbance is detected at the supposed beginning of the disease.

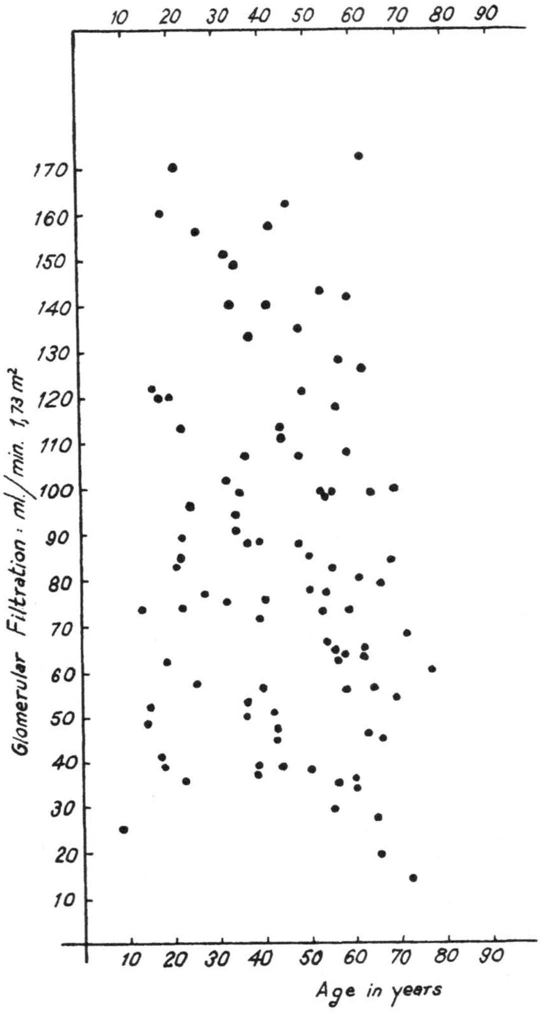

Fig. 136. Age influence on the glomerular filtration rate in diabetics (Clearance of endogenous creatinine).

b) By applying the χ^2-test to the results of Table XXVII it was found that the duration of the diabetes was associated with a significant reduction in GFR.

c) There was a statistically significant correlation between GFR and the presence of arterial hypertension ($p = 0.05$).

A further selection was made within the cases having low GFR by eliminating those ranging from 70 to 100 ml/min. The group of patients with normal GFR was then compared to this new group of patients with very low GFR.

This new selection resulted in two groups of patients with reduced GFR:

- 29 patients with a GFR of 70–99.5 ml/min. (30.2%);
- 38 patients with a GFR of 13.8–70 ml/min. (39.6%).

By eliminating the group of 29 patients with a medium GFR more suggestive evidence is obtained concerning the cases with low GFR as shown in Fig. 137. This group (GFR lower than 70 ml/min.) had an average of 46.84 ± 23 ml/min/1.73 m^2.

Several correlations were examined in the group of 96 patients, particularly those between the functional state of the renal glomerulus in the two extreme categories (normal GFR and very low GFR) and several components of the Kimmelstiel-Wilson syndrome: proteinuria, presence of oedema, arterial hypertension and concomitant diabetic retinopathy.

Table XXVII: The correlation between the diabetic's age and the values for GFR.

GFR	Duration of the diabetes		
	1–15 years	16–30 years	Total
Normal	20	9	29
Reduced	25	42	67
Total	45	51	96

Table XXVIII: The correlation between the blood pressure and GFR.

GFR	Maximal blood pressure in mm Hg		
	Under 140 mm	Over 140 mm	Total
Normal	19	10	29
Reduced	28	39	67
Total	47	49	96

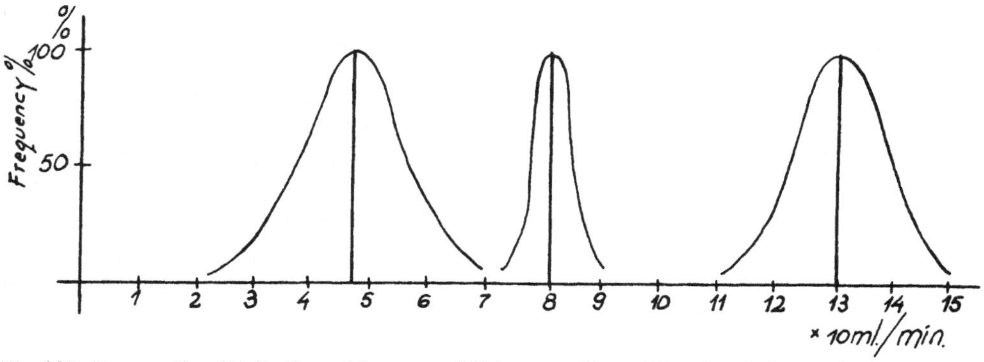

Fig. 137. Comparative distribution of the cases of diabetes mellitus with reduced glomerular filtration rate and those with normal glomerular filtration rate.

1. The significance of the presence or absence of proteinuria and cylindruria was examined by means of the χ^2-test (Table XXIX). There was a good correlation between the reduction in the GFR value and the above symptoms of diabetic renal microangiopathy (p = 0.01).

Table XXIX: The correlation between proteinuria and the values for GFR.

GFR	Proteinuria and cylindruria		
	Present	Absent	Total
Normal	8	21	29
Reduced	29	9	38
Total	37	30	67

2. Table XXX shows the distribution of oedema in the two extreme categories of diabetic patients, those with normal and very low GFR. The statistical analysis (χ^2 = 6.635, p = 0.01) shows that there is a real difference in the incidence of oedema between the two categories of patients.

3. Examination of the eye was performed in 63 of the 96 patients, but only 45 of these belonged to the two subgroups considered. The occurrence of retinopathy is shown in Table XXXI and χ^2 analysis showed that retinopathy is characteristic of the diabetic patients with low GFR (χ^2 = 7.67, p = 0.01).

Table XXX: The correlation vetween oedemas and the values for GFR.

GFR	Oedema		
	Present	Absent	Total
Normal	4	25	29
Reduced	21	17	38
Total	25	42	67

4. In 21 of the 96 investigated diabetic subjects, the fasting blood urea was higher than 45 mg%. These supranormal values ranged from 45 to 164 mg%, with an average of 74.71 mg%. Correlating these values with the respective GFR it was found that:

- in 13 uraemic patients GFR was less than 70 ml/min.;
- in 5 uraemic patients GFR was lower than 100 ml/min.;
- in 3 uraemic patients GFR was higher than 100 ml/min.

Table XXXII: The correlation between the values for blood urea and GFR.

GFR	Eye examination		
	Normal	Retinopathy	Total
Normal	15	8	21
Reduced	5	19	24
Total	18	27	45

Most of the cases of nitrogen retention also exhibited a low GFR. An inverse analysis, as shown in Table XXXII, reveals a parallelism between the average blood urea value and the GFR in all three categories considered. It seems, therefore, that under clinical conditions, the retention of urea depends to a great extent on the glomerular filtration capacity.

Table XXXIII: The correlation between the values for blood urea and GFR.

GFR	Blood urea in mg %		
	Minimum	Maximum	Average
13.8–70 ml/min	20	164	48.97
70–100 ml/min	16	108	33.48
100–172 ml/min	16	56	30.82

Similar investigations performed by Robertson et al. [124] showed that the retention of urea correlates with inulin and PAH clearances. These conclusions are consistent with the results obtained at the Clinic of Metabolic Diseases and Nutrition in Bucharest.

The complex Romeo test (the simultaneous determination of endogenous creatinine and urea clearances) enables us to calculate the following indexes, whose variations are significant in diffuse diabetic glomerulosclerosis:

- The active glomerular surface (AGS). Normal figures obtained range from 5–8 l/hour. The AGS was diminished in 84 of 118 diabetic patients with clinical symptoms of glomerulosclerosis i. e. about 3/4 of the investigated group. This reduction is also consistent with a low GFR, as obtained by the simple test of endogeneous creatinine clearance.

- The capacity of tubular diuresis of urea (CTDU) normally ranges from 25–30 %. Variable values were found in the investigated patients, depending on the respective degree of renal azotaemia.

Of the 84 patients with a low GFR:

- 58 (69%) had a CDTU higher than 30%
- 16 (19%) had a CDTU in the normal range
- 10 (12%) had a CDTU lower than 25%.

These results suggest that tubular function was satisfactory in most of the investigated patients.

- The index of water tubular diuresis (IWTD) normally ranges from 1–3 %, but was lower in the 10 patients with oedema (6 of these had a low CDTU and 4, a CDTU in the normal range). IWTD values were increased in 11 patients with polyuria due to renal insufficiency.

- The renal index (RI) normally oscillates between 0.09–0.12, but was lower in all the patients with low GFR.

The Romeo test is less adequate for functional renal explorations than inulin and PAH clearances Nevertheless, it is a valuable instrument, for studying diabetic renal microangiopathy.

4. Additional Investigation Techniques

As well as the usual routine laboratory tests, some diagnostic importance has also been given to electrophoresis and to the determination of serum enzymes and electrolytes.

Certain changes in the electrophoresis of serum proteins are significant in diabetic renal angiopathy, i. e. a reduction of the albumin fraction and an increase in alpha-globulins found in 70 % of cases [51, 75]. An increase of the beta-globulins is of no significance in this late complication of diabetes [71, 139]. The reported investigations also suggest that the serum protein pattern is important in the diagnosis of diffuse diabetic glomerulosclerosis, but of no importance for the diagnosis of nodular diabetic glomerulosclerosis. An albumin fraction of 40–43 % has been regarded as an important sign of renal diabetic angiopathy when associated with an alpha-globulin value of 15–16 %. In diabetic patients without diabetic microangiopathy, the values obtained for these two fractions may vary, but albumin never falls below 52–54 % and alpha$_2$-globulins never rise above 10 %.

An increase of the isoenzyme lactodehydrogenase 5 (LDH-5), although the enzyme is not specifically of renal origin, is said to be significant. The determination is interesting for differential diagnosis, since the above increase is not found in patients suffering from chronic pyelonephritis without diabetic glomerulonephritis [150].

The serum electrolyte picture in diabetes mellitus, is not different from that found in other renal pathological conditions. However, the water and electrolyte balance at a given stage of the disease may be useful for estimating the general condition of the patient and prescribing adequate therapy. The following deviations from the normal have been observed:

- Hypocalcaemia and hyperphosphataemia, eventually leading to "renal osteodystrophy", more so since diabetic microangiopathy shows a remarkable osteotropic tendency.

Besides diabetes, other factors, such as a low intestinal absorption of calcium, and vitamin D resistance, are likely to bring about this pathological complication.

Fluctuating hyponatraemia, associated with advanced stages of diffuse diabetic glomerulosclerosis is supposed to originate from an inability of the renal tubules to reabsorb sodium filtered by the glomerulus.

- Potassium levels are generally normal in diabetic glomerulosclerosis. Hypokalaemic states have however been reported following loss of potassium through long-lasting diarrhoea caused by a visceral diabetic neuropathy or by prolonged uraemia.
- Hypermagnesaemia has been reported in some cases but its significance is unknown [150].

D. Prognosis in Renal Diabetic Angiopathy

The prognosis is variable and closely related to the type of nephropathy. According to data reported by the Joslin clinic 9 % of diabetics die from diabetic nephropathy [127].

Death by uraemia rarely occurs in nodular glomerulosclerosis, but mostly in cases of juvenile diabetes [36]. The older patients with glomerular nephropathy die generally as a result of extrarenal vascular disease, such as cardiac infarction and cerebral vascular accidents [147].

In 50% of the deaths caused by renal failure an associated pyelonephritis is found [111, 112]. Among the renal diseases of a purely angiopathic character, death by renal failure occurs mostly with diffuse diabetic glomerulonephritis.

Research on the duration of the disease and the life expectancy of patients with renal diabetic angiopathy has shown the average duration of diabetes to be about 10 years before the onset of retinopathy and 11–13 years before the onset of nephropathy, while death due to the latter occurs after 13 years of diabetes [113]. There are no indications that renal angiopathy undergoes any regression [57]. On the contrary, most authors stress its progressive character. The long-term prognosis is worse in cases with the whole spectrum of symptoms than in cases with intermittent or persistent proteinuria as the only feature. Life expectancy is estimated to be 3.5–5 years in the former case [43, 147] and some 10 years in the latter [147].

E. Therapy of Renal Diabetic Angiopathy

Prophylaxis of diabetic nephropathy is theoretically possible by the permanent maintenance of a good metabolic control of the diabetes. There are no studies to confirm this possibility so far.

The treatment of the established renal disease is the only therapeutic aspect thoroughly studied.

1. Diet

The guiding principle of dietary prescriptions should be an individual diet for each particular case, in keeping with certain peculiarities such as:

- the stage of the renal disease
- the method of controlling the diabetic disease
- the patient's state of nutrition.

The dietary prescription should take into account several possibilities related to the development of the clinical syndrome.

a) During the stage of intermittent or permanent proteinuria, there is a trend to hypoproteinaemia, with subsequent oedema and protein starvation. Besides carbohydrate, a high protein diet should be prescribed.

b) With the onset of oedema, generally resistant to therapy, new problems arise. The high protein diet should be continued as long as no clinical or functional signs of nitrogen retention occur. Perfusions of plasma, whole blood, and human albumin may be used to raise the protein intake [133].

The dietary salt intake should be reduced. A low salt diet may keep under control, for a certain time, both the oedema and the progressive rise in blood pressure.

Insulin requirements and tolerance to glucose should be frequently tested during this period in order to reduce the doses of insulin or increase the intake of carbohydrate, as the evolution of the diabetic glomerulosclerosis brings about the characteristic improvement of glucose tolerance.

With a moderate fat intake, a reasonable proportion should be given to unsaturated lipids (see Section V, p. 165). If required by the state of nutrition, the caloric intake may be further supplemented by fat.

c) Dietary prescriptions must be fundamentally altered with the onset of nitrogen retention. The caloric requirements should be met as far as possible by raising the quota of carbohydrate. This shift becomes less difficult as glucose tolerance improves with the advance of the renal diabetic microangiopathy. At the same time, the fat ratio can also be increased. One has to disregard its possible effects on a concomitant or developing arteriosclerotic process, since the renal insufficiency cannot be excluded.

The protein intake should be reduced to the minimum tolerated, controlled by frequent determinations of nitrogen retention. For patients with a GFR between 1.5–5.0 ml/min, the protein intake should amount to 20 g daily and the caloric requirements to at least 2,000 calories daily [134]. Some authors also recommended a low potassium intake, in order to slow down the advance of azotaemia [133].

2. Drug Therapy

The drug therapy in renal diabetic angiopathy is symptomatic and aims at correcting the various disorders arising in the course of the disease.

During the stage of intermittent or persistent proteinuria, synthetic anabolic drugs may be given in order to delay or, if possible prevent the onset of hypoproteinaemia. Proteinuria can sometimes be reduced by urine alkalinizing therapy, associated with atropine or some similar preparation. To this end, small doses of corticoids have also been recommended [133]. Bed-rest often exerts a positive effect on proteinuria.

When oedema and eventually hypertension occur, the patients should be given carbonic anhydrase inhibitors or other diuretics in keeping with the response [133]. Anderson [2] stressed the potential hazard of this therapy in inducing hyponatraemia, which further enhances nitrogen retention. Ion exchange resins should be given carefully as they may cause acidosis. The concomitant arterial hypertension is generally moderate and does not require a special therapy [147].

Iron therapy and vitamins stimulating haematopoiesis should be given if anaemia occurs, but their effect is generally minor. Blood transfusion is indicated in cases with a very low haematocrit.

The administration of certain drugs reputed to reduce blood nitrogen level (e. g. the extracts of Lespedia) may be effective in the early stages of nitrogen retention, but their effect is diminished with the advance of the chronic renal insufficiency.

3. Surgical Treatment

Kidney transplants are not recommended because of the widespread diabetic angiopathy and the macroangiopathic alterations in particular [52, 96].

Surgical [96] or functional hypophysectomy, also recommended in diabetic retinopathy, results in a fall in proteinuria in most of the patients. Although the operation is followed by a fall in inulin clearance, some authors suggest that it might improve renal function [61, 62]. Concerning the pathomorphological aspects, it has been claimed that following hypophysectomy the already thickened basement membrane becomes thinner, and the cytoplasm of the renal endothelial cell grows larger [72]. The procedure is undoubtedly justified during the early phases of renal glomerulosclerosis, but one hesitates to prescribe it at that stage because of the hazards.

The results of bilateral suprarenalectomy, also recommended by some authors, are less spectacular than those of hypophysectomy.

It should be noted that, according to Anderson [2], a blood urea level higher than 75 mg% should be regarded as contraindicating both hypophysectomy and suprarenalectomy.

Chapter V Diabetic Macroangiopathy

Diabetic macroangiopathy is among the most frequent chronic complications of diabetes mellitus and one of the main causes of death. It is sufficient to remark that in the statistics of the Joslin Clinic of Boston, diabetic angiopathy accounted for 77.9% of the total number of deaths during 1960–1964. In 53.3% of these cases death was due to coronary sclerosis, in 12.4 % to cerebral macroangiopathy and in 1.3 % to peripheral ischaemic syndromes [47, 68].

The problem appears to be even more serious if one takes into account the fact that the incidence of the diabetic macroangiopathic disorders is rising in parallel with the increase in the average life expectancy of the diabetic patient subsequent to the progressive improvement of therapy (see Fig. 7 in Chapter I), which has resulted in an increase in the average duration of diabetes mellitus [116]. It is also true that there are, at present, various standpoints regarding the seriousness of the problem of diabetic macroangiopathy, and consequently, various attitudes concerning the prophylaxis and therapy of this chronic complication. While the majority of researchers admit that the incidence of arteriosclerotic disorders is much higher in diabetics than in non-diabetics [122, 175, 185], there are others who believe that there is no difference [119].

A. Pathophysiological Problems in Diabetic Macroangiopathy

Diabetes mellitus and the arteriosclerotic, or macroangiopathic disorders, are a typical example of pathological syntropism, both in the clinical and the humoral fields. They are so closely interconnected that some authors regard them not as separate conditions but as different manifestations of the same process. In fact, it is possible to distinguish between

- arteriosclerotic phenomena preceded, accompanied, or followed by, carbohydrate intolerance.
- arteriosclerotic angiopathic phenomena occurring in the absence of any disorder of carbohydrate metabolism and displaying the well known symptoms of common arteriosclerosis.

However certain pathophysiological, morphological and prognostic particularities confer a specific character on diabetic macroangiopathy and prevent its total identification with common arteriosclerosis.

It appears that the two types of macroangiopathy differ in the presence of a disturbed carbohydrate metabolism and have in common primary and secondary disorders of fat metabolism [97, 164]. The disorders of the lipid balance will be mainly dealt with, as they are pertinent to many practical, prophylactic and therapeutic aspects.

A major role has been assigned to some of the circulating lipids. Greenhalgh et al [64] find anomalies of the blood lipids in 44 % of patients with peripheral vascular disease, irrespective of the existence of diabetes. Our investigations of 7,085 normal subjects revealed the presence of dyslipaemic states in 46 % of the randomly examined individuals (see Chapter I "Frequency of global dyslipaemia" p. 8).

The studies of Albrink et al. [1, 2, 3, 138, 139] performed over intervals of more than 30 years on groups of diabetic (139 subjects) and non-diabetic patients suffering from macroangiopathy, are already classical. They demonstrated that significantly higher serum triglyceride levels are found in patients with clinical angiopathy, cardiac or peripheral than in patients free from such disorders, or showing only the symptoms of diabetic microangiopathy [106]. Greenhalgh et al. [64] found that 30% of patients with peripheral vascular disease showed increased levels of blood triglycerides, while cholesterol and pre-beta-lipoprotein levels were normal. In 5 % of patients high cholesterol with normal triglycerides levels and hyper-beta-lipoproteinaemia were found. The association of higher triglycerides and cholesterol in blood was found in 9% of the cases. (Compare this data with that of healthy subjects and newly discovered diabetics in Chapter I p. 7.)

It has been demonstrated with ^{131}I labelled triolein that diabetic patients with macroangiopathy have an abnormal tolerance to fat [148]. The fact that this phenomenon is not found in the absence of macroangiopathy emphasises the role of lipids in the prevalence of this complication.

On the other hand, many investigators have succeeded in demonstrating that serum triglyceride levels are higher in adults than in young people, a fact which coincides with the comparatively late onset of macroangiopathy. Triglyceride values have also been found to be elevated in the non-diabetic adult with signs of coronary insufficiency [1, 2] and the findings are even more obvious in diabetic subjects with diabetic macroangiopathy [16].

Cholesterol has also been assigned a role in the genesis of diabetic macroangiopathy. The followers of the hypothesis that claims an essential role for triglycerides [3] regard the alterations of serum cholesterol as too small and insignificant to be assigned an atherogenetic role similar so that of triglycerides. However, the investigations performed at Framingham [33] tend to ascribe the major cause of degenerative vascular disorders to the changes in cholesterol metabolism. Moreover, some authors [178] investigating experimental diabetes in the rat, have suggested that the diabetes plays a role in determining the vascular lesions only to the extent to which it induces a secondary hypercholesterolaemia.

The preponderant role of high serum cholesterol levels is also suggested by the fact that the course of macroangiopathy is paralleled by a gradual decrease in fibrinolytic activity and an increase of plasma fibrinogen. The latter phenomenon has often been incriminated as a secondary factor in the determination of ischaemic disorders of the small and medium vessels [99, 163].

Suggestive correlations have been made between disorders of fat and carbohydrate metabolism, and the angiopathy of large and medium vessels. A remarkable correlation was found, for instance, between the symptoms of coronary insufficiency and the presence of diabetes in its chemical or inapparent stage. On the other hand, during the first days following a myocardial infarction, there is a fall in the glucose tolerance [69, 83, 121], which in some 25 % of cases continues for 2–3 years [118].

The changes in glucose tolerance which occur subsequent to such disorders have also been related to the rise in NEFA during the first 12–24 hours following the infarction. NEFA levels gradually return to normal in the subsequent 48 hours [90, 109]. Some authors claim, nevertheless, that the phenomenon pertains not only to postinfarction hyperglycaemia, but to true inapparent diabetes or "subdiabetes" [28].

Knick [86], based on personal research and literature data up to 1968, suggests a possible sequence of disorders, which might offer a pathogenetic and clinical explanation of diabetic macroangiopathy. He found in a number of patients with macroangiopathy of mainly coronary localisation, an increased glucose tolerance, possibly due to hyperinsulinism, which may exist despite a perfectly normal glucose tolerance test [86]. In fact, this had been earlier demonstrated by Welborn [177], who found an increase in circulating insulin in patients with recent myocardial infarction, high blood pressure or with various angiopathic disorders.

It is supposed that if the abnormal rate of insulin release persists, the organism reacts by releasing a hypothetical glutathione-insulin transferase which breaks the disulphide bridges of the insulin molecule. This results in smaller, only partially active fragments, which may be still lipogenetic. Consequently, the serum NEFA level rises and glucose tolerance falls. The result is either an imbalance in a preexisting diabetes mellitus or in a preexisting chemical diabetic state, or a similar disorder in carbohydrate metabolism. All this may further bring about an alteration of fat metabolism and a secondary increase in the triglyceride and NEFA levels, as well as a further fall in glucose tolerance [136], via the glucose-fatty acid cycle [106]. Since NEFA are oxidized first a smaller consumption of pyruvate occurs, with a corresponding effect on the Krebs cycle [49].

This sequence explains on one hand the high incidence of disorders of fat metabolism found in subjects with inapparent diabetes as well as in diabetic patients, and on the other hand, the mechanism of the lipid disorders in diabetes which may occur at the onset of a macroangiopathic complication [16, 85, 86]. Experimental work with various animals has confirmed the atherogenic synergism between the lack of endogenous insulin and the disorders in fat metabolism, induced by the administration of a high fat diet and inhibition of thyroid function, i. e. by the simultaneous action of exogenous and endogenous factors [82].

The behaviour of lipids and serum lipoproteins following an acute macroangiopathic episode is highly interesting. It was found, for instance, that infarction is immediately followed by a fall in the concentration of pre-beta-lipoproteins, with a subsequent rise to levels higher than the initial ones [40, 93, 109, 157]. This change is even more conspicuous if the serum lipoprotein level is already high when the acute incident occurs [40]. In cases with initial normal values the subsequent changes are insignificant or even absent.

These findings show the importance of a preexisting disorder in carbohydrate metabolism, such as a chemical, inapparent or manifest diabetes mellitus, or some alteration in fat metabolism, in increasing the risk of a macroangiopathy. These two types of disorder potentiate one another, either during the disease, or if both exist from the start, during the respective angiopathy (see Fig. 1).

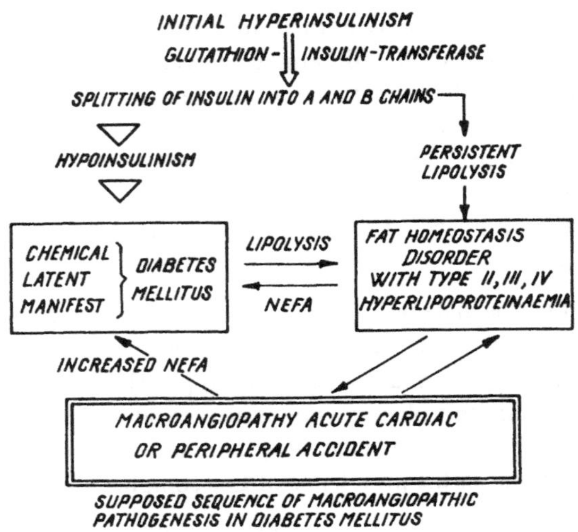

Fig. 1. Supposed sequence of macroangiopathic pathogenesis in diabetes mellitus

It may be useful to examine the present state of the investigations in the field of hyperlipoproteinaemia, both from the pathogenetic point of view and from that of efficient therapeutic or prophylactic treatment [59, 60, 73].

The following types of hyperlipoproteinaemia have been described:

Type I – an excess of chylomicrons (exogenous hypertriglyceridaemia)
Type II – a) familial hypercholesterolaemia
b) over indulgence hyperlipaemia
Type III – familial hyperlipaemia
Type IV – endogenous hypertriglyceridaemia
Type V – mixed hypertriglyceridaemia (exogenous + endogenous)

Table I shows the plasma enzymatic, electrophoretic and ultracentrifugal characteristics of the hyperlipoproteinaemic types. It should be noted that types II and III in particular and types IV and V to a lesser extent, are associated with a high incidence of macroangiopathic complications. Some of these hyperlipoproteinaemias improve with low fat diets (Type I). Others, on the contrary, improve with low carbohydrate diets (Type IV) or with combined low fat and low carbohydrate diets. Type II/a responds especially to restricted fat intake and Type II/b to the administration of drugs which restore the normal serum cholesterol level and, to a lesser extent, to diet prescriptions.

Finally, types IV and V, as well as type I, are frequently associated with low glucose tolerance while in types II and III normal or only slightly impaired glucose tolerance is found (see table I).

The mechanism which leads to a hyperlipaemic state in general and in diabetics in particular may also be important with regard to macroangiopathy. According to Thanhauser [183, 184], hyperlipaemia results from two mechanisms:

- by mobilization, and
- by retention.

Much stress has been recently put on the relationship between diet and its influence on lipaemia and the familial and/or hereditary character of certain lipaemias. All these aspects should be taken into account when speculating on the pathogenesis of diabetic microangiopathy. The existence of a familial or hereditary hyperlipaemia increases the hazard of macroangiopathy, despite faithfully observed dietary restrictions. It is most likely that the two metabolic changes, during diabetes mellitus have certain characteristics in common with the idiopathic hyperlipaemias, but without the whole clinical picture of Bürger-Grütz's disease.

It is most likely that the two metabolic alterations, when associated, potentiate one another with regard to the occurrence of macroangiopathy.

Table I

TYPE	SYNONYMS	PLASMATIC ASPECT	LIPIDAEMIC ANOMALY	LIPOPROTEINOGRAM	DENSITY ULTRA CENTRIFUGATION	LIPOPROTEIN LIPASE ACTIVITY	INGESTION EXCESS: LIPIDS	INGESTION EXCESS: CARBOHYDRATES	FAMILIAL CHARACTER	ATS TREND	CARBOHYDRATE TOLERANCE	CLINICAL FEATURES	EFFICIENT TREATMENT	SUPPOSED CAUSES
NORMAL INDIVID.	NORMAL	CLEAR	TG < 150 mg% CHOL < 220 mg%	ABSENCE OF CHYLOMICRONS	–	N	N	N	–	N	N	–	–	BALANCED FOOD INTAKE
I	EXOGENOUS HYPERTRIGLYCERIDAEMIA	MILKY	TG +++	LIPOPROT ↓ CHYLOMICRONS IN EXCESS	< 1006 SF. 100-400	↓	+	N +++	+	N	↓	ABDOMINAL PANCREATIC PAIN	FAT RESTRICTION IN DIET	INGESTED FAT PERSISTS IN BLOOD STREAM
II a	FAMILIAL HYPERCHOLESTEROLAEMIA	CLEAR	CHOLESTEROL ++	B-LIPOPROTEINS +++	1006-1013 SF. 0-12 +	N	±	N	+	++	N	XANTHOMA XANTHELASMA	CLOFIBRATE D-THYROXIN NICOTINICACID CHOLESTIRANIN	HEREDITARY METABOLIC FAILING
II b	OVER INDULGENCE HYPERLIPAEMIA	CLEAR	CHOLESTEROL + TRIGLYCERIDE +	B AND PRE B LIPOPROTEINS ++	SF. 12-100 ±	N ↓	+	+	±	+	N ↓	XANTHELASMA	DIET ± CHEMOTHERAPY	PROLONGED ALIMENTARY EXCESS ± HEREDITY
III	FAMILIAL HYPERLIPAEMIA	MUDDY	CHOLESTEROL ++ TRIGLYCERIDES ++	BROAD B	< 1006 ++ SF. 12-100 ++	N ↓	+	+	±	+++	N ↓	–	CARBOHYDRATE + LIPID RESTRICTION CHEMOTHERAPY	HEREDITARY METABOLIC FAILING
IV	ENDOGENOUS HYPERTRIGLYCERIDAEMIA	MUDDY	TRIGLYCERIDE ++	PRE-B LIPOPROTEINS +++	SF. 20-400 +++	N	–	++	++	±	↓	ERUPTIVE XANTHOMES PANCREATITIS RETINOPATHY	CARBOHYDRATE RESTRICTION	CARBOHYDRATE METABOLIC FAILING OR EXCESSIVE INTAKE
V	MIXED HYPERTRIGLYCERIDAEMIA (TYPE I + IV)	MUDDY OR MILKY	TRIGLYCERIDES +++ CHOLESTEROL +	CHYLOMICRONS ++ PRE-B-LIPOP. ++	< 1006 ++ SF. 20-400 ++	N ↓	++	+	±	±	↓	ERUPTIVE XANTHOMES PANCREATITIS HEPATOMEGALY	GLOBAL CALORIC RESTRICTION + CHEMOTHERAPY	METABOLIC FAILING

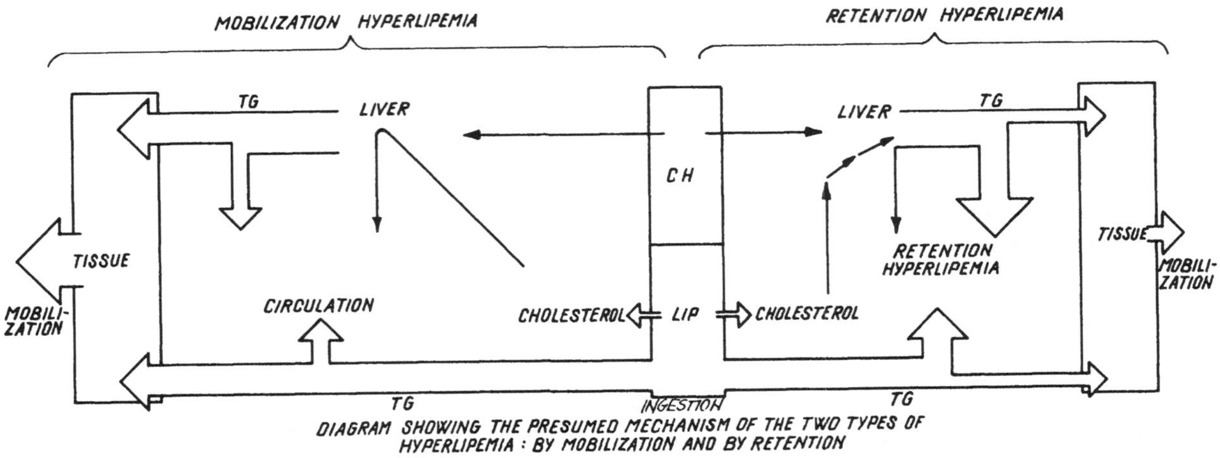

Fig. 2. Diagram showing the presumed mechanism of the two types of hyperlipaemia: by mobilization and by retention.

A schematic comparison of the two mechanisms producing hyperlipaemia – retention and mobilization – reveals the possibility of therapeutic treatment consisting of dietary prescriptions covering both disorders, and keeping under control, although not to the same extent, both the idiopathic hyperlipaemic state and that induced by the diabetic condition itself (Fig. 2):

Type I hyperlipoproteinaemia is characteristic of hyperlipaemias with retention and type V has a mixed character.

Lipoprotein activity in diabetics is usually low, according to Braunsteiner [17]. Bagdade [8], showed that a diet rich in unsaturated fats increases the lipoprotein lipase activity, which is important for the treatment of diabetic hyperlipaemia. The frequent increase of pre-beta-lipoproteins [62, 107] also relates diabetic dyslipaemia to primary hyperlipoproteinaemias. This phenomenon is more obvious in those cases where diabetic angiopathy is also present.

The connection between the circulating lipids and the metabolism of carbohydrates is indicated by a number of findings:

- minor anomalies in the glucose tolerance test in non-diabetic patients in whom hyperliaemia is induced by high carbohydrate intake.
- the fact that the reduction of sugar intake [141, 142] or the substitution of sugar by starch results, in a fall in serum triglycerides [44].
- the administration of hypoglycaemic sulphonamides raises the serum triglyceride level [161].
- the administration of biguanides such as Phenformine decreases both the triglycerides and serum cholesterol [54, 149].

The rise of serum triglycerides and, to a lesser extent, of cholesterol in the normal individual generally goes hand in hand with an increased carbohydrate consumption (particularly of the saccharose type) and is at the same time associated with hyperinsulinaemia.

All these facts stress the reciprocal relationship between diabetes mellitus and the hyperlipaemic states which bring about, or are more often associated with, macroangiopathy, as well as the reciprocal process by which hypertriglyceridaemia impairs the metabolism of carbohydrates. The interplay of these phenomena exerts a harmful effect on the vessels.

According to Stout [161] and Vallance-Owen [166] the common substratum of all these processes is to be found in the stimulation-repression interplay between glucose and insulin. Insulin is inactivated in its effect on carbohydrate metabolism by synalbumin, or, according to Knick [86] by the intervention of a hydrolysing enzyme, but continues to exert, without hindrance, its lipogenetic effect and stimulates the accumulation of fat in the liver, the fatty tissues and the vascular walls.

As regards the ischaemic heart, experimental investigations suggest that the homoeostatic disorders associated with myocardial infarction, for instance, somehow correspond to the metabolic particularities brought about by the pathological process going on ın the myocardium. It was found, during myocardial ischaemia in the dog, that the utilization of glucose rose to levels 3–4 times above the normal, probably by the mechanism of anaerobic glycolysis. The energy output of the latter process is only 1/5 of that obtained by aerobic glycolysis, representing, however, a possibility of adaptation of the myocardium to anoxia [124]. No concomitant increase, but, on the contrary, a decrease in the uptake of NEFA has been found. It might be regarded as another adaptation mechanism in the sense of decreasing myocardial oxygen consumption [124]. These findings are consistent with those observed in the human organism at the onset of a myocardial infarction, when blood NEFA levels rise to about 727 mEq/l, as compared to the normal values of about 550 m Eq/l [142]. In any case, the advent of an acute macroangiopathic accident aggravates the dysmetabolic disorders and opens the way to new accidents or prevents rapid healing of the lesions.

B. Heart Disorders in Diabetic Macroangiopathy

1. Prevalence

There is no general agreement concerning the prevalence of diabetic cardiac macroangiopathy. Some authors do not assign to diabetes any potentiating effect on the general incidence of macroangiopathic heart conditions, only admitting that it modifies their sex distribution, in favour of female [119]. Others claim, on the contrary, that besides the above effect, diabetes mellitus remarkably increases the incidence of coronaropathies and aggravates their course [183]. Table II summarizes some literature data reflecting these different points of view. The authors concerned investigated this problem during three different decades of this century and their results are compared with those obtained in our clinic.

The race differences postulated by some authors [132] in the sense of a lower incidence in negroes have not been confirmed by more recent work [4, 115].

The statistics contained in Table II concern patients admitted to hospital on whom ECGs have been performed. They are compared with the data obtained in diabetic outpatients in Bucharest (on 17,000 registered patients up to December 31, 1968). ECG anamnesic questionnaires and laboratory tests revealed evidence of

Table II

AUTHOR	NR. IN REFERENCE LIST	YEAR	MYOCARDIC MACROANGIOPATHIES %	SEX		AGE	OBSERVATIONS
				M	W		
EDEIKEN	42	1945	8-13 %	4 %	9 %	–	–
LIEBOW et. al	95	1955	10.2 %	–	–	–	–
BRYFOGLE et. al	15	1957	12.3 %	–	–	> 39	–
MIASNIKOV	108	1960	40 %	–	–	–	–
ANDERSON et. al	4	1961	33 %	–	33 %	BETWEEN 57-62	NEGROES
OAKLEY et. al	119	1968	4.5 %	4.7 %	4.2 %	BETWEEN 50-69	–
ANTIDIABETIC CENTRE IN BUCHAREST	–	1969	25.3 %	42 %	58 %	<40 (21 %) >40 (79 %)	ECG. CONTROL

angiopathy in 8.8 % of these patients. Clinical and electrocardiographic evidence of coronary disease was found in 2.3 %, and 11.1 % of the diabetics were shown to suffer from macroangiopathy. The distribution of out-patients according to sex was similar to that indicated in Table II. 79 % of the subjects were over the age of 40.

The incidence of coronary macroangiopathy in rural areas in Rumania is not known, but considering the worldwide urban preponderance of the disease, even more striking in those countries with great differences between town and village [115], it may be supposed that the incidence of this complication of diabetes mellitus is much lower in Rumanian rural areas.

In Rumania, the highest cardiovascular morbidity per 100,000 of population was found in Cluj (1,853.9 cases) and Bucharest (1,776.3 cases) but it is not possible to estimate the percentage due to diabetes [115] since the vascular alterations found in a diabetic patient are not always a consequence of the respective diabetes [66]. As a matter of fact, cardiovascular morbidity caused by diabetes is likely to change from one period to another, subsequent to the rapid evolution of economic conditions in the world and the improvement in treatment.

2. Classification

Diabetes may bring about acute and chronic angiopathic disorders of the heart.

The acute disorders are:

- associated diabetic acidosis, ketoacidosis and coma. They may depend on the interplay of diabetic angiopathy and the electrolytic disorders in the different phases of the decompensation of diabetes mellitus.
- myocardial infarction in the diabetic.

Chronic disorders may be further classified into:

- early disorders and
- late disorders,

The early disorders may acquire a characteristic or non-characteristic aspect to the extent that they suggest a more or less serious myocardial disturbance.

The acute disorders observed during the decompensation episodes of diabetes mellitus may have an angiopathic component, but do not chiefly depend on it. Therefore, they will not be dealt with in detail in the present work. The other acute diabetic macroangiopathic disorder, myocardial infarction, cannot be distinguished from myocardial infarction in non-diabetic subjects. No specific description can be made of the myocardial infarction that ends a diabetic coronary angiopathy, except a consideration of the prognosis and evolution depending on the state of metabolic balance of the diabetes.

Early chronic angiopathic disorders of the heart are already present during the chemical stage or in the mild, untreated cases of diabetes mellitus. They can be detected by an ECG and are likely to represent early signs of coronary macroangiopathy. One should remember, however, that such manifestations are also frequent in non-diabetics.

We examined 328 diabetics in the chemical stage, recording 12-lead ECGs. In order to estimate the severity of the case, the electrocardiographic alterations were divided into two large categories

a) non-characteristic and
b) characteristic

according to the information about the state of coronary circulation.

The following were classified as non-characteristic alterations:

- minor right bundle branch block (rbb)
- flat T wave in leads 1–2
- depressed segment S–T in leads 2–3
- a shift of at least 30° of the QRS axis
- the appearance of supraventricular extrasystoles
- slight signs of left ventricular hypertrophy (lvh)
- sinusal tachycardia and
- sinusal bradycardia.

The following were classified as characteristic ECG alterations:

- major right bundle branch block (RBB)
- negative T wave
- left branch block
- symmetrical T wave
- atrial fibrillation
- depressed ST segment
- flat T wave on all recorded leads
- clear signs of left ventricular hypertrophy (LVH)
- infarction sequelae.

The prevalence of both non-characteristic and characteristic ECG alterations was more frequent in chemical and mild diabetes mellitus in men (Table III).

All electrocardiographic changes were more frequent in patients over 50 than in those under 50 (Table III).

In the attempts at establishing some relationship between electrocardiographic changes and the lipaemic status of these patients, we found that, on the average, the values of all lipid fractions investigated (cholesterol, triglycerides, NEFA and $\beta + \mu$ lipoproteins) were within normal limits, irrespective of the type of electrocardiographic change (Table III).

185 of the 328 diabetics were compared with 2,326 healthy subjects (Table III, IV). No obvious correlation was observed between electrocardiographic changes and lipid fractions investigated, their values lying within the normal range in both diabetic and healthy subjects. We can say, however, that the average values of blood lipids were higher, without surpassing the normal, in diabetics. No differences were noticed in relation to age or sex.

We could therefore conclude that in the early stages of diabetes mellitus, functional or lesional

Table III

TYPE OF ECG	SEX	AGE YEARS	NR OF INVESTIGATED PERSONS. ENTIRE GROUP	DIABETICS	CHOLESTEROL mg % ENTIRE GROUP X̄±SEM.	DISP.	DIABETICS X̄±SEM.	DISP.	TRIGLYCERIDES mg % ENTIRE GROUP X̄±SEM.	DISP.	DIABETICS X̄±SEM.	DISP.	NEFA mEq ‰ ENTIRE GROUP X̄±SEM.	DISP.	DIABETICS X̄±SEM.	DISP.	β+μ LIPOPROTEINS % ENTIRE GROUP X̄±SEM.	DISP.	DIABETICS X̄±SEM.	DISP.
PATHOLOGICALLY NONCHARACTERISTIC ECG. PATTERNS	M	<50	282	15	210±3	44	236±7	28	108±6	104	241±35	140	660±11	180	830±78	312	70±0.5	9	77±3	9
		>50	453	45	224±3	48	249±9	60	159±3	64	209±13	92	650±8	167	780±30	213	70±0.44	9	75±1	7
	W	<50	331	6	216±3	51	SMALL NUMBER OF SUBJECTS		156±4	67	SMALL NUMBER OF SUBJECTS		625±8	151	SMALL NUMBER OF SUBJECTS		69±0.4	8	SMALL NUMBER OF SUBJECTS	
		>50	590	31	232±2	49	245±13	64	159±3	71	187±12	63	651±7	179	758±42	211	70±0.4	9	73±1,4	7
PATHOLOGICALLY CHARACTERISTIC ECG. PATTERNS	M	<50	73	7	228±5	45	SMALL NUMBER OF SUBJECTS		165±9	79	SMALL NUMBER OF SUBJECTS		633±16	134	SMALL NUMBER OF SUBJECTS		72±0.9	8	SMALL NUMBER OF SUBJECTS	
		>50	249	27	225±3	45	228±8	42	169±5	78	187±16	83	673±12	192	756±39	195	73±0.6	9	74±2	10
	W	<50	83	6	210±5	49	SMALL NUMBER OF SUBJECTS		170±6	59	SMALL NUMBER OF SUBJECTS		670±18	165	SMALL NUMBER OF SUBJECTS		72±0.8	7	SMALL NUMBER OF SUBJECTS	
		>50	265	27	239±3	47	230±9	48	165±0.6	10	181±16	80	655±10	165	708±33	168	73±0.6	10	73±1	6
TOTAL			2,326	164																

Table IV

AGE OF INVESTIGATED DIABETICS (YEARS)	NUMBER OF INVESTIGATED DIABETICS			PATHOLOGICALY NON CHARACTERISTIC ECG PATTERNS				PATHOLOGICALY CHARACTERISTIC ECG PATTERNS				PATHOLOGICALY NON CHARACTERISTIC + CHARACTERISTIC ECG PATTERNS			
				MEN		WOMEN		MEN		WOMEN		MEN		WOMEN	
	MEN	WOMEN	TOTAL	NR.	%	NR.	%	NR	%	NR	%	NR	%	NR	%
< 50	79	46	125	15	19	6	13	7	9	6	13	22	29	12	26
> 50	111	92	203	45	41	45	49	28	26	27	30	73	66	72	78
TOTAL	190	138	328	60	31	51	37	35	19	33	24	95	60	84	61

Table V

	SEX		AGE (YEARS)		TYPE OF DIABETES			WEIGHT			APPLIED TREATMENT		
	W	M	> 40	< 40	JUVENILE	MATURITY ONSET	SENILE	DEFICIT	NORMAL	EXCESS	DIET ONLY	DIET + INSULIN	DIET + ORAL A D
NUMBER OF CASES	587	413	218	782	103	547	350	94	454	452	302	426	272
TOTAL	1,000		1,000		1,000			1,000			1,000		

Table VI

	PRESUMED DURATION OF DIADETES						TOTAL
YEARS	> 5	6-10	11-15	16-20	21-25	< 25	
NR. CASES	438	222	187	81	28	44	1,000

electrocardiographic changes are determined by complex metabolic disturbances rather than by the existence of dyslipaemia.

The presence of electrocardiographic changes in non-diabetics, suggests that several other factors, besides diabetes mellitus are involved, perhaps the glucose ingested for the oGTT may play a certain role.

Their higher prevalence in diabetics should be taken into account, however, and carefully watched along the entire evolution of diabetes, so that their true significance may be deduced (Table V and VI).

3. Late chronic angiopathic disorders of the heart

a) Diabetic Myocardosis

Myocardosis is generally defined as a disorder, which does not result from inflammatory processes, from hypoxia caused by vascular sclerosis or from chronic overstress but occurs subsequent to long-lasting disturbance in the protein metabolism [57, 70, 179, 180]. This definition needs to be completed in the case of diabetes mellitus. In fact, the general dysmetabolic factor, which includes, as already mentioned in Chapter II, protein metabolism as well, is combined here with an alteration of the small vessels (microangiopathy) and very often with lesions of the medium and large vessels too. The resulting condition differs from plain myocardosis, as defined above, as well as from typical ischaemia, at least for a long interval in the course of diabetes mellitus.

The following, mostly non-specific, clinical symptoms, frequently found in patients suffering from diabetic myocardosis are guide lines to the clinician making a diagnosis.

a) *marked tiredness.* This must be differentiated from the state of physical asthenia caused by the metabolic unbalance of poorly controlled diabetes. The very fact that weariness persists after correction of the carbohydrate metabolism and although electrolyte metabolism is normal, points towards a possible cardiac involvement. On questioning, the patient will probably describe a notable reduction in his working ability. But the patient's statement is to be regarded as positive only if other possible causes (neurosis, renal failure, adrenal deficiency, liver involvement, etc.) are ruled out. Careful consideration and electrocardiographic control are required before assigning weariness to a heart involvement.

b) *neuro-vegetative disorders*, are often associated with chronic weariness. They consist of dizziness, sleeplessness and heavy sweating in no relation to the physical effort involved. In the case of diabetes mellitus, such symptoms can be assigned to the heart only after careful discrimination, since they are also found with visceral diabetic neuropathy. They should be correlated with clinical and ECG findings.

c) *palpitations, extrasystoles,* a trend towards *moderate tachycardia* or *bradycardia* and *arrhythmic breathing* are less frequent in other types of myocardosis, but are often associated with diabetic myocardosis. These are the symptoms which usually draw the attention of the patient and physician to a possible heart involvement.

d) the objective clinical symptomatology is usually poor before a haemodynamic deficit occurs. Slight *cyanosis* and *dyspnoea* after extreme physical effort and at high altitude may be found [32].

The size and configuration of the heart are usually normal. The intensity of the heart sounds is medium or marked. Sometimes an attenuated or double 1st heart sound is found at the apex. Gallop rhythm may also occur in the terminal stages, but usually associated with the symptoms of heart failure [32, 57, 180].

e) No firm diagnosis can be reached before recording one or several bipolar and unipolar electrocardiograms. Their appearance, although non-specific, usually leads to the diagnosis of myocardosis.

The following abnormal ECG tracings have been described:

- *alterations in the QRS complex:* lower amplitude, sometimes an increased interval and irregular tracing. They indicate myocardosis if the T wave is also flattened [57, 180].
- a *flattened or negative T wave* in leads I and II or in leads II and III [180].
- *prolonged QT interval,* predominantly on the account of the T wave [32].
- *ST-T fusion,* i. e. the difficulty in separating the ST segment from the T wave, as they trace a continuous ascending line [180].

Such electrocardiographic changes were found in 218 out of 1,000 diabetic patients admitted to our clinic (21.8 %) (see Table V). The recordings also revealed some other remarkable aspects:

- myocardosis associated with diabetes mellitus was found both in subjects with juvenile diabetes (Fig. 3) and in maturity onset diabetes (Fig. 4) or in senile diabetes mellitus (Fig. 5). The tracings are strikingly similar to those obtained in a female patient suffering from severe malnutrition caused by a syndrome of chronic malabsorbtion (Fig. 6).

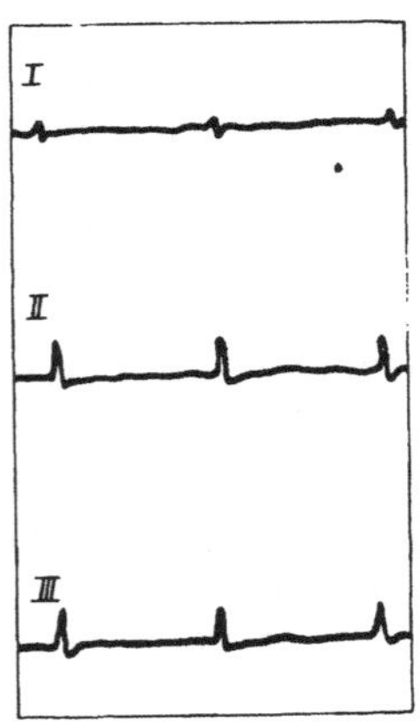

Fig. 3. S. P. Woman aged 27. Apparent onset of diabetes mellitus 5 months before. Underweight by 17% due to starvation. No treatment. Aspect of myocardosis with flat T in all standard derivations. ST and T are confluent.

- no constant relation appears to exist between the apparent onset of the diabetic condition – as judged by the history – and the onset of the electrocardiographic and clinical signs of myocardosis. The latter were found in various patients at very short as well as at very long intervals after the apparent onset of the diabetes (compare figures 5 with Fig. 3 and 4).

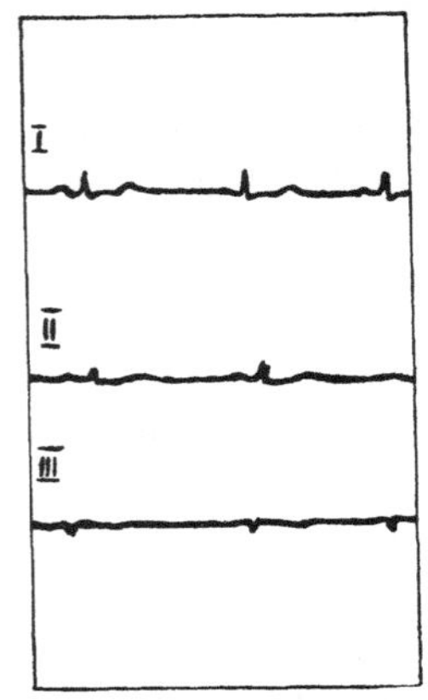

Fig. 4. B. N. Man aged 57. Apparent onset of diabetes mellitus 7 years before. Underweight by 14 % due to starvation. Treated with antidiabetic sulphonamides during the last year. Diet 200 g. carbohydrates daily, hypoproteic and comparatively hypocaloric. Flat T in all standard derivations. Negative T in D_{III}.

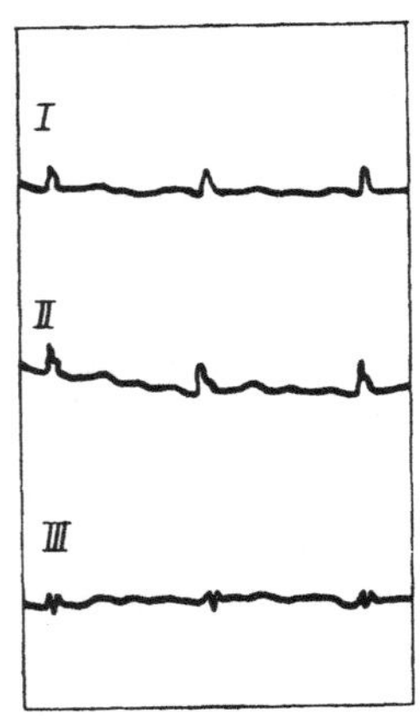

Fig. 5. S. M. Woman aged 79. Apparent onset of diabetes mellitus 14 years before. Normal weight. Treated by insulin for 14 years. Diet 200 g. carbohydrates daily. Flat T in all standard derivations. Low amplitude, QRS prolonged (0.12″) and irregular on intrinsecoid deflection.

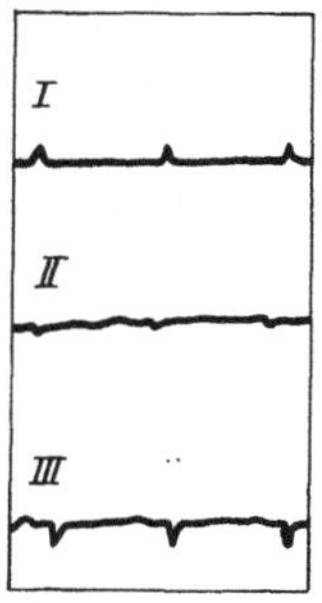

Fig. 6. M. A. Woman aged 54. Chronic starvation due to a malabsorbtion syndrome of pancreatic origin. Aspect of myocardosis.

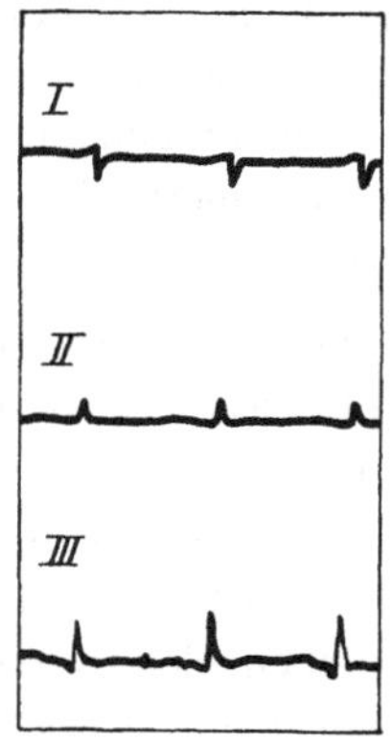

Fig. 7. L. G. Woman aged 26. Lipoatrophic diabetes mellitus and advanced starvation, hyperlipaemia with hypertriglyceridaemia, sensitive to insulin. ECG aspect of myocardosis.

- no correlation was found between the type of antidiabetic management and myocardosis. Tracings suggesting myocardosis have been recorded both in patients who had no antidiabetic therapy (Fig. 3) and in patients in whom antidiabetic management had consisted of dietary restrictions and hypoglycaemic sulphonamides (Fig. 4) or insulin (Fig. 5).
- a common feature of the majority of patients suffering from diabetic myocardosis is that they are either underweight or at the lower limit of the normal weight range. A borderline case was that of a female patient with lipoatrophic diabetes mellitus in which an early and swiftly progressive peripheric arteriopathy occurred and, at the same time, a specific myocardotic electrocardiogram was found (Fig. 7). It appears that there is no necessary concordance between the alterations of the peripheral arteries and those of the heart.
- finally the presence of a coronary deficit is suggested by the frequent sharp and symmetrical T waves (Fig. 4 and 5), even where this wave is flattened and tends to fuse with the ST interval as occurs in myocardosis.

The above findings suggest that, without being a typical symptom of coronary angiopathy in diabetes mellitus, myocardosis is frequently associated with it, thus aggravating the course of a possible acute coronary disorder. It is most likely that the deficit in the myocardial blood supply, due to diabetic macroangiopathy, creates favourable circumstances for the onset and severe course of the degenerative myocardial process, that is of diabetic myocardosis.

b) Disorders in the Coronary Blood Supply

Discrepancy between the optimal and the actual myocardial blood supply may undoubtedly occur in the diabetic in various degrees, from a relative coronary insufficiency to the absolute coronary failure. The latter presents the well-known clinical picture and is of less prophylactic and therapeutic interest for the diabetologist than relative coronary insufficiency, which is the functional stage of the myocardial diabetic macroangiopathy proper [22].

It must be noted from the very beginning that clinical symptomatology is mostly non-specific. It ranges from early weariness on physical effort to angina-like pain, from common praecordial discomfort to palpitations, which may or may not be related to physical effort and emotion. Some patients complain of respiratory disorders, which may simulate a paroxysmal dyspnoea, but careful examination reveals their neurotic character in that they only consist of a feeling of insufficient breath. It should be noted that this symptom occurs mostly at rest [172].

The only element which may deter the clinician from assigning this symptom to a simple neurosis is the presence of diabetes and a possible correlation with episodes of metabolic imbalance or therapeutical interventions.

An electrocardiogram performed on such a patient may suggest the presence of a relative coronary insufficiency, and draw attention to the heart.

An investigation performed on 1,000 electrocardiographic tracings recorded in diabetic patients admitted to hospital enabled us to establish certain parameters which appear to be related to the presence of coronary macroangiopathy. The findings are summarised in Tables III and IV.

The ECG findings could be divided into 4 groups: [101].

a) the group of patients with no outstanding ECG anomalies. It comprises the normal tracings, respiratory arrhythmia in the young and negative but asymmetrical T waves in the III-rd standard and the first praecordial leads (V-1).

b) the group of non-pathological modifications (from the point of view considered in this chapter). Ectopic rhythm, isolated and sporadic ventricular and supraventricular extrasystolic arrhythmia, small axis deviations and tracings showing prolongation of the P-R interval, have been put into this group.

c) the group of tracings of doubtful pathological significance. Their interpretation depends on the pathological background against which they occur and in our opinion they are significant in diabetes mellitus. They consist of right complete or partial blocks, left partial block, ventricular hypertrophy [153], P-R intervals exceeding 0.20″ and especially symmetrical T waves, peaked and found in at least two different leads.

d) modifications having a definite pathological significance, among which stress was laid on left branch block, atrio-ventricular block anomalies associated with recent ischaemic episodes.

Within the group of 1,000 diabetics examined, in which there was a slight predominance of females (58.7 % as compared to 41.3 % males) the age of the patients requiring an ECG because of their clinical symptomatology exceeded 40 years in 78.2% of the cases (Table V). This indicates that clinically manifest heart disorders prevail in the adult, in regard to both their subjective and particularly to their objective symptomatology.

As for body weight, 45.2% of these patients were obese, 45.4% in the normal weight range and 9.4% underweight (Table V). The group of underweight patients comprised mostly young people suffering from juvenile diabetes mellitus.

The 1,000 patients were divided into groups of 5 years' duration of diabetes, up to 25 years, and all the cases exceeding that interval were considered in a single group over 25 years. The largest group (43.8% of the total) was found to be that of diabetic patients recently diagnosed or with an apparent history of less than five years, then the patients with a history of 6 to 10 years (22.2%), 11 to 15 years (18.7%), 16 to 20 years (8.1%), over 25 years (4.4 %). The smallest group (2.8 %) was that of patients with a diabetic history of between 21 and 25 years' duration (2.8 %) (Table VI).

As far as antidiabetic therapy is concerned, most of these patients (42.6 %) were on insulin and a low carbohydrate diet (200 gm per day). A smaller group (30.2 %) was only observing diet restrictions, and in the other 27.2 % of patients, diabetes was controlled by the administration of oral hypoglycaemic drugs (antidiabetic sulphonylureas in 82% of these cases and biguanides in the other 18%) (see Table V).

The appearance of the tracings found in the groups of normal, non-pathological and obviously pathological electrocardiographic findings correspond entirely to the data generally agreed to be independent of the presence of diabetes mellitus. Particular attention should be paid, however, to the group of findings of doubtful pathological significance (see Table VII). We feel that it is possible to identify in that group certain aspects which, although not characteristic, are nevertheless relevant to the probable presence of a coronary angiopathy in a phase preceding necro-

Table VII. Electrocardiographic aspects in 1,000 diabetic inpatients.

ECG. FINDINGS	NORMAL		NON-PATHOLOGIC ANOMALIES		CONTROVERTIBLE ANOMALIES		NECROSIS		LESION		ISCHAEMIA		MYOCARDOSIS		TOTAL
TYPE OF DIABETES	JUV.	MAT.	JUV.	MAT.	JUV.	MAT.	JUV.	MAT.	JUV.	MAT.	JUV.	MAT.	JUV.	MAT.	
NUMBER OF CASES	92	144	2	85	5	201	–	7	4	132	–	110	18	200	1000

JUV = JUVENILE DIABETES ; MAT = DIABETES WITH MATURITY ONSET

sis, lesion or ischaemia. Similar investigations performed by Waitzkin et al. [173] emphasized the anomalies of the T wave, ventricular hypertrophy and intraventricular block as indicating the presence of a coronary diabetic macroangiopathy.

Distinction was made between spontaneous and induced electrocardiographic alterations, since the former are more likely to correspond to an advanced coronary vascular involvement.

Spontaneous alteration suggesting a relative insufficiency in coronary blood flow, that is the presence of an angiopathy in its late functional stage, may consist of a J point lowered by more than 1 mm and in frequent and often sharp symmetrical T waves, with no other alterations in the tracings. Such a picture was found in 24.5% of the diabetic patients complaining of a variety of subjective praecordial symptoms. In 11.5 % this was the only electrocardiographic pathological finding, while in 13% it was associated with signs indicating necrosis, ischaemic lesions and myocardosis.

The above alterations were found in all types of diabetes (juvenile, adult and senile) and in the whole range of duration.

1. In juvenile diabetes symmetrical T waves were found in patients between 4 and 36 years old (see. Figs. 8, 9, 10, 11 and 12) and at various intervals of diabetic history. In one case (Fig. 8) in which the apparent onset of the disease occurred only one month before, a fairly obvious symmetrical T wave was, however, found in the standard leads.

Lowering or raising of point J, which was less frequently found, was nevertheless, often associated with symmetrical T waves (see Figs. 9 in L-1,

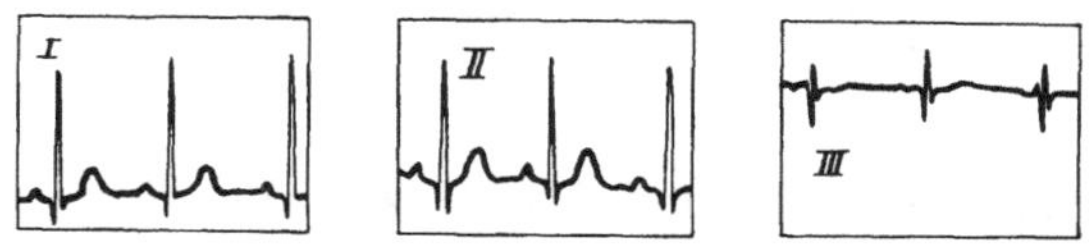

Fig. 8. B. D. aged 4. Juvenile diabetes mellitus, insulinodependent, discovered one month previously. Normal weight.

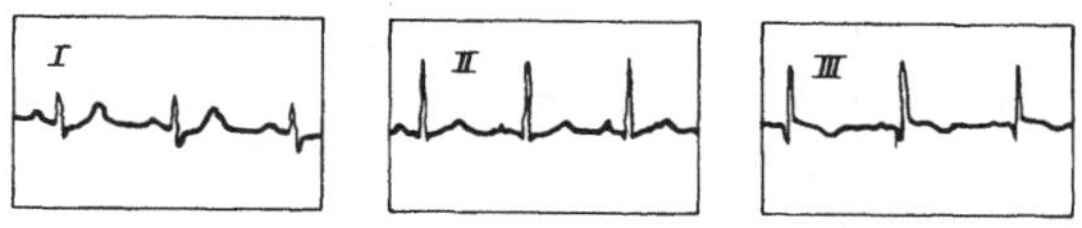

Fig. 9. G. M. Girl aged 6. Juvenile diabetes mellitus, insulinodependent. Apparent onset at the age of 3. Permanent insulinotherapy. Underweight.

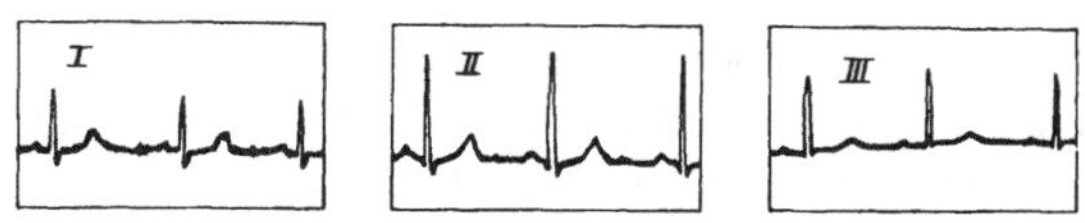

Fig. 10. F. I. Girl aged 9. Juvenile diabetes mellitus, insulinodependent. Apparent onset of diabetes 6–7 years before. Continuous insulin therapy. Moderate underweight.

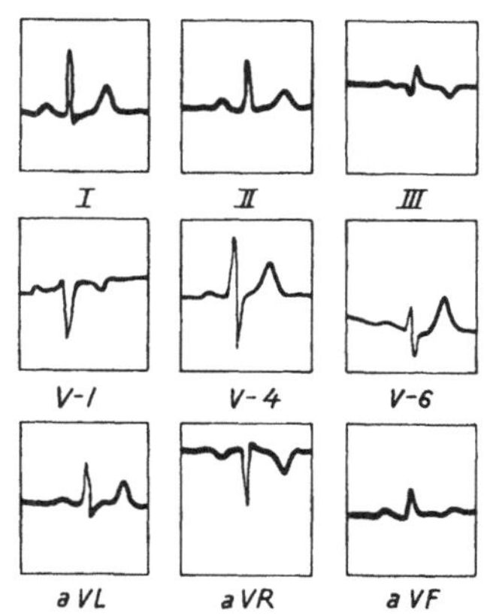

Fig. 11. M. A. Woman aged 27. Juvenile diabetes mellitus, insulinodependent. Apparent onset of diabetes 7 years before.

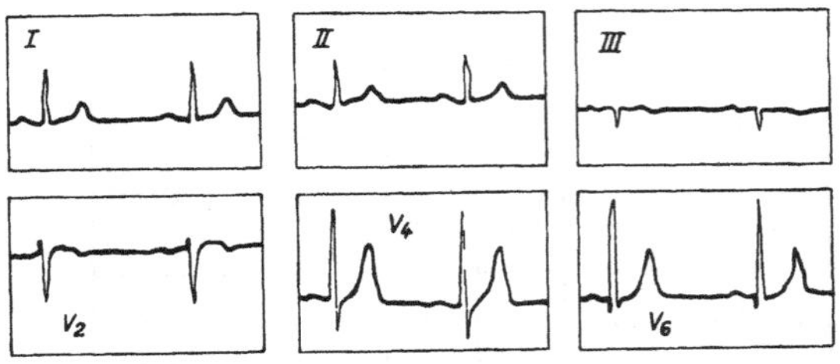

Fig. 12. L. P. Man aged 36. Juvenile diabetes mellitus, insulinodependent. Apparent onset of diabetes 18 years before. Continuous insulin therapy. Normal weight.

and L-III, Fig. 11 in L-1, L-III, V-6, aVL, aVR, and AVf).

2. Age and duration of diabetic history were also very variable in the group of adult diabetics (Figs. 13, 14, 15, 16 and 17). While all the patients in the group with juvenile diabetes were insulin-dependent, in the group of adult diabetics, symmetrical and/or sharp T waves were found both in patients receiving insulin (Figs. 15 and 16) and in patients treated only with oral hypoglycaemic sulphonylureas (Figs. 13, 14 and 17).

In the group of adult diabetics, modifications in the position of point J were less often found than in those of the T wave (Figs. 14, 15 and 17).

3. With senile diabetes, the ECG alterations may be isolated and in no relation with the apparent duration of the diabetes, but more often in association with, ischaemic and necrotic modifications.

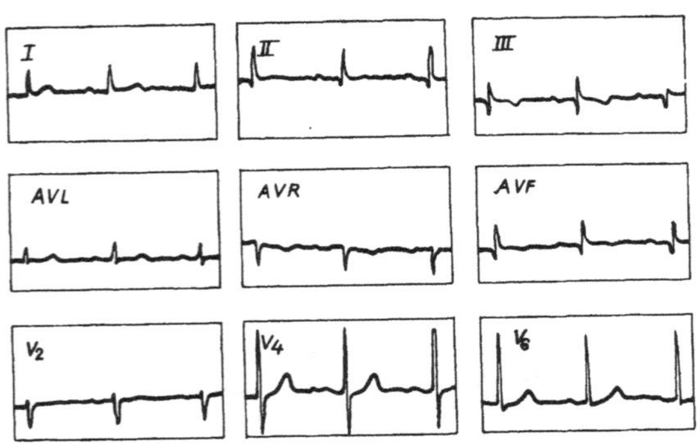

Fig. 13. G. P. Man aged 60. Mature diabetes mellitus, insulinodependent. Treated by oral hypoglycaemic drugs. Apparent onset 7 years before. Normal weight.

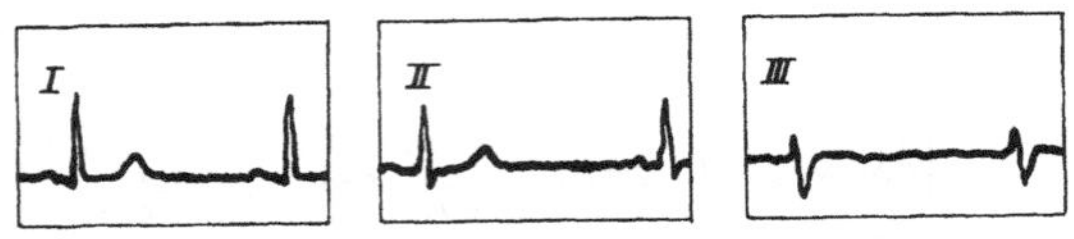

Fig. 14. V. C. Woman aged 46. Mature diabetes mellitus, insulinodependent, treated with oral hypoglycaemic drugs. Apparent onset of diabetes 2 years before. Normal weight.

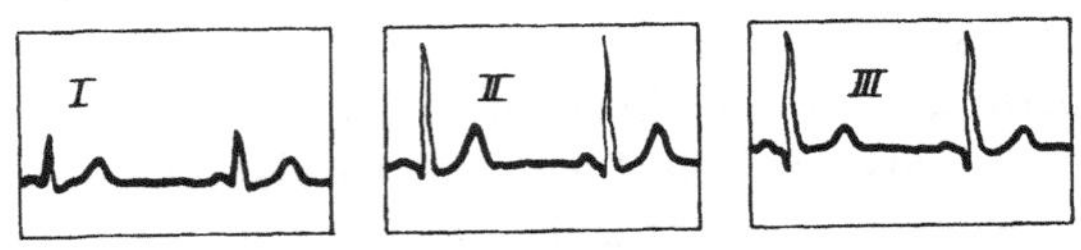

Fig. 15. F. A. Man aged 35. Mature diabetes mellitus, insulinodependent. Apparent onset of diabetes 8 years before. Continuous insulin therapy with overdosage and frequent hypoglycaemic episodes. Normal weight.

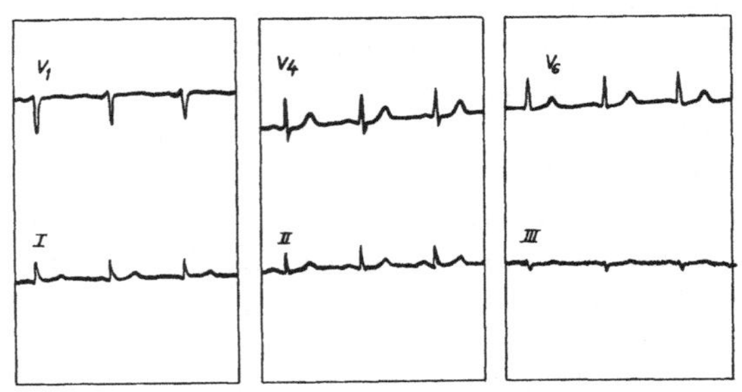

Fig. 16. N. H. Man aged 66. Onset of diabetes 11 years before. Treated with insulin for 1 year, after 10 years of therapy with oral hypoglycaemic drugs (Mature diabetes mellitus).

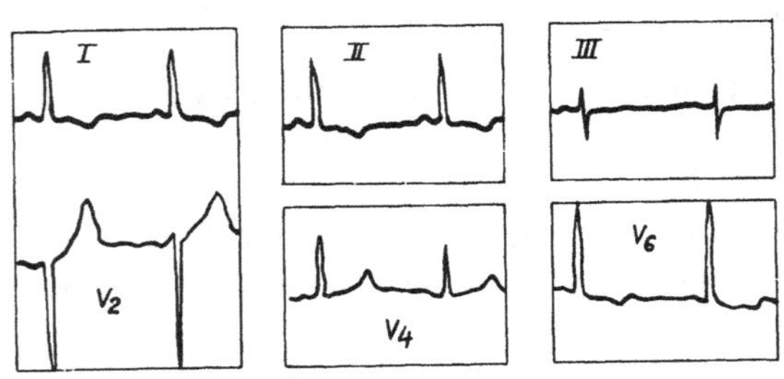

Fig. 17. H. I. Man aged 59. Mature diabetes mellitus, insulinodependent. Treated with oral hypoglycemiating drugs. Apparent onset 30 years before. Normal weight.

The latter may well be related to diabetic macroangiopathy, but are just as often found at that age in the absence of diabetes mellitus.

In summary, the electrocardiographic picture which consists of a symmetrical and/or sharp T wave, with or without a modification in the position of point J may occur in diabetics irrespective of their age, the duration of the disease and the kind of therapy applied. Most of the patients examined had been admitted to hospital for a correction of their metabolic balance and had a history of frequent episodes of decompensation or even of permanent imbalance. It might, therefore, be possible that an inadequate management of the fundamental disease creates favourable conditions for the onset of the respective ECG appearances which, in our opinion, suggest the presence of macroangiopathic involvement.

A significant case in this sense was that of a male insulin-dependent diabetic who used to take overdoses of insulin, being unable to observe the prescribed dietary restrictions and had, consequently, frequent episodes of postinsulinic hypoglycaemia followed by hyperglycaemia and acidosis. The electrocardiographic picture in this case consisted of both symmetrical and sharp T waves and modifications in the position of point J (Fig. 15).

Induced alterations of the electrocardiographic tracing in diabetics correspond, we consider, to a less advanced stage of coronary macroangiopathy, that is to say to an earlier functional stage of the condition. They can be induced by exercise of varying degree (Master's test).

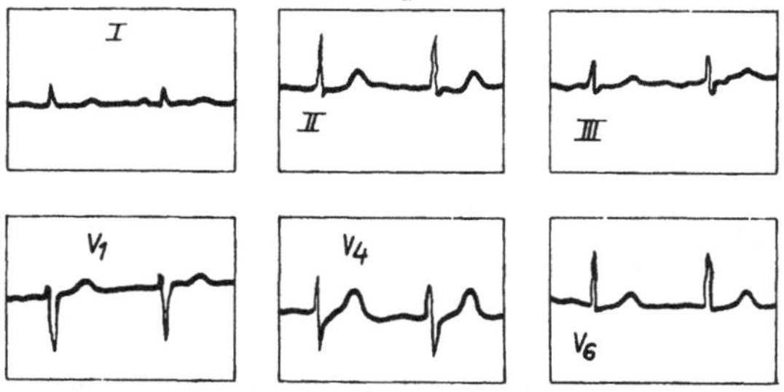

Fig. 18. P. P. Man aged 73. Senile diabetes mellitus, insulinodependent. Apparent onset 1 month before. Normal weight.

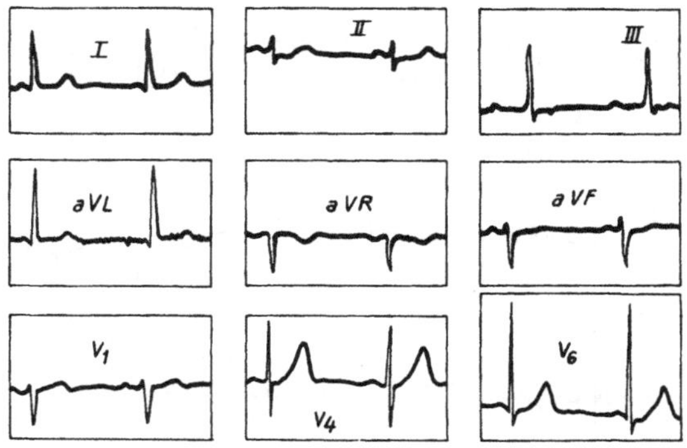

Fig. 19. B. P. Man aged 72. Senile diabetes mellitus. Apparent onset 9 years before. Treated with oral hypoglycaemic drugs. Normal weight.

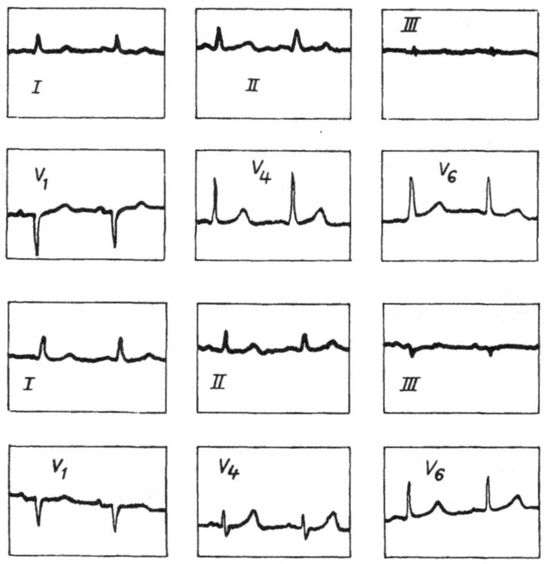

Fig. 20. D. E. Woman aged 75. Senile diabetes mellitus, insulinodependent. Apparent onset of diabetes 8 years before. Continuous insulin therapy. A = ECG aspect in clinostaying; B = changes of T wave in orthostaying.

In certain patients, standing up results in the same pointed T wave, of a more symmetrical pattern which tends to reverse, particularly in lead III (Fig. 20). In other cases, the same movement brought about a flattening of the T wave (Figs. 21 and 22). This test appears therefore to have some significance if an obvious modification ensues in

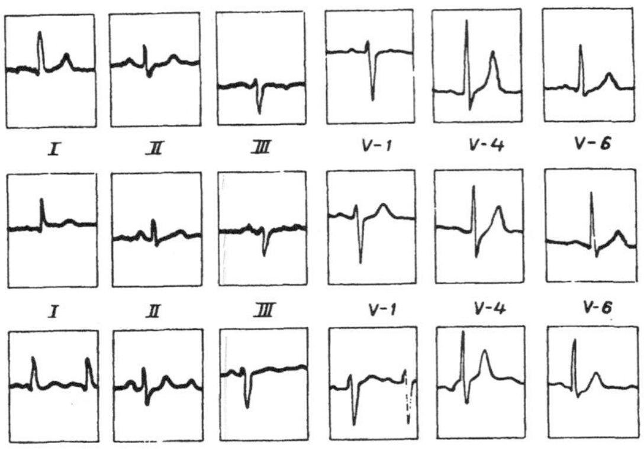

Fig. 21. P. V. Woman aged 55. Mature diabetes mellitus, insulinodependent, with diabetic retinopathy. Treated with oral hypoglycaemic drugs. Apparent onset of diabetes 15 years before. A = before exercise standing up; C = after standard exercise (Master).

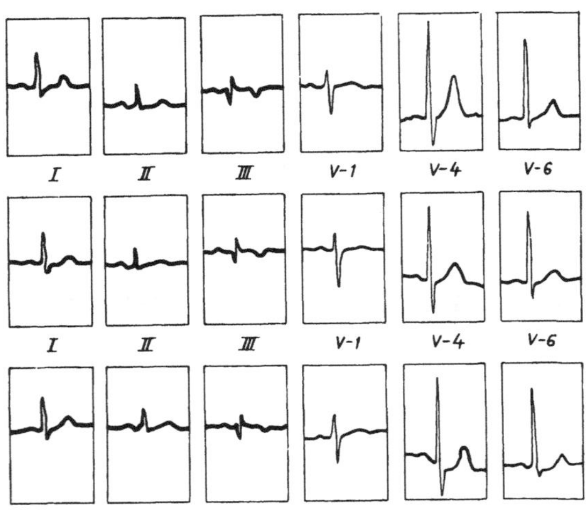

Fig. 22. B. G. Man aged 33. Mature diabetes mellitus, rerently discovered. Overweight by 12%. A = before exercise lying down; B = before exercise standing up; C = after standard exercise.

the T wave and in the position of the J point, but is otherwise only a proof of the lability of the shape of the T wave. Whether that lability might be regarded as indicating some variation in the coronary blood flow is a problem deserving further consideration.

The performance of measured exercise may result in modifications which Robb [142] classified into ischaemic and non-ischaemic. They were described as appearing in the standard leads I, II and III, as well as in aVL, aVF, V-4, V-5 and V-6.

Such alterations in the tracing, frequent in elderly diabetic patients (Fig. 23 in leads I and II, V-1, V-4, V-6 and Fig. 24 in leads V-4 and V-6) undoubtedly express some disorder in the coronary blood flow.

If these findings are associated with a sharp and symmetrical T wave (Fig. 21 in leads I and III, Fig. 22 in leads I, II and III), it is justified to suspect a coronary macroangiopathy even in the absence of corresponding clinical symptomatology.

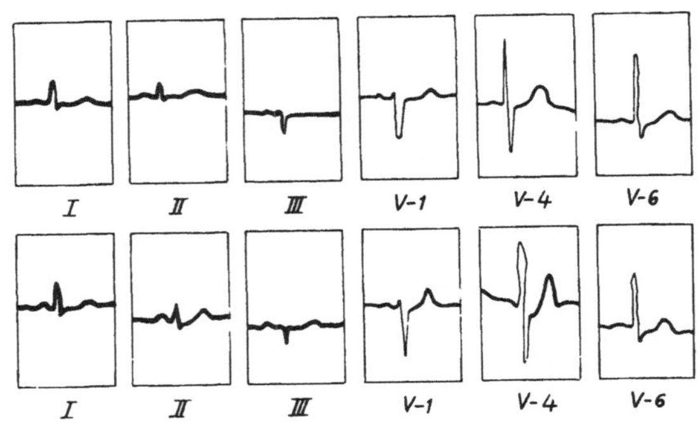

Fig. 23. M. G. Man aged 58. Mature diabetes mellitus, insulinodependent. Apparent onset of diabetes 3 years before. Treated with oral hypoglycaemic drugs. Overweight by 21 %. A = before exercise; B = after standard exercise (Master).

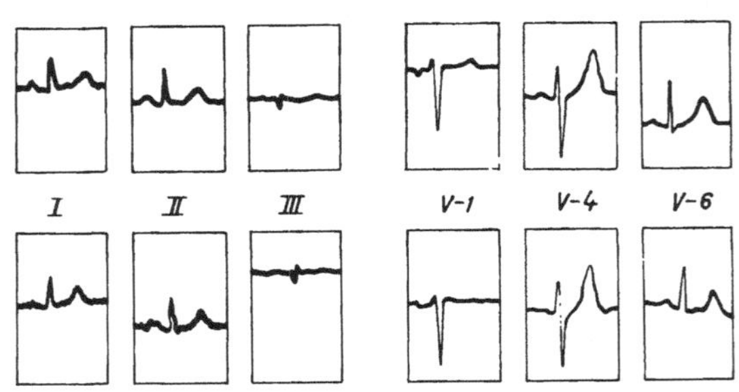

Fig. 24. T. C. Woman aged 50. Mature diabetes mellitus, insulinodependent. Apparent onset 13 years before. Overweight by 23 %. A = before exercise; B = after standard exercise (Master).

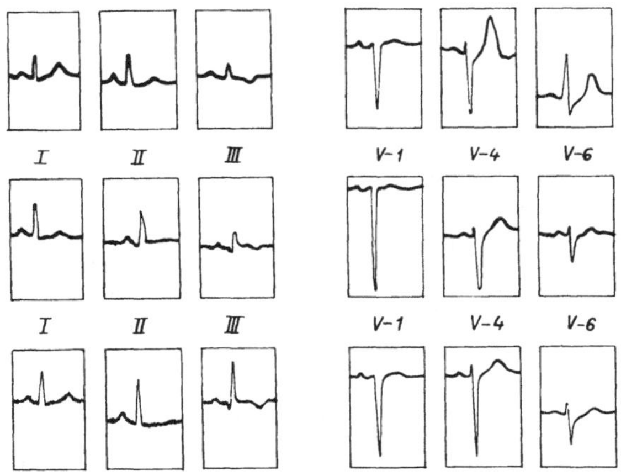

Fig. 25. C. C. Woman aged 50. Mature diabetes mellitus, insulinodependent. Apparent onset of diabetes 28 years before. Treated with insulin and oral hypoglycaemic drugs (tolbutamide). Proliferative diabetic retinopathy. Diabetic nephropathy with chronic renal failure. During the last year frequent episodos of angina pectoris, and the ECG recordings were performed in periods of frequent such attacks.

The relation between the alterations of the T wave and the coronary blood flow in the diabetic is even more obvious if electrocardiographic investigations are performed at intervals in the same patient and there is a parallel development of a clinical picture suggesting ischaemia. Fig. 25 shows the tracings from a female patient Chel. C., aged 50, a maturity onset diabetic, with an apparent history of 28 years. The first electrocardiographic record was at the beginning of 1968 when the patient started to complain of a vague and uncharacteristic praecordial discomfort. ECG changes were found and consisted of symmetrical sharp T waves in the standard leads and a low J point in the unipolar leads V-4 and V-6. At that time, diabetic retinopathy and mild glomerulosclerosis were already present (ECG, Jan. 1968).

Later in the same year, intermittent claudication began in the left leg and the praecordial discomfort turned into short attacks of angina, occurring after meals. A new electrocardiogram was recorded in May 1968, similar in many aspects to the original, but also showing a flattened T in standard lead II and a high J point and ST interval in the standard lead III. In spite of therapy, the coronary insufficiency worsened and became the main complaint of the patient. An ECG recorded in December 1968 is characterized by manifestly symmetrical and sharp T waves and a trend to crossing of ST-T in standard lead III and unipolar lead V-6.

The same correlation is suggested by the effects obtained by exercise tests in patients in which obvious symptoms of diabetic angiopathy were found at the time of the recording. Such is the case of I.I. (Fig. 26), suffering from a clinically manifest Kimmelstiel-Wilson syndrome, in which symmetrical T waves can be readily seen both before and after physical effort, and B. T. (Fig. 27) suffering from a diabetic gangrene of the lower limbs, with a similar electrocardiographic appearance.

In such cases as the above, the ECG picture under discussion tends to be associated with alterations suggesting the presence of a process of myocardosis. That was the case of patient S. E. who suffe-

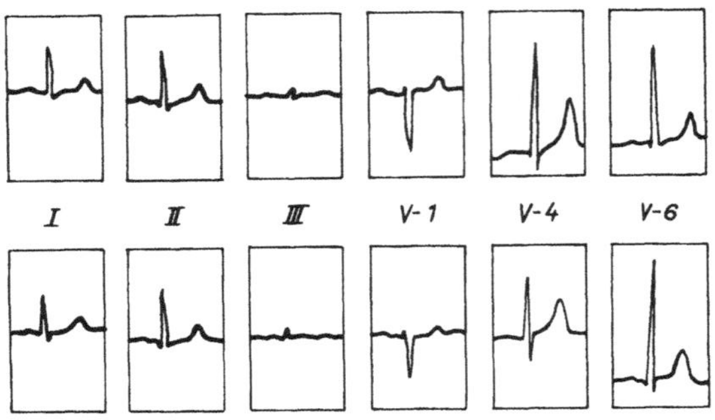

Fig. 26. I. I. Man aged 39. Mature diabetes mellitus, insulinodependent. Apparent onset of diabetes 13 years before. Continuous treatment with oral hypoglycaemic drugs. Kimmelstiel-Wilson syndrome.
A = before exercise. B = after standard exercise (Master's test).

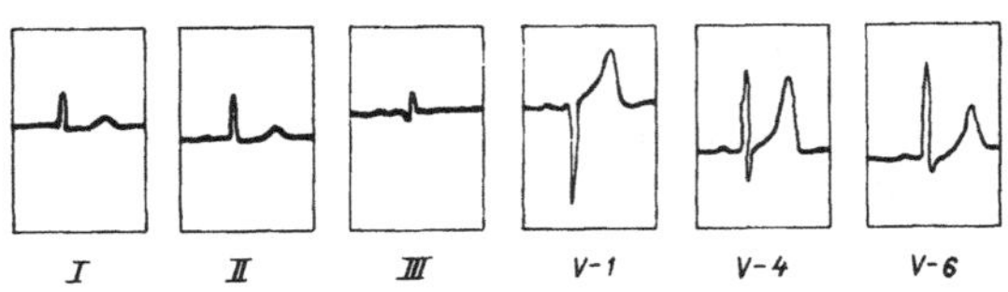

Fig. 27. B. T. Man aged 77. Mature diabetes mellitus, insulinodependent. Apparent onset 42 years before. Diabetic arteritis with gangrena of the right big toe.

red from juvenile diabetes mellitus with malignant trend. Diabetic angiopathy rapidly led to blindness and the patient died in cardio-renal failure following Kimmelstiel-Wilson syndrome (Fig. 28). The T wave, in the ECG of this patient is sharp and of very low voltage.

It might be concluded that certain modifications of the T wave and of the position of point J should serve as an indicator drawing the attention of the clinician to a possible involvement of the coronaries in the general process of diabetic angiopathy. The significance of these alterations further increases if they are enhanced by exercise tests and if, repeatedly investigated, they follow a progressive course parallel to the general evolution of the disease and the onset of certain subjective complaints indicating a relative or absolute coronary insufficiency.

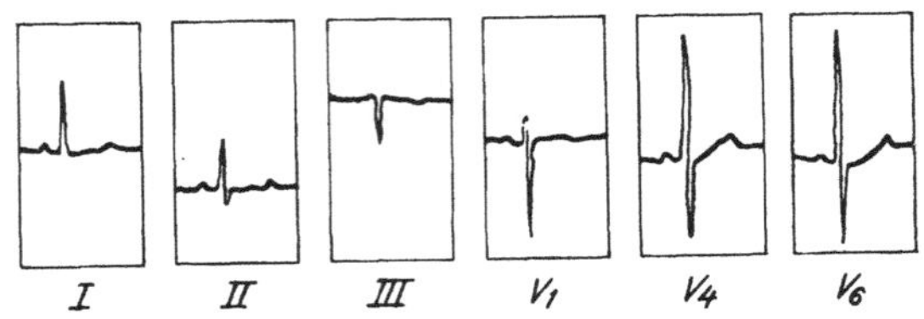

Fig. 28. S. E. Woman aged 20. Juvenile diabetes mellitus, insulinodependent. Apparent onset of diabetes 17 years before. Kimmelstiel-Wilson syndrome and diabetic retinopathy.

Ballistocardiographic investigations were normal in some 41% of the diabetic patients. This would imply that the process of coronary sclerosis develops at an early stage of the disease.

C. Clinical Laboratory Picture

Standard laboratory tests are important especially for the diagnosis of acute episodes of coronary macroangiopathy, but they yield no specific information in relation to the diabetic contribution to the aetiology.

In a case of diabetic angiopathy there are, however, certain laboratory data which make it possible to estimate the dysmetabolic background against which the respective process develops and to determine the various underlying pathogenetic mechanisms [39, 50, 159, 168, 169, 170].

1. Determination of the Serum Glycoproteins

As already mentioned in Chap. II, total serum glycoproteins increase in the diabetic.

A rise in the alpha$_2$-glycoprotein fraction frequently accompanies the degenerative vascular processes, both in common atherosclerosis and in diabetic macroangiopathy [27, 58].

Significant for diabetes mellitus are the increases in beta and gamma glycoproteins. However, if diabetes is associated with atherosclerosis, this indication loses its value and the only specific increment

Table VIII. Glycoproteins in serum in diabetics compared with atherosclerotics.

ATHEROSCLEROSIS	BLOOD GLYCOPROTEINS	DIABETES MELLITUS
DECREASE	← ALBUMIN	→ INCREASE
NORMAL VALUES	← α1-GLOBULIN	→ INCREASE
INCREASE	← α2-GLOBULIN	→ INCREASE
NORMAL VALUES	← β-GLOBULIN	→ INCREASE
NORMAL VALUES	← γ-GLOBULIN	→ INCREASE

left is that of the albuminic glycoprotein fraction. The latter decreases whenever the pathological process is due to atherosclerosis and increases in the presence of diabetes [58] (see Table VIII).

The testing of serum polysaccharides, such as glucosamine, yields no significant information about the alteration of polysaccharide metabolism in diabetes associated with angiopathy [145].

2. Determination of the Serum Lipid Fractions

Serum NEFA values are generally significantly increased in diabetic patients after fasting [86, 88, 138, 139, 162, 174] and there is a positive correlation between them and glycaemia, glycosuria and ketonuria. Therefore, serum NEFA may serve as a test for the state of control of the diabetic patient. No relation could be established with the duration of the diabetes, the age at which the condition occurred and especially with the severity of the angiopathic involvement [56], although some authors have attempted to correlate the phenomena of coronary ischaemia with increased blood NEFA [26]. One should remember that in such situations catecholamines might also interfere [120].

A study was performed in 1967–1968 in our clinic on a group of 160 diabetic patients. In 150 of these, signs of diabetic angiopathy were found. In the diabetic subjects with clinical symptoms of coronary or peripheral macroangiopathy, blood NEFA values were generally high, but did not differ significantly from those found in diabetics free from such complications. The average value obtained was 1,316 mEq/1 ± 752.3. The Dole procedure was used in this investigation, with normal values ranging between 335 and 700 mEq/l.

With the procedure of Courchaine for cholesterol, normal values range between 160 and 250 mg %. We found a high level in most of the 150 cases of diabetes mellitus associated with coronary or peripheral macroangiopathy, with an average of 318.3 ± 24,3 mg % for a P = 0.05. The cholesterol level increased both on account of the esterified cholesterol (average value obtained 231 mg % ± 45.2 for a P = 0.05) and particularly on that of free cholesterol (average value obtained 86.7 mg % ± 28.3 for a P = 0.05). As a result of the variations of the cholesterol fractions, the average free cholesterol/esterified cholesterol ratio, normally ranging between 0.25–0.40 was, in the cases of diabetes with macroangiopathy, 0.36 ± 0.031 for a P = 0.05.

A much higher blood cholesterol level, reaching 704 mg % was reported in a case of lipoatrophic diabetes in which arteriopathy of the lower limbs and myocardotic disorders associated with symptoms of coronary insufficiency progressed rapidly [127]. This case emphasizes the prognostic importance of a high serum cholesterol level in the course of diabetic macroangiopathy. Periodically repeated determinations might serve to estimate the progress of the condition and the effectiveness of therapy.

Normal serum triglyceride levels, measured according to the procedure of Galanos et al., range between 150–450 mg % in the normal subject. In the group of 150 diabetics with late complications, in which we investigated the efficiency of some laboratory tests, an average value was found of 857.9 mg % ± 373 (P = 0.05), twice as high as in the normal subject. Intermediate values were found in the 10 diabetic subjects free from late complications (see also Chapter I p. 14).

The concomitant determination of serum triglycerides, serum cholesterol and lipidograms permitted the classification of the cases of diabetes

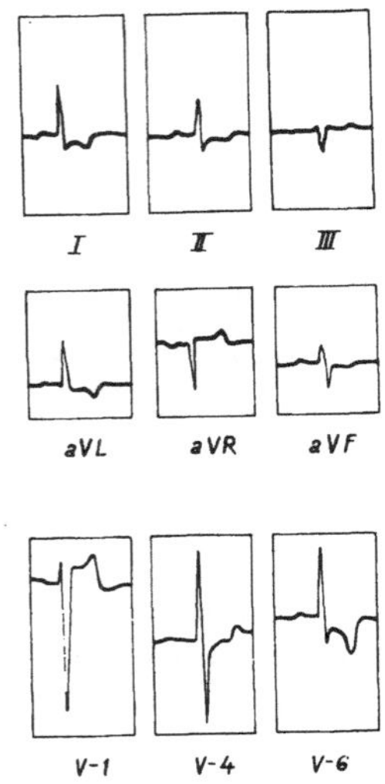

Fig. 30. B. N. Woman aged 66. Mature diabetes mellitus, insulinodependent at the beginning. Apparent onset 11 years before. Diabetic nephropathy with chronic renal failure. Clinical signs of coronary insufficiency, of the prolonged anginous type. Retinopathy. Diabetic neuropathy.

mellitus according to the hyperlipoproteinaemia groups proposed by Frederickson [59, 60]. This may serve both for diagnostic and prognostic purposes, since the patterns and trend to degenerative vascular complications differ with the type of hyperlipoproteinaemia.

The determination of phospholipids according to the procedure of Höflmeyer and Friedl, yields normal values between 150 and 250 mg %. In the 150 diabetic subjects with diabetic angiopathy, a moderate increase in phospholipids was found, with an average of 288.3 mg % ± 73.6 (P = 0.05). Such moderate increments were previously reported in the literature for both complicated and uncomplicated diabetes mellitus [11].

Kumagawa's gravimetric method of determining total lipaemia yields normal values of 5–9 g %. According to Grabner [63] an increase of total serum lipids is characteristic of diabetes. That was confirmed by our research. In the group of 150 diabetics with vascular complications, total lipaemia was 13.3 g % ± 4 (P = 0.05) on the average. No significant difference was found between diabetes mellitus without complications, and that complicated by angiopathy.

The normal paper lipidogram indicates 30–40% alpha-lipoproteins and 60–70% beta-lipoproteins. These figures change according to the type of hyperlipoproteinaemia associated with the respective cardiovascular complication. According to Grabner et al. [63] a rise of alpha lipoproteins and a decrease of beta-lipoproteins occur if the diabetes has no other complications. The association of fatty liver results in the rise of alpha$_1$-lipoproteins (Fig. 31 A, B).

In our group, average alpha-lipoproteins were 26.7% ± 6.8 (P = 0.05), while the average total beta-lipoproteins represented 73.7% ± 6.8 (P = 0.05). The appearance of most of the recorded lipidograms suggested a type II or type IV lipoproteinaemia (Fig. 31, 32).

Qualitative and quantitative immunoelectrophoresis in subjects with cardiac (Fig. 33) or peripheral macroangiopathy (Fig. 33) showed an increased beta-lipoprotein arch, which was less homogenous and appeared to divide into two components (Figs. 31, 33, 34, 35, 36, 37, 38).

3. Determination of the Serum Fibrinogen

The investigation of serum fibrinogen (II-nd phase of the coagulation) and fibrinolysis, may serve for diagnostic as well as for therapeutical purposes.

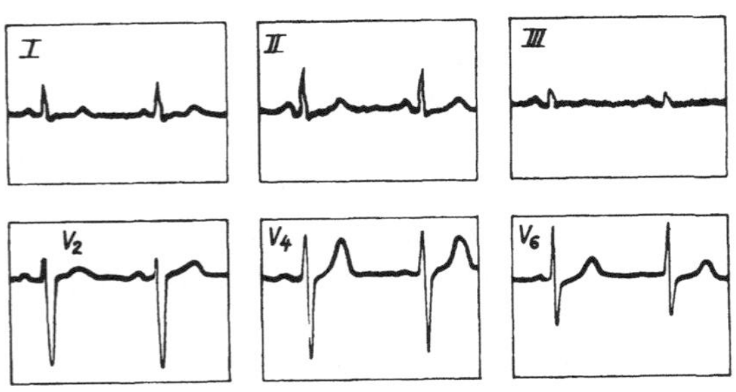

Fig. 29. S. M. Woman aged 53. Apparent onset of diabetes mellitus 20 years before. Insulinodependent. Associated diabetic retinopathy for the last ten years. Moderate obesity. Frequent episodes of acidosis.

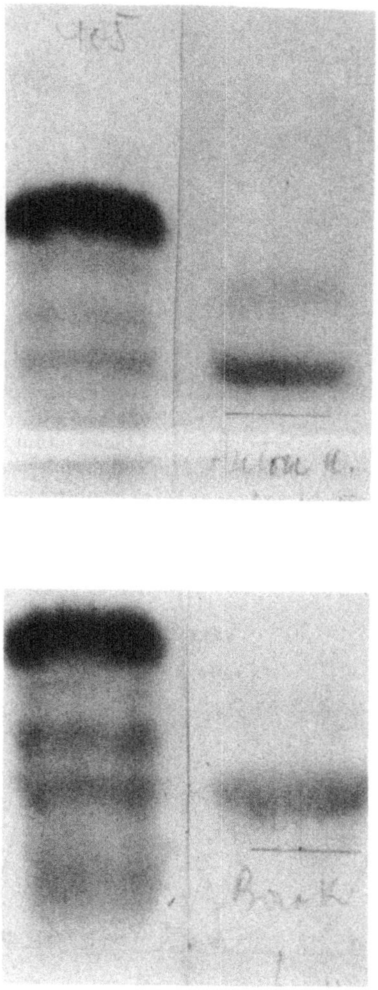

Fig. 31. A-Healthy-electrophoresis of serum proteins (1) and lipoproteins (2).
B-Diabetic-electrophoresis of serum proteins (1) and lipoproteins (2). Preponderance of the beta lipoproteins.

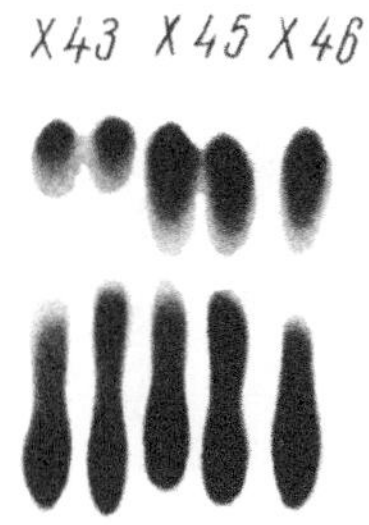

Fig. 32. Serum lipoprotein electrophoresis in agarose gel before and after a fatty meal. X43 = N. B. Woman with maturity onset diabetes. X45 = P. A. 12 years old, juvenile diabetes. X46 = normal subject. The existence of pre-β-lipoproteins is to be noticed in both diabetics.

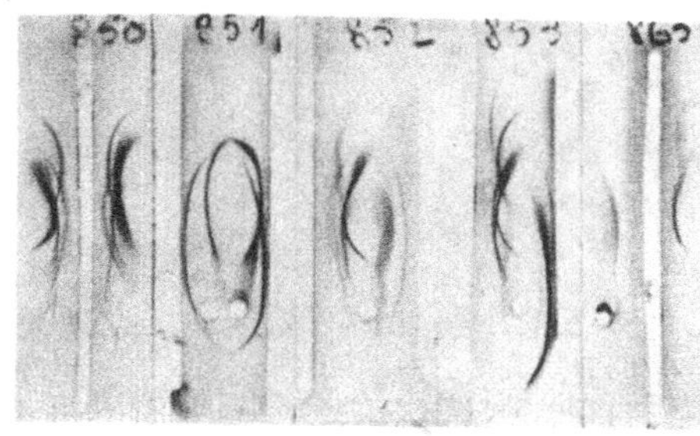

Fig. 33. 850. Diabetic with macroangiopathy at left, control serum at right, inactivated by heat. Comparatively low concentration in the serum of the patient of Ig M, a high level of the B_1 component. The macroglobulin from $alpha_2$ is identified in two bands situated below the $alpha_2M$ arch. The slow lipoproteins are normal in shape and position.
851. Control for Ig A- from the serum of the diabetic patient. It is found that Ig A are present in high concentration in the serum of the investigated patient.
852. Corroboration of the data obtained in plate 851 regarding Ig A, with the immune serum at the the right side of the plate and the topographical relations of the arch in the electrophoretic diagram.
853. Immunoelectrophoresis for Ig G, Ig M and Ig A. Quantitative increase in Ig A and anodic shift are found (diabetic patient).
863. At left-human milk, at right-diabetic serum, confirming the presence of macroglobulins in $alpha_2$.

As regards diagnosis, hyperlipaemia is often associated with a low activity of the fibrinolytic systems and increased fibrinogenaemia. On the other hand, some of the therapeutical approaches, particularly those implying the use of K antivitamins, require a continuous control of the coagulation processes. In this latter case, tests investigating the first phase of coagulation (prothrombin time, Quick test) should also be performed [72].

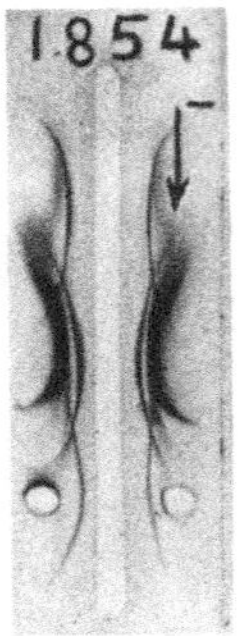

Fig. 34. Immunoelectrophoresis in normal individual. The absence of pre-β-lipoproteins is to be noticed (arrow).

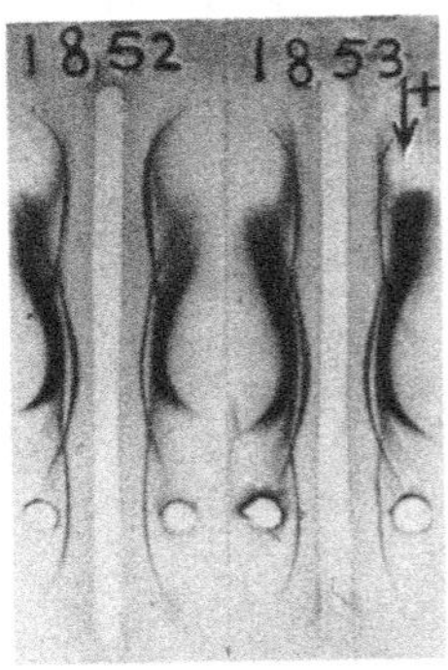

Fig. 35. Immunoelectrophoresis in diabetic subject; presence of pre-β-lipoproteins (arrow) (Diabetes with maturity onset).

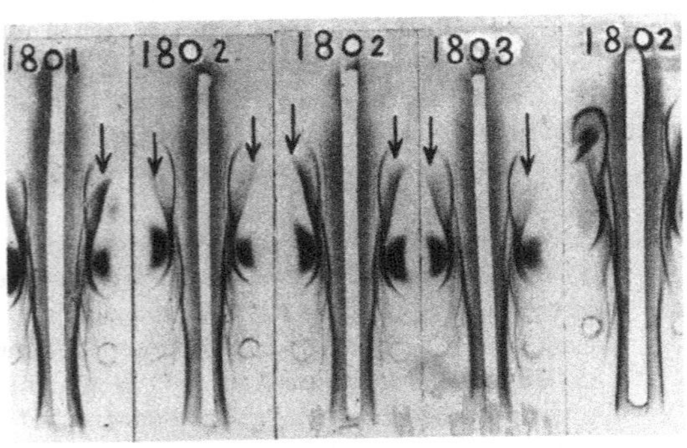

Fig. 36. Immunoelectrophoresis in a group of juvenile diabetics. Arrows indicate the presence of β and pre-β-lipoproteins.

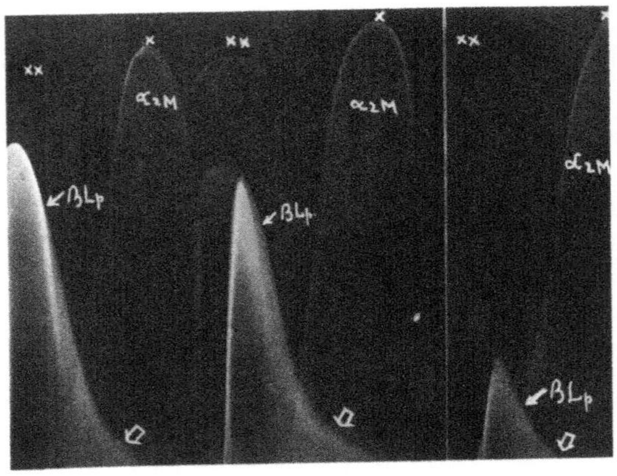

Fig. 37. Immunoelectrophoresis of blood serum in diabetics (a), non-diabetics (b) and for reference the umbilical cord (c). (x) (xx) = control levels for globulins; βLp = β-lipoproteins; a_2M = α-macroglobulins; the double arrows indicates pre-β-lipoproteins.

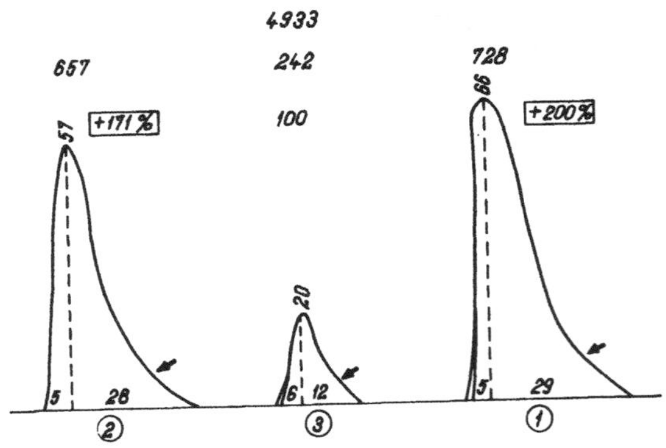

Fig. 38. Diagram for the fig. 37. Qantitative immunoelectrophoresis, for β- and pre-β-lipoproteins showing a greater increase of β-lipoproteins (200 %) in diabetics as compared with the normal individual (171 %).

D. Treatment of Heart Disorders in Diabetic Macroangiopathy

Diabetic macroangiopathy in the heart, be it clinical myocardosis or a relative coronary insufficiency, requires therapeutic measures aiming at

– controlling and maintaining under control the diabetic condition [138] and

– improvement of the subjective complaints and of the disorders in the coronary blood flow. As for the latter, their treatment is non-specific and consists of the therapy generally used with such pathological conditions.

1. Hygienic and Dietary Prescriptions

The Diet should be prescribed in each individual case taking into account the glucose tolerance of the subject and the preponderant disorders recorded by clinical, electrocardiographic and laboratory investigations [13]. Possible alterations in the blood lipid picture may also require dietary alterations [106] (see Table I).

If the dominant symptomatology is that of *diabetic myocardosis,* then proteins with a high biological value should be increased in the diet. This is important because in diabetes there may be an alteration in the metabolism of protein, with impaired ability to synthesize functional proteins. It should also be remembered that some of the patients suffering from diabetic myocardosis are aged and there is a general tendency for elderly people to reduce protein intake in favour of other food.

If the dominant symptomatology is that of attempt to reduce overweight by a low calorie intake. It may be achieved by

– reducing the share of carbohydrates, if too high, and consequently readjusting the amount of insulin or of oral hypoglycaemic drugs, and
– by reducing the intake of fat.

This will exert a favourable influence on the possible trend to acidosis and probably also on the course of the associated macroangiopathy. The daily food intake should contain some 1,000 calories, in order to bring about a gradual loss of weight, because an excessive weight loss implies consumption of the body fat, equivalent from the metabolic point of view of a high fat diet [9]. The diet should be based on various salads, green vegetables and meat.

If coronary disorders dominate the pathological picture, dietary measures should concentrate on the reduction of fat intake. Some authors doubt that a low fat diet can improve prognosis in cases of coronary or peripheral macroangiopathy [119]. Considering, however, our present knowledge of the extent to which certain hyperlipaemic states depend on exogenous fat and carbohydrate intake, it appears wiser to restrict the quantum of saturated fat in the food. One should partly or even completely eliminate fatty meat (bacon), ham, salami and sausages, lard, egg yolk, certain derivatives of milk such as cream, fatty cheese, rich, mild and whipped cream, and even some vegetable fats (coconut oil, cocoa butter, chocolate and most of the margarine varieties in which a process of hydrogenation turns fluid fats into partly saturated ones) [9, 76, 154].

Vegetable oil and fish oil rich in unsaturated fatty acids are included in the diet with a view to reducing the blood cholesterol level. They are effective only if the other fat varieties have been correspondingly restricted. The ingestion of unsaturated fats may facilitate the increase of blood serum lipoprotein lipase activity [7, 8]. It is not recommended to entirely eliminate saturated fatty acids from the diet.

It is difficult to substantially reduce the ingestion of fats in the diabetic diet, because this would imply an increase in the intake of carbohydrates and proteins. Increase of the former is practically impossible in diabetics while increase of the latter is often difficult. That is why, the usual solution is to ensure the necessary calories as follows:

45% carbohydrates,
40% fats and
15% proteins.

What can be modified and adapted is the quality of ingested fats.

According to recent studies, a serum uric acid level exceeding 7 mg per 100 ml doubles the risk of a coronary involvement. Food rich in purines (liver, calf thymus, kidneys, testicles, smoke-dried salt meat, herrings, etc.), should accordingly be restricted [9].

The prohibition of smoking is compulsory, since its effect is most unfavourable on coronary angiopathy. This often implies, particularly in heavy smokers, an effort which brings about a state of irritability. It is therefore advisable to prescribe some sort of sedative therapy. Smoking should be banned in every form (cigars, pipe, etc.).

The way of life of the patient should take into account his main pathological complaints. Stress must be avoided, as well as physical over-exertion and nervous tension. Sedentary life is dangerous since it contributes to overweight and hinders the process of formation of intercoronary anastomoses, a most useful compensating process in the functional coronary macroangiopathy [9]. In cases of juvenile diabetes, systematically performed physical exercise results in a decrease of the blood level of cholesterol, phospholipids and triglycerides. Daily exercise, especially in the young diabetic, might be a prophylactic management of diabetic macroangiopathy [92]. On the other hand, some authors have reported that NEFA blood levels increase subsequent to physical effort [139]. Exercise should therefore be maintained within reasonable limits.

It is not known whether *focal infection* is of any consequence in the course of diabetic macroangiopathy, but it certainly affects the state of metabolic balance of the diabetic. Dental granuloma, tonsil infections, sinusitis, etc., should therefore be eradicated [35].

2. Medical Treatment

Medical treatment should aim at

- preventing the progress of the coronary angiopathy by the administration of anticoagulants, of drugs correcting the lipidic imbalance and of various efficient means in the control of such aggravating circumstances as e. g. arterial hypertension.
- suppressing the subjective and objective disorders by the therapy of the main symptoms of either myocardosis or relative or absolute coronary failure.

The administration of ***anticoagulant drugs*** aims at preventing coronary thrombosis. They should be given under the cover of periodic control of the process of coagulation, to be performed at intervals no longer than one month. Hypoprothrombinaemia should be maintained around 30% in order to obtain a total blood hypocoagulability, which can be estimated by performing a thrombodynamogram.

Anticoagulant therapy is contraindicated in cachexy, renal failure, peptic ulceration and severe arterial hypertension. It was reported that the anticoagulant drugs potentiate the hypoglycaemic effect of some antidiabetic sulphonylureas (e. g. tolbutamide) by delaying their breakdown in the liver. This exerts a favourable effect on the treatment of the diabetic condition itself [89].

A close cooperation must be achieved between patient and physician, in order to detect the slightest tendency towards abnormal bleeding.

Questions related to heparin therapy are dealt with in the subsection about peripheral diabetic macroangiopathy.

There is only one drug that might be given without restriction to the diabetic, in order to correct lipid imbalance, namely clofibrate. The drug is most active in triglyceride hyperlipaemia, and less effective (in 25% of the cases only) in true hypercholesterolaemia. It should be noted that the drug interferes with the anticoagulants and during their concomitant administration, the Quick test and thrombodynamogram are to be frequently checked. Doses: 1.2–2 gm daily.

The administration of nicotinic acid or of its derivatives often results, if 1.5–3 mg per kg bodyweight are given daily, in a reduction of the serum cholesterol level even to the normal range [9]. But this therapy is hampered by its possible side-effects (skin hyperhaemia, gastric disorders) [151]. Moreover, there are other side-effects due to nicotinic acid, such as a transient hyperbilirubinaemia occurring in the hours after administration and proportional to the degree of hepatic involvement [20], a rise in serum transaminases [151], a reduction in glucose tolerance and changes in the serum glucose-6-phosphate dehydrogenase [21]. All this calls for a careful control throughout the treatment and for a judicious selection of the patients.

Sitosterol and other similar preparations have proved to be less effective. Mer 29 was abandoned because of its side-effects, particularly because of the ocular complications.

Hormonal preparations such as the thyroid hormones and especially oestrogens, were found to be inconsistently effective. When effective, they result in undesired side-effects [9] which prevent their administration in coronary insufficiency.

Anion exchange resins (cholestyramine) complex with the biliary acids and prevent the absorption of fat. This might afford a new therapeutic approach, but the procedures are still under investigation [76]. The administration of cholestyramine, for instance, in daily doses of 12–24 gm, does not bring about a significant reduction in the serum cholesterol level, but arrests the progress of certain xanthomas [9, 151]. Gastric dyspepsia and constipation have been reported as side-effects, as well as steatorrhea and symptoms of liposoluble vitamin deficiency [151] if too high a dose of the drug has been taken.

The management of arterial hypertension consists of the usual antihypertensive therapy. It should be noted, however, that insulin administration must be perfectly adapted to the requirements of individuals with coronary diabetic macroangiopathy, since certain experimental investigations [151] suggest that the hormone may bring about transient rises in the blood pressure, probably by increasing the contractility of the myocardium [103, 137], even in doses which do not result in hypoglycaemia.

The *symptomatic management* with the drugs commonly used for this purpose, aims at control of angina, congestive heart failure and of left ventricular failure.

Uricosuric therapy in cases of macroangiopathy associated with hyperuricaemia decreases serum uric acid but does not interfere with the alteration of the lipid balance [43].

3. Surgical Intervention

Surgical intervention may be indicated only if coronary insufficiency deteriorates severely. Several surgical procedures have been advocated, but only two appear to be effective [9]: the intervention of Vinebergs implantation of the internal mammary artery into the myocardium (with the aim of stimulating a collateral circulation), and direct intervention on the coronaries (coronary endarteriectomy) [100]. Prior angiography of the coronaries is required in every case for the estimation of the extent and topography of the lesions.

E. Peripheral Disorders in Diabetic Macroangiopathy

1. Prevalence

Peripheral diabetic macroangiopathy is one of the most severe chronic complications of diabetes mellitus [144]. Its incidence underwent an impressive rise during the post insulin period (see Chapter 1 Fig. 7) and it occurs in 10–63% of the diabetic population. In hospital statistics the incidence of diabetic arteriopathy ranges between 7 and 35% [150].

The problem of peripheral diabetic macroangiopathy appears to be even more serious if one takes into account that

- in 10 to 40.6% of the patients with these disorders, a chemical, inapparent or clinical diabetes mellitus is often discovered only after the onset of peripheral ischaemia, and

- that many patients in whom arteriopathy has been regarded initially as common atherosclerosis, developed in the subsequent months or years disorders of glucose tolerance that may at any time develop into diabetes mellitus.

Unlike diabetic microangiopathy, diabetic macroangiopathy is regarded by some authors as only representing an atherosclerotic process which, owing to the dysmetabolic background of the diabetic subject, takes a more rapid course than in the non-diabetic individual [34, 35, 36, 116]. Others, however, especially during the last twenty years, have assigned a certain anatomical specificity to peripheral diabetic macroangiopathy [62] consisting of a proliferation of the arteriolar endothelium up to the almost total occlusion of the lumen, and a specific staining with colloidal iron of the thickened arterial wall and basement membrane. These aspects have already been dealt with in Chapter II.

These controversies are undoubtedly theoretically important, but from a practical point of view one cannot disregard either the similarity of the diabetic and atherosclerotic angiopathies, or the specific character conferred on this condition by diabetes. This specificity results from an ensemble of data concerning prevalence, general and local symptomatology and the response to conservative management.

The distribution according to sex of diabetic macroangiopathy differs from that of atherosclerotic macroangiopathy. Males are predominantly affected by the latter and the female/male ratio in atherosclerosis without diabetes is 1:10 or even less [115, 150]. The opposite trend is found in diabetic patients. Some authors have reported an inverse ratio, that is a higher prevalence in females [116, 150], others have found a trend towards an equal distribution of the disease between the two sexes, that is a 1:1 ratio. Derot et al. [36] in a recent research found a slight preponderance of males (54 as compared to 46 females).

A statistical study was performed on 3,639 patients admitted to our clinic from 1964 to 1968; Clinical, X-ray and oscillometric symptoms of peripheral angiopathy were found in 651 patients (302 females and 349 males) (see Chapter II Table I). The overall incidence of the complication was 17.9 % (see Chapter II Fig. 4). The statistics show a slight excess of males (53.6 % v. 46.4 %). It should be noted that in the same group, the sex distribution of the cardiac diabetic macroangiopathy differed from that of the peripheral macroangiopathy in that a slight preponderance of females was found with the former condition (see Chapter II Fig. 6).

In non-diabetic individuals only 3% of patients with peripheral ischaemia occur in the 45–49 years age group, and some 7% in the 55–59 year group, while all the other cases occur at older ages, over 60 [41].

On the contrary, 14% of diabetic peripheral angiopathy according to Scheibe and 5% according to Mohnike occur before the age of 40 [150]. Scheibe also reported that 39 % of the diabetes with peripheral ischaemia occur between 40 and 60 years of age, so that by adding the above 14% cases under 40, 53% occur before the age at which the incidence of common atherosclerosis starts to rise.

In our statistics, in a group of 3,659 diabetic patients admitted to hospital, out of whom 651 suffered from peripheral macroangiopathy, the disease was found to begin before the age of 40 in 21 subjects (3.2%) (see Chapter II, Fig. 7).

The moment at which peripheral diabetic macroangiopathy begins and the rate at which the lesions progress also depends on the duration of the diabetes. It is very difficult to estimate the real duration of a diabetic history, particularly because of the high incidence of cases of chemical or inapparent diabetes. This fact probably accounts for the finding that in some 2/3 of cases diabetes mellitus is discovered because of the early signs of peripheral ischaemia [55]. This is the case of 10.4% of the subjects with diabetic macroangiopathy in the statistics of our clinic (see Table I, Chapter II and Fig. 8 in the same chapter). If one also takes into account the group of patients in which diabetes has been recognized for less than

5 years, it follows that 30% of the diabetic patients with peripheral arteriopathy are likely to have suffered for long intervals from a mild diabetes mellitus, ignored and altogether untreated.

By adding to this group all the patients with a diabetic history of less than 10 years, one may reach the conclusion that the onset of peripheral diabetic arteriopathy is in no apparent way related to the duration of diabetes itself, since the new group comprises 48% of the patients with diabetic arteriopathy. But this might be jumping to hasty conclusions since it is most likely that in all these cases diabetes started much earlier. It seems wiser to conclude that the metabolic disturbance leading to the peripheral diabetic macroangiopathy is effective even in cases of inapparent or chemical diabetes, that is to say, that the incidence of the complication depends rather on the duration of the diabetes than on its control. But this conclusion is quite the opposite to that reached by the statistical investigations based on the estimation from the history, of the duration of a case of diabetes mellitus.

In this respect, as well as the age at which the diabetic ischaemic complication occurs, one should take into account the reports suggesting that the disorders in fat metabolism which precede or accompany it are normally found with maturity onset diabetes. It seems that the lipid abnormalities are less frequent with pancreatic diabetes [115].

Most of the authors agree that *diabetes, obesity and atherosclerosis* represent one of the most typical examples of pathological syntropism. Some authors believe, however, that the stimulating effect of obesity on the onset of the syndrome of peripheral diabetic arteriopathy is only apparent because of its particular sex distribution. Since the percentage of women is high and obesity is frequent in women, the incidence of obesity appears to be high in the angiopathic group [150].

It is nevertheless true that growing statistical evidence suggests that overweight in the non-diabetic subject is a preatherosclerotic state and that the hazard of death due to an atherosclerotic condition is far greater in the obese, since peripheral arteriopathies are twice as frequent in the obese. If obesity is associated with diabetes mellitus, one should expect the hazard of a peripheral macroangiopathy to further increase.

In the group of patients suffering from diabetic peripheral arteriopathy investigated in our clinic, 59.8% were in or under the normal weight range and the remainder were obese. Such a high incidence of overweight in diabetics in which the condition is usually easy to control and does not require the administration of insulin, suggests the presence of some associated metabolic disturbance (Table IX).

Recent investigations on blood insulin levels in the obese have raised the question whether obesity might predispose to diabetes or is in itself a consequence of a diabetic or prediabetic metabolic state. The elucidation of this problem may also throw some new light on the real role played by the duration of the diabetic history on the prevalence of diabetic macroangiopathy.

Arterial hypertension is regarded as an important hazard in accelerating an atherosclerotic process in the non-diabetic patient [144]. In association with diabetes mellitus it is undoubtedly an important factor in peripheral angiopathy. This correlation was initially suggested by necropsy findings in diabetic atherosclerotic patients [62] and was recently confirmed by clinical investigations [130].

In our statistics, 57.3% of the diabetic inpatients have been found with high blood pressure (see Table X).

Table IX. Dates on 651 diabetics with peripheral macroangiopathy.

YEAR	WITHOUT ANY TRATMENT	INSULIN (I.U)		HYPOGLYCEMIATING ORAL DRUGS	DAILY DIET (CARBOHYDRATES g)		PRESENCE OF OBESITY	PRESENCE OF HYPERTENSION
		> 40	< 40		100–150 g	150–200 g		
1964	52	67	23	63	92	93	73	124
1965	36	62	21	45	79	68	67	79
1966	32	58	28	69	95	72	75	-
1967	11	23	24	37	45	39	47	75
TOTAL	131	210	96	214	311	272	262	278

Table X

	PATIENTS WITH DIABETIC AND ATHEROSCLEROTIC FAMILIAL HISTORY	SMOKERS	ALCOHOLISM	OBESITY	ARTERIAL HYPERTENSION	ELEVATED BLOOD CHOLESTEROL
GLOBAL NUMBER	799	605	820	873	2,392	1,294
PERCENTAGE	16.4 %	12.4 %	16.8 %	19.9 %	57.3 %	26.54 %

On the other hand, high blood pressure was found in 42.8% of the diabetic subjects with peripheral diabetic macroangiopathy (see Table IX). The relative independence of high blood pressure from obesity is proved by the high incidence of hypertension. This finding is consistent with several recently published reports [130].

As far as *antidiabetic therapy* before the onset of macroangiopathy is concerned, the findings (Table IX) suggest that the incidence of the arterial complication is higher in patients treated by low doses of insulin or of antidiabetic sulphonylureas, than in the group of patients receiving over 40 I. U. of insulin daily. In fact, 424 patients (65.1%) were receiving antidiabetic sulphonylureas and small doses of insulin. If one adds to this group the 131 untreated patients (20.1%), only 14.8% of the angiopathic subjects required insulin doses exceeding 40 I. U. daily. These findings challenge the alleged arteriopathic effect of insulin therapy [102, 126, 128]. Furthermore in the group under consideration, the number of patients with diabetic macroangiopathy who never received insulin exceeds (345 patients) that of the subjects who were given insulin (306 patients).

Lipaemia in the diabetic may be sensitive or resistant to the administration of insulin and it is possible that insulin has been assigned an arteriopathic role because in the cases of diabetes in which lipaemia was independent of insulin, arteriopathy occurred in spite of the administration of high doses of insulin [7, 12]. Other authors regarded the high ILA levels found in some cases of diabetes as an evidence of a possible arteriopathic role of insulin [102]. It seems, however, that there are more arguments against this point of view than in its favour [81]. Clinical findings suggest that the administration of insulin and even a slight overdosage of the drug exerts a favourable effect on the conservative management of diabetic arteriopathy [14, 34, 35, 51, 116]. The fact that favourable evolution has also been reported during the administration of antidiabetic sulphonylureas [34] suggests that in such cases of mild diabetes the major hazard in peripheral arteriopathy is represented by the diabetic condition itself. But these findings also emphasize that a satisfactory metabolic control of the diabetic state, obtained with or without insulin, is a prerequisite for the success of conservative management.

On first examining the statistical data presented by us, it appears surprising that peripheral diabetic arteriopathy was more frequently met with in diabetic subjects managed by low carbohydrate diet (100–150 gm in 311 patients) than in patients taking higher amounts (150–200 gm daily in 272 patients). Apparently this finding contradicts our present knowledge about the role played by carbohydrates in maintaining and bringing about dyslipaemic states, but it might be explained by the fact that most of the patients having been prescribed a low carbohydrate diet were overweight.

It is admitted that *hereditary factors* play a role in the prevalence of diabetes itself although the means of transmission and the information transmitted is still an object of controversy. Most of the authors agree that hereditary diabetes mellitus is transmitted by a recessive autosomal gene with an incomplete penetrance [66, 160].

According to others, heredity is multifactorial [156]. Another plausible hypothesis assumes a combination between the genetic and the environmental factors [84] and some authors, starting from this hypothesis, consider that the transmission of diabetes mellitus is dominant with graduated expressivity [129, 134]. The disagreement may be due to the fact that the investigations have been confined to the manifest stage of the condition [23] but the plurigenic mechanism seems to meet with general approval [104]. Further recent research on prediabetic subjects [19] investigating substances whose very existence is controversial (synalbumin), resulted in conclusions in which the plurigenic mechanism is also postulated [23, 166].

The investigations of Cerasi et al. [23] in this field brought a useful contribution to the problem of diabetic macroangipathy. According to these authors, there is a constant individual pattern of insulin release in response to physiological and pharmacological stimuli. This pattern may be related to the diabetic antecedents of the subject, i. e. it may be inherited. Against this background, the authors postulate the intervention of acquired factors which may act either *additively* or by disturbing a previously compensated state. Such diabetogenic stimuli are obesity, HGH or cortisol, etc.

This hereditary mechanism has also been postulated with regard to the transmission of atherosclerosis. Ilinsky [80] considers the transmission of a lack of resistance of the regulatory mechanisms, on the one hand for the functions and nutrition of the vessels, and on the other hand, for the metabolism of cholesterol [115]. Against such an inherited background one might suppose the action of either the additive or the decompensating mechanisms, or the simultaneous action of both with converging effects.

Atherosclerotic heredity in the family was ascertained in 16.4% of the diabetic patients admitted in our clinic, but only 41% of these were found to suffer from peripheral diabetic macroangiopathy.

The specific metabolic disturbance of diabetes mellitus may also interfere, either by enhancing a preexisting predisposition to atherosclerosis (the additive hypothesis), or by disturbing the compensating mechanisms controlling a trend to atherosclerosis (the compensation hypothesis). This approach might provide an explanation of the preponderance of diabetic macroangiopathy in maturity onset diabetes, in that the compensating mechanisms which protect against atherosclerosis and/or diabetes mellitus are disturbed and the two pathological conditions released.

As for the localization of diabetic macroangiopathy, the preponderance of the lower limbs is obvious in the statistics of our clinic and consistent with data reported in the literature (see Table XI and Fig. 39).

Involvement of the upper limbs is uncommon and is consistent with those findings reported by other authors [36], in spite of the fact that their statistics only comprised the cases of arteriopathy complicated by gangrene or acute obliteration [116]. The present statistics, also include patients with nonspecific symptoms, associated with oscillometric alterations and radiologically visible calcium deposits in the interdigital arteries. Sudden occlusion of the left brachial artery followed by death, occurred in one case, a diabetic and obese man.

Table XI. Principal localizations of diabetic macroangiopathy in 651 diabetic inpatients.

SUPERIOR LIMB	INFERIOR LIMB	CORONARY ARTERIES	CEREBRAL ARTERIES	GENERAL
5	251	122	120	153

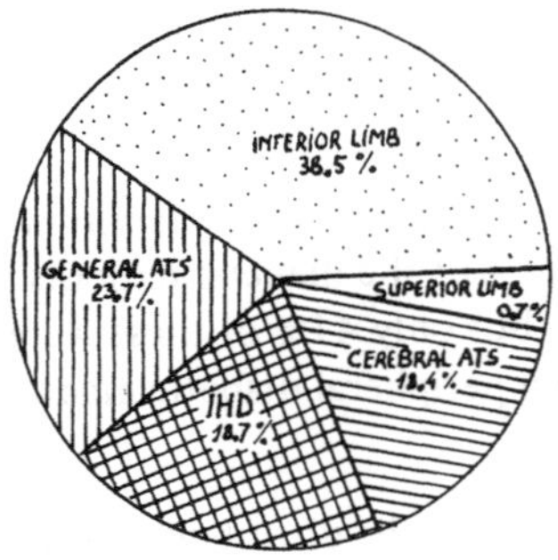

Fig. 39. Distribution in percentages of the various localizations of diabetic arteriopathy (IHD = ischaemic heart disease).

Heavy smoking plays the same role in peripheral diabetic macroangiopathy as in atherosclerosis in general, in that it further aggravates the underlying metabolic disturbances. Smoking exerts on the young organism an effect similar to that of diabetes. Its impact is heavy on the young and less severe in the elderly, but the latter suffer more often from diabetes [55]. By increasing serum cholesterol and disturbing fat metabolism in general [115], smoking becomes a factor deteriorating both the common and the diabetic arteriopathy.

Confessed and actual tabagism associated with diabetes was found in our statistics in 12.4% of the cases (see Table X). Clinical and subjective symptoms of peripheral macroangiopathy were found in 32% of the diabetic smokers.

The role of *alcoholism* in bringing about or promoting the onset of peripheral diabetic macroangiopathy is controversial. The high incidence of atherosclerotic arteriopathy among alcoholics [115] might be related to the fact that alcohol consumption is often associated with a high calorie and high fat diet. In the case of diabetic subjects, the consumption of alcohol might stimulate disregard for the prescribed dietary restrictions.

Confessed alcoholism was found in 16.8% of our diabetic patients (see Table X), but only 2.3% of these had symptoms of peripheral diabetic macroangiopathy. Alcoholism should probably also be regarded as an indirect additional element in the sense of Cerasi's hypothesis [23], or even as an agent disturbing a previous state of compensation.

It might be concluded that the conglomeration of circumstances in which diabetic macroangiopathy begins and develops confers a certain specificity on the prevalence of this complication in diabetes mellitus and differentiates it from the common peripheral atherosclerotic angiopathy.

2. Clinical Study of Peripheral Diabetic Angiopathy

The subjective and objective symptomatology of peripheral diabetic macroangiopathy shows many features different from those of the ischaemia in common atherosclerosis. These differences become even more obvious if one examines the symptomatology of diabetic macroangiopathy taking into account the division into stages that has been formulated for the description of any disorder of arterial origin of the peripheral blood supply [41].

Stage I: complete circulatory compensation.

Absent or diminished peripheral pulses may be the only clinical sign, revealed by oscillometry or oscillography with no significant alteration of the skin and muscles.

Stage II: compensation at rest.

Characterized by the onset of intermittent claudication.

Stage III: decompensation at rest.

Pain occurs even at rest and during the night in prolonged attacks which may subside if the limb is allowed to hang down below the level of the body. Paradoxically, the pain is relieved for a moment by standing up and performing small movements, probably by a momentary improvement of the circulation.

Stage IV: trophic disorders.

Necrosis and gangrene occur, indicating that the critical limit of the minimal blood flow at rest has been exceeded.

A difference in cases of diabetes mellitus [146, 150] consists in the fact that Stage II is often absent or indistinct. Intermittent claudication, the cramp-like pain, one of the most characteristic features in peripheral ischaemia of atherosclerotic origin, is often absent and the affected limb is warm and an arterial pulse is palpable [62]. Ratschow's test is often negative (if the limb is elevated it blanches rapidly and cyanosis is extreme). It may become positive only at later stages. The patient sometimes has the feeling that the limb is cold, but hisparaesthetic sensations are not severe enough to induce him to call for a doctor [150]. These differences are due on the one hand to the fact that the diabetic lesion is usually localized at the extreme periphery, in small vessels which cannot give rise to claudication because of the small tributary area, and on the other hand to the possible association of a diabetic neuropathy which results in anaesthetized areas.

Symptomatology may be minor in Stage III and the patient goes to the physician in Stage IV when peripheral gangrene occurs subsequent to slight trauma, or some neglected interdigital fungus infection. Its frequent localization is the plantar side of the big toe, the lateral sides of the other toes and also the heel [128].

Data recorded in the group of 651 macroangiopathic diabetic patients examined by us, concerning the incidence of the complication in its different stages, is shown in Table IX. It is in sharp contrast with other data reported in the literature about the evolution in stages of peripheral atherosclerosis [182].

There are undoubtedly many cases observing the classical pattern of peripheral arteriopathy, and in these "favourable" cases a prophylactic treatment is possible. Therefore any pain associated with walking should be carefully investigated, with respect to the distance covered, the rate of walking or the temperature of the environment. The localization of pain indicates the site of the vascular occlusion: if pain is felt in the thigh or the buttock, the occlusion is situated in the pelvis; in the shank if the occlusion is situated in the thigh and in the sole or toes if the occlusion is peripheral.

Once pain has begun, the diagnosis relies mostly on the medical history, but may be completed by some simple tests whilst the patient remains in bed. Clinical examination should look for modifications in the colour of the skin (pale, sometimes with a violet tint, less often with purpuric patches) (Fig. 40) [128] and for trophic modifications of the nails (thickening, friability) [171]. Superficial ulcerations which do not heal and hyperkeratosis also suggest a deficit in blood supply, to a degree approaching Stage IV. A red "slipper" is formed sometimes on the limb maintained in a low position, by the reddening of skin of the toes, sole and heel.

Palpation should be used to try to estimate local temperature, lower in the affected limb, as well as the presence, absence and comparative amplitude

Table XII. Symptomatology and stadial frequence of diabetic and atherosclerotic angiopathy.

TYPE OF PERIPHERAL ISCHAEMIA		CLINICAL STAGES OF PERIPHERAL ISCHAEMIA				
		I	II	III	IV	TOTAL
ATHEROSCLEROSIS	NR. OF CASES	40	350	7	1	398
	PERCENTAGE	10 %	87.9 %	1.8 %	0.3 %	100 %
DIABETIC MACROANGIOPATHY	NR. OF CASES	218	45	98	290	651
	PERCENTAGE	33 %	6.9 %	15 %	45.1 %	100 %

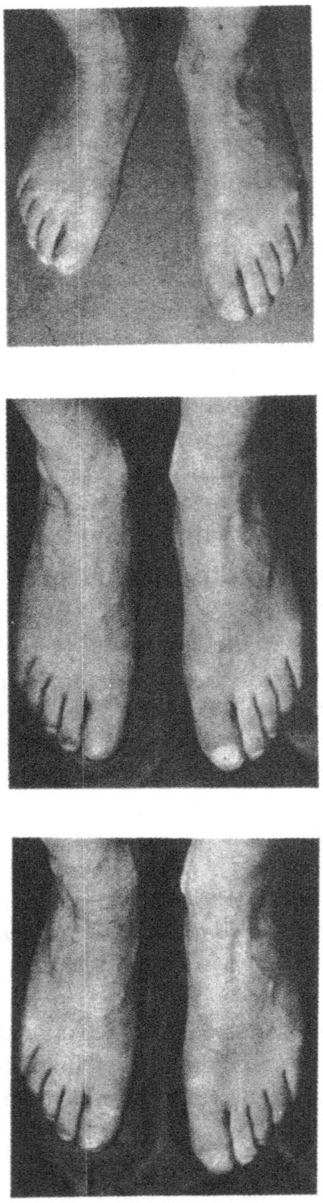

Fig. 40. Aspects of lower limbs during Ratschow's position test: 1(10') 2(20') 3(30') after lying down.

differences of the arterial pulse of the vessels supplying the respective area. In the upper limb, the subclavian artery can be felt in the supraclavicular fossa, the brachialartery on the medial side of the arm and in the sulcus bicipitalis, the radial artery in the pulse groove [38, 78]. In the lower limb, the dorsal artery of the foot can be felt on the dorsal side of the foot in normal position, the posterior tibial artery behind the medial maleolus when the foot is flexed, the popliteal artery in the popliteal fossa and the femoral artery in the groin, below Poupart's ligament, the whole limb being extended and slightly rotated outwards.

Ratschow's position test should also be performed in order to observe modifications in the colour of the skin (sock-like cyanosis) (see Fig. 40), attacks of pain, the filling of veins and reactive hyperhaemia subsequent to physical effort or high positioning of the limb. This test is performed by vertically raising both upper or lower limbs of the supine patient. In that position, the patient rotates his foot for several minutes in the tibio tarsal joint, or, in the case of upper limbs, opens or closes his fist 60 times in 60 seconds. Even in cases of mild circulatory disorders, pallor and pain occur in less than two minutes. When the limbs are laid down, the skin becomes red in 5–10 seconds in the healthy individual and much later in cases of altered blood supply (the interval should be measured and the degree of congestion noted). The veins become swollen in 6–10 seconds in the normal individual and much later in the case of a syndrome of peripheral ischaemia.

The test does not yield much information concerning digital occlusions, but temperature, pallor and pain should be looked for also at this level.

Oscillometry and oscillography are auxilliary methods which aim at obtaining some objective information concerning blood flow alterations, but their contribution to the diagnosis is only minor. Only oscillographic differences exceeding 2.5 mm between homonymous limbs should be taken into account. Values less than 15 mm found by oscillometry are also pathological.

The investigation may be supplemented by measurements of skin temperature, using a skin thermometer and comparing the findings with those obtained by oscillometry [57]. Skin temperature determinations should be performed at constant room temperature [70]. The reactivity of the vasomotor nerves may also be tested by measuring skin temperature in the suspected limb after the immersion of another limb in water at 43°C. If normal, its temperature will undergo a significant rise in 45 minutes [70].

Oscillometry and skin temperature determination may also be performed subsequent to a measured effort.

Skin thermography, recording the infra-red radiation released by the skin, yields a "thermic snapshot" of wide areas of the body surface. By correlating its results with those of angiography in cases of arteritis of the lower limbs, a map of the areas of peripheral ischaemia can be obtained, as a useful complement in the investigation of peripheral circulation [67, 176].

Sphygmography yields information concerning the rigidity of the vascular walls, indicated by the absence of a dicrotic notch in the pulse wave [41].

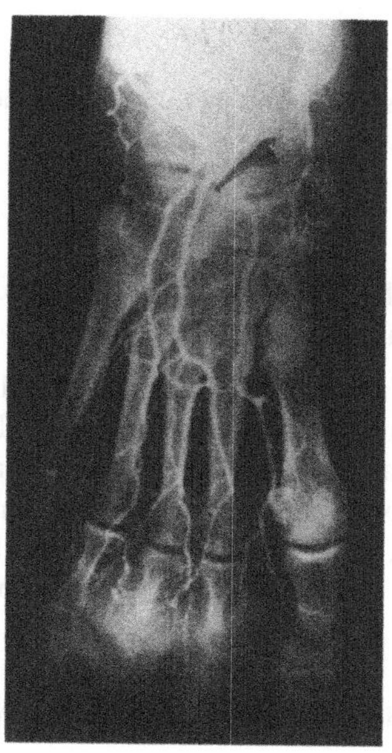

Fig. 41. Arteriography of the left lower limb. Diabetic woman aged 53. Apparent onset 14 years before. Treated by insulin and inconstant diet. Obstruction of the small arteries of the toes. Gangrenous process on the lateral and plantar faces of the IInd and IIIrd toes (see fig. 47 for clinical aspect).

The most precise method of determining the limits of ischaemic areas is arteriography. It is most useful especially when a surgical intervention is considered [41]. Figure 41 shows an arteriogram of the foot in a case of peripheral diabetic macroangiopathy, in which the small digital arteries are not obvious.

A simple X-ray examination of the limb, segment by segment, without using any contrast substance may sometimes show calcificated areas in the arteries of the region (see Fig. 42, 43, 44). The process of calcification of the media – Mönkeberg's mediocalcinosis – although evident on an X-ray, does not always result in an ischaemia.

Investigations have been performed by injecting labelled xenon into the muscle – usually of the thigh – in order to measure its diffusion and discharge from the muscle. This test yields some information concerning blood flow along the main circulatory pathways, but its results are not entirely reliable in arterioles because they depend on haemodynamic conditions. The test makes it possible for the latency interval to be estimated and gives information concerning the actual type of disturbance in blood flow [46, 117].

Finally, clinical investigations may be completed by rheography, a procedure recording the variations in the filling of blood vessels in relation to the pulse rhythm. More precise details can be obtained concerning the localization of obstructions. This test has the same indications as arteriography [115].

As far as the extent of the lesions is concerned, Goldenberg et al. [62] found gangrene extending above the ankle in 7% of the diabetic patients with angiopathy, as compared to an incidence of 50% of such gangrene in non-diabetic patients with atherosclerotic angiopathy. The final stage of diabetic macroangiopathy consisted in 70% of the cases in skin gangrene in patches situated mostly on the foot, while in non-diabetic patients with common atherosclerotic angiopathy this kind of lesion was only found in 17.5% of the cases.

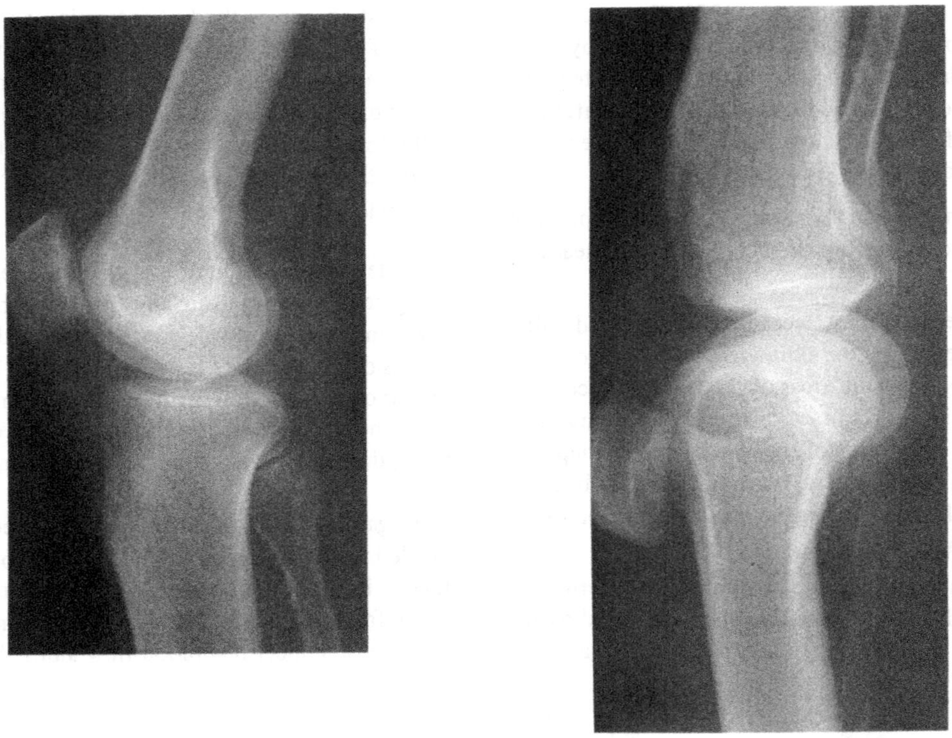

Fig. 42. S. T. 59 year old woman with a history of diabetes of only 2 years. Treatment: diet alone. Spontaneous arteriography of the femoralis, poplitea and tibialis posterior arteries.

Fig. 45, 46, 47, 48, 49 are photographic reproductions of such lesions on the lower limbs in several diabetic patients.

The investigation of the peripheral circulation should be completed by a number of procedures investigating possible signs of associated diabetic neuropathy (alterations in deep sensivity, abolished reflexes, high albumin level in the cerebrospinal fluid, etc.) [6]. The association of diabetic neuropathy once more stresses the specific character of diabetic macroangiopathy.

As a result of all these investigations it was found that in many cases of diabetes mellitus besides a major vascular obstruction there are several other points in the limbs of the diabetic patient where blood flow is diminished. It was concluded that if the general course of the arteriopathic process is slow enough, there is a tendency to build up a collateral circulation [152].

It is also of the utmost importance for the planning of a therapeutic approach whether local infection exists and whether X-rays show up any local osteolytic process. As for the general condition of the patient, other localizations of diabetic macroangiopathy or microangiopathy should be investigated.

3. Prognosis in Peripheral Diabetic Macroangiopathy

Prognosis differs in diabetic macroangiopathy from that in atherosclerotic peripheral angiopathy firstly because much smaller areas are involved in the former than in the latter, and secondly because

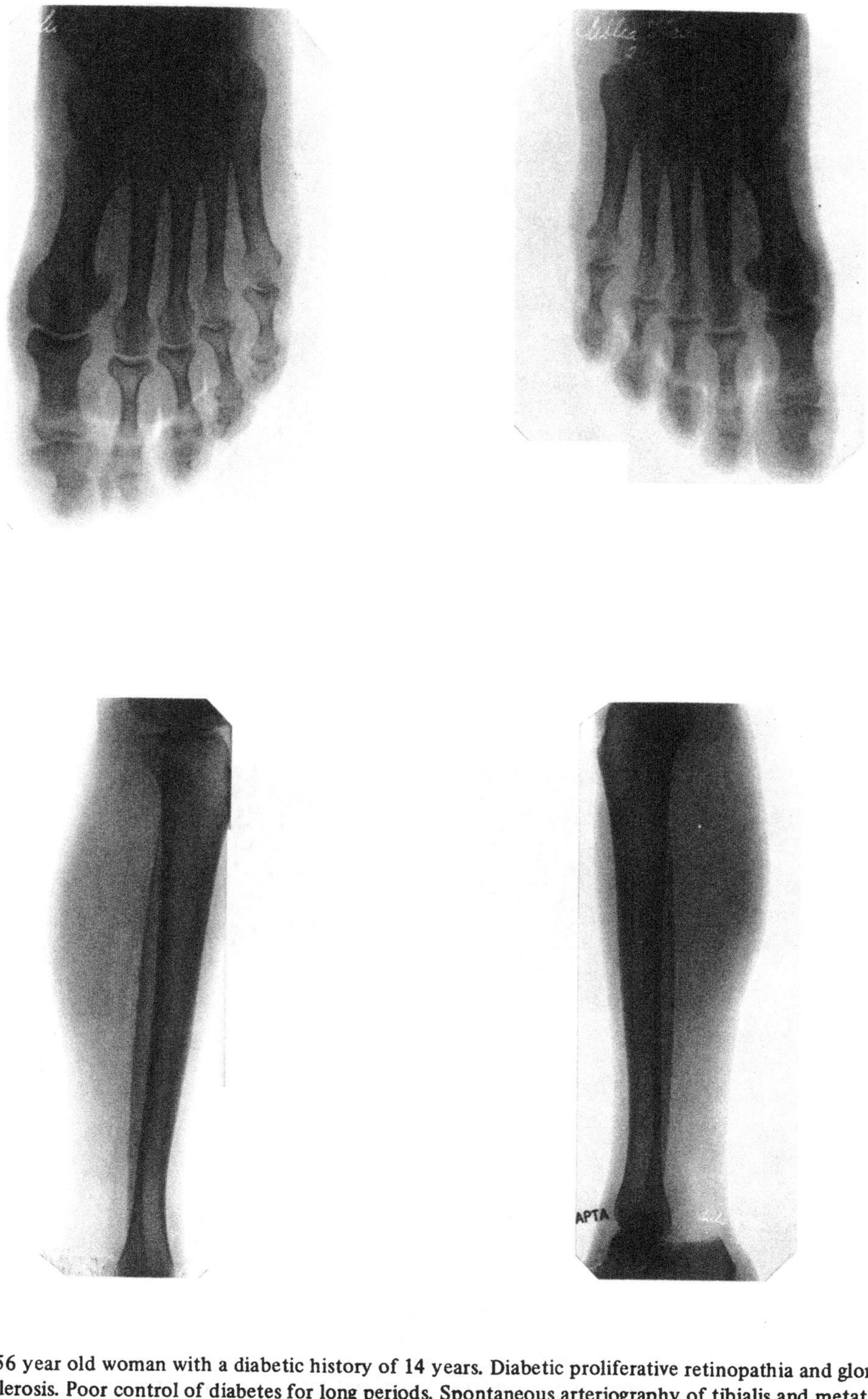

Fig. 43. M. I. 56 year old woman with a diabetic history of 14 years. Diabetic proliferative retinopathia and glomerulosclerosis. Poor control of diabetes for long periods. Spontaneous arteriography of tibialis and metatarseae plantarea arteries of the foot.

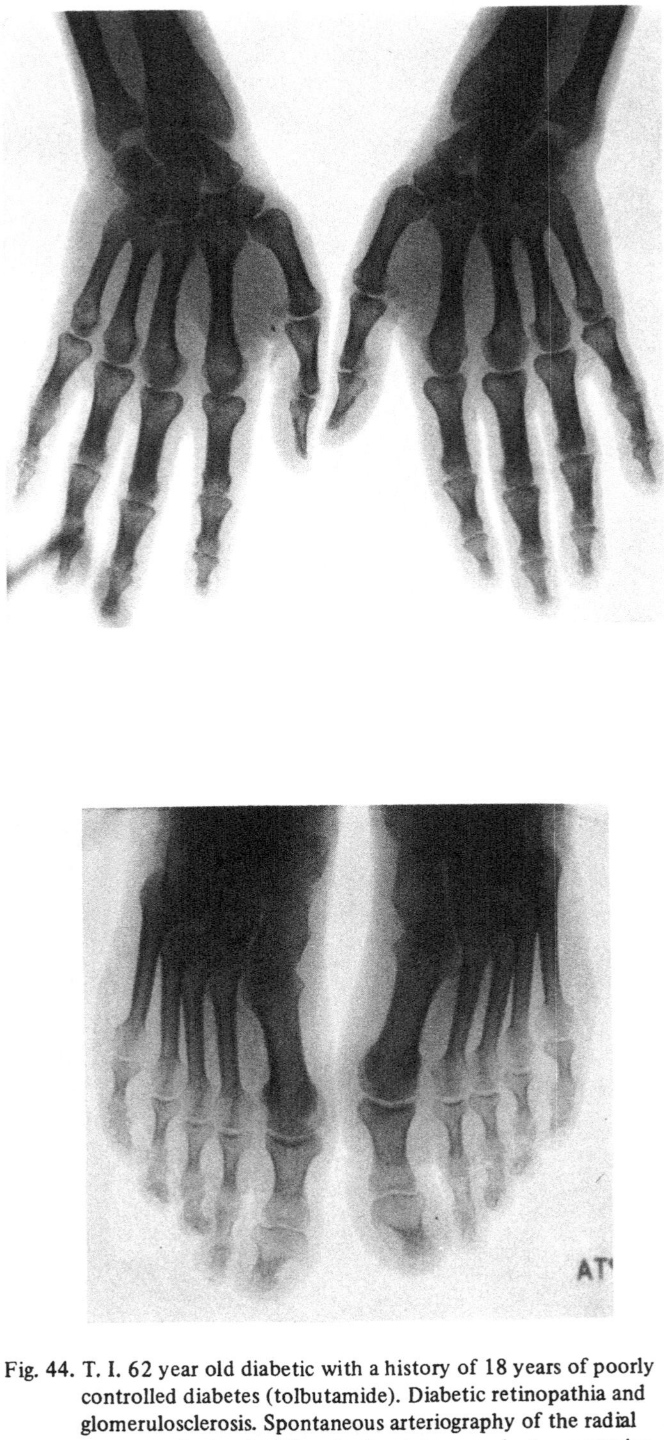

Fig. 44. T. I. 62 year old diabetic with a history of 18 years of poorly controlled diabetes (tolbutamide). Diabetic retinopathia and glomerulosclerosis. Spontaneous arteriography of the radial artery on the hands (A) and of metatarseae plantares arteries on the legs (B).

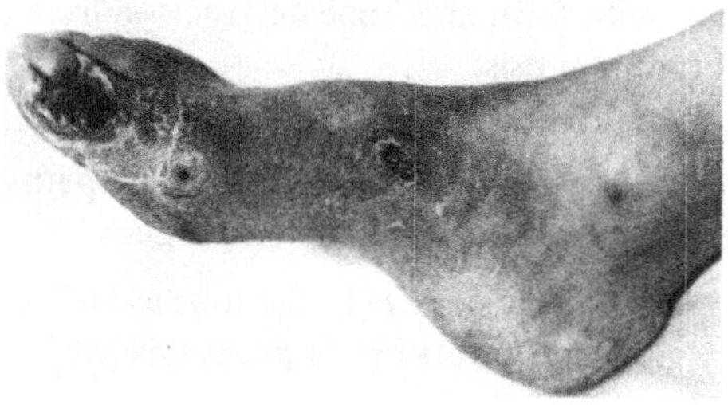

Fig. 45. Mature diabetes mellitus in a man aged 51. Insulinodependent discontinuous management with insulin. Parcelar lesions on the skin of the foot.

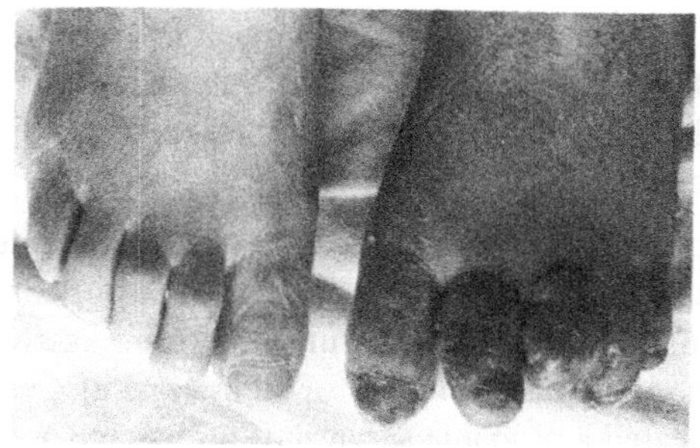

Fig. 47. Clinical aspect of the patient in fig. 41. Infected gangrene of the 3rd and 4th toes with inflammatory oedema of the leg.

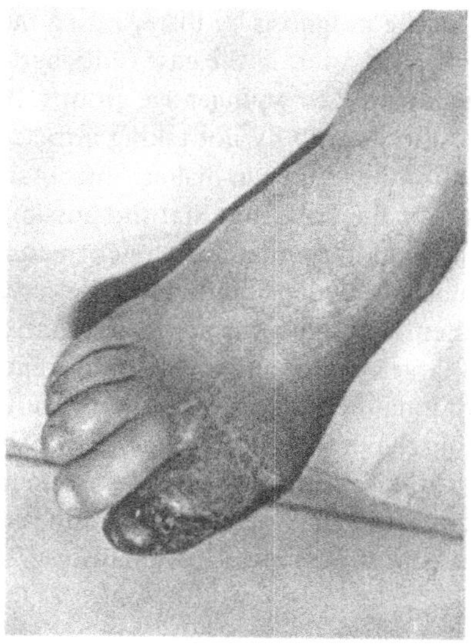

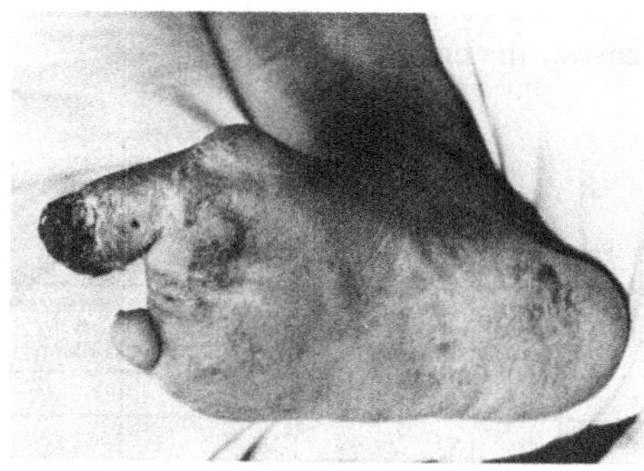

Fig. 48. B. I. Maturity onset diabetes in a man aged 50, after 10 years of poorly controlled illness. Cutaneous gangrene of the skin and deeper lesions of the thumb. Three other toes amputated following the evolution of the same process.

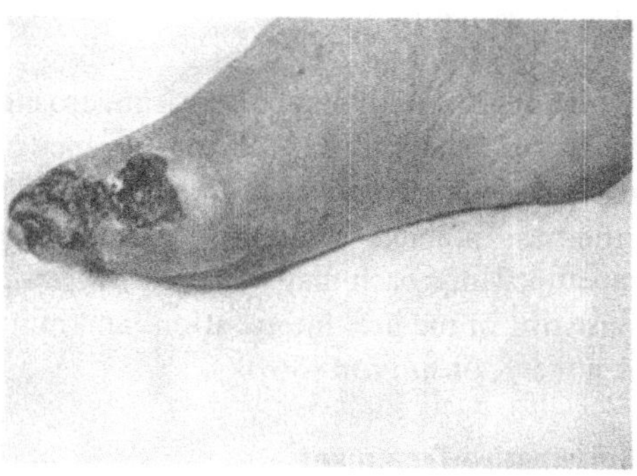

Fig. 46. (A, B) S. M. Superficial necrosis of the thumb in a 62 year old diabetic woman. Inflammatory reactions of the neighbouring areas of the leg.

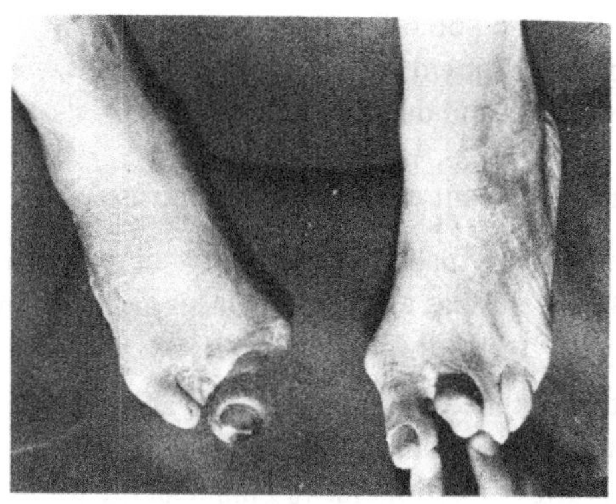

Fig. 49. Progressive gangrene of the toes in a mature diabetes (age 63 years), insulinodependent, discontinuous management with insulin.

the average age of patients is much lower with the diabetic complication. On the other hand, the diabetic condition itself is another differentiating element.

Enquiries concerning prognosis yielded variable results. Such an enquiry, performed in our clinic on 651 diabetic patients suffering from macroangiopathy and watched for an interval of 4 years, indicated a probable survival of 66.5% and a death rate of 25% (8.5% of the patients did not answer the enquiry) (see Table XIII). This data may be compared with a similar enquiry performed in patients with atherosclerotic peripheral ischaemia, in which the average death rate over 7 years was 21.26 %, and 65.8 % survived (the remainder did not answer the enquiry) [182].

Table XII. Symptomatology and stadial frequence of diabetic and atherosclerotic angiopathy.

YEAR	INITIAL NR. OF SUBJECTS	STILL LIVING AT THE END OF 1968	DELEADED TILL THE END OF 1968	NON-RESPONDING TO THE INQUIRE
1964	205	116 (56.8%)	58	31
1965	164	105 (64 %)	42	17
1966	187	131 (70 %)	50	6
1967	95	80 (84.2%)	13	2
TOTAL	651	432 (66.5%)	163 (25%)	56

If conservative treatment is applied, a recovery chance of 55–66.6% is to be expected [61]. Surgical treatment is necessary in 28.9–42.5% of the patients and death occurs in 6.6–18.5% [13].

Other important elements in prognosis:

- hereditary diabetes: appearance of gangrene in such cases has a worse prognosis and the tendency to recur is higher;
- the presence among immediate antecedents of a myocardial infarction, vascular cerebral injuries or peripheral vascular calcifications also favour a recurrence;
- in the obese, recovery is more difficult and recurrence more frequent;
- cases with fever and bone destruction have a worse prognosis;
- the presence of renal microangiopathy worsens the prognosis, while ocular microangiopathy seems to have no influence on prognosis;
- presence of pulse wave in the foot as well as dry gangrene have a better prognosis [61].

One might conclude from the above that the prognosis in diabetic macroangiopathy does not appear either better or worse than in atherosclerotic peripheral angiopathy. Such a conclusion implies both an overestimation and an underestimation of the prognosis. It underestimates the severity of the prognosis by disregarding the fact that death rates refer, in the case of diabetic macroangiopathy, to younger age groups. It overestimates the severity by not taking into account the fact that the lesions in diabetic macroangiopathy cover smaller areas and that the possibility of improving lipid dysmetabolism by correcting diabetic imbalance widens the field of conservative management and improves prognosis. Statistical study of larger groups and comparative data obtained from long-term observations are required for elucidating the problem of prognosis, which also depends on the continuous progress of therapy. New therapeutic approaches may at any time change the most pessimistic estimations.

4. Treatment of Peripheral Diabetic Macroangiopathy

The treatment of peripheral diabetic macroangiopathy should take into account the presence or absence of gangrene, as well as its extension and whether it is infected. Practically speaking, the therapeutical approach may be either *conservative* – consisting of medical interventions and minor local surgery, or *surgical* [36].

a) Conservative Treatment

The *hygiene* and *diet* prescribed in peripheral diabetic macroangiopathy, with some further indications concerning the limb affected by the obstructive process, are similar to those recommended in coronary angiopathy. Footwear should be warm, flexible and wide. Woollen stockings are indicated [75, 125, 128], excepting in cases of gangrenous wounds on the foot [35].

The use of hot-water bottles and prolonged hot baths, or of alternative hot and cold baths, may be harmful. The feet should be washed for 2–3 minutes in water at 30° C, possibly using soap but not rubbing. Much care should be given to avoid any new injury when cutting nails, corns, etc. [35].

Rest cures are recommended in severe cases with intensive pain. The position of the involved limb should be frequently changed, in order to avoid the formation of eschars.

Exercise may consist in massage, movements performed in bed, or walking, and must be prescribed taking into account the particulars of each case, since any effort requires an increased blood supply. If no lesion is affecting circulation, the exercise called "interval training" might be recommended. It consists in swift walking (two steps per second), stopping when the first pains occur, and walking on when they subside. Climbing of stairs is recommended in cases where impairment of blood supply is localized in the thigh. All these recommendations rely on the fact that the best way to improve muscular blood supply is muscular effort [105, 71].

The management of skin lesions by local thermotherapy is limited by the hazard of burns.

Peripheral blood supply may also be increased by light baths of the chest, which bring about a generalized hyperhaemia, or by hot baths of parts of the body (e. g. hot hip bath). The above and all the other vasodilatory procedures are controversial as to their efficacy.

As far as drug therapy is concerned, the recommendation made for diabetic myocardial macroangiopathy should be supplemented as follows:

The anticoagulant therapy.

Heparin is often given in peripheral diabetic macroangiopathy in intramuscular or intravenous injections of 5,000 I. U. every second day with a view to preventing the progress of vascular obliteration [105]. It is nevertheless difficult to estimate the extent to which it interferes in the vascular process of diabetic macroangiopathy. Rutstein [147] reported that the intravenous administration of heparin results in a release of NEFA from triglycerides, probably because of the activation of lipoprotein-lipase. The rise in NEFA goes hand in hand with an intracellular storage of lipids, particularly marked in the cases with high serum cholesterol. Although the process is reversible, it does not appear indicated in the treatment of macroangiopathy.

Conglomeration of red cells, a process related by some authors, to changes in the homeostasy of serum lipids, was occasionally found on capillaroscopy in diabetic patients. It was presumed that this sludging is hampering blood flow in the small vessels, and colloidal substances, such as Perison and Rheomacrodex have been recommended in order to prevent it. The results have been satisfactory in certain cases. This therapy should be used in cases of prenecrosis or even in necrosis of the tissues [35].

Vasodilator therapy. This treatment is justified only if functional spastic elements are present. But the spastic theory is regarded with ever increasing scepticism and it has even been presumed that a compensating dilation is found beyond the organic obstruction of the artery [35]. This might explain the finding that the intravenous administration of a vasodilator drug results, by its general effect, in an undesired lowering of the blood supply in the affected limb.

Recent findings suggest that in order to stimulate and develop the collateral vessels, a better approach may be the intra-arterial administration, perhaps in prolonged infusions, of vasodilator substances, such as a 0.5–1 % solution of procaine (10 ml) together with 10 mg of ATP or some calcium preparation in a 10 % concentration. The advantage consists in the fact that such a mixture, if introduced intra-arterially, is partly inactivated before it reaches the general circulation, and its undesired general vasodilator effect does not occur [71].

ATP may be used in doses of 20–40 mg in prolonged intra-arterial infusions into the femoral artery lasting for some 20 minutes. Laevulose is recommended as the solvent for the ATP [117].

Local circulation can also be improved by various procedures lowering the sympathetic tone of the affected limb, e. g. regional sympathetic block with procaine, the appliance of ultrashort waves or infra-red radiation on the paravertebral area, etc. Lumbar or perifemoral sympathectomy [36] may be performed, possibly associated with suprarenal medullosclerosis according to the procedure described by Turai, Mandache and Gerota. If, however, performed in a too advanced stage of the macroangiopathic process, this intervention may result in deterioration of the ischaemic process. Some improvement may also be expected from the application of constant galvanic current or of modulated current [35] in the neighbourhood of the ischaemic lesion.

Medical treatment modifying arterial pressure. It is not recommended to give hypotensive drugs in the fourth stage of peripheral diabetic macroangiopathy, if not required for reasons pertaining to the general condition [181]. On the contrary, the peripheral collateral vessels should be forced to open by hypertensive therapy [35].

A joint Danish and Swedish team obtained satisfactory results [5] with corticosteroids and sodium chloride, as hypertensive agents, in obtaining a lasting rise of 15–20 mm Hg in order to facilitate peripheral circulation. 9-α-fluoro-17-hydroxy-corticosterone-acetate was used for this purpose in daily doses of 10 mg, with 5–15 gm of sodium chloride, given in capsules each containing 0.25 gm. The dosage was adapted according to the individual response. This therapy was given for intervals up to 16 months and in the end the steroid dosage was progressively reduced while sodium chloride was suddenly discontinued.

Other recommendations should be: prohibition of smoking, about one hour's daily walk, lower positioning of the affected limb in bed during sleep (some 30 cm lower). In 40 subjects ulcerations subsided following the carrying out of these recommendations. Steroid therapy cannot be applied in patients with myocardial infarction, with clinical signs of left ventricular failure and with an electrocardiographic picture indicating necrosis or ischaemia. In 20% of the patients, the administration of steroids brought about oedema in the lower limbs and moderate headache, which subsided when the dosage of steroid and salt was reduced.

Trophic therapy is often recommended and consists in placenta extracts and some protein-free preparations from calf blood. Such preparations showed favourable effects on cell cultures, but their positive effect on diabetic gangrene is not yet established.

Fibrinolytic therapy aims at activating the process of fibrinolysis. It has been recently demonstrated that 52% of the vasculopathic patients under the age of 50 have a low fibrinolytic activity, as well as 34% of the patients aged between 50 and 59 years [24, 25]. The finding is of the utmost interest as far as diabetics are concerned, since the trend to vascular accidents is just as high in diabetic subjects as in non-diabetic atherosclerotic patients.

Certain preparations which activate the fibrinolytic processes, such as streptokinase, are indicated in acute arterial thrombosis and recent emboli [35]. The starting dose ranges between 200,000 and 1,500,000 units during the first 30 minutes following the accident. Subsequent doses of 100,000 units should be given at an hour's interval [74].

Favourable results can be obtained with these preparations if several rules of timing and localization are observed. Thus, for the femoral artery, it should be applied when the occlusion is not older than six weeks while for the iliac artery if the occlusion is not older than three months [102].

There are other, less effective preparations, which might be given for longer intervals, such as biguanides, which also contribute to restoring diabetic metabolic balance [25, 52, 53, 54].

Among tested biguanides, metformin and formin proved effective for short intervals in increasing fibrinolytic activity.

Sulphonamides, testosterone, corticosteroids and the anabolic steroids are effective as well. Long-term effects may be obtained by associating the administration of a biguanide preparation with ethyloestrol, an anabolic steroid. This association not only activates the fibrinolytic process, but also reduces the plasma level of fibrin and the adhesiveness of blood platelets. The association with phenformin also reduces serum cholesterol level. The following daily doses have been recommended: formin 1–1.5 gm, phenformin 100 mg and ethyloestrol 4 mg twice daily [18].

b) Surgical Treatment

Surgical intervention becomes necessary if the gangrene involves one or several phalanges and particularly if infection is present. The rate at which the arterial obstruction progresses should also be taken into account.

Surgery should be preceded by appropriate antibiotic therapy and by several perfusions with heparin, in order to control infection and thrombosis.

If there is an arteriosclerotic arteritis occurring against a diabetic background and the obliteration is situated above the knee, the only solution is amputation, since conservative surgical interventions are generally ineffective, because of the deterioration of the vascular bed below [36].

Reparatory surgical interventions are seldom possible, but they are, however, advisable in cases of progressive claudication originating in obliterations of the aorta or iliac arteries. Sympathectomy is often effective [37].

On the contrary, if the case is one of typical diabetic arteriopathy and the gangrene is small, localized and the skin of the foot is reasonably healthy, it is recommended to perform small local exeresis, with or without removing the head of the metacarpal or metatarsal bones. Lumbar sympathectomy may also be associated with local surgery.

Chapter VI Cutaneous and Muscular Angiopathy in Diabetis Mellitus

A. Cutaneous Angiopathy in Diabetes Mellitus

The great sensitiveness of the diabetic's skin is unanimously acknowledged. It was demonstrated by Bürger [7] and Knobloch [28] by the photometry of the intensity of actinic erythema in normal and diabetic subjects. The multitude of cutaneous affections in diabetics is the clinical evidence of the increased vulnerability of the skin to exogenous as well as endogenous agents. The metabolic disturbances in diabetes cannot fully account for such manifestations and recent researches seems to indicate, for some of these affections, a vascular aetiology.

Forms of diabetic cutaneous angiopathy. The numerous cutaneous manifestations of diabetes can be roughly classified into two large categories:

- primary cutaneous manifestations
- secondary cutaneous manifestations.

Secondary modifications are those pathological changes accompanying some of the late, major diabetic complications, such as, for instance, trophic ulcerations, limited skin atrophies secondary to diabetic neuropathy, the tendency for furunculosis, micosis, eczema, pruritus etc [18]. This group also includes skin changes secondary to ischaemia.

Primary cutaneous manifestations of diabetes are those that can be included in the picture of microangiopathies. Some of them are without symptoms [6, 12, 15, 32, 36, 39] their presence being shown up only by histological findings in a biopsy of the skin; others acquire a certain specificity which is reflected in their names. For example, the so-called necrobiosis lipoidica diabeticorum, which seems to be the result of a localized diabetic angiopathy. The other primary modifications, such as xanthodermia and cutaneous xanthoms have a predominantly metabolic pathogenesis, the vascular factor being of minor importance.

Necrobiosis Lipoidica Diabeticorum (NLD)

NLD is a relatively rare condition. Jung [28] found it to occur in one case out of 1,200 known diabetic patients, that is 0,08%. Most authors consider that it is not specific to diabetes mellitus [49], yet 80–90% of cases occur in diabetics, which might justify the name of diabeticorum. It is frequently met with in women. It usually appears between the ages of 20–40 although it may be found at any age. NLD is more frequent in patients with juvenile and unstable diabetes.

In our statistics the condition was found in two cases out of 3,679 diabetic patients admitted to hospital during the 1964–1967 interval (0.05%). Both patients were female, one aged 26 and suffering from a lipoatrophic diabetes mellitus [40], and the other, aged 47, suffering from an unstable, insulin dependent diabetes which began at the age of 31. In the history of both both patients several long intervals of metabolic decompensation were recorded, without coma but with high blood sugar values.

Necrobiosis lipoidica diabeticorum is often associated with other late complications of diabetes mellitus, such as retinopathy and nephropathy. This aspect will be detailed below. As for the two patients mentioned above, both had diffuse glomerulosclerosis and the younger one also had a diabetic retinopathy with multiple punctiform haemorrhages.

It was claimed by some authors [24] that arterial hypertension promotes the onset of the cutaneous complication. Blood pressure was normal in our patients.

Trauma has also been incriminated as a precipitating agent of the complication [18].

As far as *pathogenesis* is concerned, the majority of authors admit that the disease consists of microangiopathic alterations of the vessels situated at the borderline of the derma and epidermis, extracellular accumulation of lipids of the phospatide group [18] and degeneration and necrobiosis of the collagen.

The dysmetabolic, hyperlipaemic background most often underlying necrobiosis lipoidica was already discussed in Chapter II (p. 18) and Chapter V (p. 143).

The patchy distribution of the lesions on the skin is consistent with the general features of diabetic angiopathy, in that the condition, although widespread, is predominantly localized in preferential sites.

Clinical aspects of necrobiosis lipoidica diabeticorum. The disease may occur spontaneously or subsequent to trauma of variable intensity. It takes the form of circumscribed infiltrates with a yellowish shiny central area. This area often undergoes necrosis and the resulting small ulcerations heal in a few weeks leaving a pigmented scar [18]. This kind of eruption is mostly found on the lower limbs, especially on the thigh, the ankle and on the dorsal side of the foot, and sometimes on the ventral side of the leg (Fig. 1).

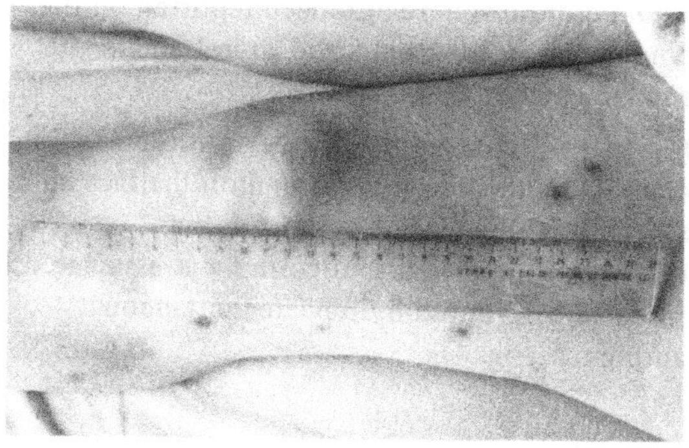

Fig. 1. B. E. 47 year old woman. Unstable diabetes with long periods of metabolic imbalance. Necrobiosis lipoidica of the lower limb.

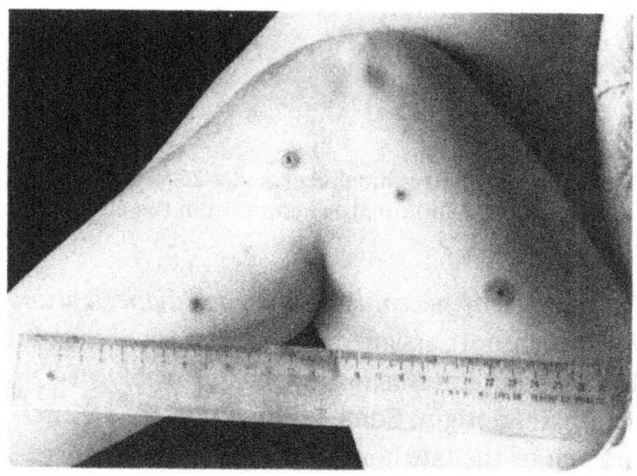

Fig. 2. Same patient as in fig. 1.

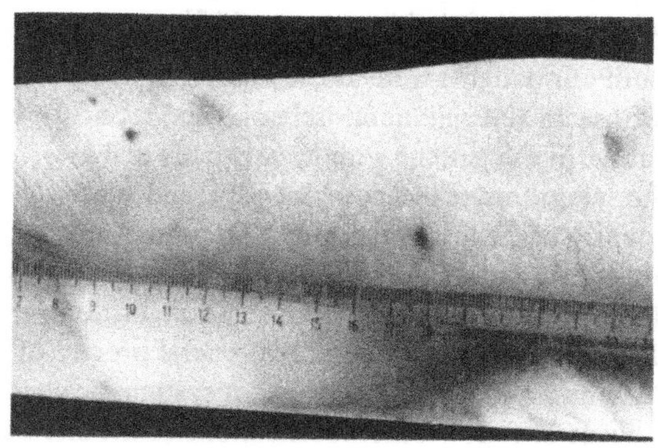

Fig. 3. Same patient as in fig. 1. Necrobiosis lipoidica on the arm and forearm.

Similar eruptions have also been reported on the shoulder, neck, breast and the lateral side of the arm and forearm (Fig. 2 and 3).

One case of lipoatrophic diabetes was reported in which such infiltrates were found on the face and especially on the nose. In this case, the necrobiosis lipoidica diabeticorum was associated, preceded or followed by repeated cutaneous xanthomas (Fig. 4).

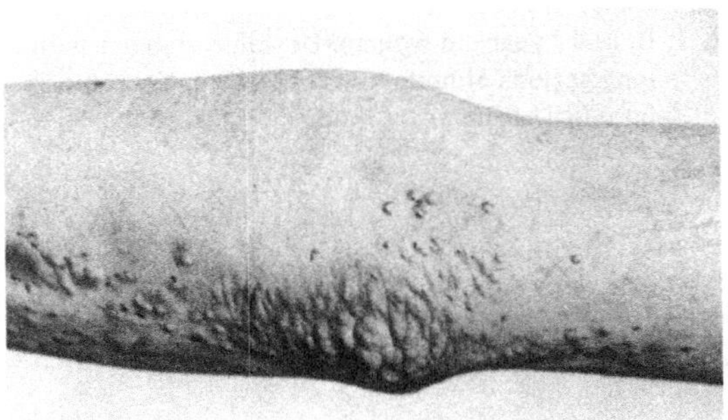

Fig. 4. L. G. Lipoatrophic diabetes in a 26 year old woman. Xanthomatous eruption in the elbow area.

Significance of necrobiosis lipoidica diabeticorum. Various authors assigned a different significance to these skin alterations, regarded as probably of angiopathic origin. Some authors consider them just one of the late complications of diabetic angiopathy [1]. According to others, they represent a sort of prelude or a warning signal indicating that the course of the disease is changing and the angiopathic process begins to affect other organs of vital importance [25].

Both our patients were already suffering from diffuse diabetic glomerulosclerosis and retinopathy. In the patient with lipoatrophic diabetes, the symptoms of macroangiopathy, and subsequently of diabetic neuropathy, appeared shortly after the onset of the necrobiosis. These two cases do not suggest different interpretation, but only that necrobiosis is a part of the general process of diabetic angiopathy, and does not systematically precede or follow other localizations of the disease. It therefore cannot display information concering the stage of the complication in other organs.

B. Muscular Diabetic Angiopathy

The place held by certain functional disorders of the striated and the smooth muscles within diabetic angiopathy is still an unsettled problem of the pathology of diabetes mellitus. On one hand, some of the muscular disorders seem to be due to diabetic neuropathy (see Chapter VII, p. 192), and on the other hand, there is no correspondence between the pathomorphological and ultrastructural alterations of the muscle fibres and clinical symptomatology. In many cases, the muscular alterations are consequently ignored throughout the course of the diabetic disease. It seems that the incidence of muscular involvement is very high if investigated by biopsy procedures, but very low if based on clinical symptoms.

There are very few data regarding the incidence of muscular angiopathy in diabetes mellitus. It was claimed, for instance, that the basement membrane of muscle supplying vessels is thickened in 98% of the diabetic patients [46] but there is some evidence that such an alteration is present already in the non-apparent stages of diabetes and, according to some authors, even in prediabetes. The atrophy of the first dorsal interosseous muscle was described as an early symptom in diabetes mellitus [5]. Since a correct diagnosis depends on systematic biopsy, it seems unlikely that extensive statistics will be obtained on this matter in the near future (see Chapter II, p. 18).

The light and electron microscopic investigations may show two kinds of histological and ultrastructural alterations in the muscle:

a) alterations in the small muscular vessels
b) alterations in the muscle cells, subsequent to ischaemia and to the general dysmetabolic state of diabetes mellitus.

As for the alterations of the small muscular vessels, typical aspects of diabetic angiopathy have been reported (see Chapter II, p. 31–32 and Figs. 17 and 18):

- thickening of the basement membrane (Figs. 5 and 6) in the small muscular vessels. According to some authors, this process represents a specific lesion of the diabetic syndrome itself and is not a consequence of hyperglycaemia [22, 46, 53, 54]. Other authors regard it as a non-specific and inconstant phenomenon [50].

hypertrophy of the endothelial vascular cells, tending to reduce and finally obstruct the vascular lumen (Fig. 5 and especially Fig. 6).

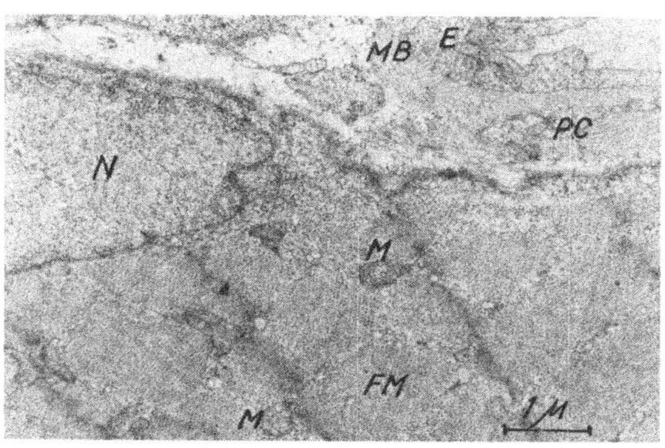

Fig. 5. S. F. 38 year old woman. Duration of diabetes about 6 years. Associated obesity. Muscle biopsy on the shank with Menghini's needle. Small vessel with thickened basement membrane (BM) which includes a pericyte (PC). Moderate hypertrophy of the vessel's endothelium (E). N = nucleus of a muscle cell. Transverse section of muscle fibres (FM) with numerous mitochondrias (M) (13,500 x).

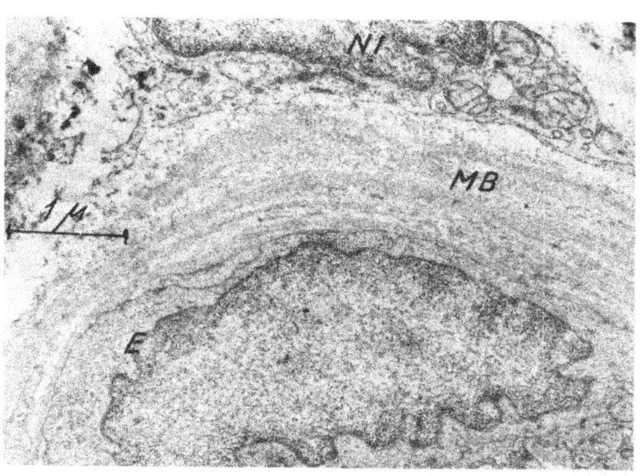

Fig. 6. Same patient as in fig. 5. Thickened basement membrane (MB) with obvious lamellar structure. Hypertrophied endothelial cell (E) which is prominent in the vascular lumen. NI = interstitial cell nucleus. M = mitochondria (20,000 x).

The modifications occurring in the muscle cells is the second element worth emphasizing. It seems likely that they are mostly a consequence of local ischaemia following the obstructive processes and the reduction of transparietal filtration in the vessels supplying the respective muscle. Other modifications were also described: an increased number of central nuclei, presence of phagocytes and necrotic fibres, and groups of isolated, thin fibres; the degenerative atrophy of muscular fibres as well as a decrease of cholinesterase and succindehydrase activity were considered of neurogenic origin [27]. But the process may also be regarded as a result of the effects exerted over a long interval by the general dysmetabolic state peculiar to diabetes meliitus, and particularly by the relative protein deficiency associated with the disease [38]. The ultrastructural findings will be further detailed since these have rarely been described in the diabetic.

In experimental studies performed on non-diabetic starved rats, it was found that in the muscle fibres of the skeletal muscles, the sarcolemma is of a sinuous, folded shape [14, 50]. The number of mitochondria is very low, especially around the nucleus.

The modifications of mitochondrial cristae as well as mitochondrial dilation were described during myocardic hypoxia. In experimental ischaemia in rats the same mitochondrial modification were noticed, associated with swelling and vacuolization of the endoplasmic reticulum [20].

Following protein deficiency induced in the monkey, it was reported that the myofibrillae become particularly thin, some sarcomeres are destroyed and the mitochondria grow large and irregular in shape [42].

In the areas of induced ischaemia, many myofibrillae preserve their integrity, but others in the I bands, including the Z strip, disintegrate. In these circumstances the A zones remain unchanged for a long interval. This appearance was named *discoid necrosis* [14].

Ultrastructure studies in the ischaemic muscle fields also showed swelling of the mitochondria and the transformation of the sarcoplasmic reticulum into vesicles.

These experimental data are reported in order to demonstrate the similarity between the ultrastructural alterations obtained in experimental pathology and those found in the muscle cells of the diabetic subjects.

A series of biopsies of the posterior muscles of the leg were performed in diabetic patients admitted to our clinic with symptoms of peripheral macroangiopathy in its functional stage.

Considering the above ultrastructural findings, certain of the observed aspects seem to be particularly significant.

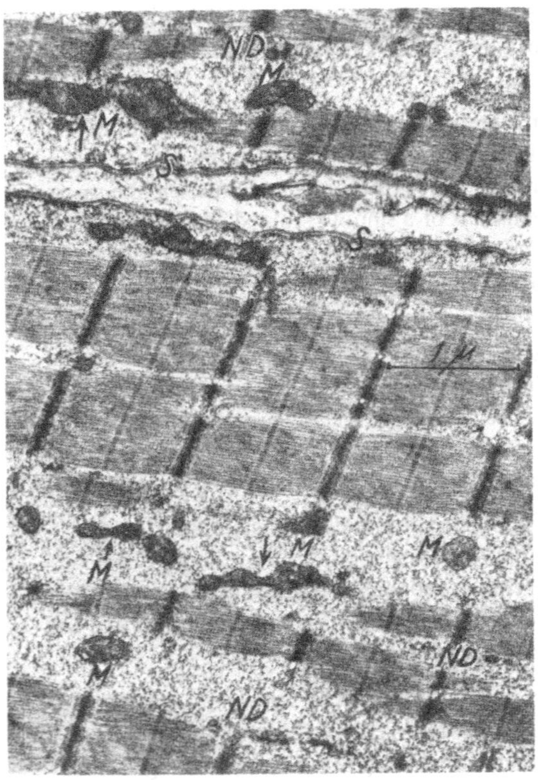

Fig. 7. L. S. diabetic man with intermittent claudication. Maturity onset diabetes mellitus. Poor control with insulin. Festooned sarcolemma (S). Decreased number of mitochondria (M) which are of various sizes and irregular form (arrow). Discoid necrosis (ND) with destruction of the "Z" band (27,000 x).

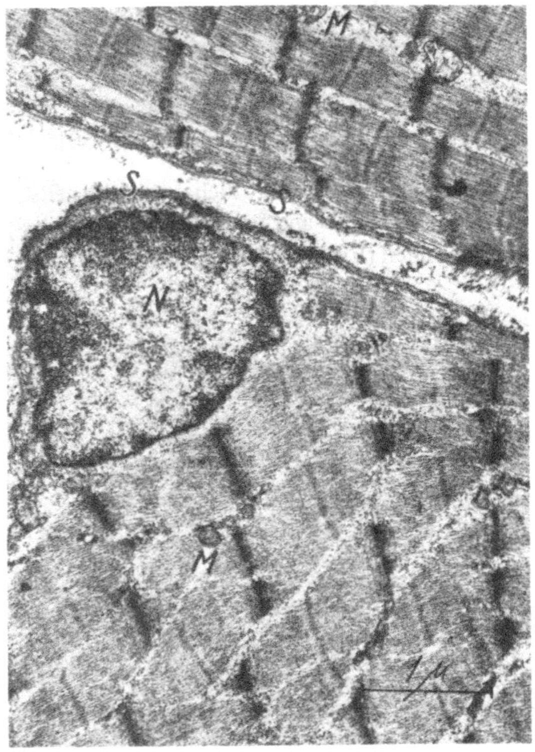

Fig. 8. Same patient as in fig. 7. Decreased mitochondrial numbers (M) especially in the perinuclear area (N). Tendency of the sarcolemma to fold (S) (27,000 x).

Sinuous and folded sarcolemma were frequently found (Figs. 7 and 8). Mitochondrial abnormalities, especially around the nucleus (Figs. 8 and 9) were observed in almost every muscle preparation. At the same time, the mitochondria situated far from the nucleus were large and irregular (Figs. 7, 9 and 10). Many of the myofibrillae were normal (Figs. 7, 9 and 10), but here and there the process of "discoid necrosis" was observed (Figs. 7, 9 and 10) sometimes completely destroying the "Z" strip (Figs. 7 and 8).

Finally, the aspects of vesicular alteration of the sarcoplasmic reticulum were quite frequent (Figs. 9 and 10).

Summarizing all these observations:

a) the diabetic angiopathy of the vessels in the skeletal muscle results in the characteristic

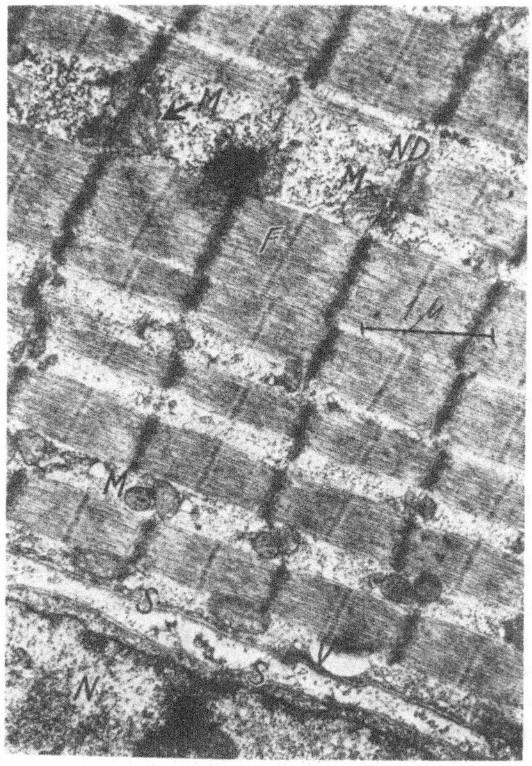

Fig. 9. Same patient as in fig. 7. Decreased mitochondrial number (M) with irregular aspect, sometimes with increased volume (arrow). Normal looking myofibriles (F). Discoid necrosis (ND). Vesicular transformation of the sarcoplasmic reticulum (V). Tendency of the sarcolemma to fold (S). Nucleus in a muscle cell (N) with a nucleolus inside (27,000 x).

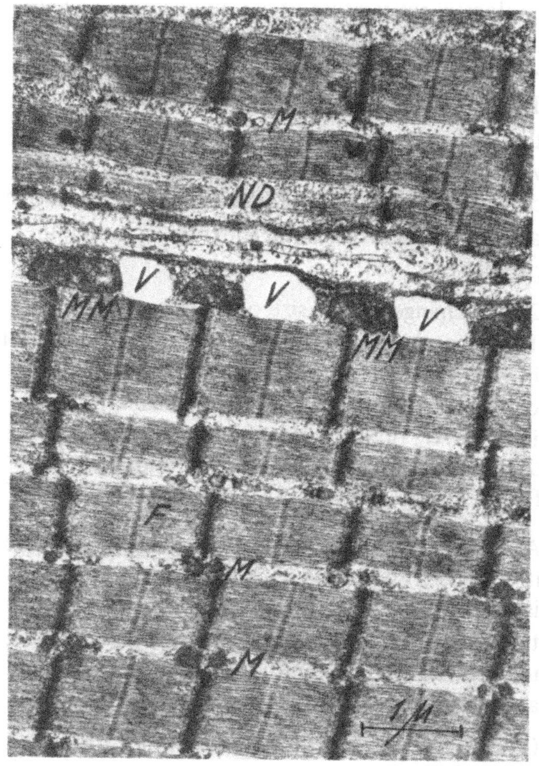

Fig. 10. Same patient as in fig. 7. Normal-looking myofibriles (F). Normal mitochondria (M) and with increased volume (MM). Vesicular transformation of the sarcoplasmic reticulum (V). Discoid necrosis (ND) (27,000 x).

appearance of total starvation and protein starvation as well as in aspects similar to those found in experimental muscular ischaemia, and

b) there is no tendency in the process to spread over all the myofibrillae, as many of them are found undamaged.

These observations are consistant with the findings reported in the human diabetic liver, where ultrastructural investigation of the parenchyma and even of the endothelial cells (see Chapter II, Figs. 48, 49, 50, 51, 52, 53, 54, 55 and 56) showed the same alterations as those found in total and in protein starvation [38]. This phenomenon seems to be a part of the integral pathology of diabetes mellitus.

Several different factors appear to intervene in the pathogenesis of the angiopathic alteration of the muscle in diabetes mellitus. These factors originate either in alterations of the supplying vessels, or in the general dysmetabolic state generated by diabetic disease.

Two main and essentially vascular processes may be regarded as acting upon the muscle fibres.

1. The alterations in the basement membrane of the small vessels. They may represent the mor-

phological substratum of certain disorders occurring in the transparietal migration of nutrients, of hormones (insulin) and of the breakdown products of muscular activity. It may be assumed that the alteration of the selective function of the vascular wall, as far as its permeability is concerned [11, 12, 13] can result in various metabolic abnormalities in all compartments, including the protein one [41].

2. The changes in the size of the vascular lumen. This second element, associated with the alteration in vascular permeability, may bring about relative or absolute ischaemia in certain areas. The resulting hypoxia or anoxia is more significant as the tissue involved requires a good blood supply for its specific activity [2, 3, 13].

As regards the metabolic state of the muscle tissue itself, and it should be remembered that the latter is one of the main sites of insulin activity [35], the diabetic state may generate disorders resulting in observable alterations in muscular morphology and function.

It may be supposed that the relative insufficiency in insulin – as in the experiments of Butterfield [8, 9, 10] or the absence of insulin activity, generates a state similar to protein deficiency Besides its effects on the metabolism of carbohydrates, insulin is known to enhance protein synthesis in muscle [30]. A relative or absolute insulin deficiency is most likely to disturb this function and even if such an alteration cannot result by itself in the classical picture of total protein deficiency, it might at least partly achieve it in conjunction with a vascular alteration consisting of ischaemia and low permeability.

Recent research shows that in experimental diabetes the ability of muscle ribosomes to synthesise proteins is disturbed at the level of information translation [48].

The turnover of glucose in the diabetic muscle is disturbed even in the presence of an adequate amount of insulin [26, 34]. This may also be related to a disorder in the metabolism of protein, since some experimental studies indicate that certain peptides can delay the breakdown of insulin in the muscle. A state of protein deficiency, caused by low intake or of dysmetabolic origin, may result in a defective utilization of insulin in the metabolism of the muscle [52].

The above processes may also be related to the disorders of growth hormone (HGH) or of the adrenocortical hormones [26, 43], and the consecutive alterations in the intracellular transport of glucose and in the phosphorylation of glucose by hexokinase [43].

The mitochondrial changes reported in the muscle cells of the diabetic subject (Figs. 7, 8, 9 and 20) may also play a role in the inadequate insulin activity, as it is considered that the intracellular metabolic activity of the hormone is preceded by a stage when it is bound to the proteins of the mitochondria [37].

All these hypotheses suggest that there are certain processes which might, in association with the ischaemia consecutive to diabetic angiopathy and with the local and general alterations of protein metabolic pathways, build up a vicious circle resulting in progressive aggravation of the disorders in the skeletal and visceral muscles.

This assumption is supported by the fact that muscular fatigue actually increases with metabolic imbalance in diabetes mellitus. In fact, this is the only clinical symptom which can be assigned to the alterations described in the skeletal muscles. There are obviously several mechanisms which may be responsible for muscular fatigue in the diabetic patient. It may originate in diabetic neuropathy (see Chapter VII, p. 192), or in endogenous hyperlactocidaemia during therapy with biguanides [4, 16], etc. The disorders in intramuscular electrolyte balance may also play a role. It was found during the ketoacidotic states induced in alloxanized rats, that there is a fall in water and potassium in the muscle cell [29]. But such a mechanism is more likely to participate in the acute disorders of diabetes mellitus than in the late complications [33].

The involvement of the muscle fibres in the long evolution of diabetes mellitus should be understood as part of a widespread process, present equally in the skeletal and in the visceral muscles. The role played by visceral diabetic neuropathy in bringing about functional disorders in the viscera is stressed in Chapter VII. It should be emphasized that besides diabetic neuropathy, the secondary muscular alterations following the angiopathic process in the supplying vessels may also be responsible for the clinical and X-ray symptomatology often assigned exclusively to the disorders in the nerve supply of the respective organs.

Chapter VII Diabetic Neuropathy

As far as pathogenesis is concerned, diabetic neuropathies are the most controversial among all the late complications of diabetes mellitus. Some authors categorically include them in the group of diabetic angiopathic disorders, others only partially agree with such a standpoint, while others deny it altogether. Unfortunately, none of the extreme standpoints can cover all the aspects of the rich and manifold picture of diabetic neuropathy, the result being that the concept itself is split in order to be explained, to the disadvantage of both therapy and prophylaxis.

Therefore, the present state of our knowledge can admit neither the purely vascular and ischaemic hypothesis, nor the exclusively dysmetabolic one for the pathogenesis of diabetic neuropathy. Neither hypothesis can wholly account for the results of the pathophysiological investigations.

Hence the inclusion of diabetic neuropathies in a study on diabetic angiopathy is fully justified even if the nervous complications are situated on the borderline between ischaemic and metabolic disorders.

In this context, the term diabetic neuropathy includes every dysfunction or pathological alteration of the central and peripheral nervous system assigned to any other preceding or concomitant pathological condition.

This complication mostly occurs in the late stages of diabetes, and possesses the following characteristics:

- preponderantly affects the lower limbs;
- higher prevalence of sensory disturbances as against motor ones, when the somatic nervous system is affected;
- higher prevalence of motor disturbances as against sensory ones when the autonomic nervous system is affected;
- relative reversibility and mobility of these disturbances.

1. Prevalence

Statistics on the prevalence of diabetic neuropathy are very variable, ranging from 5% to 60% [40, 41] when a complete clinical pattern of neuropathy is considered, while in cases of isolated criteria, such as the diminution of deep bone sensitivity, figures as high as 100% have been reported. For instance, reported data have shown that 30–50% of diabetics suffer from paraesthesia and impairment of reflexes. If disturbances of sensitivity and areflexia are considered, 20–40% of diabetics may be diagnosed as suffering from polyneuritis. If, however, the criterion for diagnosis is the presence of symmetrical paraesthetic manifestations, with motor pareses and muscular atrophy, then the diagnosis of diabetic polyneuritis can be established only in 2–10% of the cases [29].

This wide range of results obviously depends on the various methods of diagnosis and on the differences among the investigated groups with regard to age, duration of the diabetes, etc., and whether the subjects were outpatients or inpatients. It seems, for instance, that statistics from outpatient diabetic populations yield higher figures (50–60%)

[15, 82, 83] than those based on patients admitted to hospital (Figs. between 5–24%) [81].

In our statistics, diabetic neuropathy was found in 259 cases (154 males and 105 females) out of 1,813 subjects investigated and admitted to hospital between 1966 and 1968. This represents an incidence of 14.3% which is very close to that reported recently by Swedish authors (13%) [50] lying between the limits established for inpatients diabetics [87].

Correlation between the duration of diabetes and the incidence of diabetic neuropathy. Almost all statistical reports admit that the hazard of neuropathy increases with the duration of diabetes which justifies the inclusion of the condition among the late complications.

Fig. 1 represents the figures reported in the Swedish statistics [50] compared with those of the Clinic of Metabolic Diseases and Nutrition in Bucharest (Table I). The Swedish authors divided their patients into several groups, with duration of diabetes from 0–5, 6–10, 11–15, 16–20 etc., years [50]. In our statistics, unequal intervals are considered, namely, 0–5, 6–10, 11–20 and over 20 years. A comparison is however possible (Fig. 1) showing the same increase in the number of cases in relation to the duration of the disease. It should be noted that in our statistics the incidence of nervous complications, in the 5–10 years interval group, is already much higher than in the previous group.

All these observations are in contradiction with the opinions stated by Ellenberg [26], namely that there is no correlation between diabetic neuropathy and the duration of diabetes. It should nevertheless, be remembered that it is very difficult to establish the true onset moment of diabetes mellitus. For instance, in the group of patients examined at our clinic, 214 subjects were known as diabetic when the first symptoms of diabetic neuropathy occurred. In the other 45, however, diabetes was not considered at the moment when a peripheral neuritis was found for the first time. All these patients were included in the group of 0–5 years of duration, although their actual diabetic history may have been much longer.

Table I

	Duration of diabetes (yrs.)				Total
	0–5	6–10	11–20	> 21	
Nr. subjects	19	62	125	53	259
Percentage	7.8	23.9	48.2	20.1	100 %

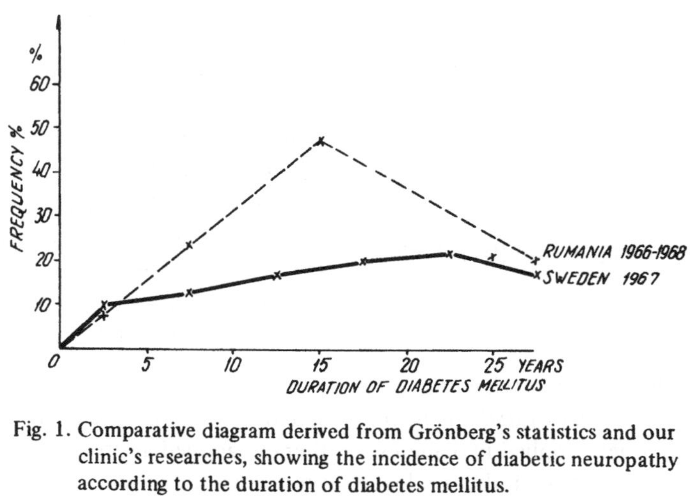

Fig. 1. Comparative diagram derived from Grönberg's statistics and our clinic's researches, showing the incidence of diabetic neuropathy according to the duration of diabetes mellitus.

Before postulating the absence of correlation between diabetic neuropathy and the duration of diabetes, the real difficulties in diagnosing the true onset of diabetes should be weighed and the possibility of error in this respect estimated.

Correlation between the age and sex of the patients and the prevalence of diabetic neuropathy. The age of the patients has no outstanding influence on the onset of diabetic neuropathy, although some authors consider that most of the subjects with diabetic neuropathy are middle-aged adults or even over the age of 40–50 years [38, 64, 85].

Age seems however to be significant as far as the clinical pattern of the complication is concerned. Chronic multineuritis is more frequently encountered in the aged, while subacute aspects occur mostly in the young [76]. Motor complications are more frequent in older patients while the sensory ones show a certain preference for young subjects [39, 40]. Alterations affecting the autonomic nervous system often occur in the young and middle-aged adults, while central neuropathy is the privilege of the old.

According to most authors, the prevalence of diabetic neuropathy [71] does not differ between the sexes. It has been claimed that the complication predominates in women [64] but this seems to correspond to the uneven distribution of diabetes itself.

Diabetic neuropathy seems to have no correlation with the type of diabetes, be it acquired or genetically determined.

In our statistics the number of males [154] exceeds that of females [105]. Similar observations were reported in England by Martin [63] and in France [8, 15].

Correlation between the type of antidiabetic management and the prevalence of diabetic neuropathy. The kind of treatment applied in diabetes seems to exert a certain influence on the incidence of diabetic neuropathy, although the severity of the diabetic condition itself does not seem to be decisive in determining the complication. Neuropathy occurs both in severe and mild cases of diabetes mellitus; the only actually important factor seems to be the degree of metabolic control achieved in the course of time, irrespective of the kind of therapy. It seems even that in mild and apparently more harmless cases, where there is a tendency towards a looser and less rigorous therapeutic control, that there is an increased hazard of secondary complications such as neuropathy. One should remember, however, the observations describing the presence of diabetic neuropathic manifestations in cases of latent diabetes mellitus [7].

The same holds true for the severe cases of diabetes undergoing long intervals of metabolic imbalance [12], but in such patients the acute diabetic accidents require more correct and persevering therapy (Table II).

The unfavourable effect of poor metabolic control over long intervals admitted by most authors is also obvious in our statistics. It seems that only 23.5% of the 259 patients suffering from diabetic neuropathy had good metabolic control, while in the other 76.5% the therapeutic results were poor, therapy was deficient or ignored, and the subjects underwent long intervals of obvious metabolic imbalance (Table II). This is valid for all types of antidiabetic management used during the last decades, namely for restrictive diet, insulin therapy, oral antidiabetic drugs and combined therapy. It also appears that in the distribution of diabetic neuropathy according to the type of therapy, the lowest incidence was recorded in the cases treated by biguanides and by high doses of insulin. These are mostly cases under satisfactory control, either because their condition is severe, requiring intensive insulin therapy, or because it is mild and responds well to biguanides.

It might therefore be concluded that, as already stated by others, none of the types of antidiabetic therapy applied at present can be incriminated as promoting the onset of diabetic neuropathy.

The data concerning the prevalence of diabetic neuropathy may be summarised as follows:

a) as in other angiopathic complications of diabetes, the incidence of diabetic neuropathy rises with the duration of the disease and the condition should be considered among the late complications of diabetes mellitus;

b) age is less influential in determining the complication than in its clinical pattern. Aspects which can be assigned to a process of arteriosclerosis appear in later years, which proves that macroangiopathy also participates in the determination of diabetic neuropathy;

c) the efficiency of metabolic control of the disease seems to bear the same influence on the hazard of diabetic neuropathy as on all varieties of diabetic micro- and macroangiopathy;

d) the influence of sex on the onset and clinical aspects of diabetic neuropathy has not yet been elucidated. Investigations on larger groups and over longer intervals are required for this purpose. The same remark holds good with respect to other factors which seem to bear an influence on the incidence of the complication. Investigations on homogenous groups of prediabetic patients are necessary in order to assess the role of duration and a possible genetical determination of the type and pattern of the angiopathic diabetic complication.

Table II

Type of treatment	Diet only			Sulphamides			Biguanides			Insulin						Total		
										> 40 I.U.			< 40 I.U.					
Type of control	G	M	B	G	M	B	G	M	B	G	M	B	G	M	B	G	M	B
Nr.Subjects	8	35	13	12	30	10	6	20	5	20	40	17	15	20	8	61	145	53
Partial percentage	14.2	62.5	23.3	23	57.8	19.2	19.3	64.6	16.1	25.8	51.6	22.6	34.8	46.6	18.6	23.5	56	20.5
General percentage		21.6			20.0			11.9			29.6			16.9				
General total		56			52			31			77			43			259	

G = Good control; M = Medium control; B = Bad control;

2. Problems of Morphology and Ultrastructure in Diabetic Neuropathy

Histological investigations performed on biopsy specimens and in post-mortem examinations in diabetic patients showed several histological and ultrastructural alterations which afford a better understanding of the pathophysiology of this late complication of diabetes mellitus.

They are characterized by the following general remarks:

a) the morphological alterations – histological or ultrastructural – occur both in the subjects with juvenile diabetes mellitus and in those suffering from maturity onset diabetes [50];

b) these alterations start and remain preponderantly located in the peripheral nerves. The morphological alterations in the brain and spinal cord are acknowledged, but many authors regard them as of secondary importance [78];

c) there is no correspondence between the morphological alterations in the nerves and the respective clinical picture. The former are generally more severe than one would suppose on the ground of clinical symptomatology [16];

d) morphological alterations – histological and ultrastructural – were described both in the nerve and in its supplying vessels – vasa nervorum.

Lesions in the nerve consist of process of segmental demyelinization or peri-axonal segmentary neuritis, of non-inflammatory character [31], possibly associated with a longitudinal proliferation of Schwann's cells. The axon is not involved in the process. If segmental demyelinization advances, axon damage also ensues [16, 59, 92]. Heavy collagen accumulation was noted to go hand in hand with this degenerative process.

The electronmicroscopic investigations revealed that the myelin sheath breaks into fragments and becomes folded. Schwann's cells are comparatively poor in cell organelles, they contain multimembraneous or lamellar inclusions – true myelin figures – and their cytoplasma appears obviously vacuolar and contains granules which seem to be of glycogen [8]. The presence of cytosomes at this level as well as in the cells of nerves with or without myelin suggests a metabolic disorder in the neuronal cells. There is no evidence as to whether this disorder is the direct or secondary result of poor blood supply.

The basement membrane of the Schwann cells is also thickened, even in the nodes of Ranvier. The evidence of neuronal regeneration and of neoformation with Schwann's cells is much less frequent.

The axon appears initially undamaged, but subsequently the density of its cytoplasm increases and the nerve filaments appear in conglomerates and sometimes with a fine granulary transformation. Such morphological findings have been reported in myelinated as well as in the non-myelinated fibres [8]. It should be noted that according to Bischoff they are more evident in the amyelinic than in the myelinic fibres.

In the vessles supplying the nerves (vasa nervorum) a process of thickening of the walls was found to occur, by the accumulation of PAS-positive material, similar to that observed in diabetic angiopathy in general. The size of the vascular lumen diminishes accordingly [31]. As a matter of fact, many of these histological aspects have often been reported in diabetic neuritis since 1901 [61].

The corresponding, electronmicroscopic appearance consists of the multiplication and thickening of the basement membrane which creates interstitial spaces subsequently filled by precipitated collagen fibres [57]. In the following stage, swelling of the vascular endothelium reduces the lumen of the vessel. Endothelial proliferation has also been reported, and subsequent obstruction in the retina or in the kidney.

The actual sequence of these structural changes is very difficult to demonstrate, but the pathogenetic correlations (Fig. 2) mentioned at the end of the subchapter on pathogenesis may be of some help in elucidating it.

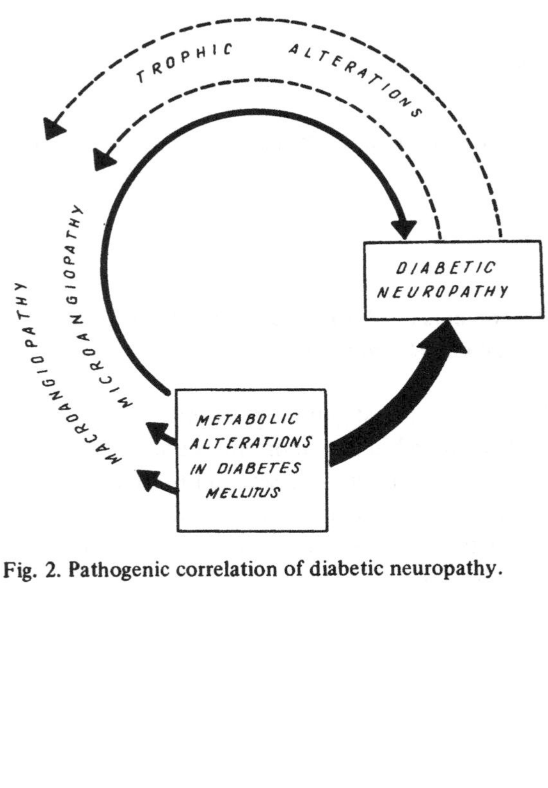

Fig. 2. Pathogenic correlation of diabetic neuropathy.

3. Problems of Pathogenesis in Diabetic Neuropathy

It was at the beginning of the 20th century (1901) that Marinescu described almost all the histological features of neuropathy in diabetes known to-day and which still underlie most of the pathogenetic interpretations advanced with regard to this complication. This author reported the considerable thickening of the walls of the small vessels in the degenerated nerves, supplying the basis for the ischaemic theory of the pathogenesis of diabetic neuropathy. He also mentioned "certain toxic substances present in the diabetic subject" which may be held responsible for the alterations in the myelinated fibres very similar to those which follow the sectioning of a peripheral nerve, and for their secondary influence on the radicular cells in the spinal cord. One may recognise in this line of thought the elements of an outlook grounded on metabolic disorders and implying that diabetic neuropathy is determined to some extent by dysmetabolic factors [61].

This point of view already implies the intervention of a vascular and of a metabolic element and subsequent research did not go very far beyond this hypothesis.

a) Ischaemic hypothesis. Many recent works, and particularly that published by Fagerberg [31], advocated the ischaemic pathogenesis of diabetic neuropathy, consisting of an angiopathic process in the vasa nervorum.

This hypothesis relies on the following arguments:

- the scattered, "multi neuritic" aspect of diabetic neuropathy [51];
- the researches of Goldenberg et al. [43] which demonstrated highly significant correlations between the angiopathic alterations in diabetes mellitus and diabetic neuropathy;
- the reported thickening of the basement membrane in the vasa nervorum;
- the concomitant reduction of the lumen of these vessels [7, 96];
- the accumulation of collagen among the lamellae of the thickened basement membrane and the presence of extensions of the fibroblast cells [57];
- the changes reported in the endothelial cells of the vasa vasorum, such as hypertrophy, multiplication of intracellular organelles and reduction of the vascular lumen [59];
- the fact that the metabolic hypothesis can account less easily for the asymmetrical and disseminated character often observed with diabetic neuropathy [59].

As for the paralysis of the seventh pair of cranial nerves in diabetics, Korczyn admits the existence of an ischaemia of the nerve itself. The great vulnerability of this nerve might be the result of poor vascular anastomosis and of the anatomical position of the nerve in its bony canal, which favours compressions through oedema [56].

A further argument consists of the correlation, admitted by most authors between the duration of the diabetic disease and the onset of diabetic neuropathy and between neuropathy and the degenerative alterations found in blood vessels situated elsewhere in the organism [74, 75, 76]. In certain cases, the nervous system seems to become involved earlier and to be more sensitive than other systems and organs, but such findings are consistent with the character of diabetic angiopathy, which is widespread but clinically predominant in a certain region of the vascular system of the body. Fagerberg [31] examined biopsy specimens of the anterior tibial nerve from 151 diabetic and 45 non-diabetic patients and reported a patchy, non-inflammatory degeneration of the medium sheath of the intraneural vessels, thickened walls, accumulation of PAS-positive matter and a reduction of the lumen, the whole picture being very similar to that described in the renal vessels in diabetic nephropathy. Such alterations in the vasa nervorum were found in 68% of the patients who had diabetic neuropathy and in only 38 % of those diabetics who did not suffer from neuropathy. The difference is statistically highly significant. Similar conclusions with regard to the role of angiopathy in the determination of diabetic neuropathy have been reached by Goldenberg et al. [43].

The following objections have been raised to the ischaemic hypothesis:

- neuropathy is comparatively rarely found in non-diabetic patients with obvious symptoms of advanced obliterating atherosclerosis;
- diabetic neuropathy starts in certain cases with an acute episode;
- marked improvement sometimes occurs in patients with obvious symptoms of diabetic neuropathy;
- the autonomic nervous system is often involved;
- diabetic neuropathy may occur in patients free from any sign of micro- or macroangiopathic vascular alteration [26, 33];
- arteriopathic complications may occur after a previous neuropathy has subsided [70, 74];
- there is no correlation between the angiopathic process in the vasa nervorum and the segmental demyelinization of the respective nerve [16, 46, 91]. Similar findings have been reported from electronmicroscopic investigations of the autonomic nervous system [65, 92].
- alterations of the vasa nervorum could be found neither in cases of human diabetes without neuropathy nor in steroid hyperglycaemia in the rabbit [55, 58];
- there are some morphological differences between the histological appearance of diabetic neuropathy and that of the ischaemic processes [43, 51]. The rich anastomotic network which unites the superficial and the deep vessels of the nerves may prevent the appearance of ischaemic alterations, since compensation by collateral pathways is possible [75, 76].

b) Metabolic hypothesis. This explains the condition resulting from degenerative alterations occurring in the peripheral nerves subsequent to the metabolic disorder of diabetes mellitus. Some of the arguments in favour of this outlook may be defined as follows:

- the characteristic lesion of diabetic neuropathy, segmental demyelinization, reflects a metabolic alteration in Schwann's cells [94];
- the abnormal uptake of labelled acetate in the cholesterol found in the spinal cord and peripheral nerves of the alloxanized rat proves that there is a metabolic disorder in the nervous system in experimental diabetes. It may be assumed to exist in spontaneous diabetes as well [19, 20].
- there is an inability of the diabetic nerve to store the excess of glucose as glycogen. Consequently, glucose is transformed to a greater extent into sorbitol, and the uptake of sorbitol and fructose increases. This metabolic deviation might be regarded as a dysmetabolic state which contributes to diabetic neuropathy [34, 35].
- the ability of the nerves to synthesize fatty acids is reduced as compared to that of triglycerides and cholesterol [35], as shown by the fact that the uptake of acetate mostly occurs into saturated hydrocarbons and phospholipids and not into the fatty acids of the triglycerides and into the esters of cholesterol.
- in many diabetics, the metabolism of pyruvic acid is arrested or delayed as part of the general metabolic disorder [53]. Pyruvataemia is increased in diabetic patients in general [53] but was claimed to reach a significant level in patients suffering from neuropathy [27, 28];
- the speed of the nerve conduction was diminished in young diabetic patients even in the absence of any retinopathy, nephropathy or capillaropathy in the skin. The finding can be correlated to the age of the subject, the duration of diabetes and to metabolic imbalance due to inadequate treatment [19, 48, 49]. The time of its onset rules out the possibility of a macroangiopathy, but not that of a microangiopathy;
- the metabolic state of the diabetic patient undoubtedly exerts an influence on the nervous

system. A basic argument of the supporters of the metabolic hypothesis is that the deterioration of the metabolic balance is often followed by objective and subjective recurrence of the neuropathy [48, 49, 50];

– neurological disorders are more frequent in diabetic patients over the age of 50 with vascular lesions than in non-diabetic patients of the same age and suffering from various vascular pathological conditions. This difference suggests that the vascular factor is unimportant and that the dysmetabolic diabetic factor is decisive;
– diabetic retinopathy and diabetic nephropathy were found in only 40 % of diabetic patients with neuropathy. Thus, diabetic angiopathy does not seem a prerequisite of diabetic neuropathy.

The above arguments prove beyond doubt that the dysmetabolic factor is at least partly responsible for diabetic neuropathy. The ischaemic hypothesis is also based on valid arguments. Therefore some authors admit the existence not of a single neuropathy, but of several neuropathies, different with regard to pathogenesis, as well as to clinical course, prognosis and therapy [91].

c) Hypothesis of vitamin deficiency. Another attempt to explain the pathogenesis of diabetic neuropathy on a different metabolic basis, resulted in the hypothesis of vitamin deficiency. According to this view, the condition is a secondary complication of a B avitaminosis, brought about by prolonged ketosis, hyperglycaemia and glycosuria [41]. Strausz [91] attempted to include diabetic neuropathy in the same group with the toxic neuritis of pregnancy, postinfectious and alcoholic neuritis, on the ground of a common assumed deficiency in vitamin B_1. It was found in experimental diabetes that cocarboxylase and the flavin enzymes decrease in the liver of enzymes diabetic animals [91].

Khan et al. [55] have found a latent vitamin B_{12} deficiency in some diabetics with diabetic neuropathy. In such cases, characterized by positive Babinski reflex, optic atrophy, etc., the treatment with vitamin B_{12} led to remarkable clinical improvements. The dificiency in vitamin B_{12} was noticed in 7 out of 87 patients with diabetic neuropathy.

A fall in free ATP has also been reported in diabetes mellitus. This substance represents the source of energy and of phosphorus required for the phosphorylation of these vitamins, in order to activate them as co-enzyme, in intermediary metabolism. Consequently, the deficiency in unbalanced diabetes does not consist of a true avitaminosis, but in a deficient phosphorylation of the B-vitamins, due to a relative deficit in ATP. Vitamin therapy (with thiamine for example) is often inefficient in diabetic neuropathy. This fact is consistent with the above assumption [68]. In fact, blood thiamine levels in neuropathic diabetic patients are in the normal range.

d) Role of prolonged undernutrition should not be disregarded. Investigations performed in our clinic demonstrated that a chronic metabolic perturbation is most likely to occur with most diabetic patients. Duncan also stressed the fact that the nutritional disorders associated with loss of weight in prolonged unbalanced diabetes occur in the history of many cases of diabetic neuropathy and may be assumed to play a role in the pathogenesis of the complication [18].

Protein starvation may intervene in two ways: on one hand the diminished synthesis of structural and enzymatic proteins in various organs seems to affect the metabolism of the nervous system, which is known for its high metabolic rate of amino-acids and proteins [79]; on the other hand, the reactivity of the organism as a whole is diminished in cases of protein deficiency [54].

Some of the symptoms of diabetic neuropathy in the autonomic nervous system may be partly explained by the state of protein disturbance and deficiency of patients having lost too much weight. Such are arterial hypotension, certain digestive disorders, oedemae, etc. The fact that diabetic neuropathy is resistant to a therapy consisting of a high calorie and high protein diet does not contradict the hypothesis, since the origin of the disorder is rather endogenous than exogenous.

It should be noted that there are also authors who maintain that it is obesity in diabetics that predisposes to diabetic neuropathy. As some varieties of obesity are associated with partial protein denutrition [11], this hypothesis may also be included in the general view that diabetic neuropathy originates in a kind of protein disturbance.

e) Localization of the disorders underlying diabetic neuropathy. Before attempting a correlation of the various pathogenetic theories of diabetic neuropathy, mention should be made of the problem of the original localization of the respective disorders in the organism of the diabetic patient and particularly in the nervous system.

The majority of authors agree that diabetic neuropathy is preponderantly localized in the peripheral nerves. Others, based on neurological findings and laboratory tests upon cerebrospinal fluid, situate the pathological alteration at a more central level, namely in the spinal cord, the nerve roots, the ganglia of the autonomic system and even higher, in the central nervous system. It has been claimed that although certain symptoms in diabetic neuropathy might be better explained by alterations of the peripheral nerves, there are symptoms, including the disorders in proprioception, ataxia and the pupillary modifications, in which the causal lesion must be located more centrally [14].

Goodman et al. [45] developed the idea set forth in 1901 by Marinescu [61] that the latter symptoms may be explained by the secondary influence exerted by the alteration of the peripheral nerves on structures situated more centrally.

According to Ellenberg and Krainer [22] the alteration may be central, peripheral or both. If the various clinical aspects of diabetic neuropathy are considered in the light of the ischaemic hypothesis, some of them can be explained by a *central lesion,* generally macroangiopathic, while others are more readily explained by *peripheral lesions* of the microangiopathic type (see subchapter, Clinical study of the diabetic neuropathy). The coexistence of both types of lesion is undoubtedly possible and most likely to exist. It corresponds to mixed cases where it is very difficult to discern whether the original disorder was central or peripheral.

As for the dysmetabolic background, it seems to contribute to the pathogenesis of diabetic neuropathy mainly in determining its course, more precisely the degree of reversibility of the clinical disorders at a given moment of the disease. The cases of diabetic neuropathy which may be regarded as *functional,* those in which there is a chance of restitutio ad integrum of the disorders, are the cases where the contribution of the metabolic element is predominant.

f) Correlation of the different pathogenetic factors of diabetic neuropathy. It may be assumed that the relationship between the ischaemic and the metabolic factors in the pathogenesis of diabetic neuropathy (Fig. 2) consists of a multiple correlation in which the specific diabetic metabolic disorder is likely to be the primum movens. The neuropathic complication may result from a direct effect of the latter on the nervous system, or as a consequence of the two types of angiopathy, macro- and microangiopathy, which may occur in any organ of the diabetic. Subsequent ischaemia, peripheral or central, promotes or accelerates the course of diabetic neuropathy. Diabetic neuropathy may in its turn enhance the angiopathic complication by means of the trophic influence of the nerves on the effector organs and through the nerves of the vessels.

The role of stress in the onset of diabetic neuropathy, particularly emphasized by Ellenberg [24], cannot represent a pathogenetic factor by itself. The alterations of the nerves and vessels described in this complication of diabetes must be the result of a much longer process than that of stress.

4. Clinical Study of Diabetic Neuropathy

Clinical classification of the aspects of diabetic neuropathy. Taking into account the pathogenetic interpretation defined above (Fig. 2) and the type of angiopathy involved in the localization of the respective process within the nervous system, three main clinical groups of diabetic neuropathy can be distinguished:

A) The group of alterations caused by a vascular diabetic complication of macroangiopathic type. They result in the clinical picture of the *central neuropathies*, and consist of transient or permanent palsies such as hemiplegia or monoplegia with or without aphasia [33]. Paralysis of the oculomotor nerves, similar to those found in non-diabetic subjects, also belong to this group. The clinical symptom is diplopia due to the involvement of the IIIrd, IVth or VIth cranial nerves and may be preceded by ocular pain [78].

B) The group of alterations caused by vascular diabetic complications of microangiopathic type. The clinical picture is of a chronic or acute diabetic multineuritis or mononeuritis, also involving in some cases the autonomic nervous system [78].

C) The group of alterations caused by vascular diabetic complications both of macroangiopathic and microangiopathic types, resulting in a mixed clinical picture.

The symptomatology of the cases in group A is not specific for diabetes, and the only peculiar element suggesting the diabetic background is the small extent of the central angiopathic process [73], which may subside and recur several times. The central neuropathic syndrome is often associated, preceded or followed by states of depression, irritability or anorexia [76].

In the case of group C the central symptomatology mentioned above is gradually joined by signs of peripheral neuropathic alteration.

The most typical case of diabetic neuropathy is that of group B, that of peripheral and visceral neuropathy. It may be *multineuritic* or *mononeuritic*, according to the number of nerves involved [7].

The multineuritic type may be, in its turn, (a) a peripheral neuritis proper or (b) a visceral disorder.

The peripheral neuritis may again be divided into (1) a chronic predominantly sensory disturbance, and (2) a subacute sensory and motor distrubance [78].

The preclinical stage of diabetic neuropathy. The characteristic clinical aspects of diabetic neuropathy, as detailed above, are preceded by a long preclinical stage, which may also be called a functional stage.

Minor disorders occur during the first years of diabetes and can be identified as changes in the impulse conduction speed in the motor nerves or as alterations in the sensitivity to vibration [7, 52], as well as in the vasomotor [63] or sudoral reactions [82].

The conduction speed in motor nerves is significantly diminished in young diabetic subjects, as compared to controls. Such changes are found mostly in the lower limbs and are regarded as objective indications of an early alteration of the peripheral nerves, as they occur much earlier than the obvious clinical symptoms of diabetic neuropathy [93].

Similar changes were reported in determinations performed on the sensitive nerves [94].

The biothesiometric estimation of the sensivity to vibration indicates a fall in the very first year of manifest diabetes mellitus, and the subsequent evolution is parallel to the course of the alterations in the peripheral motor nerves as mentioned above [48, 49].

C.S.F. examination may provide some information if a moderate rise of all proteins is present. This is a means of differentiating between diabetic neuropathy and multiple sclerosis, for instance, when the increase of proteins in C.S.F. is mainly due to gamma-globulins.

The chronic multineuritic type of diabetic neuropathy. The characteristic subjective symptom of chronic multineuritis is pain. It occurs mostly in the lower limbs and is usually unilateral and sometimes symmetrical. It is felt most often on the anterior side of the respective limb. Pain is persistent, exacerbated by rest and cold and especially during the night [18]. In rare cases it takes the subjective aspect of pseudotabetic pain attacks.

Pain is preceded, associated or followed by various paraesthetic sensations such as cold, burn, hyperaesthesia to contact with clothing the sensation of walking on a soft surface, itching, etc.

The suffering of the patient is rendered visible by the following clinical symptoms:

- the absence of certain ostheotendineous reflexes, usually found distally and often asymmetrical. In some cases this may be the only symptom of the condition;
- the diminution or absence of sensitivity to vibration, usually found in the distal parts of the lower limbs. The latency interval of the perception of the respective stimulus is increased [18].
  The age of the patient should always be taken into account when assessing this sign;
- there is a decrease in the ability to discriminate pain and temperature stimuli, which may result in various traumatisms, skin lesions, burns, etc.;
- deep pain sensation is often lost;
- trophic alterations which confer a characteristic appearance on the patient. They consist of dry, fissured and hyperkeratosic skin, deformed and thickened nails and uni- or bilateral oedema;
- neuropathic ulcerations ("mal perforant") usually localized in the lower limbs. They show no tendency to healing, and if infected, may be confused with the peripheral lesions of diabetic arteriopathy. The underlying bone may become involved and a true osteomyelitis results. These trophic ulcerations occur mostly at the level of the proximal epiphyses of the I and V metatarsal bones and on the calcaneum. The trophic ulceration may be preceded by superficial alterations of the skin. The patient rarely complains of the latter, since sensation is diminished [5];
- the alterations in the bones may take the shape of a non-specific osteoporosis (Fig. 3), with or without microgeodes [4] and reach the condition called "Charcot's foot", consisting of spontaneous fractures, dislocation and severe

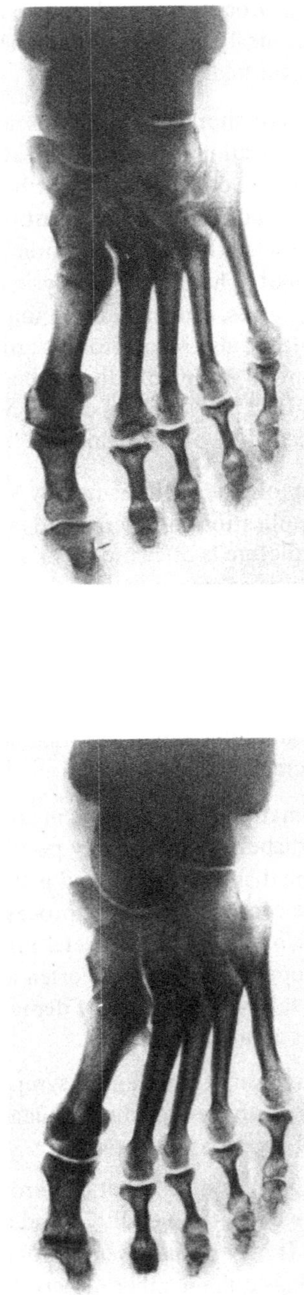

Fig. 3. (And B) Diabetic neuropathy with osseous determinations. Ostheoporotic aspect in a woman (T.C.) with maturity onset diabetes. Presumed duration of diabetes: 2 months. Familial history of diabetes. Bilateral metatarsian and phalangian lesions.

osteolysis. This process, quite similar to lepromatous osteopathy, has also been called *diabetic osteopathy* [81]. This suggests the intervention of a neurological rather than metabolical mechanism [36]. Several hypotheses have been put forward to explain the appearance of diabetic osteopathy, without, however, elucidating the problem. It has been postulated that the anaesthesia produced by diabetic neuropathy might allow some trauma and abnormal local pressures which could lie at the origin of diabetic osteopathy. The hypothesis was advocated of a real "autosympathectomy" by diabetic neuropathy, which would bring about vascular dilation and increased bone resorption, respectively [4]. This hypothesis also theorises that during simple ischaemic manifestations the bone is locally densified and only in the final stages of osteomyelitis destroyed.

Diabetic arthropathy, of the Charcot type, takes place when severe articular and periarticular destructions occur.

The incidence of diabetic osteopathy is differently estimated by various authors, from 6.8% [44, 77] to 77% of patients [36].

Diabetic osteopathy is clinically diagnosed and differentiated from osteomyelitis by the following symptoms:

a) its symmetry and location, similar to the distribution of neurological disturbances in diabetic neuropathy,
b) lack of pain,
c) association with trophic disturbances in the skin,
d) foot distortions,
e) painless local inflammatory manifestations,
f) multifocal, bilateral, peripherally located lesions.

X-ray examination shows a symmetrical thinning of the metaphysis, especially at the phalanges. X-ray examination should constitute a decisive argument in differential diagnosis of this condition from osteomyelitis (Fig. 3 and 4).

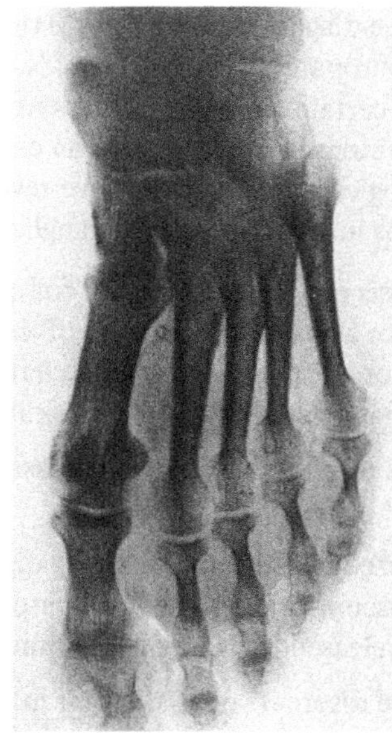

Fig. 4. C. S. 58 year old man with maturity onset diabetes. Presumed duration of diabetes: 9 years. Oral hypoglycaemics during the entire period despite their poor efficiency. Tarsian, metatarsian and phalangian osteoporosis. Moderate arterial calcifications.

The above lesions represent a particular form of the wide-spread trophic alterations caused by diabetic neuropathy.

- another objective finding in some cases is a high protein content of the cerebral fluid, but the amount of protein is not correlated with the severity of diabetic neuropathy [63].

In the autonomic nervous system, chronic multineuritis results in a varied symptomatology [83] which may overlap the symptoms enumerated above or appear as an independent picture. These are called *"the vegetative neuropathies of diabetes mellitus"* [30]. Among the many possible patterns, the following were more often reported:

- in *the skin* of approximately 30% of diabetic patients with a history longer than 5 years, symptoms of hyperhydrosis are to be found. These are frequently followed, after a variable interval, by anhydrosis [82]. The various tests used in the diagnosis of the early, latent phases of this neuropathic complication [1, 3, 68] suggest a certain similarity to experimental sympathectomy [71], and in some cases pathomorphological investigations have revealed alterations in the sympathetic ganglia [2].

Hyperhydrosis may be preceded or followed by a diminution or arrest in the activity of the sweat and sebaceous glands, which gives a characteristic atrophic appearance to the affected skin area [18].

The patients often complain of unpleasant sensations of heat or cold [69].

The generalized or localized sweating disorders cause real discomfort to the patient, especially as they are released by inadequate stimuli [30].

The digestive disorders consist either in secretory disturbances or in inadequate motor activity of the smooth muscles in cavitary organs. Among the secretory disturbances, extreme variations of salivary flow are frequent [39]. Gastric secretions may be modified in amount, in composition or in both. As regards composition, *hypochlorhydria* and even *anachlorhydria* have been reported. Hypersecretion often occurs [18, 62] hindering X-ray examination of the stomach (Fig. 5).

Is is more difficult to diagnose secretory disturbances further along the gut. Disturbed pancreatic enzyme secretion has been reported in some cases [11]. The results of these estimations have been interpreted as indicating that there is no correlation between the endocrine pancreas, damaged in diabetes mellitus, and the exocrine pancreas, which may be unaffected. This conclusion should probably be re-examined considering the possible presence of vegetative neuropathy.

The following disturbances have been more often reported in the smooth musculature of the digestive tube and organs:

- *oesophageal disorders* consisting of delayed evacuation of the oesophagus, possibly associated with a hiatal hernia and with gastro-oesophageal reflux. The corresponding clinical picture consists of regurgition and possibly dysphagia [60].
- *gastric kinetic disorders.* X-ray examination shows a distended hypokinetic stomach, evacuation is delayed and the general appearance resembles that following vagotomy [13]. No characteristic symptomatology has been described. Gastric pain has been reported in some cases, in attacks similar to those in tabes. A dyspeptic syndrome has also been reported (anorexia, nausea, vomiting) which may occur in frequent attacks at short intervals and result in a metabolic imbalance of the diabetes and/or in a state of starvation. The latter – as already mentioned above – may also contribute to diabetic neuropathy (Fig. 5).

  In other cases the tone of the stomach appears to be adequate but peristaltic movements are rare and even if efficient, the evacuation of the barium content is delayed and lasts 1–2 hours (Fig. 6).
- a low motor activity has also been reported in the *bowel,* localized at various segments. Hypo-

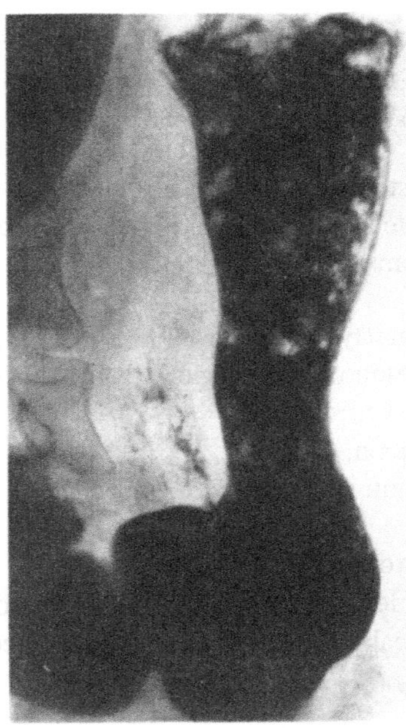

Fig. 5. C. I. Juvenile diabetes mellitus in a woman with presumed onset 13 years before. Hypotonic, hypokinetic, elongated stomach with hypersecretion. Anachlorhydria. Ingested nutriments 14 hours after meal.

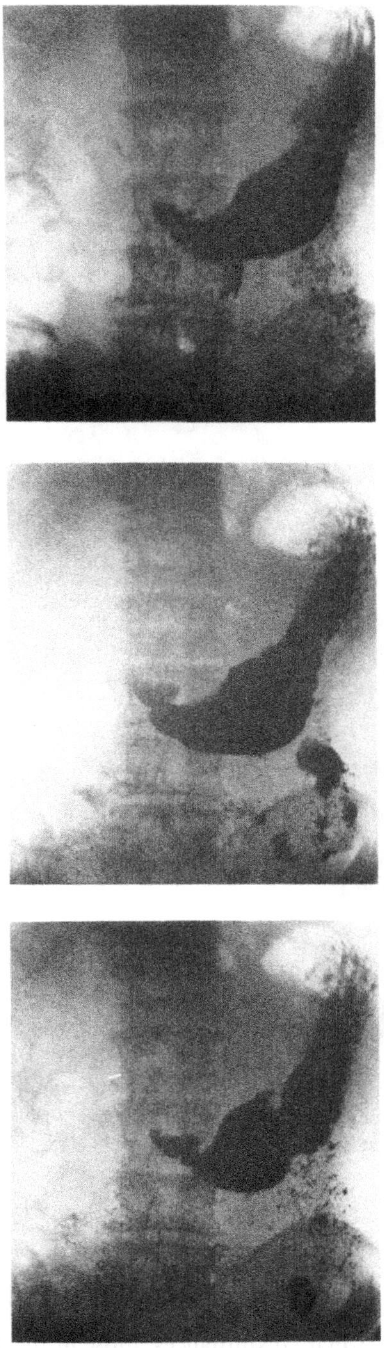

Fig. 6. S. I. 38 year old man with diabetes duration of about 12 years. Poor control with oral antidiabetics. Stomach retarded evacuation 30'(A), 60'(B) and 180'(C) after barium ingestion.

mobility in the duodenum results in prolonged stasis in its different portions (Fig. 7).

Similar findings were reported in the small intestine (Fig. 8 and 9).

Hypomobility in the large intestine usually results in constipation resistant to therapy [83]. Contrary to this is another syndrome, less frequent, but more characteristic of diabetes mellitus and bringing about more severe consequences for the patient. This is "intestinal neuropathy" which consists of intermittent or persistent diarrhoea, paroxysmal during the night, without pain, with typical watery discharges and resistant to the administration of pancreatic extracts. This complication finally results in steatorrhoea and secondary starvation. Severe and prolonged cases may also develop anal incontinence;

– multiple dystonic-dyskinetic disturbances have been reported in the *biliary tract.* Among them, hypotonia of the gall-bladder, associated sometimes with hypokinesia, appears as the most frequent [42] (Fig. 10).

Hyperkinetic states are much less frequent. They may be associated with a hypotonic or hypokinetic gall-bladder (Fig. 11, 12 and 13).

All the above dystonic-dyskinetic aspects should be assigned to diabetes only if no other elements can account for them, and especially if other aspects of multineuritis are found in the same patient. In this latter case, the whole clinical picture was called by Gitelson [42] "the diabetic neurogenic gall-bladder".

Most often, these disorders are not associated with subjective complaints. There is sometimes a non-specific biliary dyspeptic syndrome which improves with the correction of the diabetic balance;

– the *visceral diabetic neuropathy* may result in various urogenital disorders:

a) Hypotonia of the bladder is relatively common (Fig. 13).

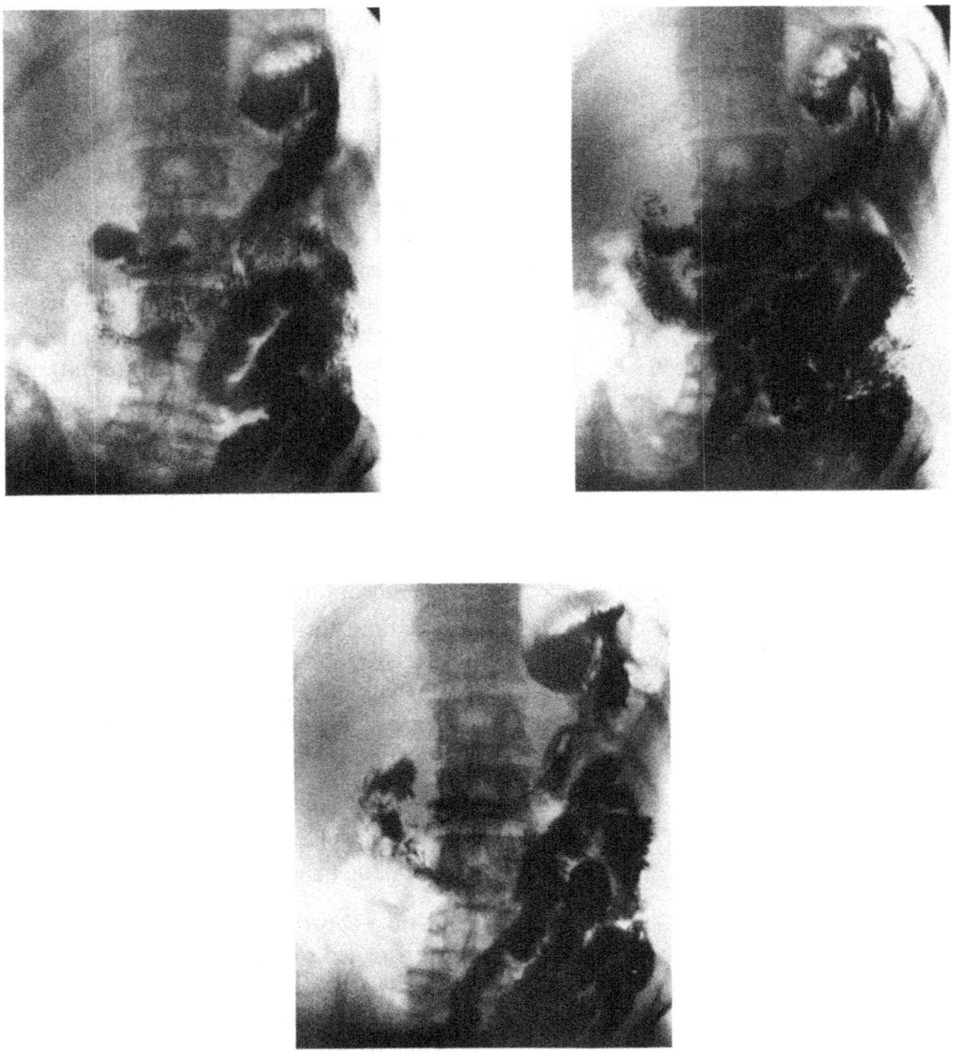

Fig. 7. D. S. 42 year old diabetic man. Poor control only by diet. After a satisfactory evacuation of the barium from stomach (A), there is a 15′retard of the meal in the first duodenal segment followed by a very slow passage in the second duodenal segment (B) and finally a bipolar stasis for 20′ (C).

b) bladder disturbances, such as hypotonia or atonia are more frequent in women and usually respond favourably to high doses of parasympathicomimetic drugs. They often subside spontaneously [69].

The interval between micturitions increases in the early stages, later, micturitions are small and frequent, as released by overdistention of the bladder.

c) unlike urinary disturbances, those in the genital sphere occur earlier and represent a permanent complaint of the patient. Impotence which was reported in 1–37% of the diabetic patients [63], is seldom transient [6] or treatable. It occurs most

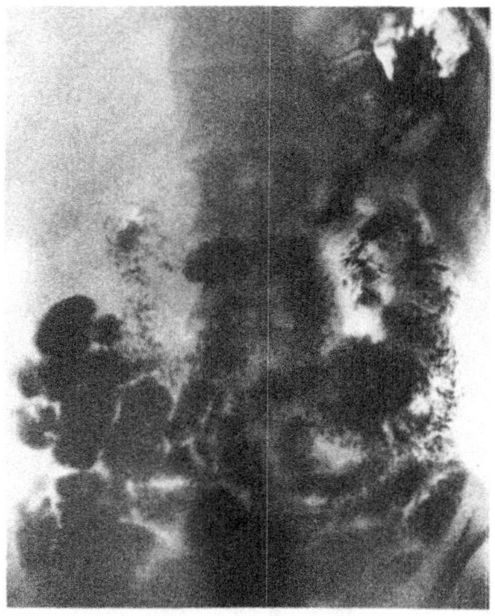

Fig. 8. Same patient as in fig. 8. Small intestinal aspect 3 hours after the barium meal ingestion.

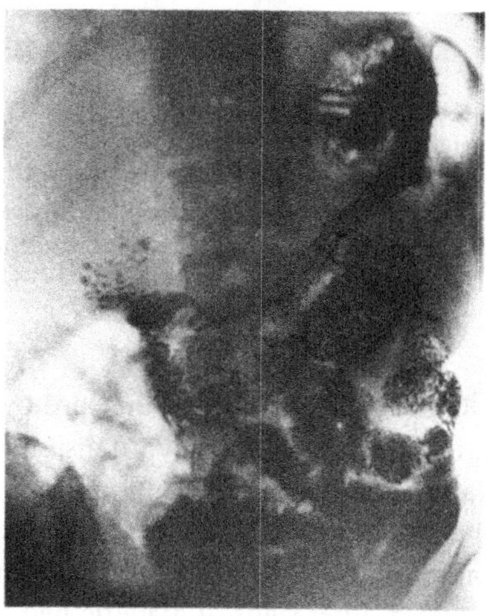

Fig. 9. Same patient as in fig. 8. Small intestinal aspect 5 hours after the barium meal ingestion.

often in young adult diabetic patients, and the fact that libido is preserved only aggravates the situation. Impotence is often the earliest symptom drawing attention to the underlying diabetes mellitus.

In some cases, the onset of impotence is preceded or accompanied by the phenomenon of retrograde ejaculation and eventually by a neurogenic bladder syndrome [25, 47].

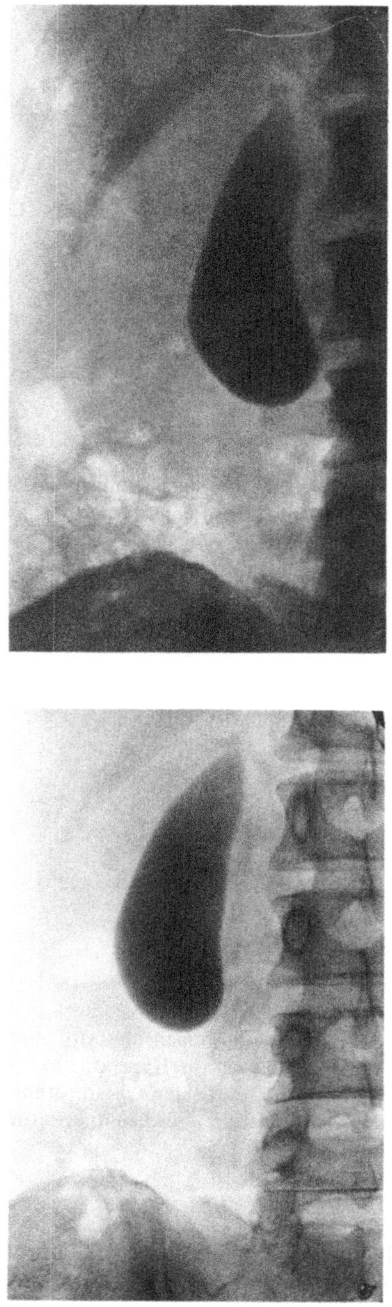

Fig. 10. N. S. 34 year old woman with juvenile diabetes. Presumed duration of diabetes about 12 years. Discontinued insulin treatment. Hypotony and hypokinesy of the gall-bladder. A = 30′after injection of radioopaque substance. B = 60′after Boyden's meal.

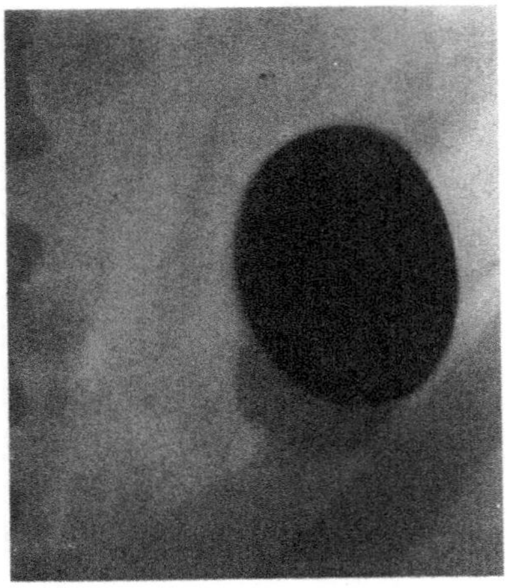

Fig. 11. V. C. 36 year old woman. Maturity onset diabetes. Biguanides treatment. Hypertonic gall-bladder.

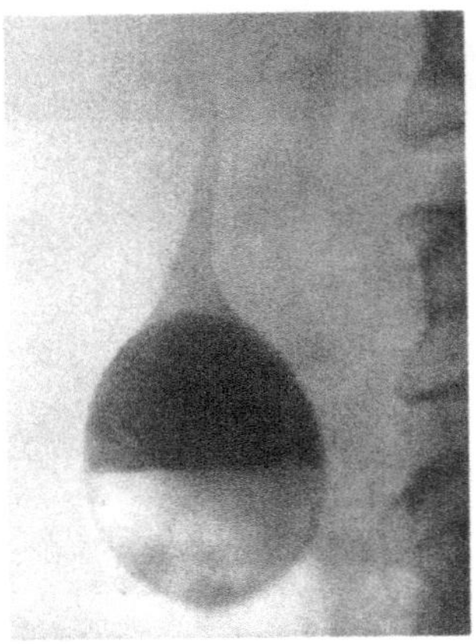

Fig. 12. B. E. 46 year old woman. Maturity onset diabetes with frequent acidosis. Hyperkinetic aspect of the gall-bladder after Beyden's meal. Although in the initial examination it seemed to be rather hypotonic.

According to certain authors, sexual impotence in the diabetic is part of a more complex endocrine picture frequently found with this pathological condition [84]. Such a view implies some hope of positive therapeutic results by hormonal therapy. Unfortunately, the practical results obtained are poor (see Subchapter V – The management of diabetic neuropathy p. 211).

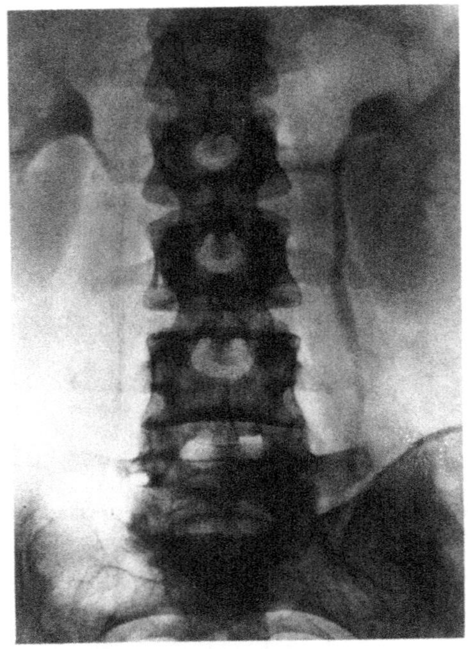

Fig. 13. C. E. 44 year old woman with maturity onset diabetes. Presumed diabetes duration: 9 years. The patient is in a poor nutritional state. Urography showing the hypotonic aspect of superior urinary tract without any mechanical obstacle in the urine evacuation.

When the neuropathy involves the cardiovascular system, it takes the form of hypotension and orthostatic tachycardia, as found in some 12% of the diabetic patients [1]. Less often subjective symptoms are associated, but are usually more frequent with other signs of diabetic neuropathy. More common complaints are vertigo, a tendency to syncope and fatigue. They require some kind of symptomatic therapy since the neuropathic complications gradually disable the patient.

Ocular involvement of the autonomic nervous system in diabetic neuropathy was also described, especially as pupillary disturbances, anisocoria, slow reaction to light and, in some cases, a positive Argyll-Robertson reaction [83].

Multineuritis. Subacute sensorial multineuritis has been regarded by many authors as an early phase of chronic multineuritis. It usually begins following long intervals of metabolic imbalance of diabetes and is often reversible. It may start or be exacerbated during the first weeks of an efficient antidiabetic therapy [21]. Here is a recent case of ours, typical of the clinical situation in which such a diabetic neuropathy may occur [91].

The patient M. Paul, aged 37, was admitted to hospital on October 18th, 1967 (Obs.Nr. 15,627), in a state of diabetic ketoacidosis. The disease had been diagnosed in 1962 and the patient attributed it to an episode of severe psychical stress. In 1962 the patient was prescribed a low carbohydrate diet (200 gm daily) and insulin therapy had been recommended. However, observance of the diet prescription was approximate and the patient gave up insulin therapy from the very beginning. On the other hand, without any medical advice, he started to take 1.50 gm tolbutamide daily. The blood sugar level of the patient had exceeded 250 mg % ever since and was accompanied by marked glycosuria. Six weeks before, the patient had complained of severe asthenia, associated with diminished working ability, sleeplesness, polyuria, polydipsia and considerable loss of weight. Appetite was generally unaffected. Biguanide therapy (metformin in doses of 1.50–1.00 gm daily) was prescribed. Initially well tolerated, this therapy subsequently resulted in digestive disorders which subsided when the drug was discontinued.

On admission to hospital, the weight deficit of the patient was 27 %(height 1.68 m, weight 49.5 kg), blood glucose level was 348 mg %, glycosuria 132 gm in 24 hours and a large amount of ketone bodies were found in the urine.

The patient was eventually controlled by 48 I. U. of Novolente insulin and discharged on November 14th, 1967 having gained 5 kg in weight, in good general condition, without glycosuria and with a blood sugar level of 120 mg%. He was recommended to observe a maximal daily intake of 200 gm carbohydrate.

Shortly after discharge, the patient started to complain of hyperaesthesia in the lower limbs, as well as of difficulties in walking, heavy nocturnal sweating and renewed loss of weight. Hyperaesthesia became paroxysmal and the patient could not tolerate the contact of clothes and even of bed sheets. He was again admitted to hospital on January 18th, 1968 (Obs.Nr. 806) with a diagnosis of subacute sensory multineuritis. He weighed 52 kg, had a blood sugar level of 141 mg%, no glycosuria and orthostatic hypotension. Insulin therapy was continued, associated with general tonic and anabolic drugs, vitamins and sedatives. The patient was discharged on the 10th of February, 1968, slightly improved, with a well balanced diabetic state, having gained 2 kg in weight. He was prescribed a daily carbohydrate intake lower than 200 g and a daily dose of 40 I. U. of insulin retard. It took several weeks and months for the sensory symptoms to gradually subside.

It should be noted that the neuropathy began after insulin therapy was started, in conditions of adequate diabetic balance, although previously, over a period of several years, management had been inadequate.

Some authors attribute such events to an idiosyncrasy to insulin, since the neuropathic manifestations sometimes subside if insulin is discontinued. Buch such disorders may occur in patients treated only by restricted diet or oral hypoglycaemic drugs. It often happens, as in the case reported above, that the subacute neuropathic disturbances subside even if the administration of insulin is not discontinued. According to other authors [21], the antidiabetic management precipitates the onset of the complication by correcting the metabolism of glucose and thereby increasing the utilization of thiamine and of other vitamins and even enzymes, which results in a relative deficiency. This hypothesis is refuted by the fact that intensive vitamin-therapy is ineffective. Another hypothesis is that a too rapid correction of the glycaemia causes a stress which precipitates the onset of a latent neuropathy [21, 22].

The fulminant pains of this form of diabetic multineuritis might be due to a disturbance of the control system, resulting in increased excitation of a group of neurons up to a level where a synchronous discharge of the spino-thalamic neurons takes place. This quasi epileptic discharge is followed by a refractory period, and by a relative lack of excitability of the respective neurone group. This might account for the acute, short, violent character of fulminant pains [10].

In summary, the clinical picture of subacute sensory multineuritis is characterized by pain and paraesthesiae, especially in the lower limbs, which may also cause difficulties in walking. Muscular asthenia is sometimes associated. The objective signs include the loss of tendon reflexes, especially the patellar and Achilles, and disturbances in all varieties of sensation, usually in the direction of hyperaesthesia.

Subacute motor multineuritis was more often reported in the past than to-day. It was initially described as a myelopathy in the diabetic, and involvement of the spinal cord was assumed. However, the characteristic amyotrophic disorders show that the alteration is situated in the nerve endings, in the muscles. The subjective symptomatic picture of this complication should be differentiated from that of diabetic arteriopathy, as one of its most frequent symptoms is pain in the leg, simulating intermittent claudication. However, it is exacerbated at night and is associated with marked muscular weakness and rapid wasting of the respective muscles.

The objective findings are amyotrophy, the absence of tendon reflexes, hyperaesthesia of the skin in the respective areas and reduction in or loss of the ability to percieve a pin prick [78].

This complication occurs in mild cases of diabetes, where therapy has been long neglected, usually in elderly patients. It is often reversible. After subsiding in one limb, the whole symptomatic picture may occur in the other one.

It is often difficult to differentiate this complication from the preceding one, when their symptoms are mixed, in a picture which may be regarded as a sensorial-motor subacute multineuritis.

In all these forms of subacute multineuritis, a high protein content of the cerebrospinal fluid is often found.

Mononeuritis manifestations in diabetic neuropathy. Peripheral mononeuritis mostly involves the VIIth cranial nerve (Bell's paralysis) the supraclavicular, common peroneal, tibial, ulnar, radial and median nerves.

It usually starts with pain localized in the area supplied by the respective nerve. A paralysis in the corresponding area follows. Mononeuritis may be the earliest sign of diabetic neuropathy [86].

Another form of diabetic mononeuritis is optic neuritis, eventually resulting in optic nerve atrophy.

Evolution and prognosis of diabetic neuropathies. The particular feature of these manifestations is that they are reversible, although almost always chronic [29]. Reversibility is relative, but it obviously occurs with this type of complication much more frequently than with any other of the late angiopathic complications of diabetes.

Considering the pathogenetic mechanism of the neuropathic complications in diabetes, the possibility of recovery increases where the dysmetabolic element plays a predominant role in their determination. If the angiopathic factor is more important, the resulting complications are less reversible. It should, however, be noted that nerve regeneration has been reported even in severe cases where at least an equal share can be attributed to both pathogenetical mechanisms. Regeneration of the oculomotor nerve was reported by Dreyfus [17], while Foster and Basset [37] described regeneration in cases of neurogenic arthropathy.

The relationship between chronically evolutive forms (C) and acutely-chronical (A–C) and acute forms (A) is

C (8) : A - C (1) : A (1) [29].

This outlook implies a more optimistic approach to the matters of prophylaxis and therapy, by insisting in all cases on the long-term correction of the metabolic disturbances. The maintenance of a metabolic balance as close to normal as possible, offers the chance of a remission or clinical improvement of the neuropathic disorders and at the same time may be assumed to prevent, or at least to delay, the onset of such complications in predisposed subjects.

5. The Management of Diabetic Neuropathy

The causal treatment. Just as in any diabetic state, the causal therapy, in these cases, consists of two elements:

a) Re-establishing the metabolic balance of diabetes by means of a high calorie, high protein and possibly even high carbohydrate diet, observing, however, a precise upper limit of the latter. This basic therapeutic prescription should be completed by the prohibition of alcohol and smoking [32, 78].

b) If a correct and observed diet does not result, over a short interval, in the correction of the metabolic imbalance, hypoglycaemic agents such as insulin or antidiabetic sulphonamides must also be prescribed.

Symptomatic treatment. It aims at easing as far as possible the subjective symptoms.

a) If intense pain is the chief complaint, powerful analgetics should be prescribed. The oral administration of pilocarpine nitrate, given three times daily in doses of 5 mg exerts a remarkable effect. Pilocarpine should be avoided in cases of atony of the digestive tract [17].

In cases of fulminant pains, some authors recomend carbomazepin (tegretol) administration, which slows transmission at the synaptic level [10].

b) Sedative drugs are frequently used, to enable quiet sleep, although their excessive use may cause further disturbances of metabolism.

c) In cases of atony or paresis of the bladder, synthetic parasympathomimetic drugs are effective. Intensive treatment by exercise and physical agents is recommended in order to facilitate an increased peripheral blood supply [10].

The auxiliary treatment.

a) Complex vitamin therapy has been recommended, especially the group of B vitamins, by those who incriminated vitamin deficiency in the pathogenesis of diabetic neuropathy. Intensive therapy with vitamin B_{12} (daily intramuscular administration of doses of 1,000 gamma and over) is still often prescribed.

b) The authors who stress the microangiopathic alterations of the vasa nervorum, recommend vasodilating drugs.

c) Impotence has been treated by the administration of chorionic gonadotrophin and testosterone [84].

Other recommendations. The application of heat should be avoided in the painful areas, since burns may result following disturbances of sensation. Such burns heal slowly and often become infected.

Local exercice or massage may exacerbate pain and paraesthesiae in the predominantly sensory cases. Such procedures also enhance the vascular disorder and prevent healing.

The removal of any infectious foci should be considered.

References

Chapter I

[1] Albrink, M. J., Man, E. B.: Serum triglycerides in coronary artery disease. – *Arch. intern. Med.* **103**, p. 4–8 (1959).

[2] Angeli, I.: Adatok a diabetes mellitus epidémiologiàjàhòz. – *Orvosi Hetilap* **111**, p. 1159–1164 (1970).

[3] Bagdade, J. D., Porte, A., Bierman, E. L.: Diabetic lipemia: a form of acquired fat induced lipemia. – *New Engl. J. Med.* **276**, p. 427–433 (1967).

[4] Bergqvist, N.: Serum lipids in an ambulatory diabetic clientele. – *Acta med. scand.* **187**, p. 213–218 (1970).

[5] Blumenthal, H. T., Hirata, Y., Owens, C. T., Berns, A. W.: A histo- and immunological analysis of the vessel lesion of diabetes in human and in the rabbit. – In *"Small blood vessel involvement in diabetes mellitus"*. Ed. Siperstein, M. A. – Amer. Inst. of Biol. Sci. Washington D. C. 1964.

[6] Blumenthal, H. T., Goldenberg, S., Berns, A. W.: Pathology and pathogenesis of the disseminated angiopathy of diabetes mellitus. – In *"On the nature and treatment of Diabetes.* – Ed. Leibel, B. S., Wreenshall, G. A. – Excerpta Med. Found. Amsterdam 1965, p. 397–408.

[7] Bürger, M.: Angiopathia Diabetica. – G. Thieme Stuttgart 1954.

[8] Butterfield, W. H. I.: Summary of results of the Bedford Diabetes Survey. – *Proc. roy. Soc. Med.* **57**, p. 169 (1964).

[9] Butterfield, W. H. I.: Priorities in Medicine. – The Nuffield Provincial Hospital Trust. 1968 p. 30.

[10] Butturini, U., Negri, A. U.: Rilevazioni clinico-staistiche sul diabete giovanile. – Atti del 1° Congr. Naz. della Soc. Ital. di Diabetologia e del Simp. Naz. sul Diabete. Catania 16–18 Feb. 1966.

[11] Carlson, L. A.: Serum lipids in normal man. – *Acta med. scand.* **167**, p. 377–387 (1960).

[12] Christensen, N. C., Hørder, M., Simonsen, E. E., Toft, H.: Serum triglyceride values in healthy adults. – *Scand. J. clin. Lab. Invest.* **23**, p. 355 (1969).

[13] Cochran, H. A. jr., Buck, N. F.: A mortality study of an insured diabetic population. – *Proc. Med. Sect. Amer. Life Convention* **49**, p. 145–171 (1961).

[14] Cohen, A. M.: Prevalence of diabetes among different ethnic jewish groups in Israel. – *Amer. Heart J.* **65**, p. 291–293 (1963).

[15] Connor, W. E., Stone, D. B., Hodges, R. E.: The interrelated effects of dietary cholesterol and fat upon human serum lipid levels. – *J. clin. Invest.* **43**, p. 1691–1696 (1964).

[16] Cullen, M. F.: Computer analysis in preventive health research. – *Meth. Inform. Med.* **6**, p. 8 (1967).

[17] Doyle, J. T., Kinsch, S. H., Brown, D. F.: Seasonal variation in serum cholesterol concentration. – *J. chron. Dis.* **18**, p. 657–664 (1965).

[18] Duncan, G. G.: Diabetul zaharat. – In *"Bolile Metabolismului"* vol. II, pp. 1162–1163. Bucureşti, Editura Medicală.

[19] Eberhardt, G.: Diagnostik und Therapie der Fettstoffwechselstörungen. – *Das öffentl. Gesundheitswesen* **33**, p. 633–641 (1971).

[20] Entmacher, P. S., Root, R. F., Marks, H. H.: Longevity of Diabetic Patients in recent years. – *Diabetes* **13**, p. 373–377 (1964).

[21] Falta, W., Högler, F.: Die Zuckerkrankheit. – Ed. IV. Carl Marhold, Halle (Saale) 1953.

[22] Freedman, L. E., Blackard, W. G., Sagan, L. A., Morikiro, I., Hamilton, H. B.: The epidemiology of diabetes mellitus in Hiroshima and Nagasaki. – *Yale J. Biol. Med.* **37**, p. 283 (1965).

[23] Fried, R., Hoeflmayr, J.: Erkennung von Fettstoffwechselstörungen. – *Med. Klin.* **64**, p. 1320–1323 (1969).

[24] Fritz, G.: Ergebnisse der Münchener Aktion zur Früherkennung von Diabetikern (1967). – Inaugural-Dissertation, München 1969.

[25] Gegesi-Kiss, P., Barta, L.: Diabetes mellitus im Kindesalter. – Ungarische Akad. f. Wissenschaft, Budapest 1957.

[26] Goldenberg, S., Alex, M., Joshi, R. A., Blumenthal, H. T.: Nonatheromatous peripheral vascular disease of the lower extremity in Diabetes mellitus. – *Diabetes* **8**, p. 261–273 (1959).

[27] Goodkin, G., Wolloch, L. B.: Longevity of Diabetics. – *J. occup. Med.* **11**, p. 522–532 (1969).

[28] Görig, G.: Statistische Untersuchungen an 17 000 Münchener Diabetikern. – Inaugural-Dissertation, München 1968.

[29] Grönberg, A., Larsson, T., Jung, J.: Diabetes in Sweden. – Stockholm 1967.

[30] Gsell, O.: Epidemiologie des Diabetes. *Dtsch. med. Wschr.* **93**, p. 2446–2450 (1968).

[31] Herman, J. B., Medalie, J. H., Kahn, H. A., Neufeld, H., Riss, E., Perlstein, I.: Diabetes incidence. A two year follow-up of 10 000 men in a survey of ischemic heart-diseases in Israel. – *Diabetes* **19**, p. 938 (1970).

[32] Hørder, M., Toft, H., Christensen, N. C., Sinomsen, E. E.: Plasma pre-beta-lipoproteins in healthy adults. – *Atherosclerosis* **14**, p. 31–37 (1971).

[33] Kannel, W. B., Castelli, W. P., Gordon, T., McNamara, P. M.: Serum cholesterol lipoproteins and the risk of coronary heart disease. – *Ann. intern. Med.* **74**, p. 1–12 (1971).

[34] Klemens, U. H., Löwis, O. F., Menar, P. V., Bremer, A., Wnuk, E. V., Schröder, R.: Hyperlipoproteinaemien und Koronarerkrankungen. – *Klin. Wschr.* **50**, p. 139–148 (1972).

[35] Leipert, Th.: Über die diagnostische Bewertung des Blutfettstatus. – *Wien. med. Wschr.* **119**, p. 23–25 (1969).

[36] Lüthy, R.: Untersuchung von Serumlipiden bei Normalpersonen und Patienten mit essentieller Hypertonie unter Berücksichtigung des Kohlenhydrat-Stoffwechsels. – *Praxis* **38**, p. 1365–1372 (1969).

[37] Mares, H. H.: Longevity and mortality of diabetics. – *Amer. J. publ. Health,* **55**, p. 416–423 (1965).

[38] Masarei, J. R., Summers, M., Curnow, D. R., Cullen, K. J., McCall, M. G., Stenhouse, N. S., Welborn, T. A.: Lipoprotein electrophoretic patterns, serum lipids and coronary heart-disease. – *Brit. med. J.* **1**, p. 78–82 (1971).

[39] McGurl, T. J., Pollack, N. A.: Diabetes mellitus experience 1951–1962. – *Trans. Ass. Life Insur. Med. Dir. Amer.* **49**, p. 126–133 (1965).

[40] Mincu, I.: Studiu critic al testelor de explorare în diabetul zaharat. – *Med. interna* (Buc.) **21**, p. 471 (1969).

[41] Mincu, I., Dumitrescu, C., Câmpeanu, S., Mihalache, N., Pirvulescu, M., Covanov, D., Georgescu, St., Nuţeanu, V., Vasilescu, V., Aron, L., Antonescu, El., Ionescu, D., Bolea-Feldman, M.: Epidemiological researches on diabetes mellitus in Rumanian urban and rural population. – *Diabetologia* **8**, p. 12–18 (1972).

[42] Mincu, I., Câmpeanu, S., Dumitrescu, C., Mihalache, N.: Echilibrul lipemic in diabetul zaharat compensat. – *Med. interna* (Buc.) **22**, p. 1050 (1971).

[43] Mincu, I., Câmpeanu, S., Dumitrescu, C., Covanov, D., Georgescu, St., Mihalache, N.: Cercetări privind unele aspecte ale epidemiologiei diabetuluin zaharat. – *Med. interna* (Buc.) **21**, p. 813 (1969).

[44] Noble, R. P.: Electrophoretic separation of plasma lipoproteins in agarose. – J. Lipid Res. **9** p. 693 (1967).

[45] O'Sullivan, J. B., Williams, R. F.: Early diabetes mellitus in perspective. – *J. Amer. Med. Ass.* **198**, p. 579–582 (1966).

[46] Pavel, I., Covanov, D., Cazacu-Dobrescu, M.: Depistarea sistematică a unor boli de nutriţie în două circumscripţii din Bucureşti. – *Med. interna (Buc.)* **16**, p. 147 (1964).

[47] Pavel, I., Pieptea, R.: Diabetul. Bucureşti, Editura Medicală 1965.

[48] Pell, S., D'Alonzo, C. A.: Factors associated with long-term survival of diabetics. – *J. Amer. med. Ass.* **214**, p. 1835–1840 (1970).

[49] Pincherle, G.: Factors affecting the mean serum cholesterol. – *J. chron. Dis.* **24**, p. 289–297 (1971).

[50] Reinheimer, W., Bliffen, G., McCoy, J., Wallace, D., Albrink, M. J.: Weight gain, serum lipids and vascular disease in diabetics. – *Amer. J. clin. Med.* **20**, p. 986–996 (1967).

[51] Ries, W.: Physiologie und Pathologie der Kapillarpermeabilität unter besonderer Berücksichtigung des Diabetes mellitus. – Carl Marhold Verlag, Halle (Saale) 1956.

[52] Rodriguez, I. L., Goana, T., Poveda, O.: Epidemiologie du Diabète. – *Cahiers de Medicine (Europa Medica)* **11**, p. 787–794 (1970).

[53] Rudas, B.: Das Verhalten der Serumlipide in verschiedenen Diabetes-Stadien der Ratte. – *Wien. klin. Wschr.* **79**, p. 372–383 (1967).

[54] Scheibe, O., Gallenkamp, H.: Die Arteriosklerose des Diabetikers als spezifische Folgekrankheit des Diabetes mellitus. – *Med. Welt* , p. 415–421 (1968).

[55] Schettler, G.: Lipids and Lipidoses. – Springer-Verlag, Heidelberg 1967.

[56] Schliack, V.: Reihenuntersuchungen beim Diabetes mellitus. – *Dtsch. med. J.* **14**, p. 716 (1963).

[57] Schliack, V.: Über die Diabetes-Morbidität. – *Dtsch. med. Wschr.* **90**, p. 2321–2327 (1965).

[58] Schlierf, G.: Diättherapie der Hyperlipidämien. – *Dtsch. med. J.* **23**, p. 17–21 (1972).

[59] Schönbeck, M., Jakob, T., Risch, D., Werning, C., Lüthy, R., Knob, M., Rosenmund, H., Siegenthaler, W.: Serumlipide gesunder Menschen. – *Med. Klin.* **65**, p. 644–649 (1970).

[60] Sharp, C. L., Butterfield, W. J. H., Keen, H.: Diabetes survey in Bedford. 1962. – *Proc. roy. Soc. Med.* **57**, p. 193 (1964).

[61] Strang, J. M.: Obezitatea. In *"Bolile metabolismului"*. – Ed. G. Duncan Editura Medicală București 1966, p. 846–847.

[62] Suchet, A. W., Suchet, A.: Glycosurie provoquée et depistage du diabète dans les collectivités. – *Presse méd.* **78**, p. 130–1312 (1970). (1309–12).

[63] Tarnowski, W.: Die Pathogenese der diabetischen Fettstoffwechselstörung. – *Med. Welt*, p. 1952–1959 (1966).

[64] Vanini, P., De Marchi, R.: Il colesterolo dell'alfa e della beta-lipoproteine nel sogetto normale in raporto all'eta. – *Rass. Fisiopat. clin. ter.* **39**, p. 1–9 (1957).

[65] Verdonk, G.: Biochimie sanguine de l'athérosclérose et influence de differents facteurs nutritionnels et pharmacologiques. – *Bruxelles Méd.* **45**, p. 1149 (1965).

[66] West, K. M., Kalbfleisch, J. M.: Glucose tolerance, Nutrition and Diabetes in Uruguay, Venezuela, Malaya and East Pakistan. – *Diabetes* **18**, p. 9–12 (1966).

Chapter II

[1] Aagenaes, O., Moe, H.: Light microscopic study of skin capillaries of diabetics. – *Diabetes* **10**, p. 253–259 (1961).

[2] Albrink, M. J., Labietes, P. H., Man, E. B.: Vascular disease and serum lipids in diabetes mellitus. – *Amer. J. intern. Med.* **58**, p. 305 (1963).

[3] Angeli, A.: Aggiornamento di fisiopatologia della secrezione di ACTH. – Ed. Il Ponte, Milano, 1969.

[4] Angervall, L., Dotevall, G., Lehmann, K. E.: The gastric mucosea in diabetes mellitus. – A functional and histopathological study. – *Acta med. scand.* **169**, p. 339–349 (1961).

[5] Angervall, L., Dotevall, G., Tillander, H.: Amelioration of diabetes mellitus following gastric resection. – *Acta med. scand.* **169**, p. 743–748 (1961).

[6] Aslan, A., David, C., Câmpeanu, S.: Die Verschiebung der Kapillar-Permeabilität bei Arteriosklerose. – *Arzneimittel-Forsch.* **9**, p. 558–560 (1959).

[7] Aslan, A., David, C., Câmpeanu, S.: Studien über die Verschiebung der Kapillarpermeabilität mit zunehmendem Alter. – *Z. ges. inn. Med.* **16**, p. 78 (1961).

[8] Aurell, M.: Estimating glomerular filtration rate. – *Lancet* **2**, p. 188 (1965).

[9] Aviram, A., Ben, D., Ishay, I., Chowers, I., Czaczes, J. W.: Low plasma creatinine in diabetes mellitus. – *J. Lab. clin. Med.* **67**, p. 473 (1966).

[10] Bagdade, J. D., Porte, A. Jr., Bierman, E. L.: Diabetic lipaemia: a form of acquired fat-induced lipaemia. – *New Engl. J. Med.* **276**, p. 427–433 (1967).

[11] Bagdade, J. D., Porte, A., Biermann, E.: Hypertriglyceridemia. A metabolic consequence of chronic renal failure. – *New Engl. J. Med.* **279**, p. 181–185 (1968).

[12] Balasse, E., Ooms, H. A.: Effect d'une élévation aiguë du taux des acides gras libres (NEFA) sur la tolérance glucidique et la réponse insulinique a l'hyperglicémie chez l'homme normal. – *Rev. Franç. Étud. clin. biol.* **13**, p. 62–67 (1968).

[13] Baron, D. N.: Hypothyroidism and diabetes mellitus. – *Lancet* **2**, p. 796 (1955).

[14] Bell, E. T.: Diabetes mellitus. A clinical and pathological study of 2529 cases. – Ed. CH. C. Thomas, Springfield, Ill., (1960).

[15] Bencosme, S. A., West, R. O., Kerr, J. W., Wilson, D. L.: Diabetic capillary angiopathy in human skeletal muscles. – *Amer. J. Med.* **40**, p. 67–77 (1966).

[16] Berger, K. G., Sprague, R. G., Bennett, W. A.: The intestinal tract in diabetic diarhoea: a pathological study. – *Diabetes* **5**, p. 299 (1956).

[17] Berge, K. G., Ellefson, R. S.: Laboratory evaluation of hyperlipaemia (Hyperlipoproteinemia). – *Med. Clin. N. Amer.* **54**, p. 1029–1035 (1970).

[18] Berns, A. W., Blumenthal, H. J.: The detection of insulin binding protein in the urine of KW patients and its identification. – *Fed. Proc.* **23**, p. 461 (1964).

[19] Bierman, E. L., Amaral, J. A., Belknap, B. H.: Hyperlipemia and diabetes mellitus. – *Diabetes* **15**, p. 675–679 (1966).

[20] Bischoff, A.: Diabetische Neuropathie. – *Dtsch. med. Wschr.* **93**, p. 237–241 (1968).

[21] Bloodworth, J. M. B.: Diabetic microangiopathy. – *Diabetes* **12**, p. 99–114 (1963).

[22] Blumenthal, H. T., Goldenberg, S., Berns, A. W.: Pathology and Pathogenesis of the disseminated angiopathy of diabetes mellitus. – In *"On the nature and treatment of diabetes"*, ed. by Leibel, B. S. and Wrenshall, G. A. – Excerpta Med. Found. Amsterdam 1965 p. 397–408.

[23] Blumenthal, H. T., Hirata, Y., Owens, C. T., Berns, A. W.: A Histo- and Immunological analysis of the small vessel lesion of diabetes in the human and in the rabbit. – In *"Small blood vessel involvement in diabetes mellitus"*, ed. by M. A. Siperstein. – Amer. Inst. of Biol. Sci. Washington F. C. 1964.

[24] Hoden, G., Soeldner, J. S., Gleason, R. E., Marble, A.: Elevated serum human growth hormone and decreased serum insulin in prediabetic males after intravenous tolbutamide and glucose. – *J. clin. Invest.* **47**, p. 729–739 (1968).

[25] Bojsen-Moller, F., Gronbaek, P., Rostgaard, J.: Light microscopic study of gastrointestinal and skin capillaries in diabetes mellitus. – *Diabetes* **12**, p. 429–432 (1963).

[26] Boulet, P., Mirouze, J.: Les ostéoses diabétiques' – *Diabète* (Le Raincy) **2**, p. 155–159 (1954).

[27] Boullet, P., Mirouze, J., Barjon, P., Dana, M.: Panhypopituitarisme aigu chez une acromégale diabétique. Guérison du diabète sucré. – *Diabète* (Le Raincy) **7**, p. 145–149 (1959).

[28] Bridwell, T., Whitehouse, F. W.: Peroral jejunal biopsy in a patient with diabetic diarrhea. – *Diabetes* **10**, p. 58–59 (1961).

[29] Bürger, M.: Angiopathia Diabetica. – G. Thieme, Verl. Stuttgart 1954.

[30] Butterfield, W. J. H.: Discussion: *On the nature and treatment of diabetes,* ed. by Leibel, B. S. and Wrenshall, G. A. – Excerpta Med. Found. Amsterdam 1965, p. 768–772, 776, 778–779.

[31] Butterfield, W. J. H., Garratt, C. J., Whichelow, M. J.: Peripheral hormone action: studies on the clearance and effect of (131-I) iodo-insulin in the peripheral tissues of normal, acromegalic and diabetic subjects. – *Clin. Sci.* **24**, p. 331–341 (1963).

[32] Butterfield, W. J. H.: Priorities in medicine. – Nuffield Provincial Hospital Trust, 1968.

[33] Butterfield, W. J. H.: The effects of phenformin on peripheral glucose utilization and insulin action in obesity and diabetes mellitus. – *Ann. N. Y. Acad. Sci.* **148**, p. 724–733 (1968).

[34] Butterfield, W. J. H., Whichelow, M. J.: Peripheral glucose metabolism in control subjects and diabetic patients during glucose, glucose-insulin and insulin sensivity tests. – *Diabetologia* **1**, p. 43 (1965).

[35] Butterfield, W. J. H., Abrams, M. E., John, St. D. J. B., Whichelow, M. J.: The intravenous glucose tolerance test: peripheral disposal of the glucose load in controls and diabetics. – *Metabolism* **16**, p. 19 (1967).

[36] Butterfield, W. J. H., Hanley, T., Whichelow, M. J.: Peripheral metabolism of glucose and free fatty acids during oral glucose tolerance tests. – *Metabolism* **14**, p. 851 (1965).

[37] Butterfield, W. J. H., Garrett, C. J., Whichelow, M. J.: Peripheral hormone action: a method for the study of the action of insulin in the forearm tissues. – *Guy's Hosp. Rep.* **111**, p. 130–144 (1962).

[38] Butterfield, W. J. H., Abrams, M. E., Sells, R. A., Sterky, G., Veall, N., Whichelow, M. J.: Insulin sensitivity of the human brain. – *Lancet,* **1**, p. 557 –560 (1966).

[39] Butterfield, W. J. H.: Metabolisme et action physiopathologique des biguanides. – In: Journées Ann. de Diabétologie de l'Hôtel Dieu, Paris, p. 139–154 (1964).

[40] Butterfield, W. J. H., Arab, M. M. H., Buckle, A. L. J., Chlouverakis, C., Hanley, T., Mahler, R. F., Whichelow, M. J.: The mechanism of action of Tolbutamide. – *Diabetes* **11**, Suppl. p. 43–49 (1962).

[41] Caird, F. I., Garrett, C. J.: Prognosis for vision in diabetic retinopathy. – *Diabetes* **12**, p. 389 (1963).

[42] Caird, F. I., Burditt, A. F., Draper, G. J.: Diabetic retinopathy. A further study of prognosis for vision. – *Diabetes* **17**, p. 121 (1968).

[43] Caird, F. I., Pirie, A., Ramsell, T. G.: Diabetes and the Eye. – Blackwell Scient. Publ. Oxford-Edinburgh 1968.

[44] Câmpeanu, S., Câmpeanu, L.: Beitrag zum Studium der Kapillar-Permeabilität für elektrophoretische Bluteiweißfraktionen. – *Z. ges. inn. Med.* **14**, p. 42 und 638.

[45] Câmpeanu, S., Bonaparte, H.: Aspecte ale permeabilitaţii capilare la diabeticii cu interesare hepatică. – *Med. interna (Buc.)* **17**, p. 1213–1223 (1965).

[46] Câmpeanu, S., Câmpeanu, L., Petrovici, A.: The ultrastructure of the liver reticula-endothelial cells in diabetics. – *Acta diabet. lat.* **6**, p. 534–547 (1969).

[47] Canivet, J., Mantel, O., Babinet, J. P., Lelouche, D.: L'hypophyséctomie dans la rétinopathie diabétique. – *Presse méd.* **77**, p. 283–286 (1969). (1969).

[48] Carlström, S.: Studies of fatty acid metabolism in diabetics during exercise. – *Acta med. scand.* **182**, p. 363–376 (1967).

[49] Chazan, B. I., Eliashar, Z., Brzezinski, A., Davis, E.: Small blood vessel changes and the chylomicron count in mothers of big babies. – *Diabetes* **13**, p. 291–295 (1964).

[50] Charib, H., Gastineau, C. F.: Coexisting Addison's disease and diabetes mellitus: report of 24 cases with review of literature. – *Proc. Mayo Clin.* **44**, p. 217–227 (1969).

[51] Chester, E. M., Banker, B. Q.: The role of lipid thrombi in the pathogenesis of diabetic retinopathy. – *Arch. int. Med.* **120**, p. 397–407 (1967).

[52] Cleve, H., Alexander, K., Mitzkai, H. J., Nissen, P., Salzmann, I.: Serumglykoproteine beim Diabetes mellitus: quantitative immunologische Bestimmung von saurem alpha$_1$-glykoprotein, Gc, Alpha$_2$-Makroglobulin und Haemopexin bei Diabetikern mit und ohne Angiopathien. – *Diabetologia* **4**, p. 48–55 (1968).

[53] Csapo, G., Szücs, S.: Diabetische Angiopathie und Arteriosklerose bei Zuckerkranken. – In *"Diabetische Angiopathie"*, ed. by Mohnike, G. – Akademie Verlag Berlin 1964, p. 165–168.

[54] Darnaud, C., Denard, Y., Moreau, G., Mimart, J.: Hormone de croissance hypophysaire et diabète. – *Diabète* (Le Raincy) **2**, p. 161–163 (1954).

[55] Darnaud, C., Denard, Y., Moreau, G., Voisin, R., Combes, P.: Rétinopathies pré-diabétiques. – *Diabète* (Le Raincy) **7**, p. 142–143 (1959).

[56] David, H.: Elektronenmikroskopische Organpathologie. – VEB Verlag Volk und Gesundheit, Berlin 1967.

[57] Derot, M., Patel, J., Cormier, J. M., Tchobroutsky, G.: L'artérite des membres chez les diabétiques. – *Presse méd.* **72**, p. 1177–1182 (1964).

[58] Dieterle, P.: Pathogenese und Therapie der diabetischen Angiopathie. – *Med. Klin.* **64**, p. 55–59 (1969).

[59] Dietzel, K.: Diabetes und Gehör. – In *"Diabetische Angiopathie"*, ed. by Mohnike, G., Akad. Verlag Berlin 1964, p. 135–141.

[60] Ditscherlein, G., Singer, P.: Untersuchungen über die fibrinoiden Glomerulum-Veränderungen bei Diabetikern. – *Arch. klin. Med.* **212**, p. 291–312 (1966).

[61] Ditscherlein, G.: Kritische Bemerkungen zur "diabetischen Nephropathie". – *Dtsch. Gesundh.-Wesen* **22**, p. 1843–1845 (1967).

[62] Ditzel, J., White, P., Duckers, J.: Changes in the Pattern of the Small Blood Vessels in the Bulbus Conjunctivae in Children of Diabetic mothers. – *Diabetes* **3**, p. 99 (1954).

[63] Ditzel, J.: Functional Microangiopathy in Diabetes Mellitus. – *Diabetes* **17**, p. 388–397 (1968).

[64] Dreyfus, P. M., Hakim, S., Adams, R. D.: Diabetic Ophtalmoplegia. – *Arch. Neurol. Psychiat. (Chic.)* **77**, p. 337 (1957).

[65] Duncan, G. C.: *Diabetes Mellitus.* – V-th Ed., W. B. Saunders, Co. Philadelphia–London, 1964.

[66] Durand, M., Durand, A.: Les altérations vasculaires dermohypodermiques des diabétiques. – Études aux microscopes optique et électronique. – *Path. Biol. (Paris)* **14**, p. 1005–1019 (1966).

[67] Elkeles, R. S., Lowy, C., Wyllie, A. H. D., Young, J. L., Fraser, T. R.: Serum insulin, glucose and lipid levels among mild diabetics in relation to incidence of vascular complications. – *Lancet* **1**, p. 880–883 (1971).

[68] Ellenberg, N., Krainer, I.: Diabetic neuropathy. Review of literature and a case report with post-mortem findings. – *Diabetes* **8**, p. 279–283 (1959).

[69] Ellenberg, N.: Diabetic complication without manifest diabetes. – *J. Amer. med. Ass.* **183**, p. 926 (1963).

[70] Engerman, R. L., Bloodworth, J. M. B.: Experimental diabetic retinopathy in dogs. – *Arch. Ophthal.* **73**, p. 205 (1965).

[71] Entmacher, P. S., Root, H. F., Marks, H. H.: Longevity of diabetic patients in recent years. – *Diabetes* **13**, p. 373–377 (1964).

[72] Ettinger, P. O., Oldewurtel, H. A., Weisse, A. B., Regan, T. J.: Diminished glucose tolerance and immunoreactive insulin response in patients with nonischemic cardiac disease. – *Circulation* **38**, p. 559–567 (1968).

[73] Fagerberg, S. E.: Recent advances in diabetic neuropathy. – In *"On the nature and treatment of diabetes"*, ed. by Leibel, B. S. and Wrenshall, G. A. – Excerpta med. Found. Amsterdam 1965, p. 522–530.

[74] Falsetti, H. L., Schnatz, J. D., Greene, D. G., Bunnell, I. L.: Lipid and carbohydrate studies in coronary artery disease. – *Circulation* **27**, p. 184–191 (1968).

[75] Falta, W., Högler, F.: Die Zuckerkrankheit. – VEB Carl Marhold Verlag, Halle (Saale) 1953.

[76] Feinberg, A. W., Lax, H.: Vascular abnormalities in children with diabetes mellitus. – *J. Amer. med. Ass.* **201**, p. 515–518 (1967).

[77] Feudell, P.: Neuropathie und Angiopathie bei Diabetes. – In *"Diabetische Angiopathie"*, ed. by. Mohnike, G., Akademie Verlag Berlin 1964, p. 131–134.

[78] Field, R. A.: Altered nerve Metabolism in Diabetes. – *Diabetes* **15**, p. 696–698 (1966).

[79] Fischer, F.: Retinopathia diabetica proliferans und Nephropathia diabetica. – *Wien. med. Wschr.* **119**, p. 285–287 (1969).

[80] Fischer, V., Lippmann, H. G.: Zum Verhalten der freien Fettsäuren in Serum bei Diabetes mellitus. – *Dtsch. Z. Verdau.- u. Stoffwechselkr.* **26**, p. 169–175 (1966).

[81] Fischer, E. R., Perez Stable, E., Morteze, A., Sarver, M. E., Danowski, T. S.: Ultrastructural renal changes in juvenile Diabetes. – *J. Amer. med. Ass.* **202**, p. 291–295 (1967).

[82] Florey, H. W.: The endothelial Cell. – *Brit. med. J.* **2**, p. 487–490 (1966).

[83] Förster, H.: Zyklisches Adenosin-monophosphat. – *Dtsch. med. Wschr.* **96**, p. 251 (1971).

[84] Frankl, W. S.: Glycoproteins in diabetes mellitus and Atherosclerosis. – *Amer. J. med. Sci.* **248**, p. 588–595 (1964).

[85] Frederici, H. R., Tucker, R., Schwartz, T. B.: Observations on small blood vessels of skin in the normal and in diabetic patients. – *Diabetes* **15**, p. 233–250 (1964).

[86] Frerichs, H., Creutzfeldt, C., Creutzfeldt, W.: Inhibitors of insulin secretion. – In *"Mechanisms and regulation of Insulin secretion"*, ed. by Levine, R. & Pfeiffer, E. P. – Il Ponte, Milano 1968, p. 105–123.

[87] Funarashi, T., Fink, A. I.: The pathology of the bulbar conjunctiva in Diabetes. – *Amer. J. Ophthal.* **55**, p. 504 (1963).

[88] Funk, H. U.: Veränderungen an kleinen Extremitäten-Gefäßen von Diabetikern. – *Schweiz. med. Wschr.* **95**, p. 487 (1965).

[89] Gamstorp, I., Shelburne, S. A., Engelson, G., Redondo, D., Traisman, H. S.: Peripheral neuropathy in juvenile Diabetes. – *Diabetes* **15**, p. 441–418 (1966).

[90] Gegesi Kiss, P., Barta, L.: Diabetes mellitus im Kindesalter. – Ung. Akad. Wiss., Budapest, 1957.

[91] Gennes, J. L., Saltiel, H., Trémolières, J., Apfelbaum, M., Laudat, Ph.: Révision de l'exploration métabolique et endocrinnienne d'un cas de diabète lipo-atrophique. – *Presse méd.* **75**, p. 2605–2611 (1967).

[92] Goldenberg, S., Alex, M., Joshi, R. A., Blumenthal, H. T.: Nonatheromatous peripheral vascular disease of the lower extremity in diabetes mellitus. – *Diabetes* **8**, p. 261–273 (1959).

[93] Gradinger, H., Zahnd, G. R.: Neuropathie diabétique avec atteinte sévère du système autonome. – *Acta Diabetol. Latina* **4**, p. 557–571 (1968).

[94] Gries, F. A., Oberdisse, K.: Fettstoffwechselstörungen und Diabetes mellitus. – *Dtsch. med. Wschr.* **95**, p. 727–734 (1970).

[95] Griffiths, J. D.: The blood supply of the colon. – *Proc. roy. Soc. med.* **59**, p. 881–890 (1966).

[96] Grönberg, A., Larsson, T., Jung, J.: Diabetes in Sweden. – Stockholm 1967.

[97] Gsell, O.: Epidemiologie des Diabetes. – *Dtsch. med. Wschr.* **93**, p. 2446–2450 (1968).

[98] Hales, C. N., Randle, P. J.: Effect of low Carbohydrate diet and Diabetes mellitus on plasma concentrations of Glucose, Non-esterified fatty acids and Insulin during oral glucose tolerance tests. – *Lancet* **1**, p. 790 (1963).

[99] Hamilton, C. R., Dorson, H. G., Marshall, I.: Diabetic Angiopathy: Clinical and Electronmicroscope studies in six patients. – *Amer. J. med. Sci.* **256**, p. 84–90 (1968).

[100] Hardy, J., Ciric, I. S.: Selective anterior hypophysectomy in the treatment of diabetic retinopathy. – *J. Amer. med. Ass.* **203**, p. 73–100 (1968).

[101] Hartcroff, W. S.: Fat emboli in glomerular capillaries of choline-deficient rats and of patients with diabetic glomerulosclerosis. – *Amer. J. Path.* **31**, p. 381–397 (1955).

[102] Hausler, R. H., Sibay, T. M., Campbell, J.: Retinopathy in a dog following diabetes induced by growth hormone. – *Diabetes* **13**, p. 122 (1968).

[103] Hauss, W. H., Junge-Hülsing, G., Kuckulies, I. I., Otto, H., Rawyt, Sch. R., Wagner, H.: Verlängerte biologische Halbwertzeit der sulfatierten Mucopolysaccharide bei Alloxan-Diabetes als Ursache der diabetischen Mesenchym-Stoffwechselstörung. – *Z. klin. Chem.* **6**, p. 241 (1968).

[104] Heinsius, E.: Augenhintergrundsveränderungen beim Diabetes im Kindesalter. – *Dtsch. med. Wschr.* **82**, p. 918–919 (1957).

[105] Houston, J. L., Joiner, C. L., Trounce, J. R.: A short textbook of medicine. – III-rd Ed. Engl. University Press Ltd., London 1968.

[106] Introzzi, P., Bernarscotic, C., Buscarini, L.: Serum proteins, lipids and protein-bound carbohydrates in vascular complications of diabetes mellitus. – *Acta med. scand.* **160**, p. 47–58 (1958).

[107] Jakobson, T.: Glucose tolerance and serum lipid levels in patients with cerebrovascular disease. – *Acta med. scand.* **182**, p. 233–243 (1967).

[108] Janert, H., Mohnike, G., Günther, L.: Augenhintergrundbefunde bei 2600 stationär kontrollierten Zuckerkranken. – *Klin. Wschr.* **24**, p. 807–813 (1965).

[109] Janert, H., Mohnike, G., Hoffmann, G., Radlewitz, Ch., Jutzi, E.: Linsen- und Augenhintergrundbefunde bei 3000 ambulant kontrollierten Zuckerkranken. – *Klin. Wschr.* **36**, p. 623–628 (1958).

[110] Jorgensen, M. B.: The inner ear in diabetes mellitus. – *Arch. Otolaryng.* **74**, p. 373–381 (1961).

[111] Jones, P., Plotkin, G. R., Arky, R. A.: Lipoprotein-lipase activity in patients with diabetes mellitus, with and without hyperlipemia. – *Diabetes* **15**, p. 565–570 (1966).

[112] Joslin, E. P., Root, H. F., Withe, P., Marble, A.: The treatment of diabetes mellitus. – 10-th Ed. Lea & Fiebiger, Philadelphia 1959.

[113] Jung, H. D.: Die Nekrobiosis lipoidica diabeticorum als morphologisches und funktionelles Substrat einer diabetischen Angiopathie der Haut. – In *"Diabetische Angiopathie"*, ed. by Mohnike, G., Akademie Verlag Berlin 1964, p. 143–150.

[114] Jütte, A.: Über die Erweiterung der Netzhautvenen bei jugendlichen Diabetikern. – In *"Diabetische Angiopathie"*, ed. by Mohnike, G., Akademie Verlag Berlin 1964, p. 13–19.

[115] Kaeding, A.: Veränderungen des Elektrophoretogramms bei diabetischer Angiopathie. – In *"Diabetische Angiopathie"*, ed. by Mohnike, G., Akademie Verlag Berlin 1964, p. 209–211.

[116] Keiding, N. R.: Protein-bound Carbohydrates and Proteins of serum from diabetic patients and the relation to the late diabetic manifestations. – Copenhagen 1957, C. Hamburgers Bogtiykkeni.

[117] Keiding, N. R., Tuller, E. F.: Protein-bound carbohydrate in serum of diabetic patients with and without vascular complications. – *Diabetes* **4**, p. 37 (1965).

[118] Kelsey, F. I., Trounce, J. R., Nichols, T. R.: Vascular lesions in diabetes mellitus. The relation of raised blood protein-bound hexose levels. – *Diabetes* **8**, p. 174–178 (1959).

[119] Kimmelstiel, P., Osawa, G., Beres, J.: Glomerular basement membrane in diabetics. – *J. clin. Pathol.* **45**, p. 21 (1966).

[120] Kimmelstiel, P.: Basement membrane in diabetic glomerulosclerosis. – *Diabetes* **15**, p. 61–63 (1966).

[121] Klimt, C. R., Knatterund, G. L., Meinert, C. L., Prout, T. E.: A study of the effect of hypoglycemic agents on vascular complications in patients with adult onset diabetes. – *Diabetes* **19** Suppl. 12, p. 747–830 (1970).

[122] Knick, B., Lange, H. G., Kössling, F., Skoulda, D., Kremer, G.: Frühdiabetische Lipidstoffwechselanomalien bei Myokardinfarkt und arterieller Verschlußkrankheit. – *Dtsch. med. Wschr.* **93**, p. 1954–1959 (1968).

[123] Knowels, H. C. jr., Guest, G. M., Kiessler, M., Skillman, T. G.: The course of juvenile diabetes tested with unmeasured diet. – *Proc. Ann. Meet. Amer. Diab. Ass.*, p. 18 (1962).

[124] Kornerup, T.: Studies in diabetic retinopathy. An investigation of 1000 cases of diabetes. – *Acta med. scand.* **153**, p. 81–101 (1955).

[125] Kornerup, T.: Retinopathia diabetica proliferans. – *Acta ophthalm. (Kbh)*, p. 87 (1958).

[126] Krecke, H. J.: Niere bei Diabetes mellitus. – *Dtsch. med. J.* **19**, p. 676–683 (1968).

[127] Kremer, G. J., Niemczyk, H., Knick, B.: Koronarsklerose und subklinischer Diabetes mellitus. – *Schweiz. med. Wschr.* **97**, p. 735–739 (1967).

[128] Labram, C.: Les microaneurismes du champ vasculaire de la conjonctive bulbaire en pathologie interne. Étude biomicroscopique. – *Ann. Oculist. (Paris)* **197**, p. 150 (1964).

[129] Landau, J., Davis, E.: The small blood vessels in the conjunctiva and nailbed in diabetes mellitus. – *Lancet* **2**, p. 731 (1960).

[130] Larsson, O.: Studies of small vessels in patients with diabetes. – *Acta med. scand.* **183**, Suppl. 480 (1968).

[131] Leipert, Th.: Über die diagnostische Bewertung des Blutfettstatus. – *Wien. med. Wschr.* **119**, p. 23–25 (1969).

[132] Lenti, G., Tosselli, C., Sirigiu, F., Serra, A., Pelegrini, A.: Rilievi di microscopia ottica ed eletronica sui capillari congiuntivali in corso di malattia diabetica. – *Acta diabet. lat.* **3**, p. 342–350 (1966).

[133] Levine, R.: Metabolismul glucidelor. – In *"Bolile metabolismului"*, ed. by G. G. Duncan, Edit. Medicala Bucureşti 1965.

[134] Levy, A.: L'origine artériolaire de l'athérosclérose artérielle. – *Presse méd.* 77, p. 427–429 (1969).

[135] Lieb, W. A., Stark, N.: Die diabetische Mikroangiopathie der Netzhaut. – *Med. Welt*, p. 851–856 (1967).

[136] Lieb, W. A.: Das Endstromgebiet des Augenhintergrundes. – *Med. Welt*, p. 599–603 (1967).

[137] Lisewski, G.: Epinephrektomie bei diabetischer Angiopathie. – In *"Diabetische Angiopathie"*, ed. by Mohnike, G., Akademie Verlag Berlin 1964, p. 333–337.

[138] Lisiecka-Adamska, H., Piotrowicz-Kasprazakowa, K., Szendzikowski, S.: Gefäßveränderungen der Extremitäten bei Diabetes. – In *"Diabetische Angiopathie"*, ed. by Mohnike, G., Akademie Verlag Berlin 1964, p. 191–194.

[139] Losert, W.: Beziehungen zwischen Elektrolythaushalt und Kohlenhydrat-Stoffwechsel. – *Dtsch. med. Wschr.* **93**, p. 1723–1732 (1968).

[140] Loubatières, A.: Stimulators and Inhibitors of Insulin Secretion. Physiological Interferences. Synergisms and Antagonisms. – In *"Mechanism and Regulation of Insulin Secretion"*, ed. by Levine, R., Pfeiffer, E. E., Ed. Il Ponte Milano 1968, p. 220–256.

[141] Lupetzki, J., Bour, H., Funk-Brentano, J. L., Royer, P., Pequignot, H.: Le diabète juvénile bien traité echape-t-il au complications tardives? – *Presse méd.* 76, p. 1957–1960 (1968).

[142] Luft, R.: Indications that human growth hormone plays a role in diabetes mellitus and diabetic retinopathy. – In *"On the nature and treatment of diabetes"*, ed. by Leibel, B. S. & Wrenshall, G. A. – Excerpta Med. Found. Amsterdam 1965, p. 496–504.

[143] Lundbaek, K.: Longterm diabetes. – E. Munksgaard 1953, p. 21, 23, 25, 31, 39.

[144] Marston, A.: Clinical features of ischaemic colitis. – *Proc. roy. Soc. Med.* 59, p. 881–890 (1966).

[145] Martin, E., Rilliet, B.: Le problème des complications vasculaires du diabète. – *Diabète (Le Raincy)* 6, p. 5–7 (1958).

[146] Maruhama, Y., Goto, Y., Yamagata, S.: Diabetic treatment and the diurnal plasma triglycerides. – *Metabolism* **16**, p. 985–995 (1967).

[147] Mazovetsky, A. G., Podtergerya, V. G., Dela Vara, F.: Lipoproteins of the blood serum in patients with diabetic angiopathy and obliterating atherosclerosisi. – *Ter. Arkch (Russ.)* 41, p. 63–66 (1969).

[148] McCullagh, E. P.: Diabetic action of pituitary: clinical observation. – *Diabetes* 5, p. 223 (1956).

[149] Megibow, R. S., Megibow, S. J., Pollak, H., Bookman, J. S., Osserman, K.: The mechanisms of accelerated peripheral vascular sclerosis in diabetes mellitus. – *Amer. J. Med.* **15**, p. 322 (1953).

[150] Mehnert, H.: Diabetische Mikroangiopathie und Stoffwechselkontrolle. – *Dtsch. med. Wschr.* **94**, p. 42–45 (1969).

[151] Meriel, P., Darnaud, Ch., Denard, Y., Moreau, G., Suc, J. M., Putois, J., Combes, P. F.: La glomérulose diabétique: étude ultrastructurale. – *Presse méd.* 70, p. 667–670 (1962).

[152] Midtgard, K.: Diabetic visceral neuropathy. – *Diabetes* **15**, p. 93–96 (1962).

[153] Milcu, S. M.: Endocrinologie Clinica. – Editura Medicala Bucharest 1967.

[154] Mincu, I., Câmpeanu, S., Georgescu, S.: Consideraţii clinice asupra arteriopatiei diabetice. – *Med. Interna (Buc.)* **20**, p. 963–973 (1968).

[155] Mincu, I., Câmpeanu, S., Rădulescu, G., Câmpeanu, L., Petrovici, A.: Contributions a l'étude étiopathogénique et histopathologique des hépatopathies chroniques dans le diabète sucré. – *Rev. int. Hepat.* **18**, p. 987–1022 (1968).

[156] Mincu, I., Mihalache, N.: Mucopolizaharidele serice şi variaţia lor în complicaţiile degenerative ale diabetului. – *Med. interna (Buc.)* **16**, p. 723–728, 803–810 (1964).

[157] Mincu, I.: Le cycle swelling-shrinking mitochondrial dans le diabète. – *Diabète (Le Raincy)* **16**, p. 27–32 (1968).

[158] Mincu, I.: Metabolismul lipidelor în diabet. – *Med. interna (Buc.)* **16**, p. 1209–1225 (1964).

[159] Missmahl, H. P., Riemann, J.: Einfacher Nachweis der Mikroangiopathie an der Capillaren der Rektumschleimhaut bei Diabetikern. – *Klin. Wschr.* **46**, p. 374–376 (1968).

[160] Mohnike, G.: Zur diabetischen Blutgefäßkrankheit. – *Dtsch. med. Wschr.* **82**, p. 1904–1908 (1957).

[161] Mohnike, G.: Regulationskrankheit Diabetes. – In *"Diabetische Angiopathie"*, Akademie Verlag Berlin 1964, p. 1–8.

[162] Molinetti, G. M., Massara, F., Messina, M.: Feocromocitome bilaterale con diabete. – *Minerva med.* 55, p. 3, 496 (1964).

[163] Montague, W., Taylor, K. W.: Regulation of Immunosecretion by short chain fatty acids. – *Nature (Lond.)* **217**, p. 853 (1968).

[164] Moore, J. M., Frew, I. D. O.: Peripheral vascular lesion in diabetes mellitus. – *Brit. med. J.* **2**, p. 19–23 (1965).

[165] Morsiani, M., Dal Fiume, E.: Les lésions rétiniennes dans le diabète. – *J. Ophthal. Soc.* **23**, p. 21 (1958).

[166] Muri, J.: Diabetic arthropathy and intercapillary glomerulosclerosis. – *Acta med. scand.* **135**, p. 391 (1949).

[167] Nataka, Y.: An Experimental study on the vascular lesions caused by obstruction of the vasa vasorum. – *Jap. Circulat. J. (Ni.)* **31**, p. 275–287 (1967).

[168] Nicolescu, P., Rouiller, Ch.: Beziehungen zwischen den Endothelzellen der Lebersinusoide und Kupfferschen Sternzellen. Elektronenmikroskopische Untersuchung. – *Z. Zellforsch.* **76**, p. 313–338 (1967).

[169] Orth, D. N., Morgen, H. E.: The effect of Insulin, Alloxandiabetes and Anoxia on the ultrastructure of the rat heart. – *J. Cell. Biol.* **15**, p. 509–523 (1962).

[170] Osterby-Hansen, R.: A quantitative estimate of the peripheral glomerular basement membrane in recent juvenile diabetes. – *Diabetologia* **1**, p. 97 (1965).

[171] Otto, H., Otto-Benfeldt, E., Degenhardt, J.: Zur Frage der Koinzidenz von diabetischer Retinopathie und Glomerulosklerose. – In *"Diabetische Angiopathie"*, ed. by Mohnike, G. – Akademie Verlag Berlin 1964, p. 153–157.

[172] Otto, H., Bennek, M., Degenhardt, I.: Über den Einfluß des Diabetes auf die Arteriosklerose. – In *"Diabetische Angiopathie"*, ed. by Mohnike, G., Akademie Verlag Berlin 1964, p. 181–185.

[173] Otto, H., Themann, H., Wagner, H.: Qualitative und quantitative elektronenmikroskopische Untersuchungen an Hautcapillaren jugendlicher Diabetiker. – *Klin. Wschr.* **45**, p. 229–237 (1967).

[174] Pappas, A.: Zur Synthropie von Diabetes und Addisonscher Krankheit. – *Med. Welt* p. 1673–1679 (1967).

[175] Parker, F., Bagdade, J. D., Odland, G. F., Bierman, E. L.: Evidence for the chylomicron origin of lipids accumulating in diabetic eruptive xanthomas: a correlative lipid, biochemical histochemical and electron microscopic study. – *J. clin. Invest.* **49**, p. 2172 (1970).

[176] Pavel, I., Pieptca, R.: Diabetul. – Ed., Medicală Bucharest 1965.

[177] Pavel, I., Câmpeanu, S., Nicolesco, M., Bonaparte, H., Petrovici, A., Stoian, N.: Le diabète lipo-trophique est-il un diabète lipidique? –*Presse méd.* **71**, p. 1279–1283 (1963).

[178] Petrides, P.: Über den derzeitigen Stand der Diabetes-Behandlung. – *Klin. Mbl. Augenheilk.* **147**, p. 777–805 (1965).

[179] Pfeiffer, E. F.: Recognized Diabetogenic hormones in diabetes in man. – In *"On the nature and treatment of diabetes"*, ed. by Leibel, B. S. & Wrenshall, G. A., Exc. Med. Found. Amsterdam 1965, p. 368–386.

[180] Phocas, E., Andriotakis, C., Kilaidonis, F., Ketseas, T.: Diabète sucré et rétinopathie. – *Presse méd.* **69**, p. 1518–1520 (1961).

[181] Pieri, A., Scarpelli, P. T., Rizzo, M.: Small blood vessels in diabetes mellitus: light microscope study of specimens obtained by ear lobe biopsy. – *Diabetologia* **1**, p. 109 (1965).

[182] Pirart, J.: Diabetic neuropathy: a metabolic or a vascular disease? – *Diabetes* **14**, p. 1–9 (1965).

[183] Prochorow, M., Romanowicz, J., Dorozynska, B.: Serum proteins and lipids in juvenile diabetes. – *Bull. pol. med. Hist. Sci.* **10**, p. 170–173 (1967).

[184] Proto, R., Nardelli, G., Tafaro, E., Giorgino, R.: Osservazioni sull'incidenza delle complicanze vasculare nei diabetici con mucoviscidosi. – *Acta diabet. lat.* **5**, p. 87–94 (1968).

[185] Pyke, D. A.: Coronary disease and diabetes. – *Postgrad. med. J.* Suppl. December 1968.

[186] Randle, P. J., Garland, P. B., Hales, C. N., Newsholme, E. A.: The glucose fatty acid cycle. – *Lancet* **1**, p. 785 (1963).

[187] Randle, P. J.: The glucose fatty acid cycle. – In *"On the nature and treatment of Diabetes"*, ed. by Leibel, B. S. & Wrenshall, G. A. – Exc. Med. Found. Amsterdam 1965, p. 361–367.

[188] Regazzini, A.: La ripartizione del colesterolo tra le alfa e beta lipoproteine nei sogetti di diversa età ed in alcune condizioni morbose. – In *"Scritti in onore di Giuseppe Pellegrini"*, Viscontea, Pavia 1966, p. 419–432.

[189] Reske-Nielsen, E., Lundbaek, K.: Diabetic encephalopathy. Diffuse and focal lesions of the brain in long-term diabetes. – *Acta neurol. scand.* Suppl. 4, p. 273–290 (1963).

[190] Ricketts, H. T.: The influence of diabetic control on angiopathy. – In *"On the nature and treatment of diabetes"*, ed. by Leibel, S. B. & Wrenshall, G. A. – Exc. Med. Found. Amsterdam 1965, p. 588–600.

[191] Ries, W.: Physiologie und Pathologie der Kapillarpermeabilität unter besonderer Berücksichtigung des Diabetes mellitus. – VEB Carl Marhold Verlag, Halle (Saale) 1956.

[192] Rifkin, H., Leiter, L.: Diabetic microangiopathy. – In *"Clinical Diabetes Mellitus"*, ed. by Ellenberg, M. & Rifkin, H. – McGrow Hill, New York, p. 360–373.

[193] Romani, J. D., Bonnet-Boutier, M., Got, O., Bernheim, R.: Manifestations angiopathiques chez les diabétiques et chez les obèses. – *Presse méd.* **77**, p. 669–672 (1969).

[194] Romani, J. D., Bonnet-Boutier, M.: Obésité et prédiabète. Recherche de la microangiopathie par biopsie cutanée et par biomicroscopie conjonctivale. – *Diabète (Le Raincy)* **4**, p. 309–318 (1967).

[195] Romani, J. D.: Les lésions pariétales des capillaires lymphatiques du derme chez les diabétiques. – *Presse méd.* **79**, p. 228–229 (1971).

[196] Rudas, B.: Das Verhalten der Serumlipide in verschiedenen Diabetes-Stadien der Ratte. – *Wien. klin. Wschr.* **79**, p. 377–382 (1967).

[197] Sailer, S., Sandhoffer, F., Braunsteiner, H.: Beziehungen zwischen Blutzuckerspiegel, Umsatzrate der freie Fettsäurenumbau in Plasmatriglyceride bei Diabetikern. – *Klin. Wschr.* **45**, p. 86–91 (1967).

[198] Schaefer, L. E.: Hyperlipemia. – *Ann. N. Y. Acad. Sci.* **148**, p. 925–936 (1968).

[199] Scheibe, O., Gallenkamp. H.: Die Arteriosklerose des Diabetikers als spezifische Folgekrankheit des Diabetes mellitus. – *Med. Welt*, p. 415–421 (1968).

[200] Scher, S. M., Lawrence, A. M.: Functional microangiopathy in alloxan diabetic rats. – *Acta Endocrinol. (Kbh.)* **66**, p. 357–367 (1971).

[201] Schrade, W., Boehler, E., Biegler, R., Harmuth, E.: Fatty acid composition of lipid fractions in diabetic serum. – *Lancet* **1**, p. 285 (1963).

[202] Schrader, W., Boehler, E., Meder, V., van Teicke, R. V.: Gas chromatographic studies on the serum acids in man. I-st Part. On the fatty acid composition of serum fats in healthy subjects, arteriosclerotics and diabetics. – *Klin. Wschr.* **38**, p. 126 (1960).

[203] Schrader, A.: Klinisch-pathogenetische Aspekte der diabetischen Polyneuropathie. – *Münch. med. Wschr.* **114**, p. 2017–2024 (1972).

[204] Schrader, A., Weinges, K.: Peripher-neurologische Erkrankungen beim Diabetes mellitus. – *Internist* **2**, p. 100–105 (1961).

[205] Singer, P., Ditscherlein, G., Natusch, R.: Der diagnostische Wert der Nierenbiopsie bei Diabetikern. – *Dtsch. Gesundh.-Wes.* **22**, p. 2321–2326 (1967).

[206] Siperstein, M. D., Unger, R. H., Madison, L. L.: Studies of Muscle Capillary basement membrane in normal subjects, diabetic and prediabetic patients. – *J. clin. Invest.* **46**, p. 1973–1999 (1968).

[207] Smith, K.: Diabetic Neuropathy. – *Postgrad. Med.* **30**, p. 223–228 (1961).

[208] Somlo, Z., Szücs, S., Csapo, G., Kovacs, K.: Beitrag zum Zusammenhang zwischen der diabetischen Angiopathie und Neuropathie. – In *"Diabetische Angiopathie"*, ed. by Mohnike, G., Akademie Verlag Berlin 1964.

[209] Spiro, R. G.: Glycoproteins: structure, metabolism and biology. – *New Engl. J. Med.* **269**, p. 566–573, 616–621 (1963).

[210] Stocks, A. E., Martin, F. I. R.: Insulin sensitivity and vascular disease in maturity-onset diabetics. – *Brit. med. J.* **2**, p. 397–399 (1969).

[211] Stout, R. W.: Insulin-stimulated lipogenesis in arterial tissue in relation to diabetes. – *Lancet* **2**, p. 702–703 (1968).

[212] Strisower, E. H., Adamson, G., Strisower, B.: Treatment of hyperlipidemia. – *Amer. J. Med.* **45**, p. 488–501 (1968).

[213] Suschke, J., Foldenauer, A.: Untersuchungen über die Beziehung zwischen Serumcholesterin und Plasmafibrinogen. – *Dtsch. med. Wschr.* **93**, p. 1705–1707 (1968).

[214] Terry, E. N., Messina, E. J., Schwartz, M. S., Redisch, W., Steele, J. M.: Manifestations of diabetic microangiopathy in nailfolds capillaries. – *Diabetes* **16**, p. 595–597 (1967).

[215] Thomsen, A. C.: The kidney in diabetes mellitus. – Munksgaard, Copenhagen, 1965.

[216] Tragl, K. H., Reaven, G. M.: Effect of experimental diabetes mellitus on protein synthesis by liver ribosomes. – *Diabetes* **20**, p. 27–32 (1971).

[217] Tuna, N., Frankhauser, S., Goetz, F. C.: Total serum fatty acids in diabetes. – *Amer. J. med. Sci.* **255**, p. 120–131 (1968).

[218] Turtle, J. R., Littleton, G. K., Kipnis, D. M.: Stimulation of Insulin secretion by theophylline. – *Nature (Lond.)* **213**, p. 727 (1967).

[219] Tzagournis, M., Seidensticker, J. F., Hamwi, G. J.: Serum Insulin, carbohydrate and lipid abnormalities in patients with premature heart disease. – *Ann. intern. Med.* **67**, p. 42–47 (1967).

[220] Unger, H. H., Unger, J.: Retinale Angiopathie juveniler Diabetiker. – *Klin. Mbl. Augenheilk.* **150**, p. 644–654 (1967).

[221] Unger, H. H.: Zur Frequenz retinaler Spätschäden bei Diabetesmanifestation im Kindesalter. – Zusammenkunft der Deutschen Ophthalm. Ges. Heidelberg 1960.

[222] Vallance-Owen, J.: Insulin Antagonists. – In *"On the nature and treatment of diabetes"*, ed. by Leibel, B. S. & Wrenshall, G. A. – Excerpta Med. Found. Amsterdam 1965, p. 340–353.

[223] Vollrath, L.: Über Bau und Funktion von Basalmembranen. – *Dtsch. med. Wschr.* **93**, p. 300 (1968).

[224] Wilber, J. F., Turtle, J. R., Crane, N. A.: Inhibition of Insulin secretion by a phaeochromocytome. – *Lancet* **2**, p. 753 (1966).

[225] Wilcox, H. G., Dishmon, G., Heimberg, M.: Hepatic lipid metabolism in experimental diabetes. – *J. biol. Chem.* **243**, p. 655–657 (1968).

[226] Wilens, S. L., Elster, S. K., Baker, J. P.: Glomerular lipidosis in intercapillary glomerulosclerosis. – *Ann. intern. Med.* **34**, p. 592–607 (1951).

[227] Zacks, S. I., Peques, J. J., Elliott, F. A.: Interstitial muscle capillaries in patients with diabetes mellitus. A light and electron microscope study. – *Metabolism* **2**, p. 381–393 (1962).

[228] Zöllner, N.: Metabolism of neutral fats and fatty acids. – In *"Thanhauser's textbook of metabolism and metabolic disorders.* – II-nd Vol. Blackwell Scient. Publ., Oxford-Edinburgh 1962, p. 541–566.

[229] Zschoch, H.: Gefäßveränderungen in der Leber bei Diabetes mellitus. – I-st Int. Symp. Diabetesfragen, Berlin 1–3 X 1962.

[230] Yalow, R. S., Berson, S. A.: Plasma insulin concentration in nondiabetic and early diabetic subjects: determination by a new sensitive immunoassay technique. – *Diabetes* **9**, p. 254–260 (1960).

Chapter III

[1] Adams, D. A., Rand, R. W., Roth, N., Dashe, A. M., Heuser, G., Hanley, J., Parker, M.: Cryoablation of the Pituitary in the Treatment of Progressive Diabetic Rethinopathy. – *Diabetes* **17**, p. 634 (1968).

[2] Adnitt, P. I., Taylor, E.: Progression of Diabetic Retinopathy. Relationship to blood sugar. – *Lancet* **1**, p. 652–654 (1970).

[3] Alterman, I., Lopez-Gomez, A. A.: Phenformin Effect on Body Weight, Lipids and Glucose Regulation. – *Ann. N. Y. Acad. Sci.* **148**, p. 884–891 (1968).

[4] Anschütz, F.: Die diabetische Angiopathie. – *Dtsch. med. J.* **17**, p. 634 (1966).

[5] Ashton, N.: Retinal Micro-aneurysms in the Non-diabetic Subject. – *Brit. J. Ophthal.* **35**, p. 189 (1951).

[6] Ashton, N.: Retinal Vascularisation in Health and Disease. – *Amer. J. Ophthal.* **44**, p. 7 (1957).

[7] Ashton, N.: Diabetic Retinopathy, a New Approach. – *Lancet* **2**, p. 625 (1959).

[8] Ashton, N.: Studies of the Retinal Capillaries in Realtion to Diabetic and other Retinopathies. – *Brit. J. Ophthal.* **47**, p. 521–538 (1963).

[9] Ashton, N., Henkind, P.: Experimental Occlusion of Retinal Arterioles (Using Graded Glass Ballotini). – *Brit. J. Ophthal.* **49**, p. 225–234 (1965).

[10] Azepad, E.: La rétinopathie diabétique. –*Mèd. et Hyg. (Genève)* **26**, p. 18 (1968).

[11] Ballantyne, A. S., Loewestein, A.: The Pathology of Diabetic Retinopathy. – *Trans. ophthal. Soc. U. K.* **63**, p. 95–115 (1944).

[12] Becker, B.: Ocular Complications of diabetes. – In *"Small Vessel Involvement in Diabetes Mellitus"*, Ed. Siperstein, M. D.

[13] Beetham, W. P.: Visual Prognosis of Proliferating Retinopathy. – *Brit. J. Ophthal.* **47**, p. 611 (1963).

[14] Beetham, W. P., Aiello, L. M., Balodimos, M. C., Koncz, L.: Ruby laser Photocoagulation of early diabetic neovascular retinopathy. – *Arch. Ophthal.* **83**, p. 261–272 (1970).

[15] Best, C. H., Taylor, N. B.: The Physiological Basis of Medical Practice. – 6 th ed., Williams and Wilkins Co., Baltimore, 1955.

[16] Bloodworth, J. M. B.: Diabetic Retinopathy. – *Diabetes* **11**, p. 1 (1962).

[17] Bloodworth, J. M. B.: Histochemistry and Electron Microscopy of Diabetic Retinopathy. – In *"Small Blood Vessel Involvement in Diabetes Mellitus"*. – Amer. Inst. of Biol. Sci. Washington, D. C., 1964, p. 81–88.

[18] Bloom, A.: The Management of Diabetes and its Complications. – *Hosp. Med.* **2**, p. 766–771 (1960).

[19] Blumenthal, H., Alex, M., Goldenberg, S.: A Non-Atheromathous Proliferative Vascular Lesion of the Retina in Diabetes Mellitus. – *Amer. J. Med.* **31**, p. 382–396 (1961).

[20] Bradley, R. F., Rees, S. B., Fager, C. A.: Pituitary ablation in the treatment of diabetic retinopathy. – *Med. Clin. N. Amer.* **49**, p. 1105–24 (1965).

[21] Brunn, C., Gormsen, H., Hilden, T., Ivensen, P., Raaschon, F.: Diabetic Nephropathy, Kidney Biopsy and Renal Function Tests. – *Amer. J. Med.* **15**, p. 187 (1953).

[22] Burditt, A. F., Caird, E. I., Draper, G. J.: The Natural History of Diabetic Retinopathy. – *Clin. J. Med.* **37**, p. 307–317 (1961).

[23] Burditt, A. F., Caird, F. I.: Natural History of Lens Opacities in Diabetics. – *Brit. J. Ophthal.* **52**, p. 433–440 (1968).

[24] Caird, F. I., Burditt, A. F., Draper, G. T.: Diabetic Retinopathy. A Further Study of Prognosis for Vision. – *Diabetes* **17**, p. 121 (1968).

[25] Caird, F. I., Garret, C. J.: Prognosis of Vision in Diabetic Retinopathy. – *Diabetes* **12**, p. 389 (1963).

[26] Caird, F. I., Hutchison, M., Pirie, A.: Cataract Extraction and Diabetes. – *Brit. J. Ophthal.* **49**, p. 466 (1965).

[27] Caird, F. I., Pirie, A., Ramsell, T. G.: Diabetes and the Eye. – Blackwell Scientific Publications, Oxford-Edinburgh 1968.

[28] Câmpeanu, S., Bonaparte, H.: Aspecte alc permeabilitaţii capilare la diabetici cu afectare hepatica. – *Med. interna (Buc.)* **17**, p. 1213–1223 (1965).

[29] Canivet, J., Mantel, O., Babinet, J. P., Lelouche, D.: L'hypophysectomie dans la rétinopathie diabétique. – *Presse méd.* **77**, p. 283–286 (1969).

[30] Canivet, J., Cathelineau, G., Beaufiis, F., Derome, P., Passa, P.: Conséquences endocrinennes de l'hypophyséctomie pour rétinopathie diabétique. – *Presse méd.* **79**, 129–32 (1971).

[31] Chazan, B. M., Balodimos, M. C.: Conjunctival vascular lesions. Classification and clinical significance with special reference to Diabetes. – *Acta Diabetol. Latina.* **2**, p. 355–370 (1959).

[32] Chester, E. M., Banker, B. Q.: The Role of Lipid Thrombi in the Pathogenesis of Diabetic Retinopathy. – *Arch. intern. Med.* **120**, p. 397–407 (1967).

[33] Cogan, D. G., Toussaint, O., Kuwabara, T.: Retinal vascular patterns. IV. Diabetic retinopathy. – *Arch. Ophthal* **66**, p. 366–78 (1961).

[34] Cogan, D. G., Kuwabara, T.: Capillary Shunts in the Pathogenesis of Diabetic Retinopathy. – *Diabetes* **12**, p. 293–300 (1963).

[35] Coleman, S. C., Becker, B., Cannan, S., Rosenbaum, L.: Fluorescent Insulin Staining of the Diabetic Eye. – *Diabetes* **11**, p. 375–377 (1962).

[36] Collier, M.: La pathologie cornèene des diabètiques. – *Bull. Soc. Ophthal. (Paris)* **1**, p. 105 (1967).

[37] Colwell, A. R. H.: Relations of Small Blood Vessel Complications to Treatment of Diabetes: a Review. – In *"Small Blood Vessel Involvement in Diabetes Mellitus"*, (Eds. Siperstein, M. D., Colwell, A. H., Meyer, K.) – Amer. Inst. of Biol. Sci., Washington D. C. 1964, p. 203.

[38] Colwell, J. A.: Effect of Diabetic Control on Retinopathy. – *Diabetes* **15**, p. 497–9 (1966).

[39] Constam, G. R., Reich, T.: Ist die "freie" oder "normale" Kost in der Behandlung Zuckerkranker harmlos? – *Schweiz. med. Wschr.* **90**, p. 14 (1960).

[40] Corcelle, L., Dabis, S.: Essai de traitment des rétinopathies diabétique. – *Bull. Soc. Ophthal. (Paris)* **67**, no. 1, p. 200–204 (1967).

[41] Cullen, J. F., Irecand, J. T., Oliver, M. F.: A controlled Trial of Atromid Therapy, in Exsudative Diabetic Retinopathy. – *Trans. ophthal. Soc. U. K.* **84**, p. 281 (1964).

[42] Danowski, T. S., Sabeh, G., Alley, R. A., Robbsons, T. S., Sarver, M. E., Parsons, J. A., Susen, A. F., Nardùlli, S. V.: Pituitary ablation insulin dosage, and course of diabetic retinopathy. – *Metabolism* **17**, p. 953–65 (1968).

[43] Daighaday, W., Boniuk, I.: Diabetic retinopathy. – *J. Amer. med. Ass.* **214**, p. 1867 (1970).

[44] Davis, E.: *"The small blood vessels in members of families of diabetics.* – Proc. 9th. Int. Cong. Life Ass. Med. Tel-Aviv 1967, p. 39–45, (Karger, Basel N. Y.) 1968.

[45] Deckert, T., Simonsen, S. E., Poulsen, J. E.: Prognosis of proliferative retinopathy in juvenile diabetics. – *Diabetes* **16**, p. 728–33 (1967).

[46] Dérot, M., Demailly, Ph.: *"Diabète et maladies de la nutrition. Complications ocularies.* – Coll. medico-chirurg. Paris, p. 318.

[47] Devill, R.: Rétinite diabétique et insulinothérapie. – *Presse méd.* **78**, p. 369 (1970).

[48] Ditzel, J.: Functional Microangiopathy in Diabetes Mellitus. – *Diabetes* **17**, p. 388 (1968).

[49] Ditzel, J., Duckers, J.: The bulbar Conjunctival Vascular Bed in Diabetic Children. – *Acta paediat. (Uppsala)* **46**, p. 535 (1957).

[50] Ditzel, J., Moinat, P.: The Response of the Smaller Blood Vessels and the Serum Proteins in Pregnant Diabetic Subjects. – *Diabetes* **6**, p. 307 (1957).

[51] Ditzel, J., Sagild, U.: Morphologic and Hemodynamic Changes in the Smaller Blood Vessels in Diabetes Mellitus. II. The Degenerative and Hemodynamic Changes in the Bulbar Conjunctive of Normotensive Diabetic Patients. – *New Engl. J. Med.* **250**, p. 587 (1954).

[52] Ditzel, J., Sargent, L., Hadley, W. B.: The Relationship of Abnormal Vascular Responses to Retinopathy and Nephropathy in Diabetics. – *Arch. intern. Med.* **101**, p. 912 (1958).

[53] Dollery, C. T. et al.: Retinal Microemboli: Experimental Production of "Cottonwool" Spots. – *Lancet* **1**, p. 1303–1305 (1965). – Focal Retinal Ischaemic Ophthalmoscopic Circulatory and Ultrastructural Changes. – *Brit. J. Ophthal.* **50**, p. 285–324 (1966).

[54] Dollery, C. T., Oakley, N. W.: Reversal of Retinal Vascular Changes in Diabetes. – *Diabetes* **14**, p. 121–127 (1965).

[55] Dollery, C. T., Hodge, I. V., Engel, M.: Studies of the Retinal Circulation with Fluorescein. – *Brit. med. J.* **2**, p. 1210 (1962).

[56] von Eck, W. F.: The Effect of Low Fat Diet on Serumlipids in Diabetes and its Significance in Diabetic Retinopathy. – *Amer. J. Med.* **27**, p. 196 (1959).

[57] Ernest, I., Linnér, E., Svanborg, A.: Carbohydrate-rich, fat-poor diet in diabetes. – *Amer. J. Med.*, **39**, 594–600, (1965).

[58] Ewing, C., Lorilla, E., Hernandez, A., Berris, R.: Diabetic Vascular Complications in Long-standing Panhypopituitarism with Diabetes. – *Diabetes* **15**, p. 419 (1966).

[59] Fager, C. A., Rees, S. B., Bradley, R. F.: Surgical ablation on the pituitary in the treatment of diabetic retinopathy. – *J. Neurosurg.* **24**, p. 727 (1966).

[60] Falta, W., Hogler, F.: *"Die Zuckerkrankheit"*, VEB Carl Marhold, V. Halle (Saale), 1953.

[61] Farquhar, M. G., Wissig, S. D., Palade, G. E.: Glomerular Permeability. I. Ferritin Transfer Across the Normal Glomerular Capillary Wall. – *J. exp. Med.* **113**, p. 47 (1961).

[62] Field, R. A., Schepens, C. C., Sweet, W. H., Appels, A.: The Effect of hypophyseal stalk section on advancing diabetic retinopathy. Report of thirteen cases. – *Diabetes* **11**, p. 465 (1962).

[63] Fischer, F.: Der erste Fall von Retinopathia diabetica. – *Wien. med. Wschr.* **107**, p. 969–972 (1957).

[64] Fischer, F.: Retinopathia diabetica proliferans mit negativem Nierenbefund. – *Dtsch. Z. Verdau- u. Stoffwechselkr.* **27**, p. 123–127 (1967).

[65] Fischer, F.: Retinopathia diabetica proliferans und Nephropathia diabetica. – *Wien. med. Wschr.* **119**, p. 285–287 (1969).

[66] François, J.: La rubéose de l'iris. – *Ophthalmologica (Basel)* **121**, p. 313 (1956).

[67] Frederici, H. H. R., Tucker, W. R., Schwartz, T. B.: Observation on Small Blood Vessels of Skin in the Normal and in Diabetic Patients. – *Diabetes* **13**, p. 233 (1966).

[68] Gass, J., McDonald, M.: A Fluorescein Angiographic Study of Maculae Dysfunction Secondary to Retinal Disease. IV. Diabetic Retinal Angiopathy. – *Arch. Ophthal.* **80**, p. 583–591 (1968).

[69] Gelman, D. D., Pirani, C. C., Soothili, S. F., Muehrcke, R. C., Kark, R. M.: Diabetic Nephropathy. A Clinical and Pathologic Study Based on Renal Biopsies. – *Medicine (Baltimore)* **38**, p. 321 (1959).

[70] Goldemberg, S., Alex, M., Joshi, R., Blumenthal, H.: Non-Atheromatous Peripheral Vascular Disease of the Lower Extremity in Diabetes Mellitus. – *Diabetes* **8**, p. 261 (1959).

[71] Gröbnerg, A., Larsson, T., Jung, J.: *"Diabetes in Sweden"*, Stockholm 1967.

[72] Guinan, P.: Treatment of Proliferative Diabetic Retinopathy. – *Brit. J. Ophthal.* **51**, p. 289 (1967).

[73] Harders, H. I.: Die diabetische Capillaropathie. Mikroangiologische Untersuchungen. Insulin-Antikörper-Konzentrationen. – *Verh. dtsch. Ges. inn. Med.* p. 112–119 (1968).

[74] Hardin, R. C., Jackson, R. I., Johnsson, T. C., Kelly, H. S.: The Development of Diabetic Retinopathy. Effects of Duration and Control of Diabetes. – *Diabetes* **5**, p. 397 (1956).

[75] Hardy, S., Ciric, I. C.: Selective Anterior Hypophysectomy in the Treatment of Diabetic Retinopathy. – *J. Amer. med. Ass.* **203**, p. 88–103 (1968).

[76] Hardy, S., Panisset, A., Marchildon, A., Lanthier, A.: Microsurgical selective anterior pituitary ablation for diabetic retinopathy. – *Canad. med. Ass J.* **100**, p. 785 (1969).

[77] Harrold, B. P., Marmion, V. S., Gouch, K. R.: A Double Blind Controlled Trial of Clofibrate in the Treatment of Diabetic Retinopathy. – *Diabetes* **11**, p. 285–291 (1969).

[78] Hart, A., Cohen, H.: Capillary Fragility Studies in Diabetes. – *Brit. med. J.* **2**, p. 89–91 (1969).

[79] Hellman, L., Zumoff, B., Kessler, G., Kara, E., Rubin, I. C., Rosenfeld, R. S.: Reduction of Serum Cholesterol and Lipids by Ethyl chlorophenoxyisobutyrate – *J. Atheroscler. Res.* **3**, p. 454–466 (1963).

[80] Henkes, H. E., Houtsmüller, A. J.: Fundus Diabeticus. – *Amer. J. Ophthal.* **60**, p. 662 (1965).

[81] Henkind, P., Wise, S. N.: Descemet's Wrinkles in Diabetes. – *Ann. Ophthal.* **52**, p. 371 (1962).

[82] Hohl, R. D., Barnett, D. M.: Diabetic hemorrhagic glaucoma. – *Diabetes* **19**, p. 944–947 (1970).

[83] Idu, S. M., Câmpeanu, S.: *"Electroforeza"*, Ed. Medicală, Bucureşti, 1957.

[84] Imre, G.: Studies on the Mechanisms of Retinal Neovascularisation: Role of Lactic Acid. – *Brit. J. Ophthal.* **48**, p. 75 (1964).

[85] Ireland, J. T., Patnaik, B. K., Duncan, L. J. P.: Effect of Pituitary Ablation on the Renal Arteriolar and Glomerular Lesions in Diabetes. – *Diabetes* **16**, p. 636 (1967).

[86] Jackson, R. C., Hardin, R. C., Walker, G. C., Hendricks, A. B., Kelly, H. G.: Degenerative change in young diabetic patients in relationship to level of control. – *Paediatrics* **5**, p. 959 (1950).

[87] Johnson, S.: Retinopathy and Nephropathy in Diabetes Mellitus. Comparison of the Effects of two Forms of Treatment. – *Diabetes* **9**, p. 1 (1960).

[88] Joplin, G. F., Fraser, R., Hill, D. W., Oakley, N. W., Scott, D. J., Doyle, F. H.: Pituitary ablatiae for diabetic retinopathy. – *Quart. J. Med.* **34**, p. 334 (1965).

[89] Joplin, G. F., Dakley, N. W., Hill, D. W., Kohner, E. M., Frase, T. R.: Diabetic Retinopathy. II. Comparison of Disease Remission Induced by Various Degrees of Pituitary Ablation by Y^{90}. – *Acta Diabetol. (Basel)* **3**, p. 406–412 (1967).

[90] Keen, H.: *Diabetic Retinopathy.* – The First Jugoslav Symposion on Diabetes, Zagreb, 20.–25. X. 1967.

[91] Keiding, N. R., Rott, H. F., Marble, A.: Importance of Control of Diabetes in the Prevention of Vascular Complications. – *J. Amer. med. Ass.* **150**, p. 964 (1952).

[92] Kimmelstiel, P.: Basement Membrane in Diabetic Glomerulosclerosis. – *Diabetes* **15**, p. 61 (1966).

[93] Kimmelstiel, P., Porter, W. B.: Medical Progress: Intercapillary glomerulosclerosis (Concluded). – *New Engl. J. Med.* **238**, p. 908 (1948).

[94] King, R. C., Dobree, J. H., Kok, D. A., Foolds, W. S., Dancerfield, W.: Exsudative diabetic Retinopathy. Symptoms Changes and Effects of a Corn-oil Diet. – *Brit. J. Ophthal.* **47**, p. 666 (1963).

[95] Kodejszko, E., Czyzyk, A.: *"Therapeutische Probleme der diabetischen Angiopathie".* – I. Internat. Symp. ü. Diabetesfragen.. – Akademie Verlag Berlin, 1962.

[96] Kohner, E. M., Dollery, C. T., Bulpitt, C. J.: Cotton wool spots in diabetic retinopathy. – *Diabetes* **18**, p. 691–704 (1969).

[97] Kohner, E. M., Henkind, P.: *"Diabetic retinopathy: comparison of fluorescence angiogram with a digest preparation of the same retina.* – VII. Conf. on Microcirculation. Ålsborg, Denmark, 22.–26. June 1970.

[98] Kornerup, T.: Retinopathia diabetica proliferans. – *Acta ophthal. (Kbh)* **36**, p. 87 (1958).

[99] Kuwabara, T., Cogan, D. G.: Studies of Retinal Vascular Patterns. – *Arch. Ophthal.* **64**, p. 904–911 (1960).

[100] Kuhlmann, H., Mehnert, H., Langer, E.: Retinopathie und Glomerulosklerose bei Diabetikern. – *Med. Klin.* **64**, p. 747–751 (1969).

[101] Larsson, O., Melin, H.: An Investigation with the Fluorescent Antibody Technique on the Occurrence of Gammaglobulin in Skin from the Lower Extremities of Diabetics. – *Acta med. scand.* **12**, Suppl., p. 423 (1964).

[102] Lawrence, R. D.: Treatment of 90 Severe Diabetics with Soluble Insulin for 20–40 years. Effect of Diabetic Control on Complications. – *Brit. med. J.* **2**, p. 1624 (1963).

[103] Lawrence, J. H., Tobias, C. A., Linfoot, J. A., Born, J. E., Gottschack, A., Kling, R. P.: Heavy particles, the Cragg curve and suppression of pituitary function in diabetic retinopathy. – *Diabetes* **12**, p. 490 (1962).

[104] Lekishvili, V. P., Scott, D. J.: Diabeticheskaja Retinopatija (Diabetic Retinopathy). – *Meditina (Moscova)* (1968).

[105] Lenti, G., Tosselli, C., Pellegrini, A. A., Sirigu, F., Serra, A.: Relievi ultrastructurali sulle arteriole congiuntivali in corso di malattia diabetica. – *Ann. Ottal.* **93**, p. 939–948 (1967).

[106] Levy, A.: L'origine arteriolaire de l'athérosclerose artérielle. – *Presse méd.* **77**, p. 427 (1969).

[107] Lieb, W. A., Stark, N.: Die diabetische Mikroangiopathie der Netzhaut. – *Med. Welt, p. 851–856* (1967).

[108] Luft, R., Olivercrona, H., Ikkos, D., Kornerup, T., Ljunggren, H.: Hypophysectomy in Man: Further Experience in Severe Diabetes Mellitus. – *Brit. med. J.* **2**, p. 712 (1955).

[109] Lundbaek, K.: *"Hypophysectomy for diabetic retinopathy".* – 6th Cong. Int. Diab. Fed. Stockholm 1967.

[110] Marble, A.: Angiopathy in Diabetes: an Unsolved Problem. – *Diabetes* **16**, p. 825 (1967).

[111] Maruhama, Y., Goto, Y., Yamagata, S.: Diabetic Treatment and the Diurnal Plasma Tryglyceride. – *Diabetes* 16, p. 985–995 (1967).

[112] Mehnert, H.: Diabetische Mikroangiopathie und Stoffwechselkontrolle. – *Dtsch. med. Wschr.* **94**, p. 42–45 (1969).

[113] Mincu, I., Dumitrescu, C., Vranceanu, M.: Cercetări epidemiologice asupra complicaţiilor oculare în diabetul zaharat. Cercetări asupra modificărilor de pol anterior. Nota I. – *Med. interna (Buc.)* **22**, p. 457–469 (1970).

[114] Mincu, I., Dumitrescu, C., Vranceanu, M.: Cercetări epidemiologice asupra complicaţiilor oculare în diabetul zaharat. Cercetări asupra modificărilor polului posterior. Nota II. – *Med. interna (Buc.)* **22**, p. 471–480 (1970).

[115] Mirouze, I., Mary, P.: Angiopathie diabétique. – *Rev. Prat. (Paris)* **18**, p. 3735 (1968).

[116] Mirsky, S., Schwartz, M.: Phenformin, Diabetic Control and Body Weight. – *J. Mt. Sinai Hosp.* **33**, p. 180–191 (1966).

[117] Mirsky, S.: Influence of Hypoglycemic Therapy on Blood Lipids and Body Weight in Diabetes Mellitus. – *Ann. N. Y. Acad. Sci.* **148**, p. 937–944 (1968).

[118] Oakley, N., Hill, D. W., Joplin, G. F., Kohner, G. M., Fraser, T. R.: Diabetic Retinopathy. I. The Assessment of Severity and Progress by Comparison with a Set of Standard Fundus Photographs. – *Diabetologia* **3**, p. 402–405 (1967).

[119] Oliveira, F.: Pericytes and Microaneurysms. – *Arch. Ophthal.* **57**, p. 151 (1957).

[120] Oliver, M. F.: Further Observations on the Effects of Atromid and of ethyl chlorophenoxyisobutyrate on Serum Lipid Levels. – *J. Atheroscler. Res.* **3**, p. 427 (1963).

[121] Oswald, W.: Fettfreie Diät. – *Ars. Med. (Liestal)* **57**, p. 778–781 (1967).

[122] Patterson, J. N.: Development of Diabetic Cataract. – *Amer. J. Ophthal.* **35**, p. 68 (1952).

[123] Phocas, E., Andriotakis, C., Kicaidonis, P., Kaklamanis, F., Ketseas, T.: Diabète sucré et retinopathie. – *Presse méd.* **69**, p. 1518–1520 (1961).

[124] Powell, E. D. U., Frantz, A. G., Rabkin, M. T., Field, R. A.: Growth hormone in relation to diabetic retinopathy. – *New Engl. J. Med.* **275**, p. 922 (1967).

[125] Ramsell, T. G.: Diabetes and cataract extraction. Age at operation. – *Acta diabet. lat.* **7**, p. 789–799 (1970).

[126] Records, R. E.: The extra-retinal ocular complications of diabetes mellitus. Current concepts of pathogenesis and management. – *Acta diabet. lat.* **7**, p. 709–759 (1970).

[127] Ray, B. S., Pazianos, G., Greenberg, E., Peretz, W. C., McLean, J.: Pituitary Ablation for Diabetic Retinopathy. – *J. Amer. med. Ass.* **203**, p. 79–87 (1968).

[128] Regenbogen, L.: *"Fundul de ochi in boala hipertensivă".* – Ed. medicala, Bucureşti 1956.

[129] Romani, J. D., Boutier-Bonnet, M., Got, O., Bernheim, R.: Manifestations angiopathiques chez les diabétiques et chez les obèses. – *Presse méd.* **77**, p. 669 (1969).

[130] Roäth, F., Mirsky, S., Ditzel, J.: Proliferative Retinopathy in Diabetes Mellitus. – *J. Amer. med. Ass.* **169**, p. 903 (1959).

[131] Ruch, T., Fulton, J.: *"Fiziologie medicala şi biofizica".* – Ed. medicală, Bucureşti 1963.

[132] Rucker, C. W., Gastineau, C. F., Svien, H. J.: Effect of section of pituitary stalk on diabetic retinopathy. – *Proc. Mayo Clin.* **42**, p. 409 (1967).

[133] Salgado, E.: *"Semeiologie vasculaire de la cononctive".* – Doin, G., Paris 1963.

[134] Salomon, M. I.: Diabetic Nephropathy: Clinicopathological Correlation. A Study Based on Renal Biopsies. – *Metabolism* **12**, p. 687 (1963).

[135] Sévin, R.: Treatments for Diabetic Retinopathy. In *"Advances in Ophthalmology".* – **24**, Editor Roper-Hall, M. J., Sautter, E. R., Streiff, S., Karger Publ. Basel 1971.

[136] Sévin, R., Cuendet, J. F.: La rétinopathie diabétique. Son traitment médical. – *Schw. Rdsch. Med. (Praxis)* **60**, p. 612–614 (1971).

[137] Simonses, S. E.: Electroretinographic Study of Diabetics. – *Acta ophthal. (Kbh)* **43**, p. 841 (1965).

[138] Skovborg, F., Ditzel, J., Lauritzen, E., Nielsen, V. A.: Quantitative Measurements of Early Changes in the Retina of Diabetics. – *Diabetologia* **1**, p. 135 (1965).

[139] Skovborg, F., Lauritzen, E.: Fluorescein Retinography: Exsudates and Microaneurysms. – *Brit. med. J.* **2**, p. 1160 (1965).

[140] Skovborg, F., Nielsen, A. C. V., Lauritzen, E., Hartkoop, O.: Diameters of the Retinal Vessels in Diabetic and Normal Subjects. – *Diabetes* **18**, p. 292–298 (1969).

[141] Skovby, A. P.: Vascular Lesions in Diabetes with a Special Reference to the Influence of Treatment. – *Acta med. scand.* **155**, Suppl. 317, p. 155 (1956).

[142] Spiro, R. G.: Glycoproteins and Diabetes. – *Diabetes* **12**, p. 223 (1963).

[143] Stohr, P., Möllendorf, W. V., Goeriler, K.: *"Lehrbuch der Histologie".* – VEB G. Fischer, Jena, 1915, p. 464–496.

[144] Striga, M., Basic, M.: *"Our Experience with the Radiations of the Hypophysis by Radioactive Cobalt in the Treatment of Diabetic Retinopathy in the Course of Four Years"* (1964–1968). – The First Jugoslav Symposium on Diabetes, Zagreb, 25.–28. X. 1967.

[145] Thiel, R., Hollwich, F.: *"Therapie der Augenkrankheiten mit diagnostischen Hinweisen"*. – G. Thieme, Stuttgart 1970.

[146] Unger, H. H., Unger, J.: Retinale Angiopathie juveniler Diabetiker. – *Klin. Mbl. Augenheilk.* **150**, p. 644–654 (1967).

[147] Vassali, P., Simon, G., Rouiller, C. H.: Electron Microscopic Study of Glomerular Lesion Resulting from Intravascular Fibrin Formation. – *Amer. J. Path.* **43**, p. 479 (1963).

[148] Verin, M. P.: Cataracte chez les diabétiques. – *Bull. Soc. Ophthal. (Paris)* **129**, p. 136 (1961).

[149] Walker, G. L.: Diabetic Retinopathy in Young Persons. – *Trans. Amer. ophthal. Soc.* **48**, p. 677 (1950).

[150] Wolfram, G.: Hyperlipidämie. Ihre Beziehung zu Gefäßkrankheiten und ihre Behandlung. – *Ann. Méd.* **59**, p. 7–9 (1969).

[151] Wolter, J. R.: Diabetic Capillary Microaneurysms of the Retina. – *Med. Ophthal.* **65**, p. 847 (1961).

[152] Wolter, J. R.: The Nature of Capillary Microaneurysms in Diabetic Retinopathy. – *Diabetes* **11**, p. 126–131 (1962).

[153] Whittington, T. H., Lawrence, R. D.: *Mod. Probl. Ophthal (Basel)* (sub red, Sorsby, A.), p. 317 (1963).

[154] Whittington, T. H.: In *"Clinical Diabetes"*, (sub red. Oakley, W. G., Pyke, D. A., Taylor, K. W.) Chap. 18, Blackwell Scientific Publications. – Oxford-Edinburgh 1968, p. 456.

[155] Wisc, G. N.: Retinal Microaneurysms. – *Arch. Ophthal,* **57**, p. 151 (1957).

[156] Zervas, N. T.: Stereotaxic radiofrequency surgery of the normal and abnormal pituitary gland. – *New Engl. J. Med.* **280**, p. 429 (1969).

[157] Yamashitta, T., Becker, B.: The Basement Membrane in the Human Eye. – *Diabetes* **10**, p. 167–174 (1961).

Chapter IV

[1] Anderson, G. S.: The Pathogenesis of Diabetic Glomerulosclerosis. – *J. Path. Bact.* **67**, p. 241 (1954).

[2] Anderson, J.: The kidney in diabetes. Chap. 21 in *"Clinical Diabetes"*, ed. by Oakley, W. G., Pyke, D. A., Taylor, K. W. – Blackwell Scient. Publ. Oxford & Edinburgh 1968, p. 562–576.

[3] Ashton, N.: Diabetic Retinopathy, Relationship to Glomerulosclerosis. – *Brit. med. J.* I, p. 1002 (1957).

[4] Bariéty, J., Druet, Ph., Lagrue, G.: Les glomérulopathies "Extra-membraneuses". – *Presse méd.* **77**, p. 1457–1458 (1969).

[5] Barrie, H. J., Aszkanazy, C. L., Smith, G. W.: More Glomerular Changes in Diabetics. – *Canad. med. Ass. J.* **66**, p. 428 (1952).

[6] Becker, D., Miller, M.: Presence of Diabetic Glomerulosclerosis in Patients with Haemochromatosis. – *New Engl. J. Med.* **263**, p. 367–373 (1960).

[7] Beiswenger, P. J., Spiro, R. G.: Human glomerular basement membrane: chemical alteration in Diabetes Mellitus. – *Science* **168**, p. 596–598 (1970). (1970).

[8] Bell, E. T.: Renal Lesions in Diabetes Mellitus. – *Amer. J. Pathol.* **18**, p. 744 (1942).

[9] Bell, E. T.: Renal Diseases. – Saunders, W. B., Philadelphia 1946, p. 373.

[10] Bell, E. T.: Renal Vascular Diseases in Diabetes Mellitus. – *Diabetes* **2**, p. 376 (1953).

[11] Bell, E. T.: Diabetes Mellitus. A clinical and Pathological Study of 2529 cases. – Thomas, Ch. C., Springfield 1960.

[12] Bencosme, S. A., Morrin, P. A. F.: Ultrastructural Pathology of the Glomerulus. In *"Ultrastructure of the Kidney"*, ed. by Dalton, A. J. & Haguenau, F. – Academic Press, New York and London 1967, p. 143–277.

[13] Bergstrand, A. F.: Electron microscopic studies of the diabetic kidney. In *"Small Blood Vessel Involvement in Diabetes Mellitus"*, ed. by Siperstein, M. D. and Colwell, A. R., Meyer, K. – Amer. Inst. Biol. Sci. Washington, D. C. 1964, p. 65–71.

[14] Berns, A. W., Owens, C. T., Hirata, Y., Blumenthal, H. T.: The Pathogenesis of Diabetic Glomerulosclerosis. II. A demonstration of Insulin-Binding Capacity of the various histopathological Components of the Disease by Fluorescence Microscopy. – *Diabetes* **11**, p. 308–317 (1962).

[15] Beroniade, V.: Aparatul urinar. In *"Ghid de date biologice"*, ed. by Paunescu-Podeanu, A. 1962. – Edit. Medicală Bucharest, p. 221–290.

[16] Blumenthal, H. T., Berns, A. W., Owens, C. T., Hirata, Y.: The Pathogenesis of Diabetic Glomerulosclerosis. I. The Significance of various histopathological components of the disease. – *Diabetes* **11**, p. 296–307 (1962).

[17] Brun, C., Gormsen, H., Iversen, P., Raaschou, F.: Diabetic nephropathy. Kidney Biopsy and Renal Function Tests. – *Amer. J. Med.* **15**, p. 187 (1953).

[18] Bittar, E. E., Misanik, L.: Renal Necrotizing papillitis. – *Amer. J. Med.* **34**, p. 82–87 (1963).

[19] Caird, F. I.: Survival of Diabetics with Proteinuria. – *Diabetes* **10**, p. 178–181 (1961).

[20] Câmpeanu, S., Câmpeanu, L., Petrovici, A.: The Ultrastructure of the Liver Reticulo-Endothelial Cells in Diabetics. – *Acta diabet. lat.* **6**, (1969).

[21] Câmpeanu, S., Bonaparte, H.: Aspekts of capillary permeability in diabetics with hepatic involvement. – *Med. interna (Buc.)* **17**, p. 1213–1223 (1965).

[22] Câmpeanu, S., Câmpeanu, L.: Die echte transkapillare Proteinfiltrierung im Verhältnis zu verschiedenen Druckhöhen. – *Zschr. f. Ges. inn. Med.* **15**, p. 495 (1960).

[23] Câmpeanu, S., Câmpeanu, L.: Beitrag zum Studium der Kapillarpermeabilität für elektrophoretische Bluteiweißfraktionen. – *Z. ges. inn. Med.* **14**, p. 42 (1959).

[24] Chimenes, H.: Etats prédiabétiques. Réalités et illusions. – *Presse méd.* **77**, no. 46, p. 1652 (1969).

[25] Collens, W. S., Silverstein, J. N., Dobkin, G. B.: Case of a diabetic with a Kimmelstiel-Wilson syndrome and a normal glucose tolerance. – *Ann. intern. Med.* **50**, p. 1282 (1959).

[26] Combes, P. F.: La glomérulose diabétique. – Thése, Toulouse 1960.

[27] Cossel, L.: Über elektronenmikroskopische Befunde bei diabetischer Glomerulosklerose. In *"Diabetische Angiopathie"*, ed. by Mohnike, G. Akademie Verlag Berlin 1964, p. 37–40.

[28] Creutzfeldt, W., Frerichs, H., Malsch, H., Moench, A.: Experimentelle Untersuchungen zur Auswirkung einer Nierenschädigung auf den Diabetes mellitus, Alloxan Diabetes und Masugi-Nierenerkrankung. – *Naunyn-Schmiedeberg's Arch. exp. Path.* **236**, p. 392 (1959).

[29] Dachs, S., Churg, J., Mautner, W., Grisham, E.: Diabetic nephropathy. – *Amer. J. Path.* **44**, p. 155 –168 (1964).

[30] Dalton, A. J., Françoise Hagueneau. Ultrastructure of the kidney. – 1967, Academic Press N. Y. and London.

[31] Danowski, T. S., Limaye, N. R., Cohn, E. R., Grimes, B. J., Narduzzi, J. V., Shelkrot, J. W.: Distribution and frequency of diabetic concomitants or complications. – *Diabetes* **15**, p. 507–510 (1966).

[32] Darnaud, C., Denard, Y., Moreau, G., Suc, J. M.: La ponction biopşie du rein chez les diabétiques. – *Sem. Hôp. Paris* **32**, p. 3935 (1956).

[33] David, H.: Elektronenmikroskopische Organpathologie. – VEB-Verlag Volk u. Gesundheit, Berlin 1967, p. 192, 206–209, 231.

[34] Daysog, A. jr., Dobson, H. L., Brennan, J. C.: Renal Glomerular and Vascular Lesions in Prediabetes and in Diabetes mellitus; a study based on renal biopsies. – *Ann. intern. Med.* **54**, p. 672 (1961).

[35] Dische, Z.: The Pattern of the chemical structure of Basement membranes. – Diabetes, Proc. VIth. Cong. Int. Diab. Fed. Stockholm 1967. – Exc. Med. Found, 1969, Amsterdam, p. 565–571.

[36] Ditscherlein, G.: Todesursachen bei diabetischer Glomerulosklerose. In *"Diabetische Angiopathie"*, ed. by Mohnike, G., Akademie Verlag Berlin 1964, p. 29–32.

[37] Ditscherlein, G.: Zu den peripheren Nierengefäßveränderungen beim Diabetes mellitus. In *"Diabetische Angiopathie"*, ed. by Mohnike, G., Akademie Verlag, Berlin 1964, p. 57–62.

[38] Ditscherlein, G.: Über Glomerulosklerose bei Diabetikern. Zur Problematik der diffusen und nodulären Glomerulumveränderung und der Beurteilung ihres Schweregrades. – *Dtsch. Z. Verdau.- u. Stoffwechselkr.* **25**, p. 27–37 (1965).

[39] Ditscherlein, G.: Häufigkeit der Glomerulosklerose bei 400 obduzierten Diabetikern. – *Dtsch. Z. Verdau.- u. Stoffwechselkr.* **25**, p. 55–63 (1965).

[40] Ditscherlein, G.: Kritische Bemerkungen zur "Diabetischen Nephropathie". – *Dtsch. Gesundh.-Wes.* **22**, p. 1843–1845 (1967).

[41] Ellenberg, M.: Diabetic Nephropathy Without Manifest Diabetes. – *Diabetes* **11**, p. 197–201 (1962).

[42] Englesson, G.: Studies in Diabetes Mellitus. – *Acta paediat. (Uppsala)* **43**, Supp. 97, p. 1–163 (1954).

[43] Epstein, F. H., Zupa, V. J.: Clinical Correlates of the Kimmelstiel-Wilson lesion. – *New Engl. J. Med.* **254**, p. 886 (1956).

[44] Fahr, T.: Über Glomerulosklerose. – *Virchow's Arch. path. Anat.* **309**, p. 16 (1942).

[45] Falta, W., Högler, F.: Die Zuckerkrankheit. – VEB Carl Marhold Verlag, Halle (Saale) 1953, p. 253–257.

[46] Farquhar, M. G., Hopper, J., Moon, H. D.: Diabetic Glomerulosclerosis. Electron and light microscopic studies. – *Amer. J. Pathol.* **35**, p. 721 (1959).

[47] Farquhar, M. G.: (1964) In Discussion of electron microscopic studies of the diabetic Kidney by Bergstrand, A. F. and Buchs, H. In *"Small Blood Vessel Involvement in Diabetes Mellitus"*, ed. by Siperstein, M. D., Colwell, A. R. and Meyer, K., p. 73. – Amer. Inst. Biol. Sci. Washington D. C.

[48] Farquhar, M. G.: Glomerular Permeability Investigated by Electron Microscopy. In *"Small Blood Vessel Involvement in Diabeted Mellitus"*, ed. by Siperstein, M. D., Colwell, A. R., Meyer, K. – Amer. Biol. Sci. Washington D. C., 1964, p. 31–38.

[49] Fiaschi, E., Naccarato, R., Scuro, L. A., Rizzo, A., Previato, G., Fagiolo, U.: La microangiopatia diabetica. – *Acta diabet. lat.* **6**, p. 87–120 (1969).

[50] Fischer, F.: Retinopathia diabetica proliferans und Nephropathia diabetica. – *Wien. med. Wschr.* **119**, p. 285–287 (1969).

[51] Franke, E.: Komplikationen und Begleitkrankheiten des Diabetes mellitus. I. Mitt. Zur Klinik der Glomerulosklerose (Kimmelstiel-Wilson). *Zschr. f. ges. inn. Med.* **26**, p. 45–48 (1971). – II. Mitt. Pyelonephritis und Arteriosklerose der Nieren bei Diabetikern. – *Z. ges. inn. Med.* **26**, p. 49–53 (1971).

[52] Fraser, R., Joplin, G. F., Steiner, R. E.: Pituitary ablation by $Yttrium_{90}$ implants for diabetic retinopathy. – *Diabetes* **11**, p. 482 (1962).

[53] Fuchs, T. G., Gutensohn, G.: Pathologische Harnbefunde bei Diabetikern. – *Münch. med. Wschr.* **111**, p. 1885–1887 (1969).

[54] Gabbay, K. H., Field, R. A.: Accumulation of Glucose, Sorbitol and Fructose in Diabetic Kidney. – 26th Annual Meeting of the American Diabetes Association June 1966, Chicago.

[55] Geller, G.: Histochemische Untersuchungen an den Glomerula bei diabetischer Glomeruloskerose. In *"Diabetische Angiopathie"*, Ed. by Mohnike, G. Akademie Verlag Berlin 1964, p. 45–49.

[56] Geiler, G.: Die diabetische Angiopathie aus der Sicht des Pathologen. – *Dtsch. med. Wschr.* **92**, p. 1640–1643 (1967).

[57] Gellman, D. D.: The Correlation Between the Pathological and Clinical Manifestations of Diabetic Renal Disease. In *"Small Blood Vessel Involvement in Diabetes Mellitus"*, ed. by Siperstein, M. D., Colwell, A. R., Meyer, K., 1964, Amer. Inst. of Biological Sciences Washington D. C., p. 13–24.

[58] Gellman, D. D., Pirani, C. L., Soothill, J. F., Muehrcke, R. C., Madukos, W., Karl, R. M.: Structure and Function in Diabetic Nephropathy. The Importance of Diffuse Glomerulosclerosis. – *Diabetes* **8**, p. 251–256 (1959).

[59] Gibbs, G. E., Wilson, R. B., Gifford, H.: Glomerulosclerosis in the Longterm Alloxan Diabetic Monkey. – *Diabetes* **15**, p. 258–261 (1966).

[60] Goetz, F. C., Hartmann, J. F., Lazarow, A.: Electron Microscopy of the Human Glomerulus in early Diabetes. – *J. clin. Invest.* **39**, p. 991 (1960).

[61] Gordon, E. S.: Surgical Hypophysectomy in the Treatment of Diabetic Nephropathy. – *J. Lab. clin. Med.* **48**, p. 8–10 (1956).

[62] Gordon, E. S., Javid, M.: Metabolic Studies in Hypophysectomy for Diabetic Vascular Disease. – *Diabetes* **11**, p. 470 (1962).

[63] Gronberg, A., Larsson, T., Juno, J.: Diabetes in Sweden. – *Acta med. scand.* Suppl. **477** (1967).

[64] Hall, G. F. M.: Factors in the Aetiology of Diabetic Glomerulosclerosis. – *Quart. J. Med.* **21**, p. 385 (1952).

[65] Hatt, P. Y.: The juxtaglomerular apparatus. In *"Ultrastructure of the Kidney"*, ed. by Dalton, A. J., Haguenau, F. – Academic Press, New York and London 1967, p. 101–141.

[66] Haugen, H. N., Blegen, E. M.: Some Clinical Observations in Diabetes Mellitus. – *Acta med. scand.* **150**, p. 291 (1954).

[67] Heintz, R., Renner, D.: Urämie. Neue Ergebnisse zur Ätiologie und Pathogenese. – *Med. Welt*, p. 1803–1807 (1967).

[68] Henderson, L. L., Sprague, R. G., Wagener, H. P.: Intercapillary Glomerulosclerosis. – *Amer. J. Med.* **3**, p. 131 (1948).

[69] Hennigar, G. R., Cohen, R. J., Katz, H. P.: Nodular Glomerulosclerosis: clinico-pathological correlation of 40 advanced cases. – *Amer. J. med. Sci.* **41**, p. 89 (1961).

[70] Huber, H., Pastner, D., Gabl, F.: Laboratoriumdiagnose hämatologischer und immunologischer Erkrankungen. – Springer Verlag, Berlin–Heidelberg–N. Y. 1972, p. 135–145.

[71] Idu, S. M., Câmpeanu, S.: Electroforeza. – Ed. Medicală, Bucharest 1967.

[72] Ireland, J. T., Patnaik, B. K., Duncan, L. J. P.: Effect of Pituitary Ablation on the Renal Arteriolar and Glomerular Lesions in Diabetes. – *Diabetes* **16**, p. 636 (1967).

[73] Ireland, J. T.: Electron Microscopy of the Glomerulus in Diabetes Mellitus. Chap. III, p. 26–30. In *"Diabetic Nephropathy"*, ed. by Syllaba, J., Praha, Universita Karlova 1968.

[74] Jahnke, K., Irmscher, K., Solbach, H. G.: Zur klinischen und morphologischen Differenzierung der renalen Komplikationen bei Diabetes mellitus. – *Klin. Wschr.* **42**, p. 251 (1964).

[75] Johnsson, S.: Retinopathy and Nephropathy in Diabetes mellitus. – *Diabetes* 9, p. 1–8 (1960).

[76] Kalliomaki, J. L., Markkanen, T. K., Sourander, L. B.: Correlation Between Insulin Requirement and Renal Retention in Diabetic Nephropathy. – *Acta med. scand.* **166**, p. 423 (1960).

[77] Kefalides, N. A.: The Chemical Basis for the Structure and Function of Basement Membranes. – *Diabetes.* – Proc. VIth. Cong. Int. Diab. Fed. Stockholm 1967, Exc. med. Found 1969, Amsterdam, p. 610–611.

[78] Keiding, N. R., Root, H. F., Marble, A.: Importance of Control of Diabetes in Prevention of Vascular Complications. – *J. Amer. med. Ass.* **150**, p. 964 (1952).

[79] Kimmelstiel, P.: Basement Membrane in Diabetic Glomerulosclerosis. – *Diabetes* **15**, p. 1 (1966).

[80] Kimmelstiel, P., Wilson, C.: Intercapillary Lesions in the Glomeruli of the Kidney. – *Amer. J. Pathol.* **12**, p. 83 (1936).

[81] Knowles, H. C.: Pancreatic Diabetes and Vascular Disease. – *Diabetes* **13**, p. 315–316 (1964).

[82] Koss, L. G.: Hyaline Material with Standing Reaction of Fibrinoid Renal Lesions in Diabetes Mellitus. – *Arch. Pathol.* **54**, p. 528 (1952).

[83] Krakower, C. A., Greenspon, S. A.: The Immunologic Properties of basement Membrane. – *Diabetes.* – Proc. VI th Cong. Int. Diab. Fed. Stockholm 1967. Exc. med. Found 1969, Amsterdam, p. 595–605.

[84] Krecke, H. J.: Niere bei Diabetes Mellitus. – *Dtsch. med. J.* **19**, p. 676–683 (1968).

[85] Kuhlmann, H., Mehnert, H., Langer, E.: Retinopathie und Glomerulosklerose bei Diabetikern. – *Med. Klin.* **64**, p. 747–751 (1969).

[86] Lambie, A. T., MacFarlane, A.: A Clinical pathological Study of Diabetic Glomerulosclerosis. *Quart. J. Med.* **24**, p. 125 (1955).

[87] Latotzki, H.: Der Einfluß unterschiedlicher Glykämie-Situationen auf die Ergebnisse renaler Clearancemessungen bei Diabetikern. In *"Diabetische Angiopathie"*, ed. by Mohnike, G. Akademie Verlag Berlin 1964, p. 81–85.

[88] Lauler, D. P., Schreiner, G. E., David, A.: Renal Medullary Necrosis. – *Amer. J. Med.* **29**, p. 322–327 (1960).

[89] Lecompte, P. M.: The Kimmelstiel-Wilson Lesion. – *Diabetes* 7, p. 495 (1958).

[90] Lecompte, P. M.: Glomerular Lesions in Diabetes: Light Microscopy and Histochemistry. In *"Small Blood Vessel Involvement in Diabetes Mellitus"*, ed. by Siperstein, M. D., Colwell, A. R. & Meyer, K. – Amer. Inst. Biol. Sci. Washington D. C. 1964, p. 1–6.

[91] Lenti, G., Pellegrini, A., Sirigu, F., Pagano: Indagini sulla nefropatia diabetica. Riproduzione sperimentale di un quadro simildiabetico in reni di conigli trattati con Protamina. – *Rass. med. sarda* **68**, p. 167–182 (1965).

[92] Levin, R., Forsham, P. H., Leopold, I., McDonald, M., Marble, A.: Les complications vasculaires du Diabète. – *Spectrum* **10**, p. 16–20 (1966).

[93] Lippmann, H. G.: Symposion zu aktuellen Fragen des Diabetes mellitus in Karlsburg. – *Dtsch. Zschr. Verdau.- u. Stoffwechselkr.* **28**, p. 369–378 (1968).

[94] Lisewski, G.: Nierenfunktion bei diabetischer Nephropathie. In *"Diabetische Angiopathie"*, ed. by Mohnike, G. – Akademie Verlag Berlin 1964, p. 87–94.

[95] Lonergan, R., Robbins, S. L.: Absence of Intercapillary Glomerulosclerosis in the Diabetic Patient with Haemochromatosis. – *New Engl. J. Med.* **260**, p. 367–369 (1959).

[96] Luft, R., Olivecrona, H., Ikkos, B., Kornerup, T., Ljunggren, H., Nilsson, L., Sjøgren, B.: Hypophysektomy vid diabetes mellitus med vaskulär komplikationen. – *Nord. Med.* **55**, p. 715 (1956).

[97] Lundraek, K.: Nephropathy in Diabetic Subjects. Chap. 30 in *"On the Nature and Treatment of Diabetes"*, ed. by Leibel, B. S. & Wernshall, G. A. 1965. – Exc. med. Found. Amsterdam, p. 436–446.

[98] Lynch, M. J. G., Raphael, S. S.: The nature of Diabetic (Kimmelstiel-Wilson) Glomerulosclerosis. – *Diabetes* 6, p. 488 (1957).

[99] Marble, A., Steinke, J.: Hämochromatose. Bericht über 42 Fälle mit Diabetes. – *Med. Welt* p. 19–23 (1959).

[100] Mehl, J.: Lichtoptische Nierenbefunde bei experimentellem Langzeit-Diabetes. In *"Diabetische Angiopathie"*, ed. by Mohnike, G. – Akademie Verlag Berlin 1964, p. 41–43.

[101] Menefee, M. G., Mueller, C. B.: Some morphological considerations of transport in the Glomerulus. In *"Ultrastructure of the Kidney"*, ed. by Dalton, A. J. & Haguenau, F. – Academic Press, New York and London 1967, p. 73–100.

[102] Meriel, P., Darnaud, Gh., Denard, Y., Suc, J. M., Putois, J., Combes, P. F.: La glomérulose diabé-

tique: étude ultra-structurale. – *Presse méd.* **70**, p. 667–670 (1962).

[103] Miatello, V. R., Machado, E., Medel, R. P.: Alteraciones cronicas de rinon del diabetico estudiadas por la biopsia renale transcutanea. – *Pren. med. Argent.* **45**, p. 1027 (1958).

[104] Michielsen, P., Creemers, J.: The structure and function of the glomerular mesangium. In *"Ultrastructure of the Kidney"*, ed. by Dalton, A. J. & Haguenau, F. – Academic Press, New York and London 1967, p. 57–72.

[105] Mincu, I., Câmpeanu, S., Radulesco, Gh., Campeanu, L., Petrovici, A.: Contributions a l'étude étiopathogénique et histopathologique des hépatopathies chroniques dans le diabète sucré. – *Rev. int. Hépat.* **18**, p. 987–1022 (1968).

[106] Mincu, I., Pieptea, R., Mihalache, N.: Nefropatia diabetica. Studiu functional. – *Med. interna (Buc.)* **21**, p. 1187 (Nota A) and p. 1271 (Nota B) (1969). (Nota B).

[107] Mirouze, J., Sagcs, A., Loubatières, R.: La Néphropathie diabétique. Analyse morphologique par ponction-biopsie et confrontation fonctionelle. In: *"Diabetische Angiopathie"*, ed. by Mohnike, G. – Akademie Verlag Berlin 1964, p. 67–80.

[108] Mogensen, C. E.: Kidney function and glomerular permeability to macromolecule in early Juvenile Diabetes. – *Scand. J. clin. Lab. Invest.* **28**, p. 79–90 (1971).

[109] Mogensen, C. E.: Glomerular filtration rate and renal plasma flow in short term and long term Juvenile Diabetes Mellitus. – *Scand. J. clin. Lab. Invest.* **28**, p. 91–100 (1971).

[110] Mogensen, C. E.: Maximum tubule reabsorption capacity for glucose infusion in normal and diabetic subjects. – *Scand. J. clin. Lab. Invest.* **28**, p. 101–109 (1971).

[111] Mohnike, G.: Zur diabetischen Blutgefäßkrankheit. *Dtsch. med. Wschr.* **82**, p. 1904–1907 (1957).

[112] Mohnike, G.: Über die diabetische Angiopathie. – *Acta diabet. lat.* **2**, p. 139 (1965).

[113] Munz, W.: Häufigkeit und zeitliches Auftreten der Organmanifestationen beim Diabetes mellitus. – *Schweiz. med. Wschr.* **90**, p. 241 (1960).

[114] Otto, H., Otto, E., Benfeldt, Degenhardt, I.: Zur Frage der Koinzidenz von diabetischer Retinopathie und Glomerulosklerose. In *"Diabetische Angiopathie"*, ed. by Mohnike, G. – Akademie Verlag Berlin 1964, p. 153–157.

[115] Patz, A., Berkow, J. W., Maumenee, A. E., Lox, J.: Studies on Diabetic Retinopathy. II. Retinopathy and Nephropathy in spontaneous Canine Diabetes. – *Diabetes* **14**, p. 700–708 (1965).

[116] Pirani, C. L., Polak, V. E., Muehrke, R. C., Kark, R. M.: Lupus nephritis. In *"Ciba Foundation Symposium on Renal Biopsy"*, London 1961, p. 218.

[117] Pyke, D. A., Oakley, W. G., Taylor, K. W.: The Prognosis of Diabetes. Chapt. 30 in *"Clinical Diabetes"*, 1968. – Blackwell Scient. Publ. Oxford & Edinburgh, p. 745–756.

[118] Rapoport, S. M.: Medizinische Biochemie, 2. Aufl. VEB Verlag, Volk u. Gesundheit, Berlin 1964, p. 669–672.

[119] Reubi, F.: Nierenkrankheiten. – Hans Huber Verlag, Bern u. Stuttgart 1960.

[120] Reubi, F.: La glomérulosclérose diabétique et le syndrome de Kimmelstiel et Wilson. – *Rev. franç. d'Études clin. biol.* **7**, p. 17–19 (1962).

[121] Ricketts, H. T., Wildberger, H. L., Regus, L.: The role of Renal Threshold for Glucose in Diabetes. – *Lancet* **2**, p. 155 (1953).

[122] Rifkin, H.: The Kimmelstiel-Wilson Syndrome and its Variants. – *N. Y. State J. Med.* **53**, p. 2947 (1953).

[123] Robert, L.: Les glycoprotéines tissulaires. – *Presse méd.* **79**, no. 50, p. 2277–2283 (1971).

[124] Robertson, W. B.: Diabetes, Hypertension and Atherosclerosis. – *Postgrad. med. J.* 1968, December-Suppl.

[125] Rogers, J., Robbins, S. L.: Intercapillary Glomerulosclerosis: A Clinical and Pathological Study. I. Specificity of the Clinical Syndrome. – *Amer. J. Med.* **12**, p. 688 (1952).

[126] Rogers, J., Robbins, S. L., Jeghers, H.: Intercapillary Glomerulosclerosis: A clinical and Pathologic study of 100 Anatomically Proven cases. – *Amer. J. Med.* **12**, p. 692 (1952).

[127] Root, H. F.: Prognosis in Diabetes. – *Med. Clin. N. Amer.* **59**, p. 1147 (1965).

[128] Root, H. F., Pote, W. H., Frehner, H.: Triopathy of Diabetes. (Sequence of neuropathy, retinopathy and nephropathy in one hundred and fifty-five patients.) – *Arch. intern. Med.* **94**, p. 931 (1954).

[129] Runyan, J. W., Hurwitz, D., Robbins, S. L.: Effect of Kimmelstiel-Wilson Syndrome on Insulin Requirements in Diabetes. – *New Engl. J. Med.* **252**, p. 388 (1955).

[130] Sabour, M. S., MacDonald, M. K., Robson, J. S.: An Electron Microscopic Study of the Human Kidney in Young Diabetic Patients with Normal Renal Function. – *Diabetes* **11**, p. 291–295. (1962).

[131] Schirmeister, J.: Fiziopatologia Rinichiului. In *"Fiziopatologie Speciala"*, ed. by Heilmeyer, L. – Ed. Med. Buc. 1968, p. 410–437.

[132] Schliack, V., Bartos, V., Ditscherlein, G.: Zur Frage klinischer Befunde bei Nierengefäßveränderungen des Sektiongutes der Berliner Diabetes-Population. In *"Diabetische Angiopathie"*, ed. by Mohnike, G. – Akademie Verlag Berlin 1964, p. 63–66.

[133] Seige, K.: Diabetes Mellitus. – VEB Georg Thieme Leipzig 1967.

[134] Sheldon, J.: The dietary management of chronic renal failure in the diabetic. – *Postgrad. med. J.* Suppl. July, p. 472–475 (1969).

[135] Sherrill, J. W.: Diabetic Retinitis. The relationship between retinal degenerative changes and the degree of diabetic control. – *Bull. Sci. Metab. Clin.* **2**, p. 1 (1951).

[136] Silberman, J. L., Kissane, J. M.: Diabetic glomerulosclerosis in renal papillary necrosis. – *Amer. J. clin. Pathol.* **40**, p. 532–536 (1963).

[137] Sims, E. A. H.: Serial studies of renal function in pregnancy complicated by diabetes mellitus. – *Diabetes* **10**, p. 190–197 (1961).

[138] Singer, P.: Diabetische Nephropathie. Clearance-Untersuchungen und ihre Beziehungen zu morphologischen Befunden. – *Med. Klin.* **61**, p. 1210–1214 (1966).

[139] Singer, P., Ditscherlein, G.: Über Glomerulosklerose bei Diabetikern. Beziehungen zwischen klinischen Befunden und dem Schweregrad der nodulären und diffusen Glomerulusveränderungen. – *Dtsch. Zschr. Verdau.- u. Stoffwechselkr.* **25**, p. 38–55 (1965).

[140] Solbach, H. G., Jahnke, K., Irmscher, K. I., Ormos, J.: Zur Differenzialdiagnose der diabetischen Nephropathie mit Hilfe klinischer und morphologischer Untersuchungsmethoden. In *"Diabetische Angiopathie"*, ed. by Mohnike, G. – Akademie Verlag Berlin 1964, p. 75–80.

[141] Spiro, R. G.: Studies on the Structure of the Glomerular Basement Membrane. – 26th Annual Meeting of the Amer. Diabetes Assoc. 1966, June, Chicago.

[142] Spiro, R. G.: Chemistry of the Renal Glomerular Basement Membrane. – *Diabetes.* – Proc. VIth Cong. Int. Diab. Fed. Stockholm 1967. – Exc. Med. Foundation 1969, Amsterdam, p. 586–594.

[143] Spühler, O., Zollinger, H. U.: Die diabetische Glomerulosklerose. – *Dtsch. Arch. klin. Med.* **190**, p. 321 (1943).

[144] Stanley, J. R.: Renal Cortical Necrosis, Diabetes and Pregnancy. – *Obstet. Gynecol.* **23**, p. 291–294 (1964).

[145] Swenson, R. S., Silvers, A., Peterson, D. T., Kohatsu, S., Reaven, G. M.: Effect of nephrectomy and acute uremia on plasma insulin 125. I. Removal rate. – *J. Lab. clin. Med.* **77**, p. 829–837 (1971).

[146] Suzuki, Y., Churg, J., Grishman, E., Mautner, W., Dachs, S.: The mesangium of the renal glomerulus. Electron microscopic studies of pathologic alteration. – *Amer. J. Pathol.* **43**, p. 555–578 (1964).

[147] Thomsen, A. C.: The Kidney in Diabetes Mellitus. – Munksgaard-Copenhagen 1965.

[148] Ussing, H. H.: The Role of the Basement Membrane in Epithelial and Endothelial Permeability. – Diabetes Proc. VIth Cong. Int. Diab. Fed. Stockholm 1967. – Exc. med. Foundation 1969, Amsterdam, p. 582–585.

[149] Wills, M. R.: Biochemical Consequences of Chronic Renal failure: a Review. – *J. clin. Pathol.* **21**, p. 591 (1968).

[150] Wilson, J. L., Root, H. F., Marble, A.: Diabetic Nephropathy, a Clinical Syndrome. – *New Engl. J. Med.* **245**, p. 513 (1951).

[151] Wilson, D. L., Rosen, D. A., Bencosme, S. A.: Steroid Nephropathy in the Rabbit. – *Diabetes* **11**, p. 402–411 (1962).

[152] Zins, E. J.: Diabetic Nephropathy. – *Amer. J. med. Sci.* **218**, p. 408 (1949).

[153] Zubrod, C. G., Eversole, S. L., Dana, G. W.: Amelioration of Diabetes and Striking Rarity of Acidosis in Patients with Kimmelstiel-Wilson Lesions. – *New Engl. J. Med.* **245**, p. 518 (1951).

Chapter V

[1] Albrink, M. J., Man, E. B.: Serum triglycerides in coronary artery disease. – *Arch. intern. Med.* **103**, p. 4–8 (1959).

[2] Albrink, M. J.: Triglycerides, Lipoproteins and Coronary artery disease. – *Arch. intern. Med.* **109**, p. 345–359 (1962).

[3] Albrink, M. J., Lavietes, P., Man, E. B.: Vascular disease and serum lipids in Diabetes mellitus. – *Ann. intern. Med.* **58**, p. 305–323 (1963).

[4] Anderson, R. S., Ellington, A., Gunter, L. M.: The incidence of atherosclerosis heart disease in negro diabetic patients. – *Diabetes* **10**, p. 114–118 (1961).

[5] Anonymous: Steroidi e clorura di sodio nelle ulcere gangrenose. – *Rass. Med. Cult.* **46**, p. 78 (1969).

[6] Aubertin, E. J., Aubertin, J.: Le syndrome douloureux polymorphe des membres inférieurs chez les diabétiques. Journées de Diabète de Lille. – *Presse méd.* **72**, p. 414 (1964).

[7] Bagdade, J. D., Porte, A., Bierman, E. L.: Diabetic lipemia: a form of acquired fat-induced lipemia. – *New Engl. J. Med.* **276**, p. 427–433 (1967).

[8] Bagdade, J. D., Hazzard, W. R., Carlin, J.: Effect of unsaturated dietary fat on plasma lipoprotein-lipase activity in normal and hyperlipidemic states. – *Metabolism* **19**, p. 1020–1024 (1970).

[9] Barillon, A., Binet, J. P., de Gennes, J. L., Hazan, E., Lenègre, J. – Le traitement de fond de l'athérosclérose coronarienne. – *Presse méd.* **77**, p. 1013–1016 (1969).

[10] Beaumont, V., Beaumont, J. L.: Les cardiopathies ischémiques precoces. – *Presse méd.* **72**, p. 3267–3270 (1964).

[11] Beyer, K., May, R., Sailer, S.: Blutlipide und Glukosetoleranz bei 100 Patienten mit arteriosklerotischem Verschluß an den unteren Extremitäten. – *Wien. klin. Wschr.* **80**, p. 392–394 (1968).

[12] Bierman, E. L., Amaral, J. A. P., Belknap, B. H.: Hyperlipemia and Diabetes Mellitus. – *Diabetes* **15**, p. 675–679 (1966).

[13] Bloom, A.: The management of diabetes and its complications. – *Hosp. Med.* **2**, p. 766–771, April (1968).

[14] Böhle, B., Schrade, W.: Über latente Störungen des Kohlehydratstoffwechsels bei nicht diabetischen Arteriosklerotikern. – *Münch. med. Wschr.* **102**, p. 565–571 (1960).

[15] Bryfogle, J. W., Bradley, R. F.: The vascular complications of diabetes mellitus. – *Diabetes* **6**, p. 159–167 (1957).

[16] Braunsteiner, H., Sailer, S., Sandhofer, F., Di Pauli, R., Gabl, F., Jung, A.: Lipidwerte bei gesunden Personen und Patienten mit Myokardinfarkt. – *Wien. klin. Wschr.* **77**, p. 859–862 (1965).

[17] Braunsteiner, H.: et al. Enzymdefekte des Fettstoffwechsels. – *Wien. klin. Wschr.* **82**, p. 724 (1970). – (Cf. from *Ars medici* **2**, p. 93 (1971)).

[18] Burstein, J., Jakobson, T., Lindell, K. A., Nikiforow, R. E.: The effect of hydrophenformin on serum cholesterol, triglycerides and body weight of nondiabetic hypercholesterolemic subjects. – *Ann. Med. intern. Fenn.* **57**, p. 15–21 (1968).

[19] Camerini-Davalos, R. A., Searle, M. D., Rees, B., Caulfield, J. B., Lozano, O., Castaneda-Marble, A.: Vascular changes in prediabetes. In *"Small blood vessel involvement in diabetes mellitus"*, ed. by Siperstein, M. D., Colwell, A. R., Meyer, C. – Inst. Amer. Biol. Sci. Washington D. C. 1964, p. 107–112.

[20] Câmpeanu, S., Câmpeanu, L.: Ein neues Verfahren der hepatischen "Clearance" gegenüber endogenem Bilirubin. – *Münch. med. Wschr.* **102**, p. 169–173 (1960).

[21] Carlsten, A., Hallgren, B., Jagenburg, R., Svanborg, A., Werkö, L.: Myocardial metabolism of glucose, lactic acid, amino acids and fatty-acids in healthy human individuals at rest and at different work loads. – *Scand. J. clin. Lab. Invest.* **13**, p. 418–428 (1961).

[22] Câmpean, S., Câmpeanu, L., Marcu, I.: Modificări induse ale glucozo-6-fosfat-dehidrogenazei sanghine prin acid nicotinic. – *Congr. Naz. Inn. Medizin (Bucharest)* **11–13**, Sept. (1969).

[23] Cerasi, E., Luft, R.: What is inherited. – What is added. Hypothesis for the pathogenesis of diabetes mellitus. – *Diabetes* **16**, p. 615–627 (1967).

[24] Chakrabarti, R., Fearnley, G. R., Hocking, E. D., Deltheos, A., Clarke, G. M.: Fibrinolytic activity related to age in survivors of myocardial infarction. – *Lancet* **1**, p. 573 (1966).

[25] Chakrabarti, R., Hocking, E. D., Fearnley, G. R.: Fibrinolytic effect of metformin in coronary disease. – *Lancet* **2**, p. 256 (1965).

[26] Christiansen, I., Deckert, T., Kjerulf, K., Midtgaard, K., Worning, H.: Glucose tolerance, plasma lipids and serum insulin in patients with ischaemic heart disease. – *Acta med. scand.* **184**, p. 283–287 (1968).

[27] Cleve, H., Alexander, K., Mitzkat, H. J., Nissen, P., Salzman, I.: Les serumglycoprotéines dans le diabète. – *Diabetologia* **4**, p. 48–55 (1968).

[28] Cohen, A. M., Shafrir, E.: Carbohydrate metabolism in myocardial infarction. – *Diabetes* **14**, p. 84–86 (1965).

[29] Coy, G. E., Taylor, O. B., Patton, D., Davis, D. jr., Blandin, N.: Origin of plasma cholesterol in man. – *Arch. Path.* **76**, p. 72–200 (1963).

[30] Csapo, G., Szücs, S.: Diabetische Angiopathie und Arteriosklerose bei Zuckerkrankheiten. In *"Diabetische Angiopathie"*, ed. by Mohnike, G. – Akademie Verlag Berlin 1964, p. 165–168.

[31] Dangerfield, W. G., Smith, E. B.: An investigation of serum lipids and lipoproteins by paper-electrophoresis. – *J. clin. Path.* **8**, p. 132 (1955).

[32] David, C.: Bolile miocardului. In *"Cardiologia"*, ed. by Theodorescu, B., Bucureşti, Editura Medicală 1960.

[33] Dawber, T. R., Moore, P. E., Mann, G. V.: Coronary heart diseases, in the Framingham study. – *Amer. J. pub. Health* **47**, p. 4 (1957).

[34] Dembowski, U.: Arterienverschlüsse an den Gliedmaßen. – *Münch. med. Wschr.* **107**, p. 1242–1246 (1965).

[35] Dembowski, U., Nielsen, A.: Konservative Therapie der arteriellen Verschlußkrankheit. – *Landarzt* **43**, p. 818–823 (1967).

[36] Derot, M., Patel, J., Cormier, J. M., Tchobroutsky, G.: L'artérite des membres chez les diabétiques. – *Presse méd.* **72**, p. 1177–1182 (1964).

[37] Dexcortes, J., Gonin, A.: Faut-il opérer les artériopathies au stade de claudication intermittente? – *Presse méd.* **79**, p. 1049 (1971).

[38] Dimitriu, V.: Mica chirurgie. – Ed. Slova, Braila 1944.

[39] Ditzel, J., Moinat, P.: Changes in serum proteins, lipoproteins and protein-bound carbohydrates in relation to pathologic alterations in the microcirculation of diabetic subjects. – *J. Lab. clin. Med.* **54**, p. 843 (1959).

[40] Dodds, C., Mills, G. L.: Influence of myocardial infarction on plasma lipoprotein concentration. – *Lancet* **1**, p. 1160–1163 (1959).

[41] Donat, K.: Diagnostik und Therapie der peripheren arteriellen Durchblutungsstörungen. – *Med. Welt* p. 2083–2090 (1965).

[42] Edeiken, J.: Diabetes Mellitus as observed in 100 cases for 10 or more years cardiac studies. – *Amer. J. med. Sci.* **209**, p. 8 (1945).

[43] Edelman, J., Kershbaum, A., Sandberg, H., Pellet, S.: The effect of Probenecid administration on blood lipids and lipid tolerance curves in subjects with myocardial infarction. – *Amer. J. med. Sci.* **241**, p. 96–102 (1961).

[44] Eden, M., Phaure, T. A.: Hyperinsulinism and carbohydrate induced hyperlipoproteinaemia. – *Lancet* **2**, p. 264–265 (1968).

[45] Editorial: Free fatty acids and heart-attacks. – *Lancet* **1**, p. 843–844 (1971).

[46] Enjalbert, A., Gédéon, A., Puec, P.: Contribution a l'étude hémodynamique des oblitérations arterielles chroniques. – *Presse méd.* **76**, p. 1625 (1968).

[47] Entmacher, P. S., Root, H. F., Marks, H. H.: Longevity of diabetic patients in recent years. – *Diabetes* **13**, p. 376–377 (1964).

[48] Epstein, E. S., Rosing, D. R., Brakman, P., Redwood, D. R., Astrup, I.: Impaired fibinolytic response to exercise in patients with type IV hyperlipoproteinaemia. – *Lancet* **2**, p. 631–634 (1970).

[49] Evans, J. R., Opie, L. H., Renold, A. E.: Pyruvate metabolism in the perfused rat heart. – *Amer. J. Physiol.* **205**, p. 971–976 (1963).

[50] Falsetti, H. L., Schnatz, D., Greene, D. G., Bunnell, I. L.: Lipid and Carbohydrate studies in coronary artery disease. – *Circulation* **37**, p. 184–191 (1968).

[51] Falta, E., Högler, F.: Die Zuckerkrankheit. – Ed. IV, VEB Carl Marhold Verlag, Halle (Saale) 1953.

[52] Fearnley, G. R., Chakrabarti, R., Hocking, E. D., Evans, J. F.: Fibrinolytic effects of biguanides plus ethyloestranol in occlusive vascular disease. – *Lancet* **2**, p. 1008–1011 (1967).

[53] Fearnley, G. R.: Phenformin as a fibrinolytic drug. – *Postgr. med. J.* **44**, p. 468–471 (1968).

[54] Fearnley, G. R., Chakrabarti, R., Evan, J. P.: Effect of ethyloestrenol combined with Phenformin or with Metformin on platelet stickiness and serum cholesterol in patients with occlusive vascular disease. – *Lancet* **2**, p. 1004–1007 (1968).

[55] Fischbacher, W.: Chronische arterielle Durchblutungsstörung der Extremitäten. – *Schweiz. med. Wschr.* **98**, p. 929–937 (1968).

[56] Fischer, V., Lippmann, H. G.: Zum Verhalten der freien Fettsäuren im Serum bei Diabetes mellitus. – *Dtsch. Z. Verdau.- und Stoffwechselkr.* **26**, p. 169–175 (1966).

[57] Fleischhacker, H., Klausgraber, F.: Herz und Gefäßkrankheiten. – J. F. Lehmanns Verl. München 1959, p. 73–76.

[58] Frankl, W. S.: Glycoproteins in Diabetes mellitus und atherosclerosis. – *Amer. J. med. Sci.* **248**, p. 588–595 (1964).

[59] Frederickson, D. S., Levy, R. I., Lees, R. S.: Fat transport in lipoproteins an integrated approach to mechanism and disorders. I–V. – *New Engl. J. Med.* **276**, p. 34–44, 94–103, 148–157, 215–225, 273–281 (1967).

[60] Frederickson, D. S., Lees, R. S.: System for phenotyping hyperlipoproteinemia. – *Circulation* **31**, p. 321 (1965).

[61] Friede, A., Kaeding, A., Wüstenberg, P. W.: Zur Wertigkeit klinischer Parameter für die Prognose der Gangrän bei Diabetikern. – *Dtsch. Z. Verdau.- u. Stoffwechselkr.* **31**, p. 57–72 (1971).

[62] Goldenberg, S., Alex, M., Joshi, R. A., Blumenthal, H. T.: Nonatheromatous peripheral vascular disease of the lower extremity in diabetes mellitus. – *Diabetes* **8**, p. 261–273 (1959).

[63] Grabner, W., Bergner, D., Peschel, W., Berg, G.: Lipid electrophoretic analysis in diabetics. – *Med. u. Ernähr.* **10**, p. 188–190 (1969).

[64] Greenhalgh, R. M., Lewis, B., Rosengarten, D. S., Calnan, J. S., Mervart, I., Martin, P.: Serum lipids and lipoproteins in peripheral vascular disease. – *Lancet* **2**, p. 947–950 (1971).

[65] Gries, F. A., Oberdisse, K.: Fettstoffwechselstörungen und Diabetes mellitus. – *Dtsch. med. Wschr.* **95**, p. 727–734 (1970).

[66] Grönberg, A., Larsson, T., Jung, J.: Diabetes in Sweden. – Stockholm 1967.

[67] Gros, C., Will, J., Vousos, C., Turpel, A.: Possibilités d'un contrôle d'action médicamenteuse circulatoire. Colloque international de Thermographie médicales. – Strasbourg. *J. Radiol. Electr.* **48**, p. 37–38 (1967).

[68] Gsell, O.: Epidemiologie des Diabetes unter besonderer Berücksichtigung von Morbidität und Mortalität. – *Dtsch. med. Wschr.* **93**, p. 2446–2450 (1968).

[69] Hagenfeldt, L., Wahlberg, F.: Comparison of intravenous glucose tolerance and intravenous Tolbutamide response in ischaemic cardiovascular disease. – *Diabetes* **16**, p. 15–17 (1967).

[70] Hegglin, P.: Differentialdiagnose innerer Krankheiten. – 9th Ed. G. Thieme Verlag Stuttgart 1963.

[71] Heinrich, F., Schultis, K.: IV. Die Therapie des arteriellen Gefäßverschlusses. – *Med. Welt*, p. 1155 –1158 (1967).

[72] Heinrich, H. G.: Praktikum der Blutgerinnungsphysiologie. – Akademie Verlag Berlin 1962.

[73] Herreman, F.: Le risque cardiovasculaire dans les diverses hyperlipoprotéinémies. – *Presse méd.* **77**, p. 860 (1969).

[74] Hess, H.: Behandlung der akuten Gliedmaßenarterienverschlüsse. – *Dtsch. med. Wschr.* **94**, p. 1194–1195 (1969).

[75] Houston, J. C., Joiner, C. L., Trounce, J. R.: A short textbook of medicine. – IIIrd Edition English Univ. Press Ltd. London 1968.

[76] Howard, A. N., Greshan, G. A.: Dietary aspects of Atherosclerosis and Thrombosis. – *Int. Z. Vitaminforsch.* **38**, p. 545–559 (1968).

[77] Hsia, D. Y. Y.: Defectele metabolice inascute. In *"Bolile metabolismului"*, ed. by Duncan, G. G., Vth Edition, Vol. I, Bucharest. – Editura Medicala 1966, p. 519–531.

[78] Iagnov, Z., Repciuc, E., Russu, G.: Anatomia omului. – Editura Medicala Bucharest 1954, Angimvologia, p. 19.

[79] Idu, S. M., Câmpeanu, S.: Electroforeza. – Editura Medicala 1957, Bucharest.

[80] Ilinsky, B. V.: Ateroskleroz. – Medghis, Moscow 1960.

[81] Jones, P., Plotkin, G. R., Arky, R. A., Lipoprotein lipase activity in patients with diabetes mellitus, with and without hyperlipemia. – *Diabetes* 15, p. 565–570 (1966).

[82] Kalant, N., Teitelbaum, J. I., Coopersberg, A. A., Harland, W. A.: Dietary atherogenesis in alloxan diabetes. – *J. Lab. clin. Med.* **63**, p. 147–157 (1964).

[83] Kingsbury, K. J.: Glucose tolerance, age and atherosclerosis. – *Postgrad. med. J.*, Supp. December, p. 944–954 (1968).

[84] Klimt, C. R., Meinert, C. L., Ho, I. O., Briese, F. W.: Study of familial patterns of reported diabetes. – *Diabetes* **16**, p. 40 (1967).

[85] Knick, B., Lange, H. J.: Graphical evaluation of the intravenous Tolbutamide test by the T-3 procedure. – *Acta diabet. lat.* **4**, Suppl. 1, p. 45–62 (1967).

[86] Knick, B., Lange, H. J., Skoluda, D., Kremer, G.: Frühdiabetische Lipoidstoffwechselanomalien bei Myokardinfarkt und arteriellen Verschlußkrankheiten. – *Dtsch. med. Wschr.* **93**, p. 1954–1959 (1968).

[87] Knittle, J. L., Ahrens, E. H.: Carbohydrate metabolism in two forms of Hyperglyceridemia. – *J. clin. Invest.* **43**, p. 485–495 (1964).

[88] Kremer, C. J., Niemczyk, H., Knyck, B.: Coronarsklerose und subklinischer Diabetes mellitus. – *Schweiz. med. Wschr.* **97**, p. 735–739 (1967).

[89] Kristensen, M., Hansen, J. M.: Potentiation of the Tolbutamide effect by dicoumarol. – *Diabetes* **16**, p. 211 (1967).

[90] Kurien, V. A., Oliver, M. F.: Serum-free-fatty acids after acute myocardial infarction and cerebral vascular occlusion. – *Lancet* **2**, p. 122 (1966).

[91] Larcan, A., Huriet, C.: L'électrocardiogramme dysmétabolique. – Masson & Cie, Edit. Paris 1959.

[92] Larsson, Y., Sterky, G., Persson, B., Claes, T.: Effect of exercise on blood lipids in juvenile Diabetes. – *Lancet* **1**, p. 350–355 (1964).

[93] Lawry, E. Y., Mann, G. V., Paterson, A., Wysocki, A. P., O'Connell, R., Stare, F. J.: Cholesterol and beta-lipoproteins in the serum of Americans. – *Amer. J. Med.* **22**, p. 603 (1957).

[94] Lehmann, H., Lines, J. G.: Hyperlipoproteinaemia classification: the optimum routine electrophoretic system and its relevance to treatment. – *Lancet* **1**, p. 557–560 (1972).

[95] Liebow, I. M., Hellerstein, H. K., Miller, M.: Arteriosclerotic heart disease in diabetes mellitus. – *Amer. J. Med.* **18**, p. 438–447 (1955).

[96] Liebow, I. M., Newill, V. A., Osesohn, R.: Incidence of ischaemic heart disease in a group of dia-

betic women. – *Amer. J. med. Sci.* **248**, p. 588–595 (1964).

[97] Lippmann, H.: Über Veränderungen der Serumlipide beim Diabetes mellitus. In *"Diabetische Angiopathie"*, ed. by Mohnike, G. – Akademie Verlag Berlin 1964, p. 253–257.

[98] Loeper, J., Tricot, R.-MUe, Loeper, J., Rouffy, J.: Valeur du lipidogramme pour le dépistage et la classification des hyperlipoprotéinémies. – *Presse méd.* **77**, p. 171–173 (1969).

[99] Lowry, A. D. jr., Borach, J. H.: Predictive values of lipoproteins and cholesterol determinations in diabetic patients who developed cardiovascular complications. – *Circulation* **17**, p. 14 (1958).

[100] Macrez, C.: Le traitement chirurgical direct de l'occlusion coronarienne. – *Presse méd.* **69**, p. 1520 (1961).

[101] Macrez, C.: Les consultations journalières en cardiologie. – 1965 Paris, Masson & Cie.

[102] Mahler, R. F.: Insulin action on arterial tissue in relation to diabetes and atheroma. In *"Diabetes mellitus"*, ed. by Duncan, L. J. P. – Baltimore, Williams and Wilkins Co. 1966, p. 41–45.

[103] Malinow, M.: The effect of insulin on the electrical activity of isolated ventricular muscle of the rat. – *Acta Physiol. Latino-Amer.* **8**, p. 125–128 (1958).

[104] Marigo, S.: Heredity of Diabetes Mellitus. – *Acta diabet. lat.* **9**, p. 115–135 (1972).

[105] Martin, M.: Die Therapie chronisch-arterieller Verschlüsse im Bereich der Extremitäten. – *Schw. Rdsch. Med. (Praxis)* **60**, p. 1409–1415 (1971).

[106] Maruhama, Y., Goto, Y., Yamagata, S.: Diabetic treatment and the diurnal triglycerides. – *Metabolism* **16**, p. 985–995 (1967).

[107] Mazovetsky, A. G., Podtergerya, V. G., de la Vara, F.: Lipoproteins of the blood serum in patients with diabetic angiopathy and obliterating atherosclerosis. – *Terap. Arkh.* **41**, p. 63–66 (1969).

[108] Miasnikow, A. L.: Ateroskleroz. – Moscow-Medghiz 1960.

[109] Milcu, S. M.: Endocrinologie Clinică. – Editura Medicala Bucharest 1967.

[110] Mincu, I., Câmpeanu, S., Georgescu, S.: Consideratiuni clinice asupra arteriopatiei diabetice. – *Med. interna (Buc.)* **20**, p. 963–972 (1968).

[111] Mincu, I.: Metabolismul lipidelor în diabet. – *Med. interna (Buc.)* **16**, p. 1209–1226 (1964).

[112] Mincu, I., Mihalache, N.: Mucopolizaharidelc serice şi variaţia lor în complicaţiile degenerative ale diabetului. – *Med. interna (Buc.)* **16**, p. 723–728 (1964).

[113] Mincu, I., Mihalache, N.: Modificările urinare ale mucopolizaharidelor acide (MPA) în diabetul complicat. – *Med. interna (Buc.)* **16**, p. 803–810 (1964).

[114] Mincu, I., Câmpeanu, S., Radulescu, G., Câmpeanu, L., Petrovici, A.: Contributions a l'étude éthiopathogénique et hystopathologique des hépatopathies chroniques dans le diabète sucré. – *Rev. int. Hépat.* **18**, p. 987–1022 (1968).

[115] Moga, A., Haraguş, S.: *Ateroscleroza.* – Edit. Acad. Rep. Pop. Rom 1963.

[116] Mohnike, G.: Zur diabetischen Blutgefäßkrankheit. – *Dtsch. med. Wschr.* **82**, p. 1904–1908 (1957).

[117] Muth, H. W.: Diabetes mellitus und Gefäßstörungen. – *Dtsch. med. Wschr.* **63**, p. 178–180 (1968).

[118] Nye, E. R.: Glucose tolerance test in hypertensive patients. – *Brit. med. J.* **2**, p. 727–730 (1964).

[119] Oakley, W. G., Pyke, D. A., Taylor, K. W.: Clinical diabetes and its biochemical basis. – Blackwell Scientific Publications Oxford and Edinburgh, 1968.

[120] Opie, L. H., Norris, R. M., Thomas, M., Holland, A. J., Owen, P., van Noorden, S.: Failure of high concentrations of circulating free fatty acids to provoke arrhythmias in experimental myocardial infarction. – *Lancet* **1**, p. 818–822 (1971).

[121] Ostrander, jr. L. D., Francis, jr. T., Hayner, N. S., Kjesslberg, M. O., Epstein, F. H.: The relationship of cardiovascular disease to hyperglycemia. – *Ann. intern. Med.* **62**, p. 1188 (1965).

[122] Otto, H., Bennek, M., Degenhardt, I.: Über den Einfluß des Diabetes auf die Arteriosklerose. In *"Diabetische Angiopathie"*, ed. by Mohnike, G. – Akademie Verlag Berlin 1964, p. 181–185.

[123] Otto, H., Brinck, U. C., Niklas, L.: Aktuelle Probleme der Diätbehandlung des Diabetes mellitus. – *Med. Welt*, p. 819 (1971).

[124] Owen, P., Thomas, M.: Relative changes in free-fatty acid and glucose utilization by ischaemic myocardium after coronary artery occlusion. – *Lancet* **1**, p. 1187–1190 (1969).

[125] Pavel, I.: Prophylaxie de l'artériopathie diabétique. – Internat. Symposium ü. Diabetesprobleme. – 1.–3. Oct. 1962, Karlsburg-Greifswald.

[126] Pavel, I., Ceausi, G., Pirvulescu, M., Vasilescu, V., Ciocau, L.: Insulin therapy and diabetic arteritis, etiological role of insulin. – *Presse méd.* **69**, p. 912 (1961).

[127] Pavel, I., Câmpeanu, S., Nicolescu, M., Bonaparte, H., Petrovici, A., Stroian, N.: Le diabète lipoatrophique est-il un diabète lipidique? – *Presse méd.* **71**, p. 1279–1282 (1963).

[128] Pavel, I., Pieptea, R.: *Diabetul.* – Edit. Medicală Bucharest 1965, p. 148–167.

[129] Pavel, I., Pieptea, R.: *Ereditatea in Diabet.* – Edit. Acad. RSR 1968.

[130] Pell, S., d'Alonzo, C. A.: Some Aspects of Hypertension in Diabetes mellitus. – *J. Amer. med. Ass.* **202**, p. 10–16 (1967).

[131] Pereda, S. A., Eckstein, J. W., Abboud, F. M.: Cardiovascular responses to insulin in the absence of Hypoglycemia. – *Amer. J. Physiol.* **202**, p. 249–252 (1962).

[132] Peters, N., Hales, L. N.: Plasma insulin concentration after myocardial infarction. – *Lancet* **1**, p. 1144–1145 (1965).

[133] Phillips, J. H., Burch, G. E.: Cardiovascular diseases in the white and negro races. – *Amer. J. Med.* **238**, p. 97, 124 (1959).

[134] Pieptea, R., Pavel, I.: Le rôle protecteur de l'allele non porteur dans le diabète héréditaire. – *Acta diabet. lat.* **6**, p. 74–86 (1969).

[135] Rakel, R. E., Skillman, T. G., Braunstein, J. R.: The ballistocardiogram in juvenile diabetes mellitus. – *Circulation* **18**, Part. I, p. 637–639 (1958).

[136] Randle, P. Y., Garland, P. B., Hales, C. N., Newsholme, E. A.: The glucose-fatty acid cycle. – *Lancet* **1**, p. 785–790 (1963).

[137] Regan, T. J., Lehan, P. H., Henneman, D. H., Behar, A., Hellmens, H. K.: Myocardial metabolic and contractile response to glucagon and epinephrine. – *J. Lab. clin. Med.* **63**, p. 638–647 (1964).

[138] Reinheimer, W., Bliffen, G., McCoy, J., Wallace, D., Albrink, M. J.: Weight gain, serum lipids and vascular disease in diabetics. – *Amer. J. clin. Med.* **20**, p. 986–996 (1968).

[139] Reinheimer, W., Davidson, P. C., Albrink, M. J.: Effect of moderate exercise on plasma glucose, insulin and free fatty-acids during oral glucose tolerance tests. – *J. Lab. clin. Med.* **71**, p. 429–437 (1968).

[140] Rickets, H. T.: Does rigid control of the blood sugar prevent the cardiovascular complications of Diabetes? – *Illin. med. J.* **115**, p. 267–268 (1959).

[141] Rifkind, B. M., Lawson, D. H., Gale, M.: Effect of short term sucrose restriction on serum lipid levels. – *Lancet* **2**, p. 1379–1381 (1969).

[142] Rifkind, B. M.: Plasma free-fatty acid levels and intravenous glucose tolerance after myocardial infarction. – *J. Atheroscler. Res.* **6**, p. 26–35 (1966).

[143] Robb, P., Marks, H. H.: Postexercise ectrocardiogram in atherosclerotic heart disease. – *J. Amer. med. Ass.* **200**, p. 918–926 (1967).

[144] Robertson, W. B.: Diabetes, hypertension and atherosclerosis. – *Postgrad. med. J.*, Suppl. Decemb. p. 939–943 (1968).

[145] Rodriguez-Minon, J. L., Larrodera, L.: Estudios de la glucosamina en la diabetes. – *Rev. Clin. Espan.* **104**, p. 103–105 (1967).

[146] Rüsch, H., Schwilbe, R.: Zur Diagnostik der peripheren Durchblutungsstörungen. – *Dtsch. med. Wschr.* **83**, p. 873–877 (1958).

[147] Rutstein, D. D., Castelli, W. P., Nickerson, R. J.: Heparin and human lipid metabolism. – *Lancet* **1**, p. 1003–1008 (1969).

[148] Sandberg, H., Min, B. S., Feinberg, L., Bellet, S.: I^{131}-triolein tolerance curves in patients with diabetes mellitus. – *Arch. intern. Med.* **105**, p. 866 (1960).

[149] Schaefer, L. E.: Hyperlipidemia. – *Ann. N. Y. Acad. Sci.* **148**, p. 925–936 (1968).

[150] Scheibe, O., Gallenkamp, H.: Die Arteriosklerose des Diabetikers als spezifische Folgekrankheit des Diabetes mellitus. – *Med. Welt*, p. 415–421 (1968).

[151] Schlierf, G., Kahlke, W.: Die Therapie der primären Hyperlipidämien. – *Dtsch. med. Wschr.* **94**, p. 329–332 (1969).

[152] Schoop, W., Gerhard, D., Roth, V.: Häufigkeit klinisch nachweisbarer Lumeneinengungen großer Arterien bei Diabetikern. – *Med. Klin.* **62**, p. 825–828 (1967).

[153] Schwartz, W.: Diabetes mellitus, idiopathic myocardial hypertrophy and paroxasmal atrial flutter. – *J. Amer. Geriat. Soc.* **8**, p. 472–477 (1960).

[154] Seymour, A.: Diabetes, Atherosclerosis and Hypercholesterolaemia: a preliminary report on the study of dietary control. – *Postgrad. Med.* **28**, p. 112–120 (1960).

[155] Shapiro, A. P., Perez, E., Stable, E., Moutsos, S.: Coexistence of renal arterial hypertension and diabetes mellitus. – *J. Amer. med. Ass.* **192**, p. 813–817 (1965).

[156] Simpson, N. E.: Multifactorial inheritance: a possible hypothesis for Diabetes. – *Diabetes* **13**, p. 462 (1964).

[157] Smith, E. B.: Lipoprotein patterns in myocardial infarction. – *Lancet* **2**, p. 910 (1957).

[158] Stănescu, M.: Inima şi tulburările de nutriţie şi metabolism. In *"Cardiologia"*, ed. by Theodorescu, B., vol. II, p. 503–512. – Edit. Medicală Bucharest 1961.

[159] Stearns, S., Schlessinger, M. J., Rudy, A.: Incidence and clinical significance of coronary artery disease in diabetes mellitus. – *Arch. intern. Med.* **80**, p. 474 (1947).

[160] Steinberg, A. G., Wilder, R. M.: A study of the genetics of diabetes mellitus. – *Amer. J. hum. Genet.* **4**, p. 113 (1952).

[161] Stout, R. W., Vallance-Owen, J.: Insulin and Atheroma. – *Lancet* **1**, p. 1078–1080 (1969).

[162] Sullivan, J., Neu, L. T., Coyle, M. J.: Serum lipids in diabetic and in coronary artery disease. – *Amer. J. med. Sci.* **243**, p. 57–62 (1962).

[163] Suschke, J., Foldenhauer, A.: Untersuchungen über die Beziehung zwischen Serumcholesterin und Plasmafibrinogen. – *Dtsch. med. Wschr.* **93**, p. 1705–1707 (1968).

[164] Szücs, S., Csapo, G.: Vergleichende Serumlipoid-Lipoprotein- und Cholesterinuntersuchungen bei 700 Zuckerkranken mit und ohne nachweisbare Angiopathie und Arteriosklerose. In *"Diabetische Angiopathie"*, ed. by Mohnike, G. – Akademie Verlag Berlin 1964, p. 247–251.

[165] Tournigand, P., Vovan, L., Kreitmann, P.: Les artériopathies athéromateuses des membres inférieurs. – *Presse méd.* **79**, p. 2453 (1971).

[166] Vallance-Owen, J., Ashton, W. L.: Inheritance of essential diabetes mellitus from studies of Synalbumin-Insulin antagonist. – *Diabetes* **12**, p. 356 (1963).

[167] Vallance-Owen, J.: The inheritance of essential diabetes mellitus from studies of the Synalbumin Insulin antagonist. – *Diabetologia* **2**, p. 248 (1968).

[168] Verdonk, G.: Biochimie sanguine de l'athérosclérose et influence de différents facteurs nutritionnels et pharmacologiques. – *Bruxelles Méd.* **45**, p. 1149–1182 and 1191–1221 (1965).

[169] Verdonk, G.: Différences entre les pertubations sanguines du métabolisme lipidique chez les diabétiques et chez les athéromateux. – *Méd. et Hyg. (Genève)* **23**, p. 475–502 (1965).

[170] Vernet, A., Smith, E. B.: Lipoprotein pattern in diabetes and changes occuring during pregnancy. – *Diabetes* **10**, p. 345–350 (1961).

[171] Visineanu, N.: Bolile arterelor periferice. In *"Cardiologia"*, ed. by Theodorescu, B., II-nd Vol., p. 874–875. – Edit. Medicala Bucharest 1961.

[172] Voiculescu, V.: Inima şi sistemul nervos. In *"Cardiologia"*, II-nd Vol. – Ed. by Theodorescu, B., Editura Medicala Bucharest 1961.

[173] Waitzkin, L., Rosenberg, C. H.: Nonspecific electrocardiographic abnomalities and unknown Diabetes. – 6-th Ann. Meet. Assoc. Diabetes 1960.

[174] Warembourg, H., Biserte, G., Jaillard, J., Sezille, G.: Les variations des acides gras libres dans le diabète. – *Ét. Clin. Biol.* **9**, p. 956–965 (1964).

[175] Wasjukova, B. A., Piassetzkij, N. R.: Einige Besonderheiten des Zustandes des Herz- und Gefäßsystems bei Diabetes mellitus. In *"Diabetische Angiopathie"*, ed. by Mohnike, G. – Akademie Verlag Berlin 1964, p. 195–196.

[176] Weill, F., Bonneville, J. F., Prevota, N., Ricette, J. P., Japy, C., Francois, J.: Sémiologie thermographique des ischémies chroniques des membres. – *Presse méd.* **77**, p. 629–632 (1969).

[177] Welborn, T. A., Deckenbridge, A., Rubinstein, A. N., Dollery, C. T., Fraser, N. T.: Serum insulin in essential hypertension and peripheral vascular diseases. – *Lancet* **1**, p. 1336–1337 (1966).

[178] Wilson, R. B., Martin, J. M., Bartroft, W. S.: An evaluation of the relative pathogenic roles of diabetes and serum cholesterol levels in the development of cardiovascular lesions in rat. – 26-th Ann. Meet. Am. Diab. Assoc. 1966.

[179] Wuhrman, G., Wunderly, C.: Die Bluteiweißkörper des Menschen. – Benno Schwabe Verlag, Basel 1953.

[180] Wuhrmann, F., Niggli, S.: Die Myokardose. – *Dtsch. med. Wschr.* **90**, p. 1261 (1965).

[181] Zagreanu, J., Haragus, S., Uza, G., Vlaicu, R., Schneider, E. R.: Therapic-Versuche mit Ismelin bei Angioorganopathien. – *Münch. med. Wschr.* **111**, p. 421–424 (1969).

[182] Zipp, H., Schreiber, B.: Progeß und Verlauf des chronischen Arterienverschlusses der unteren Extremität. – *Med. Klin.* **62**, p. 1697–1701 (1967).

[183] Zöllner, N.: Metabolism of Neutral Fats and Fatty acids. In *"Thanhauser's Textbook of Metabolism and Metabolic disorders"*, 2nd Ed., vol. II., Oxford: Blackwell Scientific Publications 1964.

[184] Zöllner, N.: Metabolism of steroids and carotinoids. In *"Thanhauser's Textbook of Metabolism and Metabolic disorders"*, 2nd Ed., vol. II., 603–645., Oxford: Blackwell Scientific Publications 1964.

[185] Zschoch, H.: Über die Häufigkeit der Arteriosklerose bei Diabetes mellitus. In *"Diabetische Angiopathie"*, ed. by Mohnike, G. – Akademie Verlag Berlin 1964, p. 99–104.

[186] Zuckermann, R.: Grundriß und Atlas der Elektrokardiographie. – VEB Georg Thieme, Leipzig 1959.

Chapter VI

[1] Aagenaes, O., Moe, H.: Light- and Electronmicroscopic study of Skin Capillaries of Diabetics. – *Diabetes* **10**, p. 253–259 (1961).

[2] Aslan, A., David, C., Câmpeanu, S.: Studien über die Verschiebungen der Kapillarpermeabilität mit zunehmendem Alter. – *Z. ges. inn. Med.* **16**, p. 78 (1961).

[3] Bencosme, S. A., West, R. O., Kerr, J. W., Wilson, L.: Diabetic capillary Angiopathy in Human Skeletal Muscles. – *Amer. J. Med.* **40**, p. 67–77 (1966).

[4] Bertrand, C. M., Duwoos, H.: Syndrome musculaire a l'effort révélatue d'un début d'intoxication par l'acid lactique endogène, consécutif à l'administration de phenformin. – *Ann. Endocr. (Paris)* **30**, p. 570–575 (1969).

[5] Bienstock, H., Davidson, S., Forschner, T. T.: First dorsal interosseus muscle atrophy: clinical sign of impaired glucose metabolism. – *N. Y. State J. Med.* **71**, p. 851 (1971).

[6] Bojsen-Moller, F., Granbaek, P., Rostgaard, J.: Light microscopic study of gastrointestinal and skin capillaries in diabetes mellitus. – *Diabetes* **12**, p. 429–432 (1963).

[7] Bürger, M.: *Angiopathia Diabetica.* – Georg Thieme Verlag, Stuttgart 1954.

[8] Butterfield, W. J. H., Garratt, C. J., Whichelow, M. J.: Peripheral hormone action: a method for the study of the action of insulin in the forearm tissues. – *Guy's Hospital Reports* **111**, p. 130–144 (1962).

[9] Butterfield, W. J. H., Hanley, T., Whichelow, M. J.: Peripheral metabolism of glucose and fatty acids during oral glucose tolerance tests. – *Metabolism* **12**, p. 851 (1965).

[10] Butterfield, W. J. H., Abrams, M. E., St. John, B. J. B., Whichelow, M. J.: The intravenous glucose tolerance test. Peripheral disposal of the glucose load in controls and diabetics. – *Metabolism* **16**, p. 19 (1967).

[11] Câmpeanu, S., Câmpeanu, L.: Beitrag zum Studium der Kapillarpermeabilität für elektrophoretische Bluteiweißfraktionen. I. Quantitative Bestimmung der sichtbaren und verschleierten Filtrierung von elektrophoretischen Eiweißfraktionen. – *Z. ges. inn. Med.* **14**, p. 42 (1959).

[12] Câmpeanu, S., Raudlescu, M., Câmpeanu, L.: Beiträge zum Studium der Kapillarpermeabilität für die elektrophoretischen Bluteiweißfraktionen. II. Die sichtbare und verschleierte Filtrierung der elektrophoretischen Fraktion in Arteriosklerose und Arthrosis im Vergleich zum normalen Individuum. – *Z. ges. inn. Med.* **14**, p. 638 (1959).

[13] Câmpeanu, S., Câmpeanu, L.: Die echte Transkapillare Proteinfiltrierung im Verhältnis zu verschiedenen Druckhöhen. – *Z. ges. inn. Med.* **15**, p. 495 (1960).

[14] David, H.: *Elektronenmikroskopische Organpathologie.* – VEB Verlag Volk und Gesundheit, Berlin 1967, p. 547–573.

[15] Durand, M., Durand, A.: Les altérations vasculaires dermo-hypodermiques des diabétiques. Etudes aux microscopes optique et électronique. – *Path. Biol. (Paris)* **14**, p. 1005–1019 (1966).

[16] Duwoos, H., Bertrand, C. M., Husson, A., Cramer, J., Tayot, J.: Hyperlactatémie réversible induite par la phenphormine avec asthénie musculaire et signes cardio-respiratoires. – *Presse méd.* **78**, p. 23–26 (1970).

[17] Fuchs, U.: Elektronenmikroskopische Untersuchungen menschlicher Muskelkapillaren bei Diabetes mellitus. – *Frankfurt. Z. Pat.* **73**, p. 318 (1964).

[18] Falta, W., Högler, H.: *Die Zuckerkrankheit.* – VEB Carl Marhold Verlag, Halle (Saale) 1953, p. 280.

[19] Fardeau, M.: Ultrastructure des fibres musculaires squelettiques. – *Presse méd.* **77**, p. 1341–1344 (1969) and ibid. **77**, p. 1563–1566 (1969).

[20] Fidzianska, A.: An electron-microscopic study of the muscles of rabbits subjected to chronic anaemia during foetal life. – *Europ. Neurology* **4**, p. 237–252 (1970).

[21] Friederici, H. H. R., Tucker, R., Schwartz, T. B.: Observation on small Blood Vessels of Skin in Normal and in Diabetic Patients. – *Diabetes* **15**, p. 233–250 (1966).

[22] Fuchs, U.: Elektronenmikroskopische Befunde an den Muskelkapillaren bei Langzeitdiabetikern. In *"Diabetische Angiopathie"*, ed. by Mohnike, G. – Akademie Verlag, Berlin 1964, p. 119–121.

[23] Goldstein, M. S.: Muscular Exercise and subsequent glucose utilization. – Chapt. 21 in *"On the Nature and Treatment of Diabetes Mellitus"*, ed. by Leibel, B. S. & Wrenshal, G. A. 1965. – Exc. Med. Found. Amsterdam, p. 308–320.

[24] Gottron, H. A.: Krankheitszustände des subkutanen Fettgewebes. – *Med. Welt*, p. 1211 (1952).

[25] Jung, H. D.: Die Necrobiosis Lipoidica Diabeticorum als morphologisches und funktionelles Substrat einer diabetischen Angiopathie der Haut. In *"Diabetische Angiopathie"*, ed. by Mohnike, G. – Akademie Verlag, Berlin 1964, p. 143–150.

[26] Kahil, M. E., Simons, E. L., Brown, H.: Magnesium Deficiency and Sugar Transport in Muscle.

Effect of Acute Insulin Deficiency. – *Diabetes* **17**, p. 673 (1968).

[27] Kakimoto, K.: Neuromuscular lesions in diabetes mellitus. – *J. Tokyo-Worm. Med. coll.* **39**, p. 157–167 (1969).

[28] Knobloch, U.: *Die Kapillarresistenz bei Diabetikern.* – Inaugural-Dissertation 1953, Leipzig.

[29] Knowles, H. C., Guest, G. M.: Changes of Tissue Electrolytes and Water in Diabetic Acidosis: Observations on Alloxandiabetic Rats with Ketoacidosis. – *Diabetes* **3**, p. 107 (1964).

[30] Krahl, M. E.: *Action of Insulin on Cells.* – Lts Ed. Academic Press New York 1961, p. 183.

[31] Krokowski, E., Haasner, E.: Die Osteoporose in heutiger Sicht. – *Kurz und Gut* **1**, no. 8, p. 2–4 (1967).

[32] Larsson, O.: Studies of Small Vessels in Patients With Diabetes. – *Acta med. scand.*, Suppl., p. 480 (1967).

[33] Lichtfield, J. A.: Biochemical Changes in Skeletal Muscle in Patients with Uncontrolled Diabetes Mellitus. – *Diabetes* **8**, p. 257–260 (1959).

[34] Magyar, I., Lehoczky, D., Marton, I.: Sugar Consumption in Vitro of the Muscle Tissue of Diabetic Patients. – *Diabetes* **14**, p. 716 (1965).

[35] Manchester, K. L.: Insulin and Protein Metabolism in Muscle. In *"On the Nature and Treatment of Diabetes"*, ed. by Leibel, B. S. & Wrenshall, G. A. – Exc. Med. Foundation Amsterdam 1965, p. 101–115.

[36] Mc-Millan, O. E., Breithaupt, D. L., Rosenau, W., Lee, J. C., Forsham, P. H.: Forearm Skin capillaries of Diabetic, Potential Diabetic and Nondiabetic Subjects. – *Diabetes* **15**, p. 251–257 (1966) (15).

[37] Mincu, I., Vieru, S.: *Mitochondrial Swelling-Contraction Cycle in Diabetes.* A new site of Insulin Action Mitochondrial Level.-*Rev. Roum. Med. Int.*, p. 409 (1967).

[38] Mincu, I., Câmpeanu, S., Radulescu, G., Câmpeanu, L., Petrovici, A. L.: Contributions a l'étude étiopathogénique et hystopathologique des hépatopathies chroniques dans le diabète sucré. – *Rev. int. Hépat.* **18**, p. 987 (1968).

[39] Moore, J. M., Frew, I. D. O.: Peripheral Vascular Lesions in Diabetes Mellitus. – *Brit. med. J.* **2**, p. 19–23 (1965).

[40] Pavel, I., Câmpeanu, S., Nicolescu, N., Bonaparte, H., Petrovici, A., Stoian, N.: Le diabète lipo-atrophique est-il un diabète lipidique? – *Presse méd.* **71**, p. 1279–1282 (1963).

[41] Palade, G. E., Bruns, R. R.: Structure and Function in Normal Muscle Capillaries. In *"Small Blood Vessels Involvement in Diabetes Mellitus"*, ed. by Siperstein, M. D., Colwell, A. R. & Meyer, K. – Amer. Inst. of Biol. Sci. Washington D. C. 1964, p. 39–49.

[42] Racela, A. J., Grady, H. J., Higginson, J., Svoboda, D. J.: Protein deficiency in rhesus monkeys. – *Amer. J. Path.* **49**, p. 419–443 (1966).

[43] Riddick, F. A., Reisler, D. M., Kipnis, D. N.: The Sugar Transport System in Striated Muscle. Effect of Growth Hormone, Hydrocortisone and Alloxan Diabetes. – *Diabetes* **11**, p. 171 (1962).

[44] Ries, W.: *Physiologie und Pathologie der Kapillarpermeabilität unter besonderer Berücksichtigung des Diabetes mellitus.* – 1956, VEB Carl Marhold Verlag, Halle (Saale).

[45] Romani, J. L.: Les lésions pariétales des capillaries lymphatiques du derme chez les diabétiques. – *Presse méd.* **79**, p. 228 (1971).

[46] Siperstein, M. D., Unger, R. H., Madison, L.: Studies of Muscle Capillary Basement Membranes in Normal Subjects, Diabetics and Prediabetic Patients. – *J. clin. Invest.* **47**, p. 1937 (1968).

[47] Taylor, K. W.: Insulin and the Control of Metabolism. – Chapt. 3 in *"Clinical Diabetes and its Biochemical Basis"*, ed. by Oakley, W. G., Pyke, D. A., Taylor, K. W. – Blackwell Scientific Publ. Oxford and Edinburgh 1968, p. 53–75.

[48] Tragl, K. H., Reaven, G. M.: Effect of experimental diabetes mellitus on protein synthesis by liver ribosomes. – *Diabetes* **20**, p. 27–32 (1971).

[49] Wagner, G., Tchoubroutsky, G., Rousselie, F., Cormier, J. M.: Etude des artérioles du rein et de la peau chez 38 sujets diabétiques et 66 sujets nondiabétiques. – *Presse méd.* **75**, p. 2091 (1967).

[50] Wechsler, W.: Veränderungen an der Skelettmuskelfaser bei neurogener Inaktivitäts- und Hungeratrophie im elektronenmikroskopischen Bild. – *Zbl. allg. Pathol. u. pathol. Anatomie* **107**, p. 77–78 (1965).

[51] Wiedmann, A.: Haut- und Geschlechtskrankheiten. In *"Diabetes mellitus"*, ed. by Boller, R., Wien. Urbau & Schwarzenberg 1950.

[52] Wohltmann, H. J., Narahara, H. T., Wesley, M. E.: Specificity of the Effect of Insulin on Permeability of Frog Sartorius Muscles to Sugar. – *Diabetes* **16**, p. **26** (1967).

[53] Zacks, S. I.: Basement Membrane Thickening in Muscle Capillaries. In *"Small Blood Vessel Involvement in Diabetes Mellitus"*, – Amer. Inst. of Biol. Sci. Washington D. C. 1964, p. 119–121.

[54] Zacks, S. I., Pegues, J. J., Elliott, F. A.: Interstitial muscle capillaries in patients with Diabetes Mellitus: a light and electron microscope study. – *Metabolism* **11**, p. 381 (1962).

[55] Yodaiken, R. E., Seftel, H. C., Kew, M. C., Lilienstein, M., Ipp, L.: Ultrastructure of Capillaries in South African Diabetics. II. Muscle Capillaries. – *Diabetes* **18**, p. 164–175 (1969).

Chapter VII

[1] Aagenaes, O.: Neurological complications in younger diabetics with special reference to the autonomic disturbance. – IV-th Cong. Diabetes Fed. Genève, 1961.

[2] Appenzeller, O., Richardson, E. P.: The sympathetic chain in patients with diabetic and alcoholic polyneuropathy. – *Neurology (Minneap.)* **16**, p. 1205–1209 (1966).

[3] Baranyi, F. Z.: Abnormal vascular reactions in Diabetes Mellitus. – *Acta med. scand.* **152** (Suppl. 204) (1955).

[4] Bauman, J. H., Girling, J. P., Brand, P. W.: Plantar pressures and trophic ulceration. – *J. Bone. Joint. Surg.* **42**, p. 684–690 (1960).

[5] Belser, F. G.: Der neuropathisch-diabetische Fuß. Die diabetische Osteoarthropathie. – *Praxis* **58**, p. 1088–1095 (1969).

[6] Benaroch, I. J.: Fructose behaviour in the course of sexual impotency in diabetic patients. – V-th Cong. Int. Fed. Diabetes, Toronto 1964.

[7] Berkman, M., Farkas, E., Faure, M., Tabet, J., Chiche, P.: Neuropathie et angiopathie diabétique. – *Sem. Hôp. Paris* **47**, p. 194–204 (1971).

[8] Bertram, F.: Carbohydrate metabolism. Clinical Section. In *"Thanhauser's Textbook of Metabolism and Metabolic Disorders"*, ed. by Zöllner, N. – Vol. I, Chap. 4, p. 255–329, Blackwell Scient. Publ. Oxford-Edinburgh (1962).

[9] Bischoff, A.: New morphologic and pathogenetic aspects in diabetic Neuropathy. In *"Diabetes"*, ed. by Östman, J. – Excerpta Med. Found. Amsterdam 1969, p. 627–632.

[10] Cambier, J., Dehen, H.: Les douleurs fulgurantes. – *Presse méd.* **71**, p. 1419–1422 (1971).

[11] Câmpeanu, S.: Aspecte fiziopatogenice şi metabolice ale obezitaţii. – *Viaţa medicala* **11**, p. 1675–1686 (1964).

[12] Casey, E. B., Harrison, M. J. G.: Diabetic Amyotrophy: a Follow-up Study. – *Brit. med. J.*, **1**, p. 656–659 (1972).

[13] Colby, A. O.: Neurologic disorders of diabetes mellitus. – *Diabetes* **14**, p. 424–429 (1965).

[14] de Jong, R. N.: The nervous system complication of diabetes mellitus with special reference to cerebrovascular changes. – *J. Neurol. ment. Dis.* **111**, p. 1181 (1950).

[15] Desmaroux, J. M.: Contribution à l'étude des neuropathie diabétiques. – *These (Paris)*, (1958).

[16] Dolman, C. L.: The morbid anatomy of diabetic neuropathy. – *Neurology (Minneap.)* **13**, p. 135–142 (1963).

[17] Dreyfus, P. M., Hakim, S., Adams, D.: Diabetic Ophthalmoplegia. – *Arch. Neurol. Psychiat. (Chic.)* 77, p. 337 (1970).

[18] Duncan, G. G.: Diabetul zaharat. In *"Bolile metabolismului"*, vol. II, Chap. 14. – Edit. Medicala, Bucureşti 1966, p. 1263–1267.

[19] Eliasson, S. G.: Change in Nerve Lipid Metabolism in Experimental Diabetes. In *"Diabetes"*, ed. by Östman, J. – Excerpta Med. Found. Amsterdam 1969, p. 620–626.

[20] Eliason, S. G.: Nerve conduction changes in experimental diabetes. – *J. clin. Invest.* **43**, p. 2353 (1964).

[21] Ellenberg, M.: Diabetic neuropathy precipitating after institution of diabetic control. – *Amer. J. med. Sci.* **236**, p. 466–471 (1958).

[22] Ellenberg, M., Krainer, L.: Diabetic neuropathy. Review of Literature and a case report with postmortem findings. – *Diabetes* **8**, p. 279–283 (1958).

[23] Ellenberg, M.: Diabetic neuropathy following stress situation. – *Amer. J. med. Sci.* **238**, p. 386–426 (1959).

[24] Ellenberg, M.: Diabetic neuropathy: evaluation of factors of onset. – *N. Y. Acad. Sci.* **82**, p. 245–250 (1959).

[25] Ellenberg, M., Weber, H.: Retrograde ejaculation in diabetic neuropathy. – *Ann. intern. med.* **65**, p. 1237–1246 (1966).

[26] Ellenberg, M.: Present status of diabetic neuropathy. In *"Diabetes"*, editor Östman J. Exerpta med. Foundation 1969, p. 615–616.

[27] Endtz, L. J.: Pathogénie de la neuropathie diabétique. – Journées ann. de Diabétologie de l'Hôtel-Dieu, May 2–4th 1968. – Ed. Flammarion Paris, p. 115–124.

[28] Endtz, L. J., Ghata, J., Azerad, E.: Le métabolisme de l'acide pyruvique dans le diabète et la neuropathie diabétique. – *Diabète (Le Raincy)* **11**, p. 229–231 (1963).

[29] Erbslöh, F.: Die polytopen Erkrankungen des peripheren Nervensystems. In *"Almanach f. Neurologie und Psychiatrie"*, ed. by Schretzenmayr, A., München 1967. – Ed. J. F. Lehmanns Verlag, p. 55–58.

[30] Fabre, J.: Les expressions periphériques de la neuropathie végétative du diabète sucré. – *Montpellier méd.* **47**, p. 196–206 (1965).

[31] Fagerberg, S. E.: Recent advances in diabetic neuropathy. In *"On the Nature and Treatment of Diabetes"*, ed. by Leibel, B. S. and Wrenshall, G. A., Chap. 38. – Excerpta Med. Found. Amsterdam 1965, p. 522–530.

[32] Falta, W., Högler, F.: Die Zuckerkrankheit, Chap. 4. – VEB Carl Marhold, Halle (Saale) 1953, p. 238–241.

[33] Fattoruso, V., Ritter, O.: Vademecum clinique. – Masson & Cie. Paris, p. 1118–1119 and ibid. 1616–1618.

[34] Field, R. A.: Altered nerve metabolism in Diabetes. – *Diabetes* **15**, p. 696–698 (1966).

[35] Field, R. A.: Altered nerve metabolism in Diabetes. In *"Diabetes"*, ed. by Östman, J. – Excerpta Medica Foundation, Amsterdam 1969, p. 617–619.

[36] Friedman, S. A., Rakow, R. B.: Oseous lesions of the foot in diabetic Neuropathy. – *Diabetes* **20**, p. 302–307 (1971).

[37] Foster, B., Basset, R. C.: Neurogenic arthropathy (Charcot Joint) associated with diabetic neuropathy. – *Arch. Neurol. Psychiat. (Chic.)* **57**, p. 173 (1947).

[38] Gamstorp, I., Shelburne, S. A., Engleson, G., Redondo, A., Traisman, S.: Peripheral neuropathy in juvenile diabetes. – *Diabetes* **15**, p. 411–418 (1966).

[39] Garcin, R., Lapresle, E.: Complications périphériques et centrales du diabète sucré. – *Ann. Méd.* **14**, p. 6 (1956).

[40] Garland, H.: Diabetic Angiopathy. – *Brit. med. J.* **2**, p. 1287 (1955).

[41] Gegesi-Kiss, P., Barta, L.: Diabetes Mellitus im Kindesalter. – Ungarische Akad. der Wissenschaft, Budapest 1957, p. 209–211.

[42] Gitelson, S., Schwartz, A., Fraenkel, M., Chowers, I.: Gall-bladder dysfunction in diabetes mellitus. The diabetic neurogenic gall-bladder. – *Diabetes* **12**, p. 308–312 (1963).

[43] Goldenberg, S., Moris, A., Joshi, R. A., Blumenthal, H. T.: Nonatheromatous peripheral vascular disease of the lower extremity in diabetes mellitus. – *Diabetes* **8**, p. 261–273 (1959).

[44] Gondos, B.: Roentgen observations in diabetic ostheopathy. – *Radiology* **91**, p. 6–13 (1968).

[45] Goodman, J. I., Baumoel, S., Frankel, J., Marcus, L. J., Wasserman, S.: The diabetic neuropathies. – Charles C. Thomas, Springfield 1953.

[46] Greenbaum, D.: Observation on the homogenous nature and pathogenesis of diabetic neuropathy. – *Brain* **87**, p. 215–232 (1964).

[47] Greene, L. F., Kelalis, P. P., Weeks, R. E.: Retrograde ejaculation of semen due to diabetic neuropathy. – *Fertil. and Steril.* **14**, p. 617–625 (1963).

[48] Gregersen, G.: Vibratory perception threshold and motor conduction velocity in diabetes and nondiabetics. – *Acta med. scand.* **183**, p. 61–65 (1968).

[49] Gregersen, G.: Variation in motor conduction velocity produced by acute changes in the metabolic state in diabetic patients. – *Diabetologia* **4**, p. 273 (1968).

[50] Grönberg, H., Larsson, T., Jung, J.: Diabetes in Sweden. – Stockholm 1967, p. 189–194.

[51] Harriman, D.: The ischaemic factor in diabetic neuropathy. – IV-th International Congr. of Neuropathology, München 1961. Georg Thieme Verlag, Stuttgart 1962.

[52] Jersild, M., Lauritzen, E.: Senibilité vibratoire chez les diabétiques. – *Diabète (Le Raincy)* **2**, p. 235 (1957).

[53] Kelsey Fry, I., Butterfield, W. J. H.: Carbohydrate metabolism in Diabetics: a possible intracellular block. – *Lancet* **2**, p. 235 (1962).

[54] Keys, A.: Subnutriţia. In *"Bolile metabolismului"*, Edited by Duncan, G. G., Chap. IX. – Edit. Medicala bucureşti 1966, p. 790–823.

[55] Khan, M. A., Wakefield, G. S., Pugh, D. W.: Vitamin B_{12} deficiency and diabetic neuropathy. – *Lancet* **2**, p. 768–770 (1969).

[56] Korczyn, A. D.: Bell's palsy and diabetes mellitus. – *Lancet* **1**, p. 108 (1971).

[57] Lapresle, J.: Étude anatomique des neuropathies périphériques du diabète sucré. – Journées Ann. de Diabétologie de l'Hôtel-Dieu, May 2–4th 1968. Flammarion Publ. House, Paris, p. 101–113.

[58] Luse, J., Moon, T. R.: An ultrastructural study ot peripheral nerves in human diabetes mellitus and in steroid induced hyperglycemia in the rabbit. – *Anat. Rec.* **154**, p. 380 (1966).

[59] Man, H.: Aspects neuro-ophtalmologiques du diabète sucré. – Journées Ann. de Diabétologie de l'Hôtel-Dieu, May 2–4th 1968. Flammarion Publ. House, Paris, p. 83–100.

[60] Mandelstam, P., Lieber, A.: Esophageal dysfunction in diabetic neuropathic gastro-enteropathy. – *J. Amer. med. Ass.* **201**, p. 582–586 (1967).

[61] Marinescu, G.: Étude d'un cas de paraplégie diabétique. – *Rev. neurol. (Paris)* 9, p. 719–721 (1901).

[62] Marshak, G., Maklansky, D.: Diabetic gastropathy. – *Amer. J. dig. Diseases* 9, p. 366–370 (1964).

[63] Martin, M. M.: Diabetic neuropathy: a clinical study of 150 cases. – *Brain* 76, p. 594 (1953).

[64] Michon, P., Larcan, A., Huriet, C., Vert, P., Vicari, F.: Les neuropathies diabétiques. – *Diabète (Le Raincy)* 9, p. 231–245 (1961).

[65] Midtgaard, K.: Diabetic visceral neuropathy. – *Diabetes* 15, p. 93–96 (1966).

[66] Mincu, I., Câmpeanu, S., Radulescu, G. H., Câmpeanu, L., Petrovici, A.: Contribution a l'étude étiopathogénique et histopathologique des hépatopathies chroniques dans le diabète sucré. – *Rev. int. Hépat.* 18, p. 987–1022 (1968).

[67] Mirsky, A., rutterman, P., Brohn-Kahn, H. R.: The quantitative measurement of vibratory perception in subjects with and without diabetes mellitus. – *J. Lab. clin. Med.* 41, p. 221 (1953).

[68] Moorhouse, J. A., Carter, S. A., Doupe, J.: Vascular responses in diabetic peripheral neuropathy. – *Brit. med. J.* 1, p. 883–885 (1966).

[69] Morel-Maroger, A.: Les neuropathiea végétatives du diabète sucré. – Journ. de Diabétol. de l'Hôtel-Dieu, May 2–4th 1968. Flammarion Publ. House Paris, p. 73–82.

[70] Needles, W.: Vitamin B_1-therapy in diabetic neuritis. *J. Amer. med. Ass.* 121, p. 914–916 (1943).

[71] Odel, H. M., Roth, G. M., Keating, F. R.: Autonomic neuropathy simulating the effects of sympathectomy as a complication of diabetes mellitus. – *Diabetes* 4, p. 92–98 (1955).

[72] Olofson, E. O., Petersen, I.: Childhood diabetic neuropathy. A clinical and neurophysiological study. – *Acta paediat. (Uppsala)* 55, p. 163–176 (1966).

[73] Pavel, I., Pieptea, R.: Diabetul. – Edit. medicala Bucharest 1965, p. 170.

[74] Pirart, J.: Diabetic neuropathy: a metabolic or a vascular disease? – *Diabetes* 14, p. 1–9 (1965).

[75] Pirart, J.: Données récentes sur la pathogénie des neuropathies diabétiques. – *Presse méd.* 77, p. 1205–1206 (1969).

[76] Pirart, J., Coers, Ch.: Diabetic neuropathy. A critical appraisal. In *"Diabetes"*, ed. by Östman, J. – Excepta Med. Found. Amsterdam 1969, p. 633–645.

[77] Pogonawska, J. J., Collins, L. C., Dobson, H. L.: Diabetic osteopathy. – *Radiology* 89, p. 265–271 (1967).

[78] Rackow, F.: Diabetic neuropathy. In *"Clinical Diabetes"*, ed. by Oakley, W. G., Pyke, D. A., Taylor, K. W., Chap. XX. – Blackwell Sci. Publ. Oxford-Edinburgh 1965, p. 542–561.

[79] Rapoport, S. M.: Medizinische Biochemie. – II-nd Edition, VEB Volk und Gesundheit, Berlin 1964, p. 700–701.

[80] Redfern, E. W., Eisenbrey, B. I.: *J. Amer. med. Ass.* 192, p. 231 (1965).

[81] Riordan, D. C.: The hand in leprosy. Part II. Orthopedic aspects of leprosy. – *J. Bone Joint Surg.* 42A, p. 684–690 (1960).

[82] Roth, G. M., Foerster, D. K., Sprague, R. G.: Skin temperature, sweating and postural blood pressure in diabetic patients with autonomic neuropathy. – XX-th Ann. Meet. Am. Diabetes Ass. 1960, p. 30.

[83] Rundles, R. W.: Diabetic Neuropathy: general review with report of 125 cases. – *Medicine (Baltimore)* 24, p. 111–160 (1965).

[84] Schöffling, K., Federlin, K., Ditschuneit, H., Pfeiffer, E. F.: Disorders of sexual function in male diabetics. – *Diabetes* 12, p. 519–527 (1963).

[85] Seige, K.: *"Diabetes Mellitus"*, VEB Georg Thieme, Leipzig 1967.

[86] Shahani, B., Spalding, J. M. K.: Diabetes mellitus presenting with bilateral foot-drop. – *Lancet* 2, p. 930–931 (1969).

[87] Smith, K.: Diabetic neuropathy. – *Postgrad. med. J.* 30, p. 223–228 (1961).

[88] Somlo, Z.: Über die Beziehungen zwischen diabetischer Angiopathie und Neuropathie. – *Dtsch. med. Wschr.* 89, p. 2040–2044 (1964).

[89] Somlo, Z., Csapo, G., Szücs, S.: Neurological complications of diabetes mellitus. – *Med. Welt* p. 2463–2465 (1962).

[90] Steiness, I.: Vibratory perception in normal subjects. vibratory perception in diabetics. – *Acta med. scand.* 158, p. 315–327 (1957).

[91] Strausz, M. B.: Therapeutic use of vitamin B_1 in polyneuritis and cardiovascular conditions. Clinical indications. – *J. Amer. med. Ass.* 110, p. 953–956 (1938).

[92] Thomas, P. K., Lascelles, R. G.: The pathology of diabetic neuropathy. – *Quart. J. Med.* 35, p. 489–509 (1966).

[93] Thompson Khalouf, S., Olsen, K. J.: Motor nerve conduction studies in young patients with diabetes mellitus. – *Cleveland Clin. Quart.* 34, p. 27–33 (1967).

[94] Vacek, J., Drugova, B., Pav, J., Platinova, H.: Periferni neuron u diabetu. Klinikoelektromyogra-

fica studie vedeni konektinovich nervu s sezretele-kykytu a patogenezi diabetikich neuropatii. – *Cs. Lek. Ces.* **106**, p. 441–448 (1967).

[95] Vague, J., Vague, Ph.: Le complication tandive du diabèt et leur prophilaxie, *Gaz. méd. Fr.* **73**, p. 1953 (1966).

[96] Vital, D., Bergodignan, Lepennec, J. J.: A propos de 12 cas de neuropathies périphériques du diabète: répartition clinique contrôles anatomiques en microscopie optique et en microscopie électronique. – C. R. du Congr. de Psychiatrie et de Neurologie de Langue Franc. 64-ème Session, Grenoble 1966, p. 690–702.

Index

Appendix

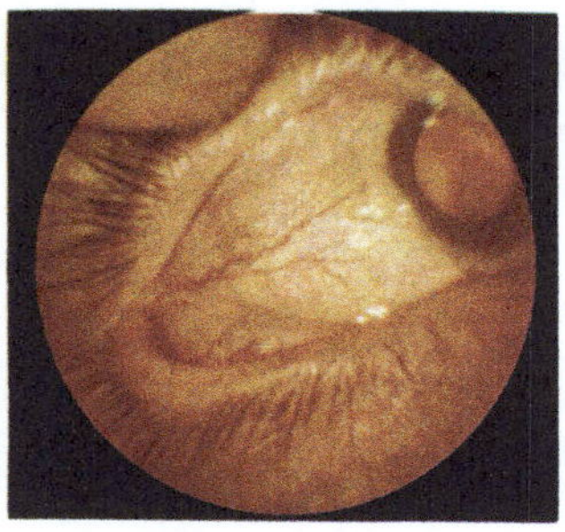

Fig. 7. M. P. Maturity onset diabetes in a man. Irregular and tortuous venules with modification of the arteriolarvenule ratio.

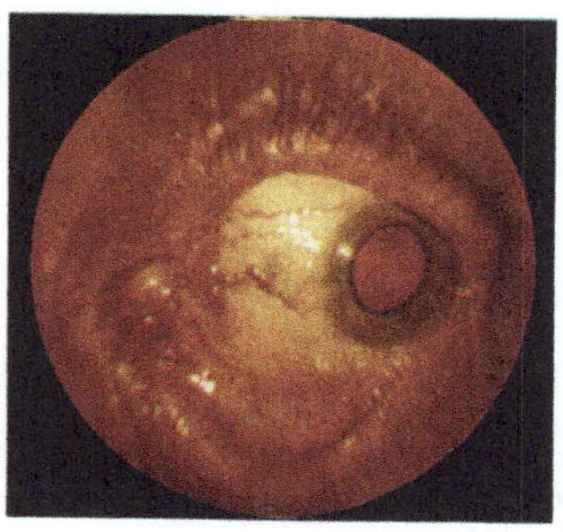

Fig. 8. L. A. Maturity onset diabetes in a female. Tortuous and enlarged venules.

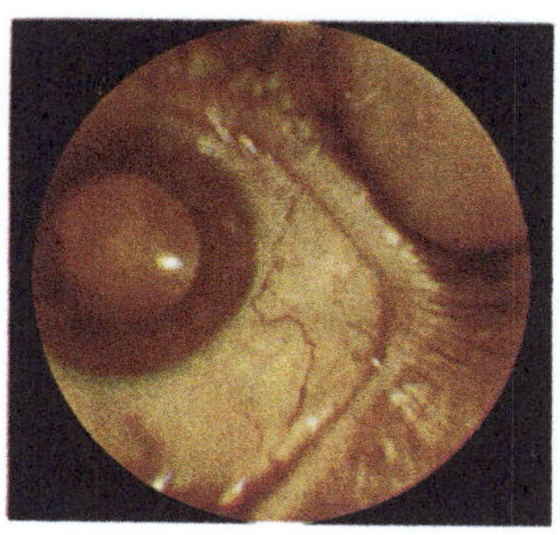

Fig. 9. R. A. Maturity onset diabetes in a man. Irregular and tortuous venules with modification of the arteriolo/venule ratio.

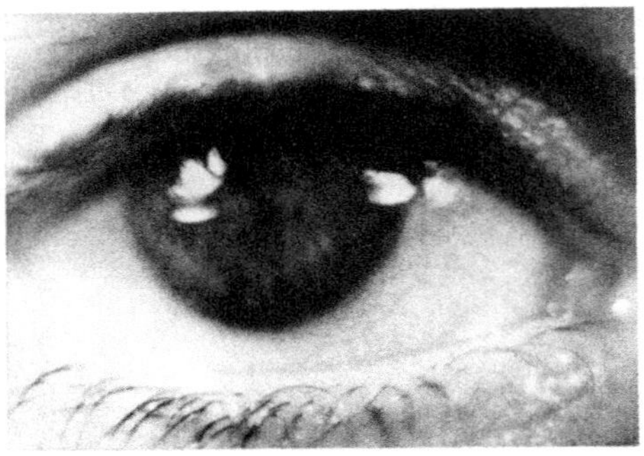

Fig. 10. L. G. Lipoatrophic diabetes in a girl. Duration of diabetes 8 years. Minor enlargement and tortuosities of the conjonctival venules.

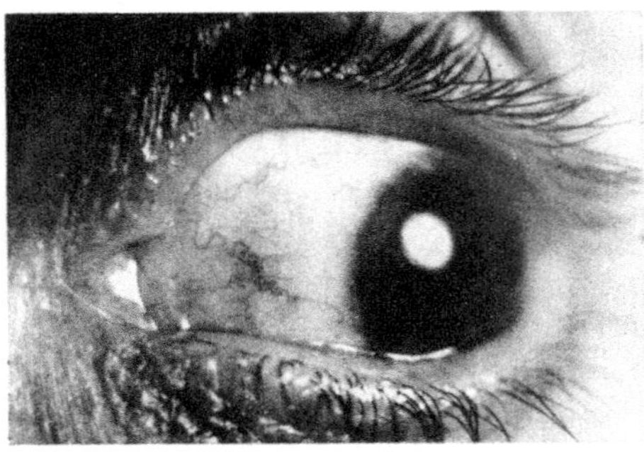

Fig. 11. A. G. Juvenile diabetes in a man. Insulin treatment. Conjonctival tortuosities and irregularities of the venules.

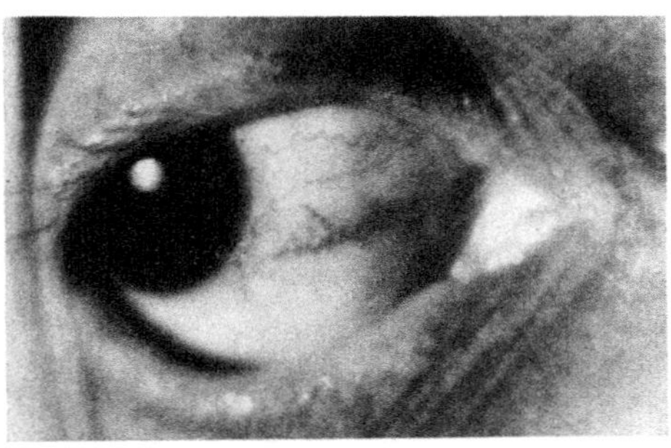

Fig. 12. L. L. Senile diabetes mellitus in a man. Insulin treatment. Irregularities, enlargements and tortuosities of the conjonctival venules. Here and there anevrismal dilatations.

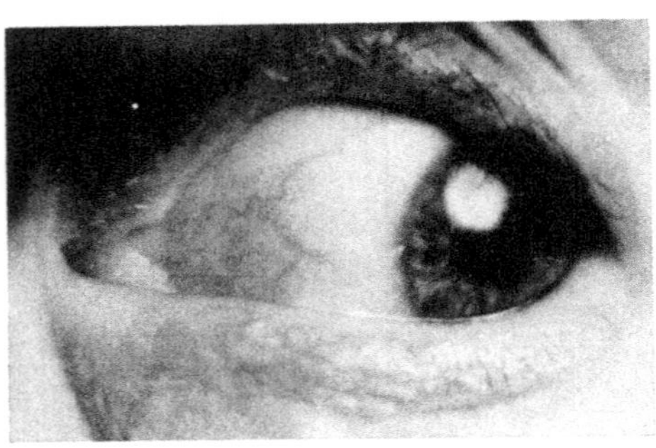

Fig. 13. I. M. Senile diabetes mellitus in a woman. Insulin treatment. Enlargements and tortuosities of the conjonctival venules.

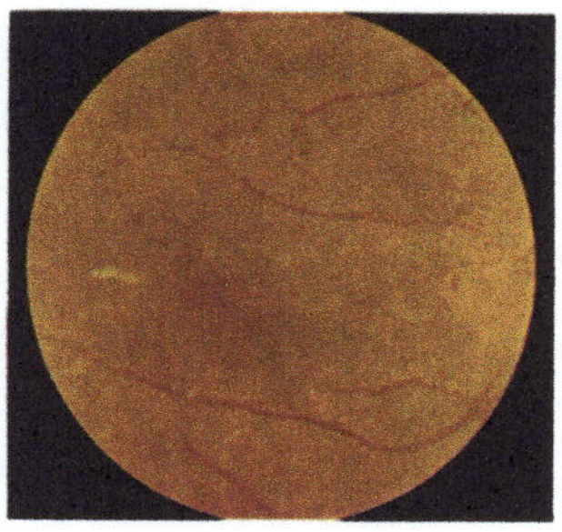

Fig. 35. C. F. 52 year old woman. Duration of the diabetic disease about 3 years. Microanevrysms.

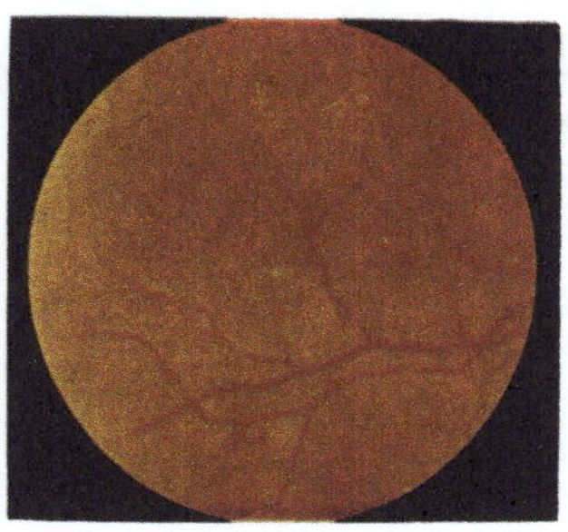

Fig. 36. L. A. 69 year old man with duration of diabetic diseases of about 9 years. Microanevrysms. Punctiform haemorrhages. Very small hard waxy exudates.

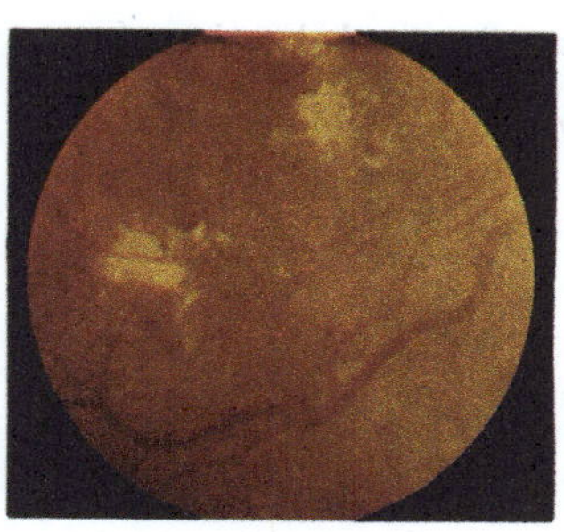

Fig. 37. B. E. 36 year old woman. Microanevrysms. Punctiform haemorrhages. Waxy exudates.

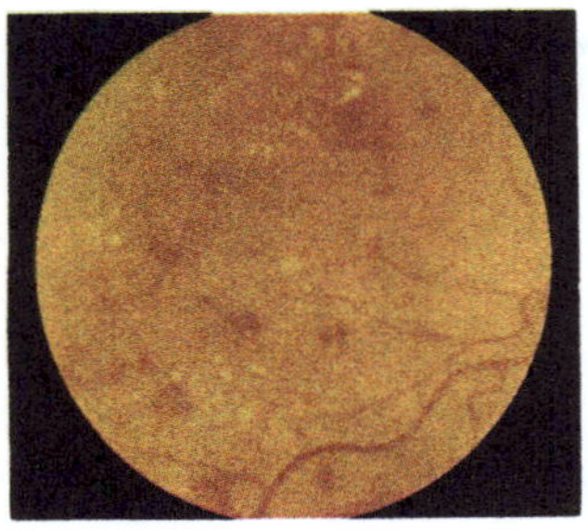

Fig. 38. S. C. 38 year old man. Duration of diabetes about 15 years. Microaneyrysms. Haemorrhages of different sizes. Waxy exudates.

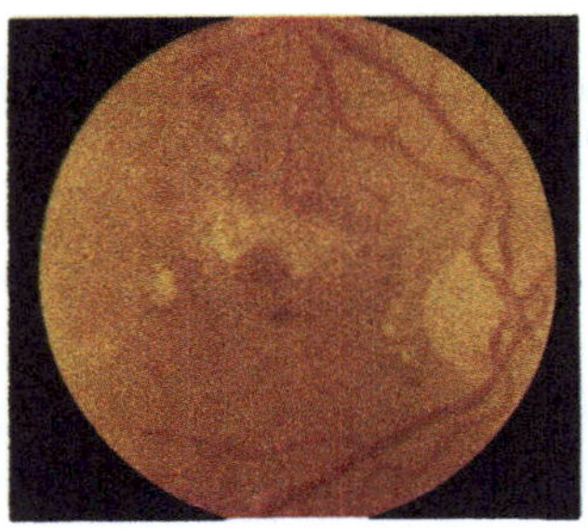

Fig. 39. Same patient as in Fig. 38. Enlarged, tortuous vessels. Few microanevrysms, large haemorrhages and many waxy exudates.

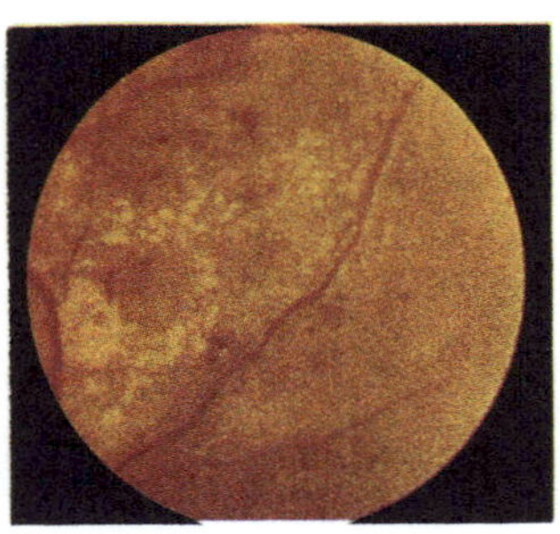

Fig. 40. S. M. 59 year old man. Supposed duration of the diabetic disease 4 years. Coexistence of small haemorrhages with cotton wool exudates.

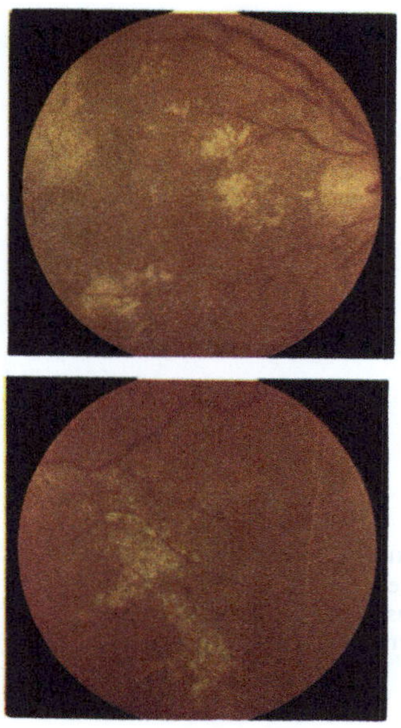

Fig. 41. B. E. Juvenile diabetes in a girl. Supposed duration of diabetes about 12 years. Many microanevrysms, and small haemorrhages simultaneously with cotton wool and hard exudates.

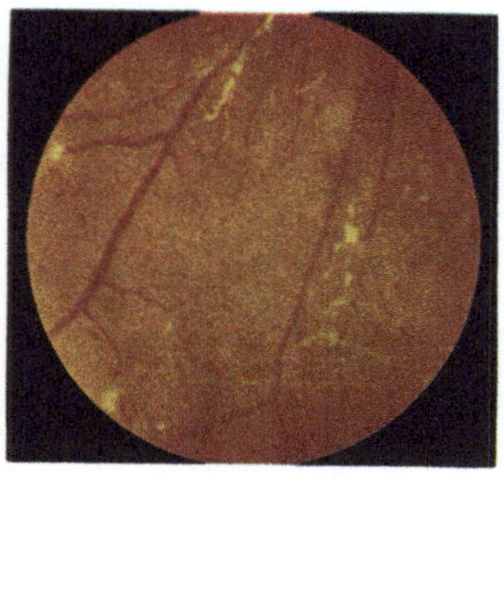

Fig. 42. G. V. 20 year old woman. Duration of diabetic. disease about 6 years. Malignant retinopathy (see Fig. 43) with seeming benign aspect.

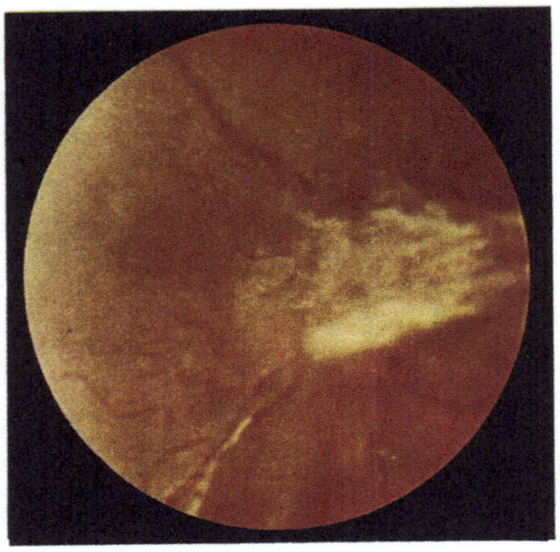

Fig. 43. Same patient as in Fig. 42. Proliferative retinitis with delicate new vessels growing forward into the globe.

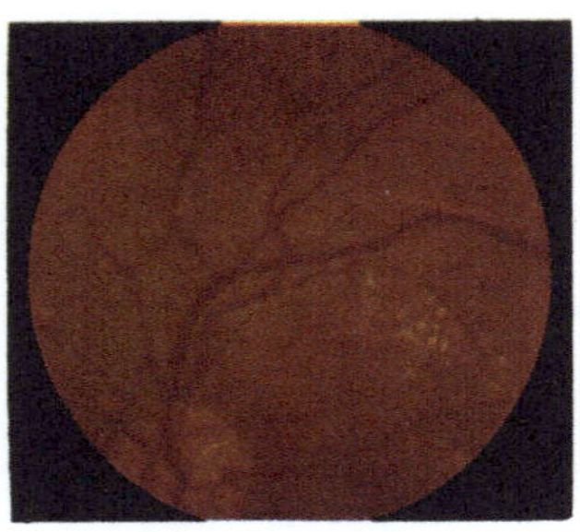

Fig. 44. B. A. 56 year old man with duration of diabetes of about 17 years. Mixed retinopathy. Rectilinear arterioles with thickened walls. Salus-Gun. Punctiform haemorrhages and small circular exudates.

Printed and bound by CPI Group (UK) Ltd, Croydon, CR0 4YY
16/09/2026
14963009-0001

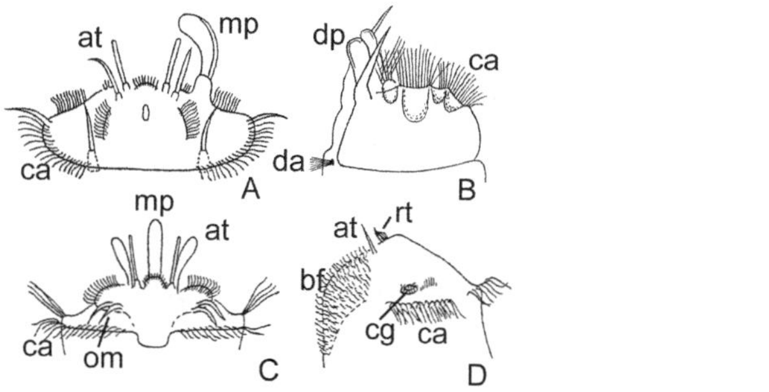

Fig. 4.22: Palps and sensory organs on apical field. (A) *Ascomorpha ovalis*, (B) *Trichocerca stylata*, (C) *Trichocerca capucina*, and (D) *Pleurotrocha petromyzon*. Abbreviations: at, apical tentacle; bf, buccal field; ca, circumapical band; cg, ciliated groove; da, dorsal antenna; dp, dorsal palp; mp, median palp; om, oral membranel. (A, C, D, From Remane 1933; B, from de Beauchamp 1965.)

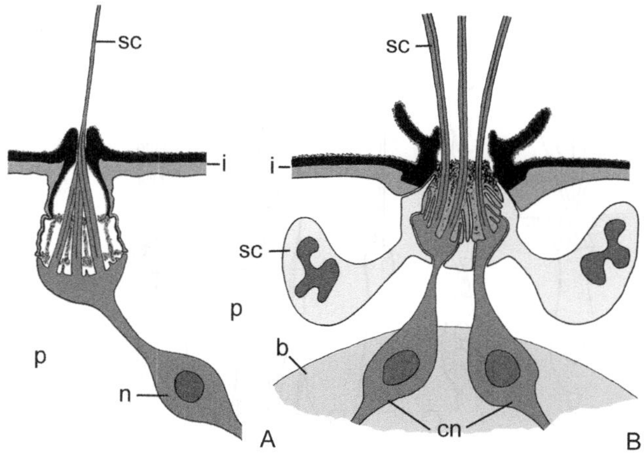

Fig. 4.23: Lateral (A) and dorsal antenna (B) in *Trichocerca rattus*. Abbreviations: b, brain; cn, cerebral neuron terminating at multinucleate, symmetrically arranged supporting cell (sc); i, integument; n, simple neuron in direct contact with integument; p, pseudocoelom. (Modified from Clément & Wurdak 1991, with permission.)

Clément & Wurdak 1991). Non-ciliary sensory endings in the form of microvilli are present inside the lumen underlying the pore (*Brachionus calyciflorus, B. sericus*) or the pore continues internally through a muff-shaped underlying epithelial cell, the cavity of which contains cilia and microvilli borne by a sensory nerve ending (*Brachionus plicatilis, Notommata copeus*).

Ciliated pits with chemoreceptor function and resembling chemoreceptive pores consist of an external cavity enclosing epithelial cilia, and an internal cavity lined with specialized cilia and sensory membranes (Clément et al. 1983, Wurdak et al. 1983). There are paired structures located on the apical field in, e.g., *Asplanchna*.

The prominent sensory organs of the body are mostly the dorsal and lateral antennae and to a lesser extent the caudal antenna. The dorsal antenna is found in all taxonomic groups of rotifer and generally situated medially on the head or neck but displaced to the anterior part of the trunk in *Testudinella*. In monogononts, it is a more or less long cylindrical projection bearing tufts of cilia or consists of tufts of cilia or styles projecting through a pore in the integument; occasionally, it is reduced to an unciliated pit. The dorsal antenna is paired in the embryonic stage, and becomes fused into an unpaired organ in most of the full-grown species; it is rarely absent (e.g., *Conochilus*). It consists of 2 cerebral nerve fibers with ciliated ends supported by an epithelial cell, which forms a subsurface pocket containing the bases of the sensory cilia (Fig. 4.23 B). The dorsal antenna is most prominent and of greater complexity in bdelloids, where it forms a long tube, telescopically retractable by paired muscles cells contained within it. The dorsal antenna of bdelloids has 3 pairs of nerve endings and several epithelial supporting cells (Clément 1977, Clément & Wurdak 1991).

Paired lateral antennae (Fig. 4.24) are present in monogononts, but lacking in bdelloids. They are usually situated laterally and symmetrically in the posterior half of the trunk but may be displaced ventrally or dorsally, or more anteriorly up to the apical field in *Conochilus*; in *Hexarthra*, they are situated on the ventral arms; they rarely lie on the caudal lorica spines (e.g., *Plationus patulus macracanthus*). In numerous Trichocercidae, the lateral antennae are in very asymmetrical positions. Partial to complete fusion of the apically displaced antennae occurs in some *Conochilus*. The lateral antennae are of similar shape as the dorsal antenna, but usually smaller (Fig. 4.23 A). They consist of a single sensory neuron in direct contact with the integument, with which it forms a pocket containing the bases of the sensory cilia (Clément 1977, Clément & Wurdak 1991).

A single, rarely paired, small dorsal caudal antenna, consisting of a ciliated pit or a more or less shallow projection tipped with a tuft of cilia, is generally present on the distal foot pseudosegment, between or above the base of the toes in Ploima (Fig. 4.25). In some species (e.g., *Notommata, Proales*), there is an unciliated papilla between the toes, and the distal foot pseudosegment of Collurellidae and *Cotylegaleata* bears a dorsal sensory pit, apparently lacking cilia.

Photoreceptors, called eyes, eyespots, or ocelli, are commonly present in monogononts and bdelloids, which most of the species retaining the eyes throughout their life. Eyespots are often lacking in adults of sessile orders, but present in their free-swimming juvenile stages (e.g., Hlava 1908, Hochberg et al. 2010). Eyespots contain a red to black pigment; the intensity of the color largely

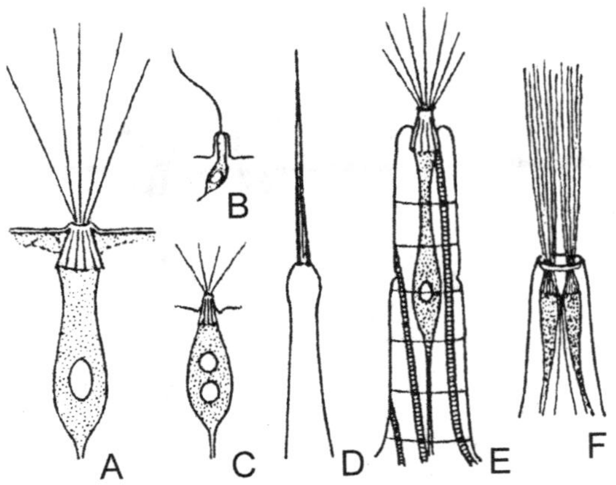

Fig. 4.24: Forms of lateral antennae in Monogononta. (A) Basic type, (B) *Lecane ligona*, (C) *Synchaeta tavina*, (D) *Tetrasiphon hydrocora*, (E) Flosculariidae, scheme, and (F) *Conochilus unicornis*. (From Remane 1933.)

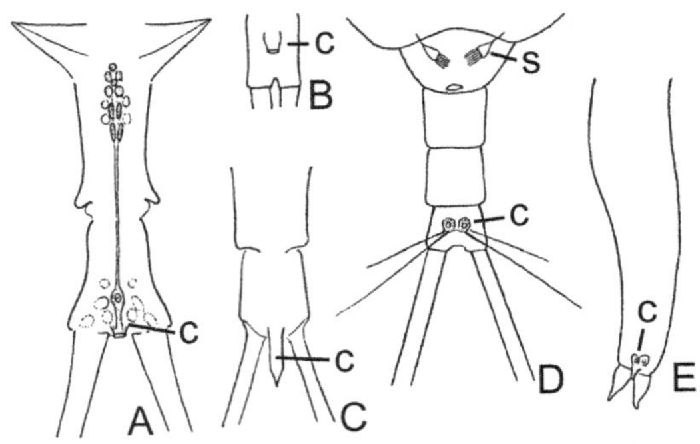

Fig. 4.25: Forms of caudal antennae in Monogononta. (A) *Trichotria tetractis*, (B) *Lepadella ovalis*, (C) *Trichotria pocillum*, (D) *Euchlanis*, and (E) *Brachionus*. Abbreviations: c, caudal antenna; s, sense organ. (Modified from Remane 1933.)

depends on the food, i.e., the carotenoids assimilated (Birky 1964). Light-refracting globules without pigment have been referred to colorless eyes (e.g., *Encentrum*) and may represent photoreceptive structures that lack a pigment cup containing screening pigment. The eyes are usually situated frontally or dorsally (rarely ventrally, e.g., *Hexarthra*) on the apical field, rostrum, and lateral sides of the corona or on the brain. According their specific location, they are called apical, frontal, rostral, or lateral eyespots, etc., and cerebral eyes. Cerebral eyes lie on the brain and are mostly single or sometimes paired but often fused (e.g., Notommatidae, Synchaetidae), unlike the other eye types, which are usually paired. Some species show a combination of frontal, lateral, and cerebral eyespots, e.g., *Eosphora najas* has 5 eyespots. The ultrastructure of the ocelli and cerebral eyes has been studied by, e.g., Clément et al. (1983) and Clément & Wurdak (1991). The frontal eyespots of *Rhinoglena frontalis* and apical eyespots of *Filinia longiseta* consist of anterior ciliated cells forming a cup with screen pigment, and enclosing a nerve ending from which microvilli containing the photosensitive pigment emanate. The paired lateral eyes of *Asplanchna brightwellii* and the paired median ones of *Trichocerca rattus* show sensory nerve endings bearing ampulla-shaped photoreceptive cilia (Fig. 4.26), separated from the outside medium by a thin cuticle. A light-refracting lipid globule in front of the microvilli of the ocelli is present in many species and referred to as lens in the older literature (Remane 1933).

The cerebral eye is integrated into the brain and associated with the epithelial cells surrounding the latter. The ultrastructure of the cerebral eyes (Fig. 4.27) of the 5 species studied to date is unique for each of them (Eakin & Westfall 1965, Clément 1980, Clément

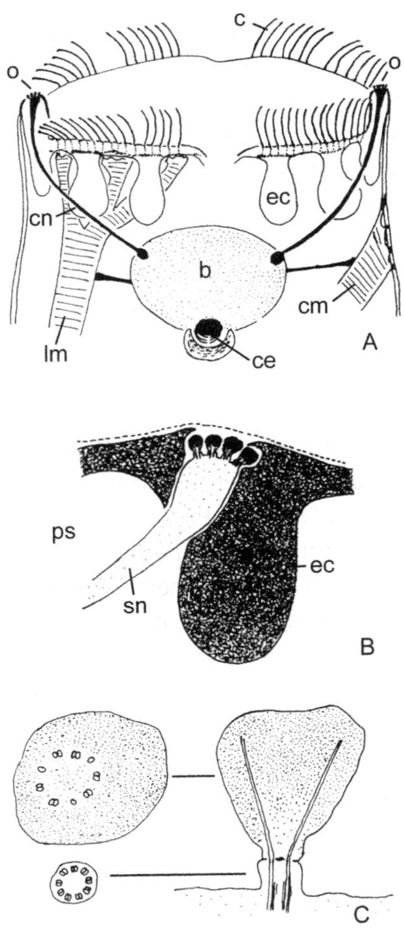

Fig. 4.26: Ocelli and cerebral eye of *Asplanchna brightwellii*. (A) General scheme of head, (B) Detail of ocellus, and (C) Detail of ampulla-shaped cilium with cross sections. Abbreviations: b, brain; c, corona; ce, cerebral eye; cm, circular skeletal muscle; cn, cerebral neuron; ec, epithelial socket cell; lm, longitudinla skeletal muscle; o, ocellus; sn, sensory nerve ending with ampulla-shaped cilia; ps, pseudocoel. (From Clément & Wurdak 1991, with permission.)

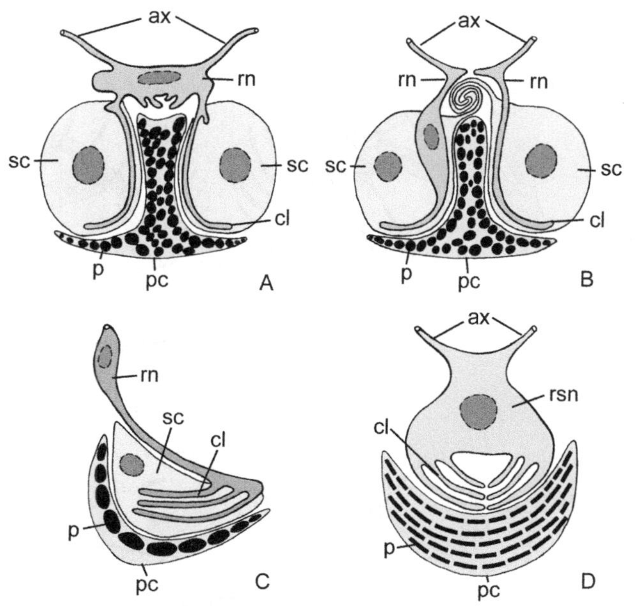

Fig. 4.27: Cerebral eyes of monogonont rotifers. (A) *Brachionus calyciflorus*, (B) *Brachionus plicatilis*, (C) *Trichocerca rattus*, and (D) *Asplanchna brightwellii*. Abbreviations: ax, axon; cl, cytoplasmic lamella of relay neuron; pc, epithelial cell with pigment cup or cavities containing pigment granules or platelets (p); sc, sensory neuron lacking axon; rn, relay neuron with axon leading to the neuropile of the brain; rsn, relay neuron becoming sensory neuron with stacked lamellae. (From Clément & Wurdak 1991, with permission.)

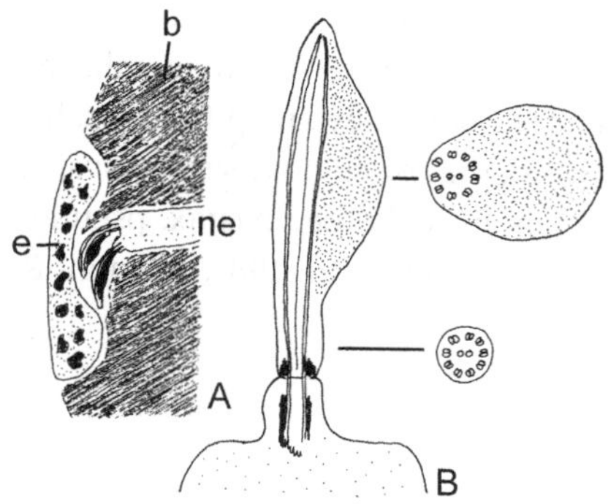

Fig. 4.28: Cerebral eye of the bdelloid *Philodina roseola*. (A) Location of the eye at periphery of brain and (B) detail of ampulla-shaped cilium in longitudinal and cross section. Abbreviations: b, brain, e, epithelial cell with pigment granules; ne, nerve ending with 2 ampulla-shaped cilia. (From Clément & Wurdak 1991, with permission.)

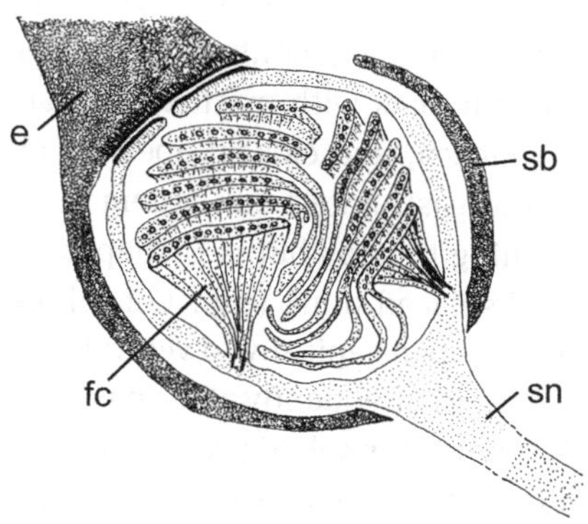

Fig. 4.29: Phaosome of the bdelloid *Philodina roseola*. Abbreviations: e, epithelial cell; fc, stacks of flattened cilia; sb, spherical bulb; sn, sensory nerve. (From Clément & Wurdak 1991, with permission.)

et al. 1983, Clément & Wurdak 1991). The monogononts (*Asplanchna brightwellii, Brachionus calyciflorus, B. plicatilis, Trichocerca rattus*) show an unpaired median epithelial cell containing the red screening pigment composed of pigment granules (*Brachionus, Trichocerca*) or platelets (*Asplanchna*). This epithelial cell is cup-shaped (*Trichocerca, Asplanchna*) or has 2 lateral cavities (*Brachionus*), which are responsible for its x-shape observed *in vivo*. The cavities and cup lodge a sensory neuron lacking axons (*Brachionus, Trichocerca*); they are connected to a single (*B. calyciflorus, T. rattus*) or 2 (*B. plicatilis*) relay neurons sending off axons to the brain. In *Brachionus*, each of the relay neurons sends a single cytoplasmic lamina into the sensory neuron; in *Trichocerca*, the relay neuron forms stacked lamellae penetrating into the unpaired sensory neuron. The structure of the cerebral eye of *Asplanchna* consists of a relay neuron that becomes the sensory neuron, forming stacked lamellae in the pigmented epithelial cup; 2 axons penetrate into the brain. A median cerebral eye is absent in bdelloids, but paired ones, located on either side of the brain, are present in, e.g., *Philodina, Dissotrocha, Embata, Habrotrocha collaris*, and *Abrochtha*. The ultrastructure of the cerebral eye of the only bdelloid studied (*Philodina roseola*) shows that it consists of a nerve ending bearing 2 ampulla-shaped cilia and lodged in an epithelial cell containing granules of screening pigment (Fig. 4.28). The presumed components for photoreception that contain the visual pigment of the above 5 species are different as well: tubular formations of the endoplasmic reticulum (*B. calyciflorus*), a stack of plasma and ER membranes (*B. plicatilis*), stacks of intracytoplasmic plasma membrane (*T. rattus*), lamellar rhabdomeres (*A. brightwellii*), and electron-dense ampulla-shaped cilia (*P. roseola*).

A photoreceptive function was also suggested for the phaosome (Fig. 4.29) of the bdelloid *Philodina roseola* (e.g., Clément 1980, Clément & Wurdak 1991). The unpaired phaosome is located at the base of the rostrum, near the outlets of the retrocerebral apparatus. It consists of a sensory nerve, ending in a spherical bulb containing a stack of fan-shaped flat cilia bearing lateral membrane expansions. The bulb is supported by an epithelial cell.

Other receptors, consisting of ciliated sensory cells, occur in the mouth region, buccal tube, mastax, pseudocoel, penis, cloaca, etc. (Clément et al. 1983, Clément & Wurdak 1991).

4.2.6 Intestinal system

4.2.6.1 Intestinal system of the female

The anatomy of the intestinal system is thoroughly documented in Remane (1933). For studies of its ultrastructure relying on TEM, see, e.g., Clément et al. (1980a, b, c, 1983) and Clément & Wurdak (1991). The digestive system is similar in most bdelloids and monogononts and consists of a mouth, buccal tube, pharynx with mastax, esophagus, stomach, intestine, cloaca, and cloacal aperture or anus. In most species, the gastrointestinal system runs straight from mouth opening to anus but is U-shaped in species with anteriorly displaced anus (e.g., Conochilidae). The mouth commonly opens apically to ventrally in the centre of the buccal field and frequently at the base of a more or less strongly developed funnel (Fig. 4.30). Several sensory receptors, supposed to participate in food intake, are present in the mouth region (Wurdak et al. 1983). The mouth leads to the buccal tube or opens directly into the pharynx. The buccal tube is formed by a simple epithelium, consisting of mushroom-shaped cells with the caps organized in an imbricate way forming the tube wall, and the stalks representing the cell bodies containing nuclei and most of the cytoplasm (Clément et al. 1980b). Sheaths of circular and longitudinal muscles surround the buccal tube (e.g., Clément et al. 1980c). The buccal tube is short and devoid of cilia or absent in raptorial species (e.g., *Asplanchna, Dicranophorus*) and more or less long and cylindrical and covered with cilia in filter feeders (e.g., *Brachionus, Philodina*). The buccal cilia are characterized by an electron-dense tip. In many rotifers, the buccal tube ends in a supple myelin-like structure, the buccal velum, separating the buccal lumen from the pharynx or mastax lumen, thus preventing rejection of the ingested food (Clément et al. 1980a, 1983). The buccal epithelium is provided with several sensory receptors (Wurdak et al. 1983).

The pharynx is short and usually ciliated but may be lacking in species with trophi that can be thrust out through the mouth opening (e.g., Dicranophoridae). Pharyngeal cilia have a classical $9 \times 2 + 2$ configuration

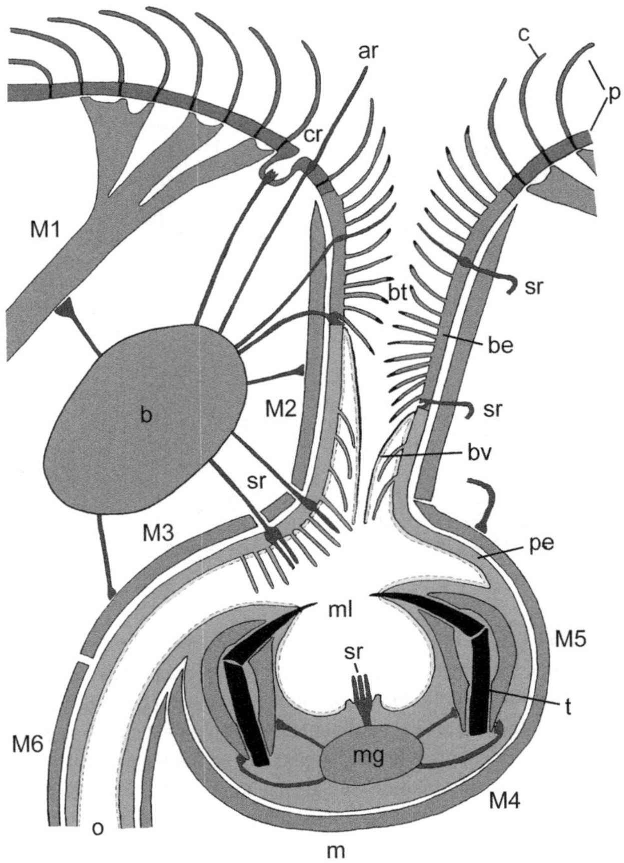

Fig. 4.30: Diagram of oral apparatus: mouth, mastax, and esophagus. Abbreviations: ar, anterior coronal mechanoreceptor; b, brain. be, buccal epithelium; bt, buccal tube; bv, buccal velum; c, cilium; cr, chemoreceptor; m, mastax; mg, mastax ganglion; ml, mastax lumen, M1–M6, muscles and their innervations; o, esophagus; p, pseudotrochus; pe, pharyngeal epithelium; sr, sensory receptor; t, trophi. (Modified from Clément & Wurdak 1991, with permission.)

but are surrounded by a double membrane that is an extension of the double membrane around the pharyngeal lumen (Clément & Wurdak 1991). The pharynx leads to the cavity of a muscular masticatory apparatus, the mastax (Figs. 4.30 and 4.31). This cavity occupies the anterior, dorsal, or anterodorsal part of the mastax and opens posteriorly into to the esophagus. The epithelial wall of the mastax cavity is lined with a thin cuticle. The cuticle is lamellar ("myelinic cuticle") and formed by the superimposition of cellular unit membranes coalescing in 2 to 30 and more bilayers (Clément 1993). The basal part of the mastax ventrally contains the sclerotized jaws or trophi and their associated muscles, epithelial cells, salivary glands, sensory receptors, and a small nerve ganglion.

The trophi comprise a set of hard, cuticularized extracellular elements formed by various epithelial cells

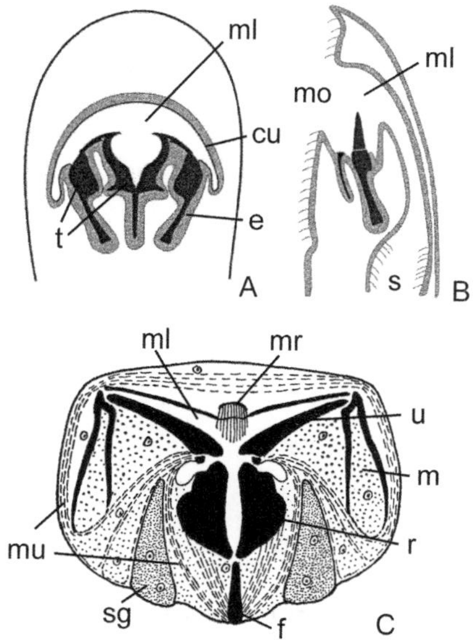

Fig. 4.31: Diagram of mastax. (A) Dorsal view, trophi forcipate, (B) lateral view, trophi forcipate, and (C) cross section, trophi malleate. Abbreviations: cu, cuticle; e, epithelium; f, fulcrum; m, manubrium; ml, mastax lumen; mo, mouth; mr, mastax sensory receptor; mu, muscles; r, ramus; s, stomach; sg, salivary gland; t, trophi; u, uncus. (Modified from de Beauchamp 1965 and Riemann & Ahlrichs 2008.)

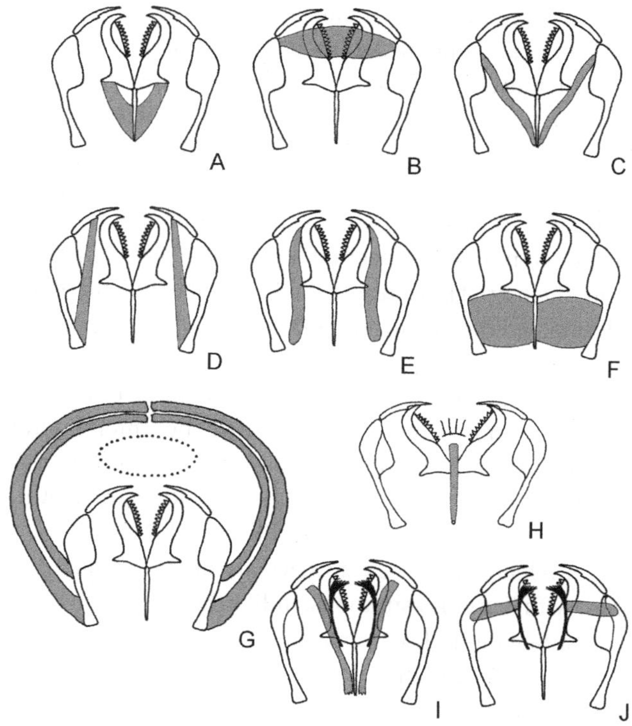

Fig. 4.32: Diagram of the musculature of the trophi apparatus of *Dicranophorus forcipatus*: (A–G) dorsal and (H–J) ventral. (A) Musculus fulcro-ramicus, (B) Musculus transversus manubrii, (c) musculus fulcro-manubricus, (d) musculus manubrico-uncus, (e) musculus caudo-ramicus, (f) musculus circumglandis, (g) musculus manubricus perioralis, (h) mastax receptor retractor, (i) musculus hypopharyngeus, and (j) musculus manubrico-hypopharyngeus. (Modified from Riemann & Ahlrichs 2008.)

(e.g., Koehler & Hayes 1969a, b, Clément & Wurdak 1991). Each element is build up of tubular sclerite bodies composed of an electron-dense core surrounded by electron-lucent material (e.g., Rieger & Tyler 1995). Some elements (ramus and manubrium) are hollow and contain the nucleus and perinuclear cytoplasm of an epithelial cell(s); others (uncus and fulcrum) are solid, lying next to their epithelial cell nucleus and cytoplasm. The main trophi elements (Fig. 4.31 C) consist of an unpaired median fulcrum, and 3 paired elements: ramus, uncus, and manubrium, connected by ligaments and moved by muscles connecting the different elements with each other and with the wall of the mastax. The development of the different elements and associated muscles is considerably modified in the different families or species, in relation to their mode of life and feeding habits (see below for a detailed description of the different trophi types).

The highly complex musculature of the different trophi types is poorly known and relies on histological observations (e.g., Martini 1912, Seehaus 1930, Stossberg 1932, Remane 1933, de Beauchamp 1909, 1965), and TEM and/or CLSM of the monogononts *Bryceella stylata, Dicranophorus forcipatus, Notholca acuminata, Pleurotrocha petromyzon, Proales tillyensis Trichocerca rattus, Asplanchna brightwellii, Notommata copeus, Brachionus calyciflorus*, and the bdelloid *Philodina roseola* (Clément 1987, Clément & Wurdak 1991, Sørensen et al. 2003, Riemann & Ahlrichs 2008, Wilts et al. 2010, Wulfken et al. 2010). There usually is a series of paired muscles (e.g., 13 in *T. rattus*, 6 in *B. stylata*) joining specifically paired trophi elements or trophi elements and mastax wall (Fig. 4.32). Paired muscles found in several mastax types studied to date are, e.g., abductor muscles interconnecting cauda of manubria with base of rami, muscles interconnecting the distal end of the fulcrum with the head of the manubria, malleus flexors interconnecting the cauda of the manubria with the unci, muscles connecting manubria to both the median and peripheral mastax floor, etc. The number of unpaired muscles is restricted: e.g., a strong hypopharynx muscle connects the enlarged dorsodistal end of the fulcrum with the opposite wall of the mastax lumen in species with virgate trophi; a weak retractor lies on the dorsal edge of the fulcrum and terminates in the mastax sensory receptor in species with forcipate and modified malleate trophi; the rami adductor muscle connects both rami distally in, e.g., malleate and incudate trophi, and a transversal manubrium adductor connects the heads of both manubria in, e.g., malleate, modified malleate, forcipate, and virgate trophi. Comparison of the musculature in different species, and identification of homologous muscles is difficult. Possible homologous muscles are: the paired muscle connecting fulcrum and caudal part of rami, the paired muscle attached to the caudal end of the fulcrum and the dorsal edge of the head of the manubria, the paired muscle joining the distal end of the manubria and the unci, the paired muscle interconnecting the distal end of the manubria with the anterolateral part of the rami, and the unpaired hypopharynx muscle/ fulcrum sensory receptor retractor (e.g., Riemann & Ahlrichs 2008, Wilts et al. 2010, Wulfken et al. 2010).

In bdelloids, mastax muscles are often laminar, and short with few cross-striations, unlike the longer and regularly striated muscles observed in monogononts (Clément & Wurdak 1991, Clément 1993). In *T. rattus*, all muscles proved unicellular, except one. The attachment of the muscles to the trophi elements and their adjacent epithelial cells is by desmosomes. The flexible ligaments connecting the trophi elements contain electron-dense cuticular material. The muscles are innervated by the mastax ganglion situated at the mastax floor. Several sensory receptors, such as ciliated pits and ciliated cells, occur between the trophi and the mastax floor, and on the roof of the mastax (Clément et al. 1983, 1991, Wurdak et al. 1983).

A variable number of mononucleate or multinucleate salivary glands are generally present, closely associated with the mastax ventrolaterally (Fig. 4.33), or incorporated in the mastax wall (Fig. 4.31 C); apparently, they also may be lacking. Their anterior part is often transformed into a large reservoir (e.g., *Asplanchna*, Flosculariacea, median salivary gland of several bdelloids). The ducts open anterior to the trophi or in the buccal tube.

The esophagus is short to long. de Beauchamp (1909), and later confirmed by Clément et al (1980b, 1991), distinguished 2 sections: the cuticular and the ciliary esophagus. The cuticular esophagus is the tube emanating from the mastax toward the stomach. It is an expansion of the dorsal pharyngeal wall of the mastax, composed of a thin epithelial layer surrounded by a thicker muscular layer and lined by a fine cuticle. The ciliated esophagus is the section between the cuticular esophagus and the stomach and made of ciliated cells, the cilia of which end in the stomach lumen. The cilia are long and form a vibratile flame, helping to move down the food and preventing regurgitation. The periesophageal musculature may consist of longitudinal and circular muscles or a reticular muscle layer and appears

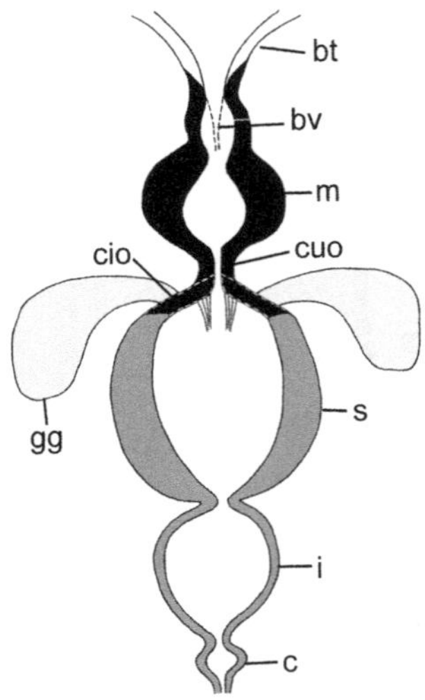

Fig. 4.33: Diagram of the intestinal system in rotifers. Abbreviations: bt, buccal tube; bv, buccal velum; c, cloaca; cio. ciliary esophagus; cuo, cuticular esophagus; gg, gastric gland; i, intestine; m, mastax; s, stomach. (Modified from Clément & Wurdak 1991, with permission.)

correlated with different modes of feeding (Remane 1933). Several types of esophagus have been recognized, based on its total length, length and width of cuticular and ciliary sections, presence of a vibratile flame, etc. (Remane 1933).

The stomach wall is syncytial in bdelloids and cellular with usually clearly defined cells in monogononts. In bdelloids (*Philodina roseola, Habrotrocha rosa*), the stomach lumen is lined by a thick, dense fibrillar terminal web (Fig. 4.34), lying directly under the plasma membrane (Mattern & Daniel 1966a, Schramm 1978a, Clément & Wurdak 1991). This web is perforated by large pores containing invaginations of the stomach cell membrane, pinching off digestive vesicles and vacuoles toward the cytoplasm. In monogononts, a thin fibrous terminal web, pierced by pores, may be present (*Asplanchna*) or lacking (*Brachionus, Filinia, Notommata copeus, Rhinoglena, Trichocerca rattus*). Digestive vacuoles are formed by endocytosis as well (Wurdak 1987, Clément & Wurdak 1991). The stomach is enveloped by a mesh of circular and longitudinal muscles or by syncytial muscle fibers. The anterior part of the stomach may be provided with an offset proventriculus (e.g., many *Encentrum* and *Proales*). Blind sacks of the stomach wall often occur in species showing intracellular digestion and/or symbiotic zoochlorellae (e.g., *Ascomorpha, Birgea, Dicranophoroides caudatus, Gastropus, Itura*).

Usually, there is a pair of syncytial gastric glands opening at the junction of ciliated esophagus-stomach by a pore directly or by a more or less long duct. The shape of the glands is variable and may be ovate, rounded, lobate, kidney-shaped, tubular, etc. The glands are rich in rough

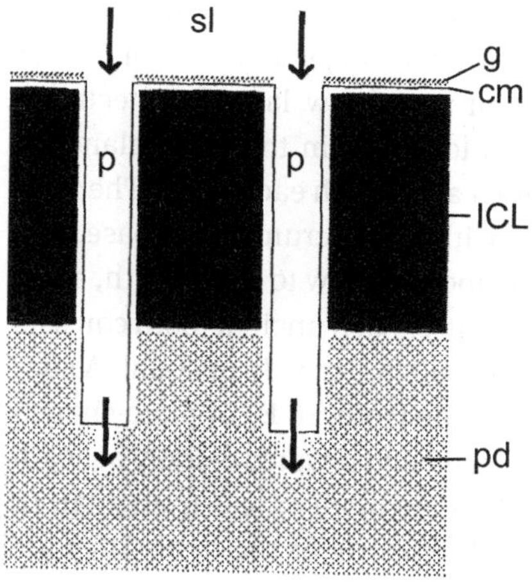

Fig. 4.34: Diagram of the apical part of the syncytial wall of the stomach in Bdelloidea. Abbreviations: cm, cell membrane; g, glycocalyx; ICL, intracytoplasmic lamina; p, pore; pd, part of cytoplasm with digestive vacuoles; sl, stomach lumen. (From Clément 1993, with permission.)

endoplasmic reticulum and Golgi complexes; secretory granules accumulate in the basal part of the glands next to the stomach (e.g., Clément & Wurdak 1991). The secretions of the gastric glands play a primary role in the extracellular digestion. Other gland-like structures of variable shape and number (Remane 1933), remembering gastric glands by structure and inclusions (de Beauchamp 1909), and mostly situated on the dorsal stomach wall occur in several species (e.g., *Enteroplea lacustris, Epiphanes clavulata, Microcodon clavus, Tetrasiphon hydrocora*). Gastric glands are rarely absent (e.g., *Albertia typhlina*), but mostly lacking in species with stomach blind sacks and/or symbiotic zoochlorellae.

The stomach either is distinctly constricted off from the intestine by a muscular sphincter, or merges gradually into it. The syncytial intestine is thin-walled and provided with motile cilia and microvilli; the latter may be replaced by atypical flattened cilia containing microtubules (Clément 1977, Clément & Wurdak 1991). In bdelloids, the microvilli show submembrane helicoidal filaments, which are lacking in monogononts. Externally, the intestine is provided with a continuation of the musculature of the stomach.

The intestine empties in a short, contractile cloaca, opening dorsally at the base of the foot. In species with ventrally displaced foot, it opens terminally or even ventrally (*Ploesoma*); in Flosculariidae, it opens on a papilla. The lumen of the cloaca is lined by a thin epithelial syncytium surrounded by a reticular muscle layer. The cloacal wall (*Asplanchna brightwellii*) includes a multicellulary sensory receptor, with cilia and microvilli projecting toward the cloacal opening. The sensory cells are near the cloacal ganglion innervating the cloacal muscles. The syncytial wall of the cloaca merges imperceptibly into the syncytial integument, and is seldom ciliated (e.g., Clément et al. 1983, Clément & Wurdak 1991, Ahlrichs 1993). Oviducts, bladder, or protonephridial ducts open in the cloaca as well. In some species, there is no cloaca or cloacal aperture, and fecal matter is ejected through the mouth (e.g., *Asplanchna*) or stored as defecation pellets in the stomach (e.g., *Ascomorpha*).

There are many variations (Fig. 4.35) on the general scheme of the intestinal system as outlined above (see Remane 1933). In Collothecacea, the anterior end is transformed into a large buccal funnel. A semicircle of cilia in this funnel separates an anterior part or vestibulum, from a posterior chamber, the infundibulum. The mouth is at the base of the infundibulum, and leads to a narrow esophagus hanging freely in a very large cavity, the proventriculus. The small trophi are situated at the bottom of the proventriculus. The proventriculus is homologous to the mastax with its lumen enlarged into a food-storage organ.

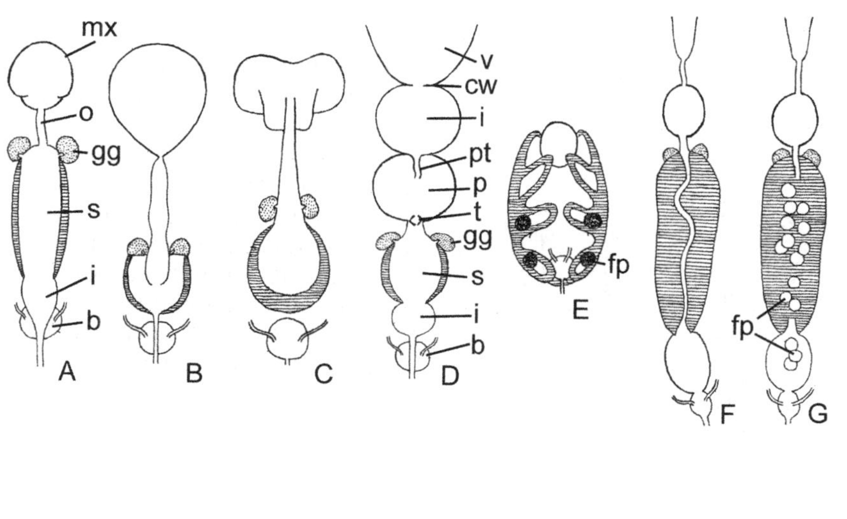

Fig. 4.35: Variation of the intestinal system in Monogononta (A–E) and Bdelloidea (F, G). (A) *Encentrum*, (B) *Synchaeta*, (C) *Asplanchna*, (D) *Collotheca*, (E) *Ascomorpha ecaudis*, (F) *Philodina*, and (G) *Habrotrocha*. Abbreviations: b, bladder; cw, ciliary wreath; fp, fecal pellet; gg, gastric gland; i, intestine; if, infundibulum; mx, mastax; o, esophagus; p, proventriculus; pt, pharyngeal tube; s, stomach; v, vestibulum. (From Donner 1956, 1965.)

Digestion is generally extracellular, although intracellular digestion can take place (*Asplanchna*) after an initial extracellular digestion (Wurdak 1987). In some monogonont genera (e.g., *Ascomorpha*) and the bdelloid family Habrotrochidae, digestion is intracellular. In Habrotrochidae, the stomach is a syncytial protoplasmic mass without lumen. The food is formed into pellets or food vacuoles in a short chamber behind the mastax; the vacuoles become digested when circulating in the stomach protoplasm.

4.2.6.2 Trophi

The trophi (Figs. 4.36–4.39) may be organized in a strictly bilaterally symmetrical (most species) to highly asymmetrical way (*Aspelta*, Trichocercidae). The fulcrum (absent in bdelloids) serves as an attachment for the 2 rami; together, these 3 elements are referred as incus. Adjoining them on each side are an uncus and manubrium, which hinging together form the malleus. The fulcrum is of variable length and can be plate- or rod-shaped and distally tapering, expanding, or forked, or provided with a basal plate. The rami are tall or flat in cross section, and their shape varies from roughly triangular to strongly elongate and almost parallel-sided. Their inner margin can be smooth or bears elongate sclerite bodies, the rami scleropili, which may fuse into a ridge and/or a series of tooth-like projections. At the outer part of their base, rami may show lateral projections, the alulae. Rami and fulcrum lie in the same plane, or form a more or less great angle with each other. The rami operate like a forceps with the fulcrum as the base. The unci consist of a single tooth, or few to many teeth, often firmly fused into rigid plates. Each uncinal tooth consists of a head and shaft; the teeth are mostly unequal. A subuncus, composed of minute teeth, rods, or plate-shaped elements, is mostly present, and situated distally beneath the uncus. The manubria are more or less triangular, or crescent- or rod-shaped supports of the unci. They are composed of an expanded head or clava, connected to the uncus, and a more or less strongly elongate shaft terminating in a handle-like distal end, the cauda, which is present in Ploima but absent in Gnesiotrocha and Bdelloidea. The head or clava is composed of 3 chambers that may be strongly reduced or absent. The malleus lies in the same plane as the incus, or the unci and manubria stand in different planes to each other and/or to the incus. A variable number of diverse accessory elements, e.g., epipharynx, hypopharynx, suprarami, etc., is often present in monogononts.

Studies by SEM of the embryonic development of the malleate trophi (Fig. 4.37) show that the first observable

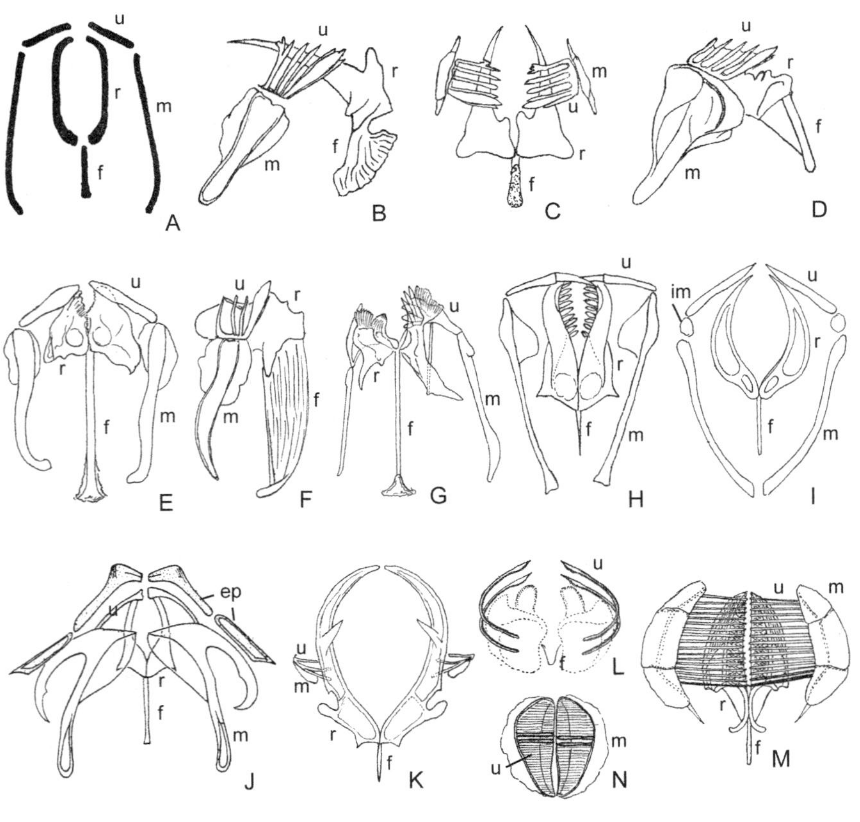

Fig. 4.36: The main trophi types. (A) Basic plan, (B–D) malleate (*Euchlanis*: B, right; C, ventral view); *Proales decipiens*, (D) right; (E–G) virgate (*Notommata copeus*: E, ventral; D, right; G, *Trichocerca rattus*, ventral), (H–I) forcipate (H, *Dicranophorus epicharis*, ventral; I, *Encentrum*), (J) cardate (*Lindia janickii*, ventral), (K) incudate (*Asplanchna*), (L) uncinate (*Collotheca*), (M) malleoramate (*Filinia*, ventral), and (N) ramate (*Macrotrachela*). Abbreviations: ep, epipharynx; im, intramalleus; f, fulcrum; m, manubrium; r, ramus; u, uncus.

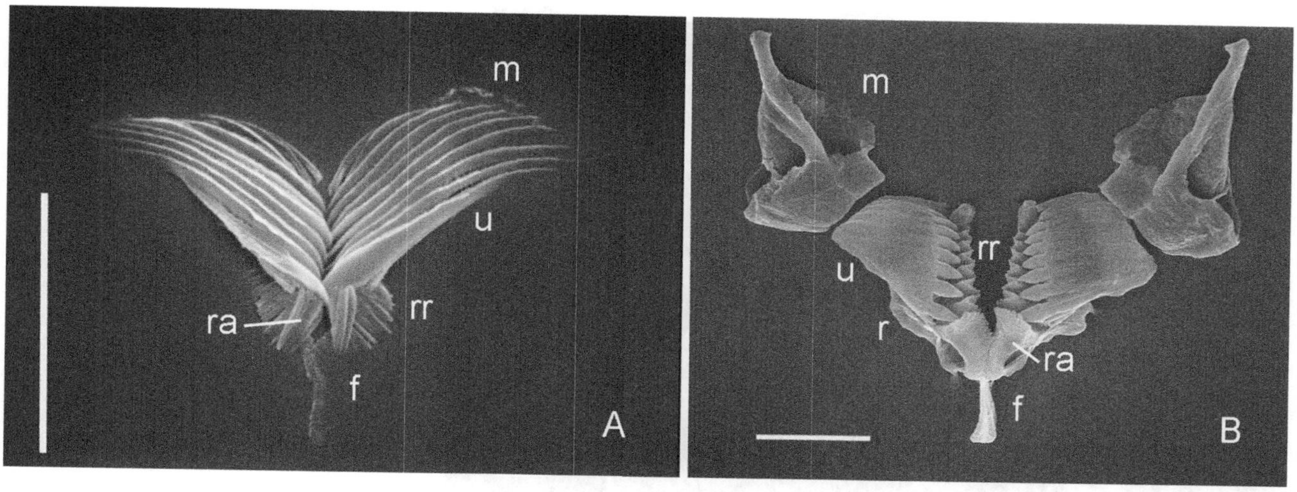

Fig. 4.37: Development of malleate trophi. (A) Early embryo and (B) adult. Abbreviations: f, fulcrum; m, manubrium; r, ramus, ra, rami apophysis; rr, reinforced ramus ridges; u, uncus. Scale bar=10 µm.

and distinctly sclerotized structures are a double row of elongate sclerite bodies along the longitudinal axis, wherein the future unci, reinforced ramus ridges, rami apophyses, and fulcrum are recognizable (De Smet, personal observation). By addition of sclerite bodies and apposition of amorphous sclerite material, the trophi attain their definitive shape and size in the fully grown embryo. After hatching ramate, malleate, virgate, forcipate, malleoramate, and uncinate trophi apparently do not change in size or shape and remain constant during the life of the rotifer (Fontaneto et al. 2003, Fontaneto & Melone 2005, 2006), although some post-embryonic growth cannot be ruled out in some taxa with incudate trophi, viz. *Asplanchna* (Fontaneto & Melone 2005).

Nine main types of trophi are recognized (Fig. 4.36), based on the shape and size of the elements, the presence of any accessory parts, and the way they operate. Several transitional types are known, and some other types are that specialized and modified that they cannot be classified into any of the main types. Shape of trophi is an utmost important character in rotifer taxonomy (Wallace et al. 2006), and even subtle differences in trophi shape may be useful in solving complexes of cryptic species; in monogononts, small details on the trophi shape can distinguish the species of the *Epiphanes senta* complex (Schröder & Walsh 2007) and between *Brachionus manjavacas* and *B. plicatilis* (Fontaneto et al. 2007). In bdelloids, the newly described *Abrochtha* from the USA have statistical differences in the number of minor teeth (Birky et al. 2011).

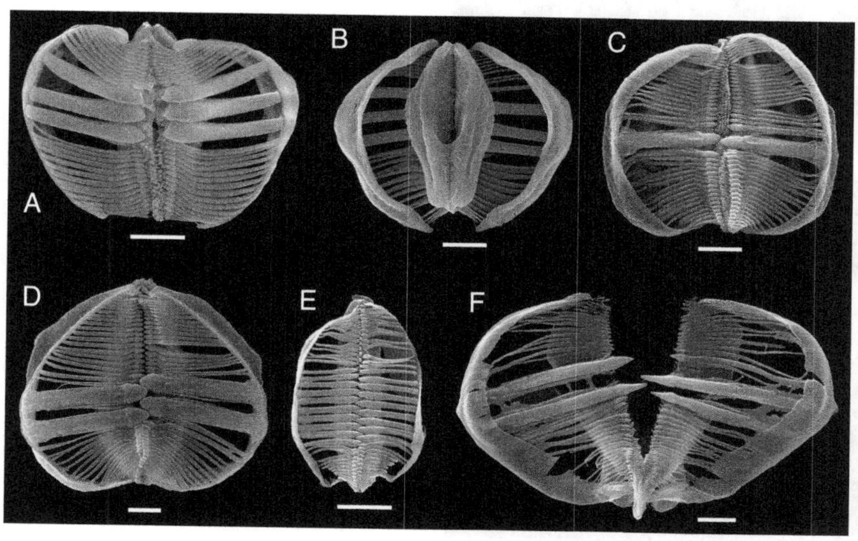

Fig. 4.38: SEM pictures of the ramate trophi in Bdelloidea. (A, B) *Dissotrocha aculeata*, (C) *Anomopus telphusae*, (D) *Rotaria tardigrada*, (E) *Otostephanos donneri*, (F) *Abrotrochtha carnivora*. (A, C–F) Dorsal view and (B) ventral view. Scale bar = 5 µm.

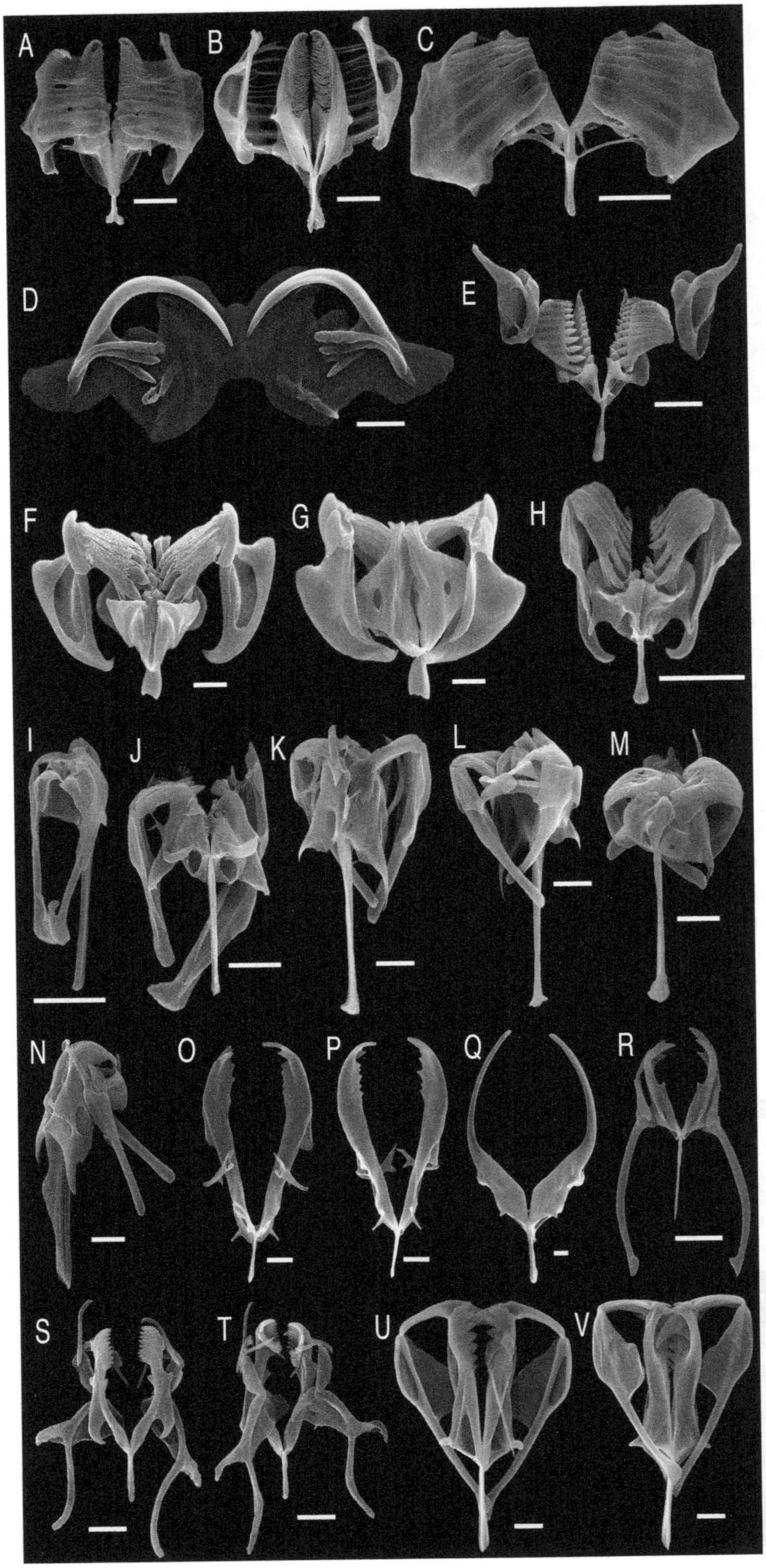

Fig. 4.39: SEM pictures of trophi types in Monogononta. (A, B) *Floscularia ringens*, (C) *Hexarthra* sp., (D) *Cupelopagis vorax*, (E) *Cyrtonia tuba*, (F, G) *Brachionus manjavacas*, (H) *Proales similis*, (I) *Cephalodella* sp., (J) *Pleurotrocha atlantica*, (K, L) *Notommata glyphura*, (M) *Notommata codonella*, (N) *Eothinia elongata*, (O, P) *Asplanchna priodonta*, (Q) *Asplanchnopus multiceps*, (R) *Encentrum algente*, (S, T) *Lindia deridderae*, and (U, V) *Dicranophorus forcipatus*. Scale bar = 10 µm.

SEM pictures of the trophi can be found in the references mentioned below for the different types and in Figs. 4.38 and 4.39.

Ramate. Rami sickle-shaped, flat. Fulcrum absent. Unci broad, usually with numerous teeth, occasionally broad semi-circular striated plates, usually with broad and narrow teeth. Manubria sickle-shaped, as lateral bands. Grinding. In subclass Bdelloidea only (e.g., Melone et al. 1998b, Melone & Fontaneto 2005).

Malleoramate. Rami more or less triangular, flat. Fulcrum short. Unci broad, with numerous teeth, occasionally resembling striated plates, proximal teeth usually enlarged. Manubria crescent-shaped with 3 superimposed major chambers, without shaft. Grinding. In order Flosculariacea only (e.g., Nogrady & Segers 2002, De Smet 2005a).

Uncinate. Similar to malleoramate type, but all trophi elements except unci strongly reduced. Unci teeth 2 or from 4 to 5, and only the first or first 2 of stout build, elongate and curved, forming supporting rods for mastax. Tearing. Only in Order Collothecacea: Atrochidae, Collothecidae.

Malleate. All parts of stout build. Rami more or less triangular, flat, inner margin usually toothed. Fulcrum short. Unci with several (4–12) firmly connected teeth, often fused into plate. Manubria provided with a fairly short shaft. The malleate trophi are adapted for gripping, grinding, and pumping. In Order Ploima: e.g., Epiphanidae, Brachionidae, Euchlanidae, Mytilinidae, Trichotriidae (e.g., Segers et al. 1994b, De Smet & Gibson 2008).

The submalleate type of Lecanidae is characterized by manubria showing a relatively long and incurved shaft (e.g., Segers 1995).

Virgate. All parts can be of slender build and/or thin. Rami broad, more or less triangular, recurved dorsally forming hemispherical dome. Fulcrum strongly elongated, distal end usually more or less expanded or strongly bent dorsally. Unci with few teeth, often only the first of stout build or teeth reduced. Manubria mostly with elongate shafts. Often strongly asymmetrical (e.g., *Trichocerca*). The virgate trophi type is the most variable of all. Used for swallowing food by pumping without crushing or piercing and sucking. The pumping action is produced by a powerful hypopharyngeal muscle. In Order Ploimida, e.g., Gastropodidae, Trichocercidae, Synchaetidae (e.g., Nogrady & Segers 2002).

The malleovirgate type showing many uncinal teeth is a transition between the malleate and virgate type. In Proalidae (e.g., De Smet 1996).

Incudate. Rami strongly elongate, curved, pincer-like. Fulcrum short. Unci and manubria strongly reduced. Specialized for seizing. Only in Asplanchnidae (e.g., Gilbert et al. 1979).

Cardate. Rami lyrate. Fulcrum medium long. Unci a few distinct teeth, first largest, or a striated plate. Manubria with well developed head and shaft, head with characteristic crescent- or rod-shaped ventral apophysis. Species-specific accessory trophi elements present, often numerous. Adapted for pumping; the pumping action is produced without the hypopharyngeal muscle: the lumen is widened by a rolling motion of the trophi. Only in Lindiidae (e.g., Nogrady & Segers 2002, De Smet 2005b).

Forcipate. Rami strongly elongate, straight, or curved, pincer-like, with toothed tips, inner margins often with few to numerous teeth. Fulcrum usually short to medium long. Unci strong, a single or few teeth only. Manubria rod-shaped, long, head reduced; often with intramalleus between uncus and manubrium. Seizing; rami and unci can be thrust out from mouth (Dicranophoridae). In Dicranophoridae and Ituridae (e.g., De Smet & Pourriot 1997).

In the hemiforcipate type, rami lack apical and medial teeth. In Asciaporrectidae (De Smet 2006).

Fulcrate. Fulcrum long, well developed. Rami short with strong, characteristic alulae. Unci small. Manubria absent. Pumping action performed by hypopharynx muscle attached to fulcrum. Only in Order Seisonacea (e.g., Segers & Melone 1998).

4.2.6.3 Intestinal system of the male

The intestinal system of the male shows transitions from fully developed to completely absent. To date, *Rhinoglena frontalis* is the only species studied in which the males possess a fully developed and functional system similar to the female (Melone 2001). The male trophi are similar to the female but display fewer uncinal teeth and a reduction of the size to about 70%. In several species, e.g., *Asplanchnopus multiceps*, *Eosphora najas*, and *Lacinularia flosculosa*, the male intestinal system is well developed, but trophi are apparently lacking (Hamburger 1907, de Beauchamp 1965). In other males, the digestive tract consists of a strand of stomach cells with distinct lumen and indications of gastric glands (e.g., *Mytilina*, *Synchaeta*) or it is a strand without lumen (e.g., *Asplanchna priodonta*); the cellular strand supports the testis. The digestive tract may be further reduced to a globular mass of cells without lumen (e.g., *Asplanchna brightwellii*, *Encentrum martes*), supposed to form an energy source. The intestinal system is completely absent in males of, e.g., *Conochilus*, *Filinia*,

Hexathra, Keratella, Polyarthra, Pompholyx, and *Trichocerca* (e.g., Wesenberg-Lund 1923). The sensory receptors in the mouth region of the female, involved in feeding, are absent (Wurdak et al. 1983).

4.2.7 Body cavity

The body cavity of the rotifers is considered a pseudocoel, as it is not lined by an epithelium, but by extracellular matrix. It is usually a spacious cavity, apparently lacking fibrils or microfilaments of collagen (Clément & Wurdak 1991, Clément 1993). The pseudocoel of several taxa, e.g., *Asplanchna, Proales, Synchaeta*, and Collothecacea, contains free amoeboid cells or amoebocytes (Nachtwey 1925, Remane 1933, Baumann et al. 2000); these cells could not be demonstrated in *Brachionus, Notommata*, and *Trichocerca* (Clément 1980). The amoebocytes form a highly dynamic, 3-dimensional polygonal network of filopodia. The cytoskeleton of the filopodia contains F-actin and microtubules that are often organized in bundles. Filopodial motion types include lateral junction displacement, formation and extension of free-ending filopodia, and fusion of filopodial strands, resulting in enlargements, diminutions, and extinctions of the filopodial polygons, and in the formation of new polygons (Baumann et al. 2000). An intense and fast particle transport takes place in the filopodial strands. The amoebocytes are often vacuolated, and contain inclusions, "bacteroids", pigments, oil droplets, etc. In some species (e.g., *Cupelopagis vorax*, adult sessile *Collotheca, Proales*), specialized immobile amoeboid cells, the excretophores, apparently accumulate catabolites as excretion particles. The excretophores often pile up symmetrically near, e.g., the longitudinal and circular muscles, and the anterior part of the protonephridial tubule; their number and size increases with age (Remane 1933).

Salt composition and volume of the pseudocoelomic fluid are regulated by the protonephridia (e.g., Braun et al. 1966, Pontin 1966). The pseudocoel functions as a hydrostatic skeleton, and supposedly as respiratory and circulatory system, its pseudocoelomic fluid being replenished by the oxygen carrying water taken in by the digestive tract, and subsequently eliminated through the protonephridia.

4.2.8 Excretory system

4.2.8.1 Excretory system of the female

The excretory system of rotifers has been studied by LM (e.g., Remane 1933, Brakenhoff 1937, Pontin 1964) and TEM (e.g., Braun et al. 1966, Mattern & Daniel 1966b, Warner 1969, Schramm 1978b, Clément & Wurdak 1991, Ahlrichs 1993, Riemann & Ahlrichs 2010). It consists of 2 similar protonephridia lying ventrolaterally in the pseudocoel. The protonephridial apparatus is formed by 3–4 multinucleate cells and consists of few to several flame bulbs or terminal organs, attached to collecting tubules or capillary canals, which are connected to the main canals; the main canals discharge in an unpaired and contractile urinary bladder, or in a contractile cloaca (Fig. 4.40).

The flame bulbs (Fig. 4.41) are conical and laterally flattened, appearing cylindrical or fan-shaped depending on their orientation (e.g., *Asplanchna priodonta, A. brightwelllii, Dicranophorus forcipatus, Notommata copeus*) or almost cylindrical and round in cross section (e.g., *Encentrum mucronatum, Erignatha clastopis, Proales reinhardti*). They are hollow, and their lumen drains into the capillary canals of the syncytium. The distal end of each flame bulb is closed by a protoplasmic cap. In monogononts, the lateral wall of the flame bulb usually consists of cytoplasmic columns and electron-dense microvilli (pillars), arranged in concentric rings around a central

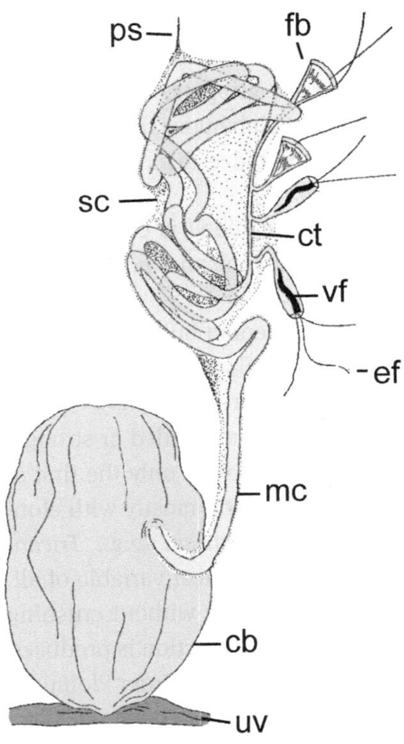

Fig. 4.40: Protonephridium and contractile bladder of *Asplanchna priodonta*. Top 2 flame bulbs shown frontally; other 2 shown from the side. Abbreviations: cb, contractile bladder; ct, collecting tubule; ef, external filament; fb, flame bulb; mc, main canal; ps, protoplasmic strand; sc. syncytial cytoplasm; uv, uterovesicular duct; vf, vibratile flame. (Modifed from Pontin 1964.)

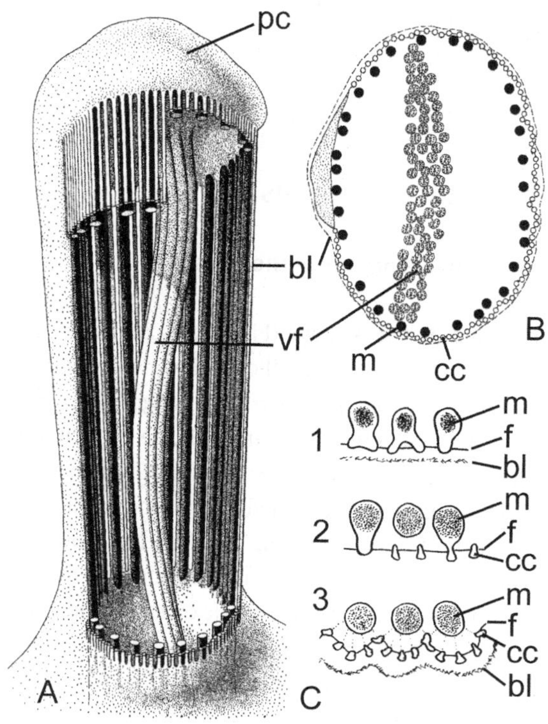

Fig. 4.41: Flame bulb. (A) Flame bulb partly opened to show internal organization, (B) cross section, and (C) detail of the filtering membrane in (1) bdelloids, (2) the monogonont *Trichocerca rattus*, (3) other monogononts (*Asplanchna, Brachionus, Notommata copeus, Rhinoglena*). Abbreviations: bl, basal lamina; cc, cytoplasmic columns; f, filtering membrane; m, microvilli; pc, protoplasmic cap; vb, vibratile flame. (A, B, From Braun et al. 1966; C, from Clément & Wurdak 1991, with permission.)

lumen with vibratile flame. Columns, and occasionally microvilli, are connected by a filtering membrane. In bdelloids and some monogononts (*Proales reinhardti*), microvilli are absent or not distinct from columns, and the filtering membrane is sustained by both. The cilia of the vibratile flame are connected with each other and inserted on the protoplasmic cap containing their basal bodies. Ciliary rootlets extending into the filter region are usually absent in monogononts, but present in bdelloids (see, e.g., Riemann & Ahlrichs 2010). The basal membrane is often present at the outside. The distal cap of the flame bulbs is connected to the integument by protoplasmic strands, maintaining the position of the protonephridial apparatus. The number of flame bulbs on each side of the body varies from 2 to 100 according to the species and appears positively correlated with the surface area of the species (Pontin 1964); the number is fairly constant for any one species.

The lumina of the flame bulbs are connected to the hollow cells of the protonephridial collecting tubule, and the latter joins with the intracytoplasmic lumen of the main canal syncytium. The intracytoplasmic lumen of the collecting tubules may be ciliated. The collecting tubules are mostly straight, whereas the main canals are straight, coiled, looped, or branched and often connected by a transversal canal, the Huxley anastomose, above the brain (e.g., *Epiphanes, Lacinularia, Stephanoceros*). Several protonephridium types (Fig. 4.42) have been described (for a review, see Remane 1933).

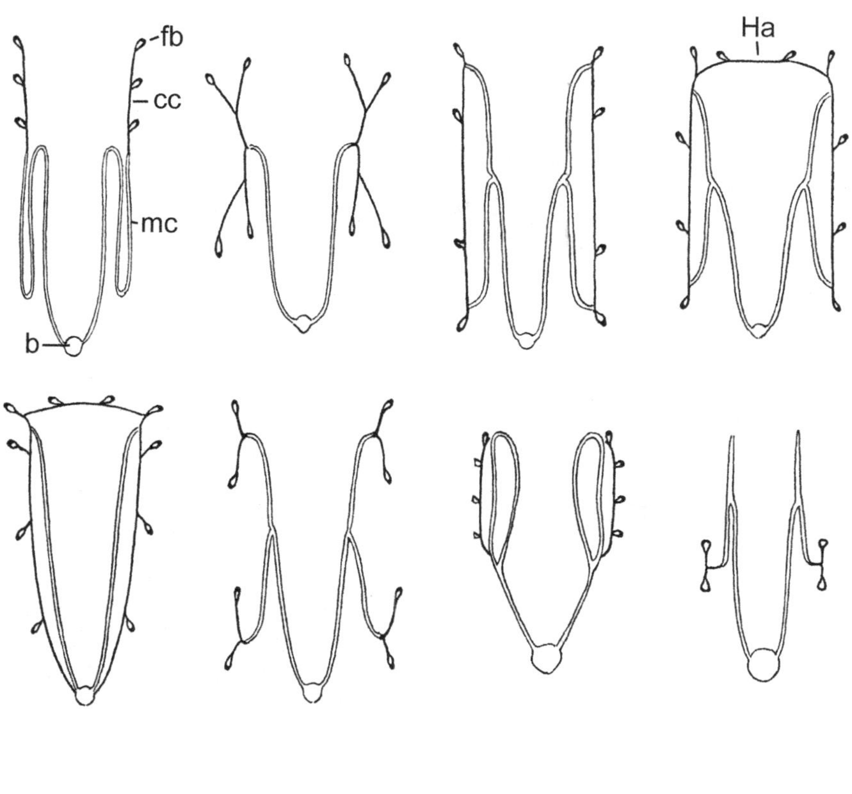

Fig. 4.42: Variation of the protonephridial system in Monogononta. Abbreviations: b, bladder; cc, capillary canal; fb, flame bulb; Ha, Huxley anastomose; mc, main canal. (From Remane 1933.)

A urinary bladder is only found in monogononts. It opens ventrally in the cloaca, or when occasionally absent, the protonephridia empty directly in the contractile cloaca (e.g., *Conochilus, Lacinularia, Testudinella*). The bladder syncytium is surrounded by a binuclear syncytial muscle, enabling the bladder to contract. In bdelloids, a separate urinary bladder is absent, and the protonephridia discharge in the terminal section of the intestine functioning as a bladder.

The protonephridial system of the rotifers has both an excretory and osmoregulatory function (e.g., Braun et al. 1966, Pontin 1966).

4.2.8.2 Excretory system of the male

Very little is known on the excretory system of the male (Wesenberg-Lund 1923), and results must be considered with caution (Remane 1933). Protonephridia have been found in most of the males described but appear absent in the strongly reduced ones. In several species flame bulbs, capillary ducts, and main canals are distinct (e.g., *Asplanchna, Asplanchnopus, Epiphanes*); the Huxley anastomose is present in male *Epiphanes*. The numbers of flame bulbs of the male and the female are identical (e.g., *Epiphanes senta, Asplanchna priodonta, Mytilina*) or apparently reduced in the male (Collothecacea). A contractile urinary bladder is usually absent but has been found in, e.g., *Asplanchna, Asplanchnopus, Cyrtonia, Stephanoceros*, and *Cupelopagis*. The protonephridia may discharge into the urinary bladder, into the vas deferens by a common duct, to the outside *via* separate pores near the genital opening, or into a bladder-like structure lying dorsally from the testis.

4.2.9 Reproductive organs

4.2.9.1 Reproductive organs of the female

The female reproductive system (Fig. 4.43) comprises the ovarium, the vitellarium, and a follicular layer surrounding both completely (bdelloids) or partly (monogononts) and continuing as an oviduct (e.g., Remane 1933, de Beauchamp 1965, Bentfeld 1971a, b, Amsellem & Ricci 1982, Clément & Wurdak 1991). In most species, the oviduct opens into the cloaca beyond the urinary bladder, or when the cloaca is reduced or absent, it directly leads to the outside. The female organs of monogononts consist of a single ovarium and vitellarium, whereas both organs are always paired in bdelloids, with the 2 oviducts joining into a single duct. They lie ventrally under the stomach and are mostly displaced to one side in monogononts.

The syncytial ovarium is small; it lies close to the vitellarium and contains the oocytes. In full-grown females, the syncytial vitellarium is a very large, yolk-producing gland with large polyploid nuclei, the number of which is usually constant within a species. The most frequently observed number is 8, but 4, and a multiple of 4 up to 32, occurs. Individual variations in number of nuclei in function of diet and doses of vitamin E have been described (e.g., Birky & Field 1966, Amsellem & Ricci 1982). The

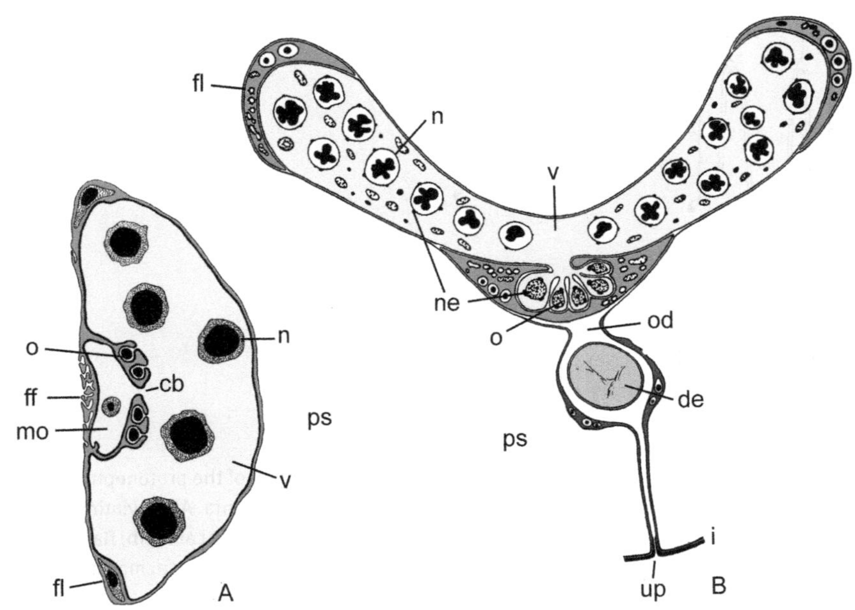

Fig. 4.43: Diagram of the female genital apparatus. (A) The bdelloid *Philodina roseola* and (B) the monogonont *Asplanchna brightwellii*. Abbreviations: cb, cytoplasmic bridge; de, developing embryo; ff, follicular folds; fl, follicular layer; i, integument; mo, maturing oocyte; n, nucleus with large nucleolus; ne, nucleolar extrusion; o, oocyte in ovarium; od, oviduct; ps, pseudocoelom; u, urogenital pore; v, vitellarium. (Modified from Clément & Wurdak 1991, with permission.)

shape of the vitellarium is rounded, lobed, band-shaped, horseshoe-shaped, cylindrical, etc., and often characteristic of the species.

4.2.9.2 Reproductive organs of the male

The male reproductive system (Fig. 4.44) consists of the unpaired, large, globular to pyriform testis, one to several accessory or prostate glands, the short to long, and mostly ciliated vas deferens, the copulatory organ or penis, and the dorsally lying genital aperture that is usually surrounded by a ring of cilia (e.g., Wesenberg-Lund 1923, Remane 1933, de Beauchamp 1965). If a digestive tract or its rudiments are present, the testis lies ventral to it. The wall of the testis is syncytial. The tip of the testis bears a wreath of cilia and often tufts of sensory cilia and several openings (*Brachionus, Asplanchna*); its inside is lined by integument (Aloia & Moretti 1974, Clément et al. 1983, Clément & Wurdak 1991). The testis is filled up with spermatids, spermatozoa, and testicular rods. The penis is protrusible (e.g., *Brachionus, Euchlanis, Gastropus*) or projecting continually (e.g., *Anuraeopsis, Keratella, Notholca*). In some species, the penis is absent, and the evertable vas deferens acts as penis (e.g., *Ascomorpha, Asplanchna, Epiphanes, Rhinoglena*), or the tube-shaped posterior extremity of the male is specialized for copulation (e.g., *Filinia, Hexarthra, Polyarthra*). Two pairs of cutaneovisceral muscles may insert on the vas deferens and act as retractores penis.

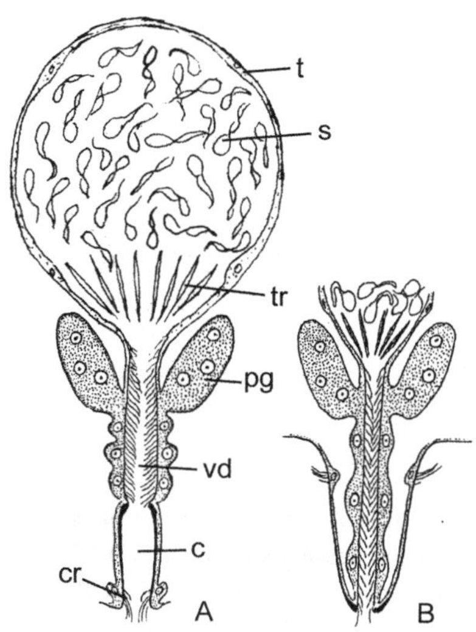

Fig. 4.44: Male reproductive system. (A) Scheme of male genital organ in Monogononta, penis redrawn and (B) penis everted. Abbreviations: c, cloaca; cr, ciliary ring at genital opening; pg, prostate glands; s, spermatozoa; t, testis; tr, testicular rods; vd, vas deferens. (Modified after Remane 1933 and Koste 1978.)

4.2.10 Gametes

Oogenesis was studied by, e.g., Nachtwey (1925), Lehmensick (1926), Bentfeld (1971a, b), and Clément & Wurdak (1991) for monogononts and by Hsu (1956a, b), Clément & Wurdak (1991), and Pagani et al. (1993) for bdelloids. The number of oocytes is fixed at birth (e.g., Buchner et al. 1965, Pagani et al. 1993). Maturation of the oocytes is by 2 subsequent equatorial divisions in bdelloids, with the extrusion of 2 polar bodies. Oogenesis of mononogonts is likewise by 2 equatioral divisions and extrusion of 1 polar body for the production of amictic eggs and 2 for the production of mictic ones (Gilbert 1993, Hsu 1956a, b). Important nucleolar extrusions are present in the cytoplasm of the immature oocytes of monogononts, but absent in bdelloids. During maturation, the volume of the oocyte increases considerably by the transfer of cytoplasm from the vitellarium through a cytoplasmic bridge; each oocyte has its own bridge (e.g., Bentfeld 1971b, Amsellem & Ricci 1982, Clément & Wurdak 1991). Subsequently, at the end of the growth period oocytes become detached from the ovary. After deposition of a shell in the oviduct, eggs are laid in oviparous species (most monogononts and bdelloids) or develop in the oviduct in ovoviviparous species. The term "viviparous" is often used for species who give live birth (e.g., the monogononts *Albertia, Asplanchna, Lindia, Rhinoglena, Trochosphaera*, and the bdelloids *Rotaria*), unlike the species who lay eggs enclosing a full-grown embryo that leaves the shell immediately after egg deposition. At hatching, juvenile females of free-swimming species usually have the adult shape. In sessile species, the females hatch as free-swimming larvae of typical rotifer appearance (Fig. 4.45), attaining the characteristic shape of the sessile stage after attachment and development into adults (e.g., Hochberg et al. 2010, Fontaneto et al 2003). Males are sexually mature at hatching and do not grow.

Three types of eggs are commonly produced in monogononts. The asexual or amictic egg (also called subitaneous egg) is a thin-shelled diploid egg produced by amictic females. The amictic egg develops into either amictic or mictic females. The sexual or mictic egg, also called male egg, is a small, thin-shelled haploid egg produced by mictic females; if unfertilized, it develop into males. Resting or dormant eggs are thick-shelled, fertilized mictic eggs, hatching into amictic females (Fig. 4.46). Resting eggs are actually resting embryos and not eggs (Boschetti et al. 2011a; see Section 4.3.3, Development). A fourth type of egg is the pseudosexual egg (e.g., in *Keratella hiemalis, Synchaeta*), an unfertilized resting egg produced *via* parthenogenesis in the absence of males (Ruttner-Kolisko 1946, 1974). Bdelloidea lack males, and their diploid eggs develop into females by parthenogenesis.

Eggs are spherical, ellipsoid, ovate, kidney-shaped, etc. They may be free floating, glued by a short stalk to the substrate, carried attached to the body of the female by a gelatinous thread, etc.; in several species, the resting egg is retained within the lorica. Amictic and mictic eggs are usually smooth, unlike the resting eggs, which are mostly ornamented with spines, ridges, pits, gas-filled vacuoles, etc. The ornamentation is often characteristic of the genus and/or species (e.g., Pourriot et al. 1983). The resting egg is mostly provided with a groove at one pole, where the shell opens on hatching of the young female. The shell of the amictic egg in *Trichocerca* consists of an external shell underlain by a thin internal envelope, joined to short microvilli at the periphery of the egg cytoplasm (Clément & Wurdak 1991). The shell of the resting egg of *Asplanchna* is composed of 3 coats: an external shell consisting of 2 coats separated by a space from an inner coat, which in its turn is separated by a space from the embryo (Wurdak et al. 1977).

During spermatogenesis, the primordial germ cells produce the spermatozoa, and atypical germ cells, which produce the testicular rods, formerly described as rudimentary, non functional, or atypical spermatozoa (e.g., Whitney 1917, 1918, Tannreuther 1919, Koehler 1965, Koehler & Birky 1966, Aloia & Moretti 1974).

The spermatozoa of a few monogononts, belonging to the genera *Asplanchna*, *Brachionus*, *Cephalodella*,

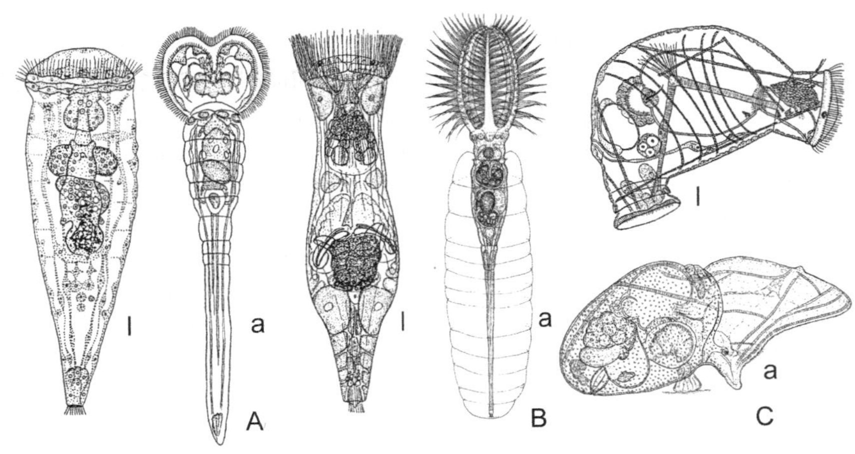

Fig. 4.45: Free-swimming larvae and sessile adults. (A) *Sinantherina socialis*, (B) *Stephanoceros fimbriatus*, and (C) *Cupelopagis vorax*. Abbreviations: a, adult female; l, larva. (From Remane 1933, Koste 1978, and Kutikova 1970.)

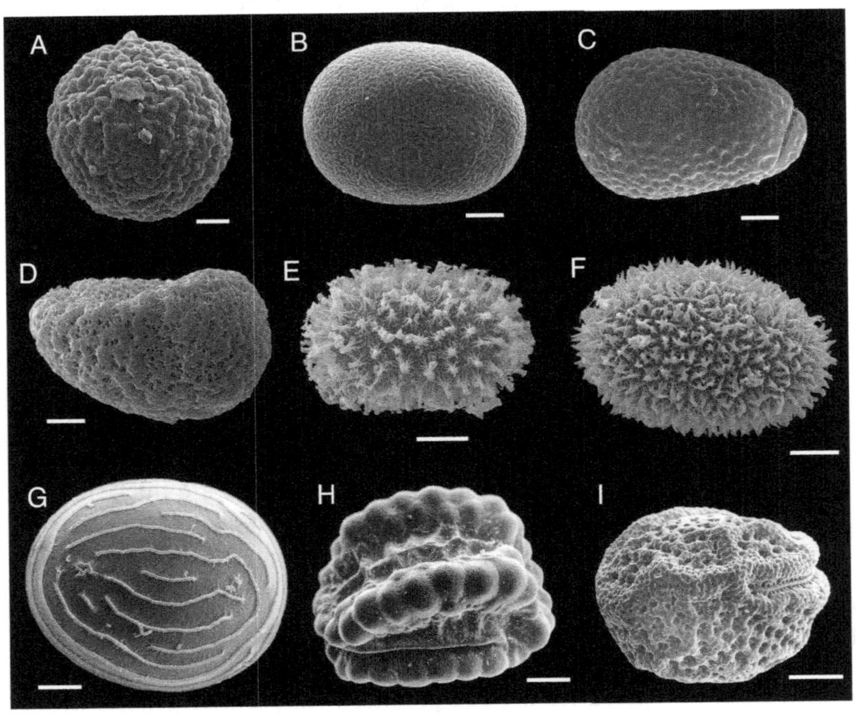

Fig. 4.46: SEM pictures of resting eggs of Monogononta: (A) *Asplanchna priodonta*, (B) *Brachionus plicatilis*, (C) *B. calyciflorus*, (D) *Epiphanes brachionus*, (E) *Rhinoglena frontalis*, (F) *Notommata codonella*, (G) *Conochilus natans*, (H) *Filinia longiseta*, and (I) *Hexarthra mira*. Scale bar = 20 µm, except for (G) 10 µm. (A–F, Photo courtesy of Giulio Melone; G–I, Photo courtesy of Hendrik Segers.)

Epiphanes, and *Lacinularia*, have been described with LM (Hamburger 1907, Whitney 1917, 1918, Tannreuther 1919, Tauson 1927). Ultrastructural studies are limited to *Asplanchna brightwellii* (Koehler 1965, Koehler & Birky 1966, Aloia & Moretti 1974), *A. sieboldii* (Koehler 1965), *Brachionus plicatilis* (Melone & Ferraguti 1994), *B. sericus* (Clément 1977, Clément & Wurdak 1991), and *Epiphanes senta* (Melone & Ferraguti 1999). The general organization of the spermatozoon is similar for the species studied, except for some minor differences concerning shape and size (Fig. 4.47). The spermatozoon is an elongated cell with a posterior cell body containing the nucleus and an anterior complex composed of a flagellum and undulating membrane; an acrosome is absent. The single axoneme is intracellular and shows the usual 9 × 2 + 2 tubules, in which the inner dynein arms only are present (Melone & Ferraguti 1994, 1999). The elongate nucleus is lobate and located anteriorly behind the flagellar region (Koehler 1965, Melone & Ferraguti 1994, 1999). The cytoplasm contains randomly distributed elongate mitochondria, different types of vesicles, free ribosomes, dense granules, etc.

The shape and length of the spermatozoa studied by EM is as follows: *Asplanchna*: gourd-shaped, 15–20 µm; *Brachionus plicatilis*: filliform, 70–80 µm (flagellum 40–45 µm, cell body 30–35 µm); *Epihanes senta*: sausage-shaped, bent, and weakly twisted, 12–15 µm (cell body 8–10 µm).

The testicular rods are rod-shaped structures developing late in embryonic life, i.e., in essentially mature males, from atypical germ cells showing intense secretory activity (Koehler 1965, Koehler & Birky 1966, Clément 1977, Melone & Ferraguti 1994). The rods contain dense material originating from Golgi vesicles and are organized as densely packed microtubules; a nucleus and flagellum are lacking. They are extruded from the cell within 2 membranes, one derived from the Golgi vesicle and one from the cell membrane. Testicular rods occur in almost all monogonont families and are supposed to assist, mechanically or enzymatically, in the penetration through the female integument during copulation (Remane 1933, Koehler 1965). They are always much smaller than the spermatozoa, e.g., 15 × 2 µm in *Asplanchna*, 16 × 1.5 µm in *Brachionus plicatilis*, and 14 × 1 µm in *Epiphanes senta* (Melone & Ferraguti 1999).

4.3 Reproduction and development

4.3.1 Reproductive biology

Rotifers are a textbook example of the different types of reproduction in animals. Seisonacea are characterized by sexual reproduction, which is in common with most animals (see chapter on Seisonacea). Monogononta can

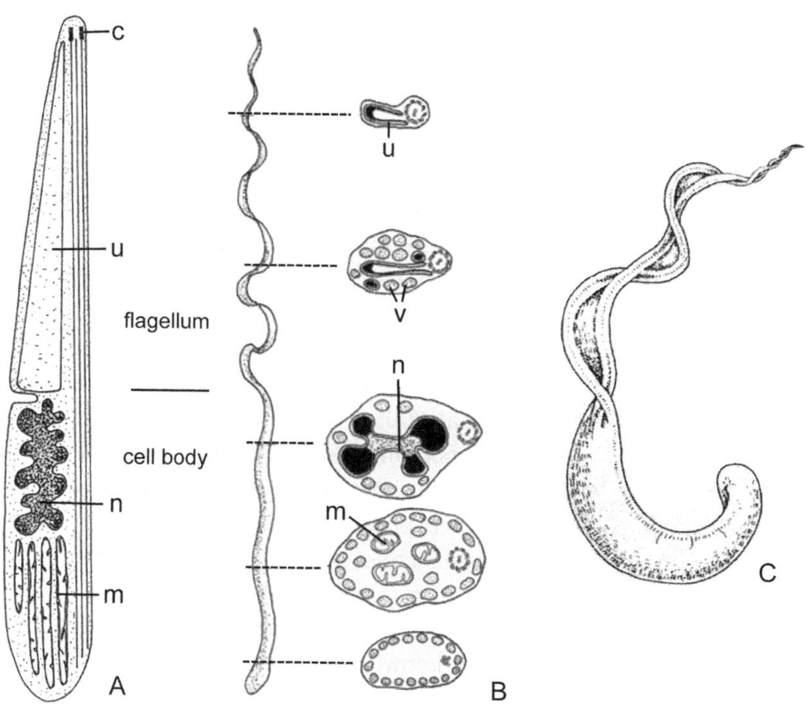

Fig. 4.47: Spermatozoon. (A) Diagram of spermatozoon of Monogononta, (B) spermatozoon of *Brachionus plicatilis* with representative cross sections, and (C) Spermatozoon of *Epiphanes senta*. Abbreviations: c, centriole; m, mitochondrion; n, nucleus; u, undulating membrane; v, vesicles containing tubules. (A, Modified from Melone & Ferraguti 1999; B, C, modified from Melone & Ferraguti 1994.)

alternate parthenogenesis, both through the development of diploid eggs producing females and through the development of haploid eggs producing males, to sexual reproduction (Serra & Snell 2009). Bdelloidea are the most famous case of ancient asexuals and the whole group diversified and persisted in the absence of any known form of sexual reproduction (Mark Welch et al. 2009).

Clear absence of sex in Bdelloidea cannot be proven unambiguously, as hidden sex may always occur. Yet, a large amount of observation on Bdelloidea never produced any evidence of meiosis, males, hermaphrodites, or vestigial genital structures (Birky 2010). Moreover, all the available indirect cytological and genetic evidence concurs in supporting their actual asexuality (Normark et al. 2003, Mark Welch et al. 2009): high sequence divergence between gene copies, functional divergence of former alleles, and multiple functionally divergent and conserved copies have been found (Mark Welch & Meselson 2000, Pouchkina-Stantcheva et al. 2007, Eyres et al. 2012), there is lack of high-copy-number retrotransposons (Arkhipova & Meselson 2000, 2005), an accumulation of deleterious mutations has been found (Barraclough et al. 2007, Swanstrom et al. 2011), and the diversification rates in Bdelloidea are clearly different from those in Monogononta (Fontaneto et al. 2012b). According to our current knowledge, Bdelloidea produce only diploid eggs that hatch into females that can lay eggs that hatch into females, without any form of sexual recombination. Thus, the whole genome of the mother is inherited by all the daughters, producing clonal lines. Because of the evolutionary success of Bdelloidea in the absence of sexual reproduction, Maynard Smith (1986) dubbed them as an "evolutionary scandal". This makes bdelloids an excellent study system for the origin of sex in animals (Bell 1982) by understanding how these peculiar organisms thrive in the absence of sex. One caveat is nevertheless present due to the possibility of horizontally transferred genes, which are abundant and functional in Bdelloidea (Boschetti et al. 2012) and may represent an alternative mechanism to sexual recombination to maintain genetic variability (Gladyshev et al. 2008).

A rather peculiar reproductive behavior is present also in the other group of Rotifera, the Monogononta, characterized by cyclical parthenogenesis. Cyclical parthenogenesis is a combination of asexual, parthenogenetic, and sexual reproduction (Serra & Snell 2009). The conditions thought to favor cyclical parthenogenesis are seasonal and/or unpredictable temporal heterogeneity (Carmona et al. 1995, Serra et al. 2003, Ricci 2001), typical of the ephemeral habitats where most Monogononta thrive. In Monogononta, asexual females, called amictic females, produce asexual daughters by ameiotic (apomictic or amictic) parthenogenesis. In response to certain environmental cues such as population density, photoperiod, or chemical triggers (Pourriot & Clément 1981, Stelzer & Snell 2003, Snell 2011), asexual females produce sexual daughters, called mictic females (Gilbert 1963b). These sexual females produce meiotic eggs, which, if not fertilized, develop into haploid males. If fertilized by a male, eggs develop into cysts, called resting eggs, which undergo diapause. When resting eggs hatch, the cycle starts again and asexual females reproduce by parthenogenesis until the next round of sexual reproduction. Variations to this life cycle have been described, including amphoteric females producing both ameiotic and meiotic eggs (Gilbert 1974, King & Snell 1977), parthenogenetic resting eggs (Gilbert 1995, Gilbert & Schreiber 1998), and sexual females hatched from resting eggs (Schröder et al. 2007). The mechanisms involved in mating behavior in monogononts has been studied mostly for those species used in aquaculture (Hagiwara et al. 1995b, Rico-Martínez & Snell 1996, 1997), and a set of molecules potentially involved in mate recognition have already been tested and described (Snell 2011) (see Section 4.4, Physiology).

4.3.2 Cleavage

Most Rotifera are oviparous, but several ovoviviparous species retain the developing embryos inside the body (Gilbert 1989). Oviparous species may carry the eggs, attach them to the substrate, or simply release them in the water column (Wallace et al. 2006).

Rotifera possess a deterministic cleavage that follows a modified spiral pattern (Gilbert 1989). The fate of the cells is established very early in the development (Pray 1965). Moreover, Rotifera are eutelic (Clément & Wurdak 1991); cell divisions occur only during embryogenesis, whereas the newborn already possesses the same number of cells of the adult. Embryo development follows the 3 typical steps of cleavage, gastrulation, and organogenesis (Boschetti et al. 2005).

Eggs are poor in yolk; they are laid unsegmented and extrude the polar body before undergoing cleavage (Hsu 1965a, b, Gilbert 1989). During cleavage, subsequent divisions produce smaller and smaller cells of unequal size and amount of cytoplasm, called blastomeres. Cleavage is holoblastic and cell divisions are unequal. For a review of the current knowledge on cleavage, see Boschetti et al. (2005). A typical 16-blastopore stage is present with 4 rows of 4 cells each, and at this stage, gastrulation starts (Gilbert 1989, Boschetti et al. 2005).

4.3.3 Development

Gastrulation in Rotifera occurs by epibolic movements and consequent involution; the resultant gastrula is a stereogastrula without a recognizable internal cavity. Lechner (1966) described 2 stages in the gastrulation process, a first epibolic growth of the blastoderm cell and a second stage with a further epibolic growth coupled with the involution of the blastoderm to form the blastopore. Not all authors agree on this 2-stage process, on the position of the blastopore and the origin of the mouth, and on the origin on the digestive system (Boschetti et al. 2005). Modern analyses should be performed to obtain a clear description of the embryo development in Rotifera.

Cell lineage mapping has been performed only on few species (Zelinka 1892b, Pray 1965, Lechner 1966), and organogenesis is not well known, with discrepancies in the scattered available information. The main differences concern the origin of the digestive and the reproductive systems (Boschetti et al. 2005). According to Gilbert (1989), the stomodaeum, the pharynx, the nervous system, the excretory system, and the muscles originate from the ectoderm; the reproductive system, the germarium, and the vitellarium from the mesoderm; the digestive system from the endoderm.

It has to be reminded that Rotifera are eutelic (Clément & Wurdak 1991) and possess a constant number of cells (or better, of nuclei) throughout all life because several tissues are syncytial. Cell divisions occur during embryogenesis only, and the fixed number of cells is supposed to be species specific (Boschetti et al. 2005). The newborn possesses the same number of cells of the adult, and the cells will only increase in size during life.

In sessile Rotifera, the juveniles that hatch from the eggs are very different from the adults, and undergo radical developmental changes (Fontaneto et al. 2003, Wallace et al. 2006). Such changes include formation of the adult corona and elongation of the foot (see Section 4.2.1.2, Coloniality).

Development of resting eggs is also poorly understood (Wurdak et al. 1978, Hagiwara et al. 1995a, Boschetti et al. 2011a). The so-called resting eggs are actually diapausing embryos that will resume their development after being activated by external and/or internal stimuli (Gilbert 1974, Pourriot & Snell 1983, García-Roger et al. 2006).

4.4 Physiology

Very few studies deal with the general physiology of Rotifera. For example, almost nothing is known on the digestive system; we only know some of the enzymes involved and the absorptive process (Lindemann et al. 2001). More efforts have been implemented to analyze the triggers of the switch between sexual and asexual reproduction in Monogononta (Snell 2011), the physiological aspects of dormancy in Bdelloidea (Tunnacliffe & Wise 2007), hormone-induced phenotypic plasticity (Gilbert 1999), and the ecotoxicological and ecophysiological mechanisms (Dahms et al. 2011).

No rotifer hormones have been yet described (Snell 2011), but the rotifers that have been tested respond to a variety of hormones and neurotransmitters from vertebrates and insects (Gallardo et al. 1997, 1999, 2000, Snell & DesRosiers 2008), including growth hormone, human chorionic gonadotropin, triiodothyronine, juvenile hormone, serotonin, GABA, and progesterone. Several putative endocrine disruptors, sufficiently similar to hormones that they interfere with normal endocrine signaling in aquatic animals have effects on rotifers (Snell & Joaquim-Justo 2007). Moreover, rotifers indeed produce growth-promoting substances (Ohmori et al. 2011).

Evidence that rotifers use chemical signals as pheromones is available in rotifers, especially to regulate their reproduction (Snell 2011). These include compounds excreted in the medium that trigger the switch from sexual to asexual reproduction (Gilbert 1963a, Stelzer & Snell 2006), and mate recognition pheromones (Snell et al. 1995, Snell & Stelzer 2005, Snell et al. 2009). Also, environmental triggers have been described, such as dietary α-tocopherol, photoperiod, and crowding (Gilbert 1981, Pourriot & Clément 1981, Stelzer & Snell 2003).

The mechanism that switches asexual to sexual reproduction in Monogononta is controlled by the accumulation of a signaling molecule produced by the rotifers themselves (Gilbert 2004). Such population-level metabolic synchrony, regulating gene expression in response to fluctuations in population density, is similar to what known as quorum sensing in bacteria (Miller & Bassler 2001).

Rotifera, together with other microscopic aquatic animals such as tardigrades and nematodes, are able to withstand lack of water, in a desiccated and/or frozen state, entering dormancy. Bdelloidea may enter dormancy in any stage of their life cycle (Ricci & Fontaneto 2009), whereas Monogononta produce resting eggs that can remain dry and/or frozen for extended periods before hatching (Gilbert 1974, Schröder 2005). In the dry state, there is little or no evidence of metabolic activity (Clegg 1986, 2001). The desiccating process in Bdelloidea is influenced by the nature of the substrate and the humidity; the process involves morphological changes such as the contraction of the body into a tun shape and the packing of internal structures (Ricci et al. 2003, 2008).

The biochemical mechanisms used to survive by microscopic animals during dormancy are not fully understood (Clegg 2001, Oliver et al. 2005, Tunnacliffe & Wise 2007, Lubzens et al. 2010), but the main actors are thought to be specific molecules that protect the intracellular and extracellular environment against the various damages induced by the lack of water (Crowe et al. 1998, Rebecchi et al. 2007). Sugars such as trehalose and sucrose were, for a time, considered the main molecules involved in the process in plants and animals (Alpert 2006). Yet, trehalose, present in nematodes and tardigrades, is absent in Bdelloidea (Lapinski & Tunnacliffe 2003) and found only in traces in Monogononta (Caprioli et al. 2004). It has been recognized that other molecules are important as well in the physiology of dormancy (Tunnacliffe & Lapinski 2009): these include heat shock proteins, late embryogenesis abundant proteins, chaperones, antioxidants, and others (Goyal et al. 2005, Denekamp et al. 2009, Clark et al. 2012). Intriguingly, even foreign genes, acquired through horizontal gene transfer, seem to be involved in the desiccation response of Bdelloidea (Boschetti et al. 2011b).

Whereas Bdelloidea recover from their dormant stage as soon as water becomes available (Ricci 1998a), hatching of resting eggs of Monogononta is triggered by a more complex mechanism, with temperature and/or light conditions, interacting with the length of desiccation (Minkoff et al. 1983, Schröder 2005).

Several planktonic rotifers exhibit considerable environmentally controlled variation in spine development and body size. The most striking case is the elongation of spines in loricated rotifers in response to the presence of specific predators (Gilbert 1999, 2011). Such elongation of spines occurs due to chemical compounds, called kairomones, identified in the environment by rotifer mothers, which produce daughters with longer spines (Gilbert 1967).

The physiological response to chemical changes in the environment is studied in detail in Rotifera, and ecotoxicological analyses have been performed both in the laboratory and in the field (Snell & Janssen 1995). Rotifers are used in the risk assessment of pharmaceuticals, endocrine disruptors, and heavy metal pollution, through whole-animal bioassays and gene expression studies (Dahms et al. 2011). Responses regarding growth condition, reproduction, population dynamics, and toxicity are well known, especially for the laboratory model of the genus *Brachionus* (Yúfera 2001, Sarma et al. 2001, 2005, 2009).

4.5 Phylogeny

The close relationship between the 3 traditional groups of Rotifera (Bdelloidea, Monogononta, and Seisonacea) and Acanthocephala is well accepted in traditional morphological studies; Rotifera and Acanthocephala share a peculiar syncytial epidermis with an ICL (Clément 1993, Wallace et al. 1996, Garey et al. 1998) and a similar morphology of the sperm cell (Melone & Ferraguti 1994, Ferraguti & Melone 1999). In addition, phylogenetic analyses using several molecular markers support their close relationship (Garcia-Varela & Nadler 2006), so that they have been grouped in the taxon Syndermata (Ahlrichs 1997).

The monophyly of the 3 major groups of Rotifera is not debated (Herlyn et al. 2003, Sørensen & Giribet 2006). Nevertheless, their evolutionary relationships are still unclear, and different analyses usually provide discordant results regarding their position and the position of Acanthocephala (Lasek-Nesselquist 2012). This latter group can be supported either as a sister group of monophyletic Rotifera, or at different positions within Rotifera (Herlyn et al. 2003, Sørensen & Giribet 2006, Fontaneto & Jondelius 2011). The 6 hypotheses regarding the possible phylogenetic relationships within the clade Rotifera+Acanthocephala (Syndermata) are, in historical order,

(a) Bdelloidea, Monogononta, and Seisonacea (traditionally named Rotifera) as a monophyletic clade, sister to Acanthocephala (Fig. 4.48 A): This hypothesis is based on general morphological similarities and supported by morphological cladistic analyses (Melone et al. 1998b, Sørensen & Giribet 2006), but never supported by molecular phylogenies.

(b) Lemniscea (Fig. 4.48 B): The hypothesis of Bdelloidea and Acanthocephala as sister groups is based on the supposed presence of a proboscis and lemnisci in Bdelloidea (Lorenzen 1985). Ricci (1998b) argued that the morphological basis of the hypothesis was false, due to a misinterpretation of the rostrum and the hypodermic cushions of Bdelloidea as homologous to the proboscis and lemnisci of Acanthocephala. Notwithstanding the unreliability of the morphological basis, this first analysis brought attention to the Rotifera+Acanthocephala relationship. Moreover, the first phylogenetic studies on

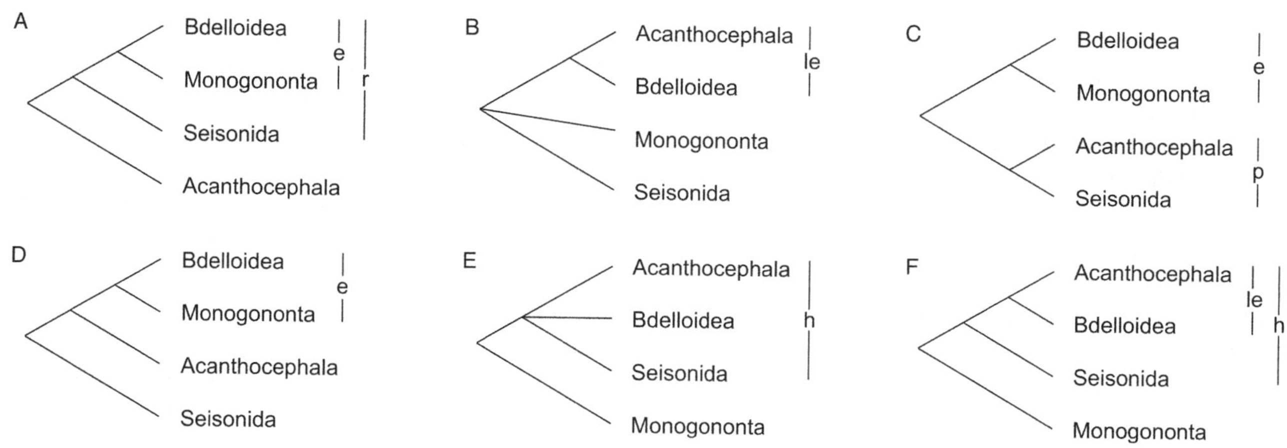

Fig. 4.48: Alternative phylogenetic hypotheses for the clade Rotifera+Acanthocephala: (A) classic theory of a monophyletic origin of the Rotifera, (B) Lemniscea hypothesis, (C) Pararotatoria hypothesis, (D) Acanthocephala as Eurotatoria sister group, (E) Hemirotifera hypothesis, and (F) Seisonacea as Lemniscea sister group. Abbreviations: e, Eurotatoria; h, Hemirotifera; le, Lemniscea; p, Pararotatoria; r, Rotifera. (Modified from Fontaneto & Jondelius 2011.)

16S and 18S rDNA supported such relationship (Garey et al. 1996). The position of Seisonacea and Acanthocephala was not included in the discussion on Lemniscea.

(c) Pararotatoria (Fig. 4.48 C): The hypothesis of Eurotatoria (Bdelloidea+Monogononta) as a sister group of Pararotatoria (Acanthocephala+Seisonacea) is based on morphological characters such as sperm morphology and epidermal ultrastructure (Ahlrichs 1997). Moreover, this relationship was supported by the inclusion of Seisonacea in the 18S molecular data set (Herlyn et al. 2003).

(d) Acanthocephala as a sister group to Eurotatoria (Bdelloidea+Monogononta) (Fig. 4.48 D): This hypothesis is supported by a phylogenetic analysis of the nuclear gene hsp82 (Mark Welch 2000) and from a combined analysis of hsp82+18S (Mark Welch 2005). Seisonacea were not included, as no hsp82 was available for them.

(e) Hemirotifera (Fig. 4.48 E): In this hypothesis, Monogononta are the sister group of Hemirotifera (Acanthoc ephala+Bdelloidea+Seisonacea), based on combined molecular and total evidence analyses of 74 morphological characters and DNA sequence data from 18S, 28S, histone H3, and COI (Sørensen & Giribet 2006).

(f) Monogononta as a sister group of the other 3 groups, and Seisonacea as a sister group of Lemniscea (Fig. 4.48 F), inferred from a phylogenetic analysis of concatenated 18S+28S+COI (Garcia-Varela & Nadler 2006) and supported by EST phylogenomics (Witek et al. 2008).

Almost any plausible relationship among Acanthocephala, Bdelloidea, Monogononta, and Seisonacea has been suggested, with no agreement between different analyses (Fontaneto & Jondelius 2011, Lasek-Nesselquist 2012). Two main patterns emerge from all the analyses performed until now: (i) the traditional hypothesis of Acanthocephala as a sister clade of monophyletic Rotifera has never been supported by molecular phylogenies and (ii) the most recent analyses even split the clade Eurotatoria (Min & Park 2009, Witek et al. 2009). Nevertheless, Seisonacea, Bdelloidea, and Monogononta share many morphological and ecological features, and there is no morphological support for the splitting of Eurotatoria (Melone et al. 1998b). The only unambiguous pattern is that each of the 3 groups of Rotifera (Bdelloidea, Monogononta, and Seisonacea) is a monophyletic clade. But the relationships between them are still not clear.

4.6 Systematics

Classically, 3 groups are recognized within Phylum Rotifera: Seisonacea, Bdelloidea, and Monogononta. The classification we report here is that of Segers (2002), based on morphology alone, given that the phylogenetic relationships have not been solved yet for rotifers using molecular approaches (see Section 4.5, Phylogeny).

4.6.1 Classification

Class Pararotatoria Sudzuki, 1964
    Order Seisonacea Wesenberg-Lund, 1899
Class Eurotatoria De Ridder, 1957
  Subclass Bdelloidea Hudson, 1884
    Order Adinetida Melone & Ricci 1995
    Order Philodinavida Melone & Ricci 1995
    Order Philodinida Melone & Ricci 1995

Subclass Monogononta Plate, 1889
Superorder Pseudotrocha Kutikova, 1970
Order Ploima Hudson & Gosse, 1886
Superorder Gnesiotrocha Kutikova, 1970
Order Flosculariacea Harring, 1913
Order Collothecacea Harring, 1913

Subclass Bdelloidea (Fig. 4.49) is a group of completely asexual animals, reproducing by apomictic thelytoky. Ovaries and vitellaria paired. Body composed of telescopically retractable pseudosegments. Usually illoricate. Corona characteristic, composed of 2 trochal discs, may be reduced to buccal field. Head bears dorsal antenna and ciliated rostrum. Lateral antennae lacking. Number of toes 2, 3, or 4 or adhesive disc. Penultimate pseudosegment with spurs. Stomach syncytial. Trophi ramate.

The bdelloids comprise 4 families in 3 orders (Melone et al. 1998b), to accommodate 19 genera and about 460 species (Segers 2007): order Adinetida with family Adinetidae (2 genera), order Philodinida with families Habrotrochidae (3 genera) and Philodinidae (11 genera), and order Philodinavida with family Philodinavidae (3 genera). Species count for bdelloids is done considering all subspecies as valid species; given the problems in defining species in asexual taxa, we here follow the rule that every morphological variability described at the subspecies level has the validity of species.

Order Adinetida is a group of bdelloids with fusiform to vermiform body, mostly compressed dorsoventrally, characterized by a corona of the *Adineta* type, without trochus and with a ventral ciliated field with rake of teeth at its base or at its lateral sides. Only 1 family, Adinetidae, with 20 species.

Order Philodinavida is a group of bdelloid rotifers characterized by trophi close to the mouth opening and extruded when animal is feeding. The corona is poorly developed, reduced to small ciliated field. Only 1 family, Philodinavidae, with 9 species.

Order Philodinida is the richest and most diverse group of bdelloids, characterized by a *Philodina*-type corona, deep and not protrusible trophi. Two families with about 435 species.

Subclass Monogononta shows cyclic parthenogenesis, interrupted by sexual reproduction. Males usually strongly reduced. Fertilization internal, resulting in dormant (resting) eggs. Single ovary, vitellarium, and testis. Body pseudosegmented, shape very various, usually with distinct head, trunk, and foot. Loricate or illoricate. Foot and

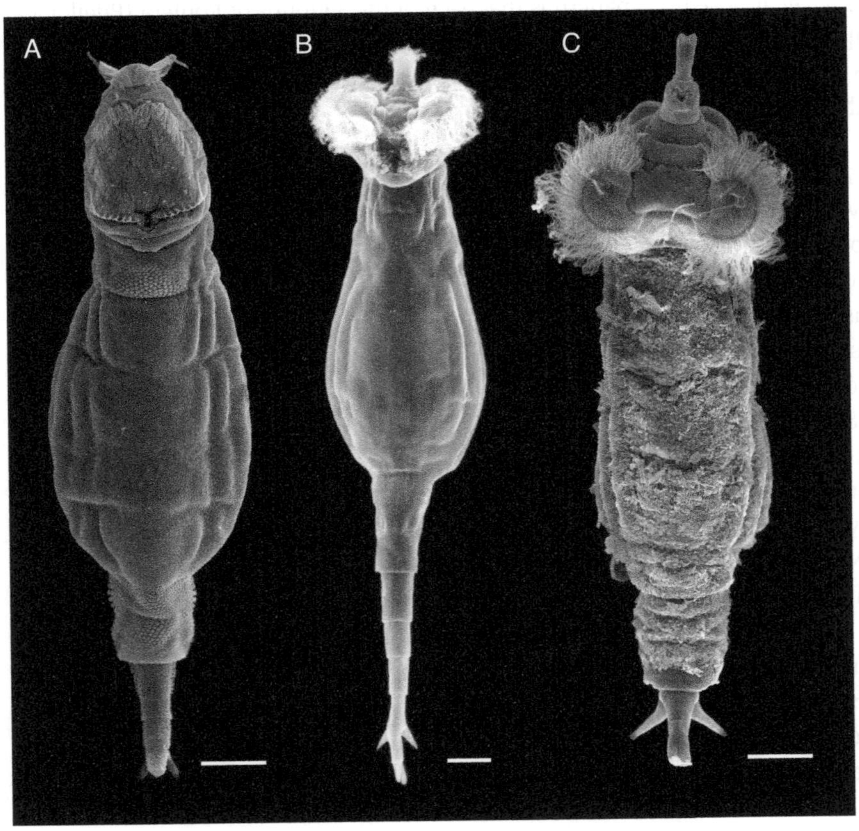

Fig. 4.49: SEM pictures of Bdelloidea. (A) *Adineta tuberculosa*, (B) *Rotaria macrura*, and (C) *Dissotrocha aculeata*. Ventral view. Scale bar = 20 µm. (Photo courtesy of Giulio Melone.)

toes very various, usually 2 toes, or adhesive disc; toes may be absent. Lateral antennae always present. Corona and trophi of various types. Dorsal antenna present, ciliated rostrum absent. Stomach cellular.

About 1,600 species are recognized in 3 orders: Ploima, Flosculariacea, and Collothecacea, comprising 23 families and 113 genera.

Order Ploima (Fig. 4.50) is extremely varied in body plan, corona, toes, and trophi. Never sessile permanently. Trochus never surrounding apical field; corona often with pseudotrochus differentiated by the buccal field. Usually 2 toes, rarely single toe, toes often absent in planktonic species. Trophi forcipate, incudate, malleate, or virgate. About 1,410 species.

Order Flosculariacea (Fig. 4.51) is a group of monogonont rotifers, characterized by malleoramate trophi. Body plan variable; free-swimming juveniles differ in shape from adult females. Foot, if present, without toes; in juveniles and free-swimming species terminating in ring of cilia or ciliated cup. Loricate or illoricate. Corona of *Hexarthra* or *Conochilus* type. About 140 species.

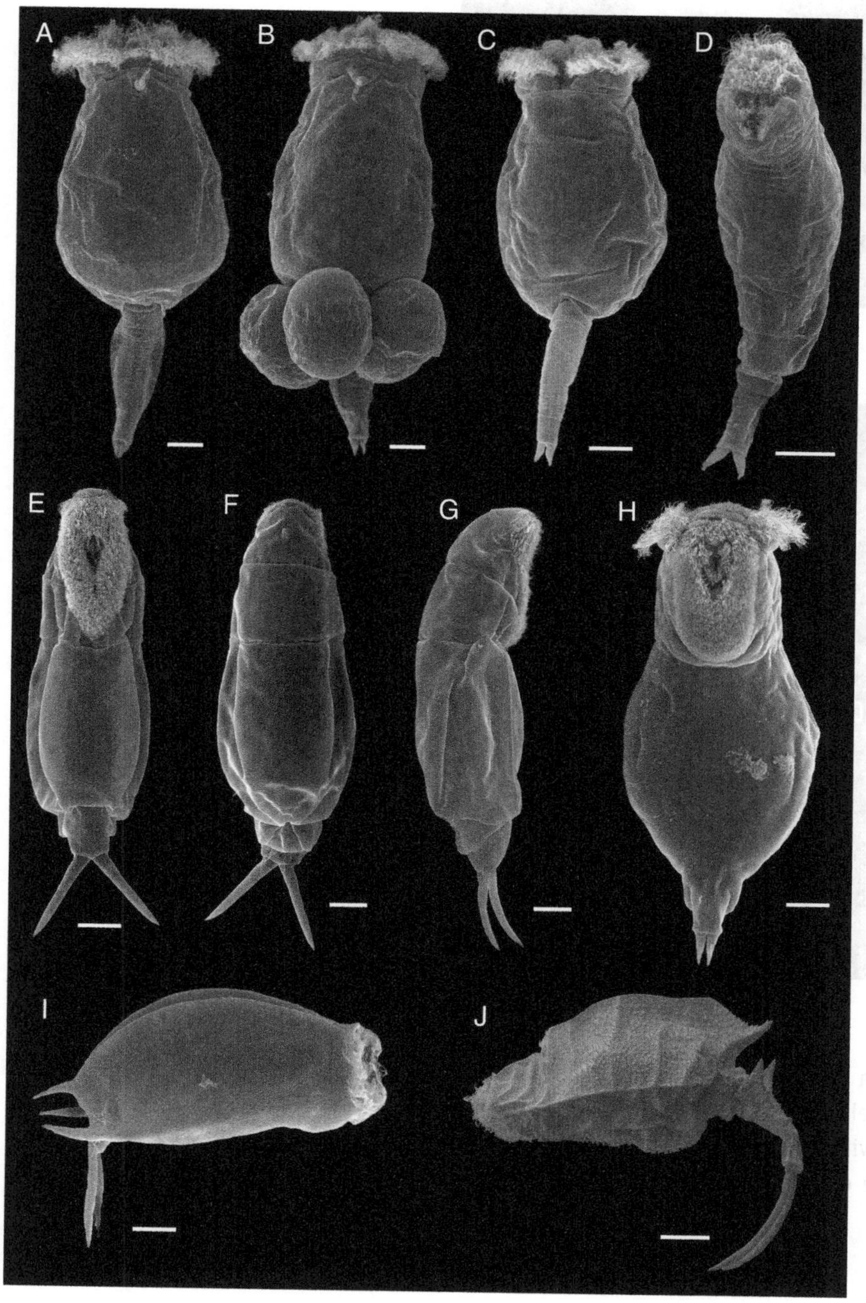

Fig. 4.50: SEM pictures of Ploima. (A–C), *Brachionus manjavacas*, (D) *Proales theodora*; E–G, *Dicranophorus forcipatus*, (H) *Notommata glyphura*, (I) *Mytilina ventralis*, and (J) *Trichotria tetractis*. Scale bar = 25 μm. (A–I, photo courtesy of Giulio Melone; J, photo courtesy of Eike F. Wiltz.)

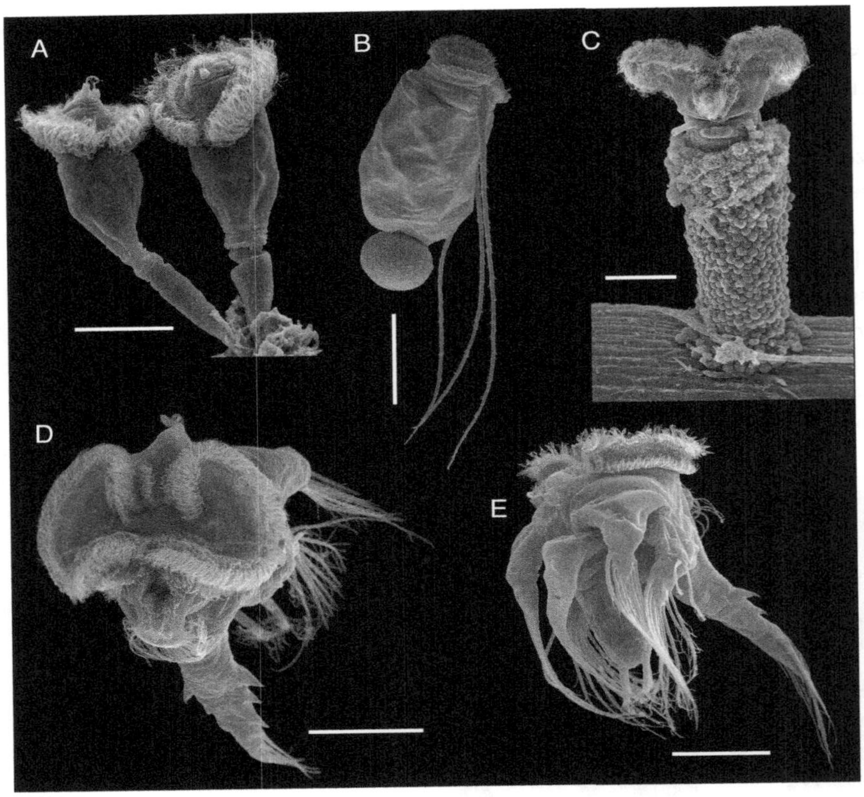

Fig. 4.51: SEM pictures of Flosculariacea, (A) *Conochilus hippocrepis*, (B) *Filinia longiseta*, (C) *Flosculariacea ringens*, and (D, E) *Hexarthra mira*. Scale bar = 50 µm. (A, C–E, photo courtesy of Giulio Melone; B, photo courtesy of Eike F. Wiltz.)

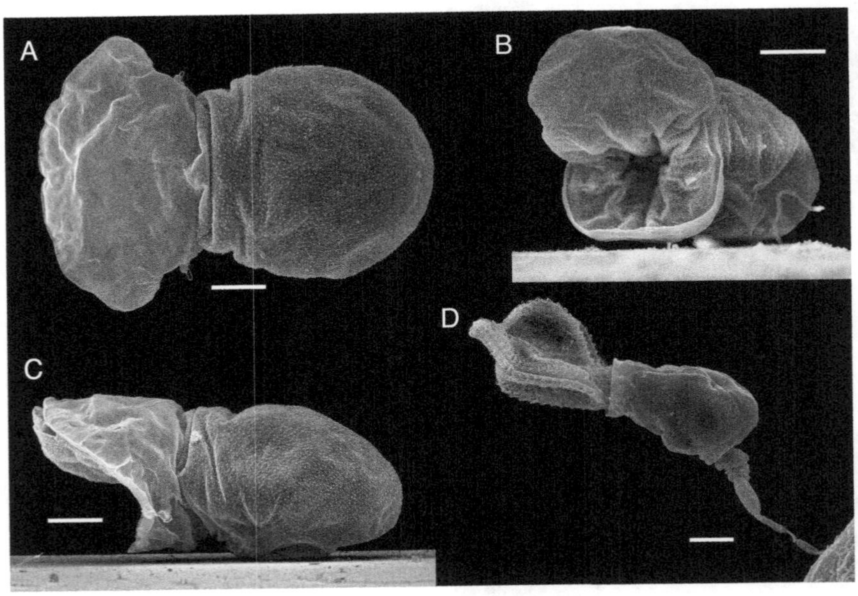

Fig. 4.52: SEM pictures of Collothecacea. (A–C) *Cupelopagis vorax* and (D) *Stephanoceros fimbriatus*. Scale bar = 50 µm. (Photo courtesy of Giulio Melone.)

Order Collothecacea (Fig. 4.52) is a group of rotifers characterized by uncinate trophi. Body elongate conical or saccate; foot always without toes, long with small adhesive disc, or modified into ventral adhesive disc, or reduced; foot of free-swimming juveniles with ciliary ring. Illoricate. Corona of *Collotheca* type, a modified funnel with or without long setae, and often lacking cilia. Most species are sessile, but several live in the plankton. About 51 species.

4.6.2 Keys

4.6.2.1 Key to higher taxa

01a – Trophi fulcrate. Corona rudimentary. Body with small oval head, long slender neck, fusiform trunk, and stalk-like foot terminating in adhesive disk. Epizoic on marine crustaceans of the genus *Nebalia*. Males and females in equal numbers. Paired ovaries ... **Class Pararotatoria, Order Seisonacea**

01b – Trophi not fulcrate. Corona mostly well developed. Body not as above. Not epizoic on *Nebalia*. Mostly or only females. Ovaries paired or single ovary **02**

02a – Paired ovaries. Trophi ramate ...... **Class Eurotatoria, Subclass Bdelloidea**

02b – Single ovary. Trophi not ramate (Class Eurotatoria, Subclass Monogononta) **03**

03a – Trophi malleoramate. Corona elliptical to round, heart-shaped, horseshoe-shaped, or 4-lobed, without long setae. Free-swimming or sessile .... **Order Flosculariacea**

03b – Trophi uncinate. Corona funnel-like with tentacles, lobes, or knobs bearing long setae; there may be cilia between the tentacles, lobes, etc. Usually sessile, a few planktonic species .... **Order Collothecacea**

03c – Trophi otherwise: cardate, forcipate, incudate, malleate, or virgate .... **Order Ploima**

4.6.2.2 Key to families of Bdelloidea

01a – Esophagus short; trophi usually close to the mouth opening, generally extruded when animal is feeding. Proximal minor teeth of uncus plate usually reduced or absent. Corona reduced to small ciliated field, trochi absent, or small ...... **Philodinavidae**

01b – Esophagus long, trophi deeper, never extruded. Proximal and distal minor teeth of uncus plate always present. Corona otherwise, with trochi absent or present **02**

02a – Corona modified to a ventral ciliated field, no trochi. Foot long and extensible, with 3 toes and 2 spurs, or short and plump, with disc-shaped distal pseudosegment, and spurs absent. Common behavior is scraping and browsing the substratum .... **Adinetidae**

02b – Corona frontal, with trochi, mostly elevated on pedicels. Foot with 2 spurs of variable length. Toes present (2, 3, or 4) or absent. Vortex feeding **03**

03a – Stomach without recognizable lumen, with round pellets in its wall ...... **Habrotrochidae**

03b – Stomach with thick wall and visible lumen, not filled with round pellets .... **Philodinidae**

4.6.2.3 Key to families of Ploima

01a – Anterior half of body composed of 16 pseudosegments with finely denticulate distal margin. Endoparasitic in earthworm *Pheretima* .... **Clariaidae**

01b – Anterior half of body not composed of 16 pseudosegments. Not parasitic in *Pheretima* **02**

02a – Vitellarium strongly elongate, cylindrical, wound around intestine, with 20–30 nuclei. Connection between stomach and intestine narrow, surrounded by wreath of ca. 6 spherical glands ...... **Tetrasiphonidae**

02b – Vitellarium spherical, ovate, U-shaped, lobed, etc., not cylindrical and wound around intestine, usually with 8 nuclei. No wreath of glands between stomach and intestine 03

03a – Mouth opening ventral, surrounded by hollow cup-shaped structure. Head covered by non-retractile shield. Trophi specialized virgate with 2 stiletto-shaped elements ...... **Cotylegaleatidae**

03b – Not as above 04

04a – Trophi highly modified, manubria heart-shaped, 2 large hook-shaped accessory elements. Stomach with blind sacks, stomach wall with green zoochlorellae. Gastric glands absent .... **Birgeidae**

04b – Not as above 05

05a – Trophi hemiforcipate, manubria with long rod-shape shaft and small axe-shaped head. Free-living or symbiotic in shells of testate amoebae ...... **Asciaporrectidae**

05b – Trophi not hemiforcipate with long manubria, if hemiforcipate with medium long manubria with broad head, and 2 trapezoid epipharyngeal plates. Free-living or symbiotic with organisms other than testate amoebae 06

06a – Trophi cardate. Illoricate .... **Lindiidae**

06b – Trophi not cardate. Loricate or illoricate 07

07a – Trophi forcipate or hemiforcipate with medium long manubria. Illoricate 08

07b – Trophi not forcipate. Loricate or illoricate 09

08a – Trophi with hook-shaped alulae, not protrusible. Stomach and intestine mostly greenish, filled with zoochlorellae .... **Ituridae**

08b – Trophi without alulae or with differently shaped alulae, protrusible. Stomach and intestine rarely with zoochlorellae ...... **Dicranophoridae**

09a – Trophi incudate. Illoricate .... **Asplanchnidae**

09b – Trophi otherwise. Loricate or illoricate 10

10a – Trophi virgate 11

10b – Trophi strictly malleate, submalleate, or malleovirgate 16

11a – Foot and toes very long, combined longer than body .... **Scaridiidae**

11b – Foot shorter, toes variable, combined shorter than or as long as body 12

12a – Body more or less strongly asymmetrical. Trophi very asymmetrical, asymmetry concerns all trophi elements. Foot terminally, a short single pseudosegment bearing several bristles (substyli) and elongate spine-like toe(s) of unequal length. Trunk usually cylindrical with dorsal crest (usually asymmetrical); ventral fissure absent .... **Trichocercidae**

12b – Body symmetrical. Trophi usually symmetrical, sometimes weakly asymmetrical (asymmetry most pronounced in rami and unci). Toes absent or present and usually of equal length, never substyli; occasionally, a single toe. Body sacciform, fusiform, conical, etc., never with dorsal crest, or if indication of dorsal, crest lorica with ventral fissure 13

13a – Stomach colored yellowish or brownish, with blind sacs. Body saccate to ovate, weakly loricate .... **Gastropodidae**

13b – Stomach without blind sacs. Trunk fusiform, conical, vasiform, or cylindrical and illoricate, or ovate to bean-shaped and distinctly loricate 14

14a – Corona with stiff setae and sensory palps. Strongly developed V-shaped hypopharynx muscles. Illoricate or loricate. With or without 6 sword-shaped paddles .... **Synchaetidae**

14b – Not as above 15

15a – Body conical, dorsum strongly arched, head continuous with trunk. Foot long, narrow. Single toe. Mouth opening bordered by long stiff cilia forming pseudotrochus ...... **Microcodonidae**

15b – Body more or less strongly fusiform, head usually distinctly offset. Foot usually short and broad. Toes usually paired, rarely a single toe. Corona of *Notommata*-type ...... **Notommatidae**

16a – Trophi submalleate, number of unci teeth reduced, usually composed of 3 stout subequal fused teeth, shaft of manubria elongate. Foot short, a single pseudosegment, inserted ventrally on ventral plate. Toes 2 or fused (partly or completely) to 1. Usually loricate with dorsal and ventral plate separated by lateral furrows (sulci); dorsal and ventral plate not distinguishable in illoricate species .... **Lecanidae**

16b – Trophi strictly malleate, or malleovirgate, unci with many teeth, gradually decreasing in length, shaft of manubria not particularly elongated; when number of teeth reduced, foot absent or composed of 2–5 pseudosegments in line with trunk. Loricate or illoricate. Dorsal, ventral and/or lateral sulci present or absent 17

17a – Head shield present, retractile or non-retractile .... **Lepadellidae**

17b – Head shield absent 18

18a – Loricate, lorica of 1 piece with longitudinal dorsal sulcus or dorsal keel (not part of polygonal facets). Foot present .... **Mytilinidae**

18b – Loricate or illoricate, without dorsal sulcus or keel (if present part of polygonal facets). Foot absent or present 19

19a – Illoricate or very weakly loricate 20

19b – Distinctly loricate 21

20a – Mouth set at end of shallow or deep, large funnel-shaped buccal field. Corona usually with conspicuous series of tufts of long cirri. Foot distinct with 1 or 2 toes or rudimentary and toes lacking. Trunk occasionally with several protruding transversal folds; without lateral sulci. Trophi strictly malleate .... **Epiphanidae [illoricate Brachionidae may key out here]**

20b – Mouth superficial, no large funnel-shaped buccal field. Corona usually without tufts of long cirri [except in *Bryceella*]. Foot distinct with 1 or 2 toes. Trunk without protruding transversal folds; usually without lateral sulci [shallow ones in *Bryceella*]. Trophi malleate to malleovirgate .... **Proalidae**

21a – Conspicuous lateral sulci present. Foot with 2 stout toes .... **Euchlanidae**

21b – Lateral sulci absent, shallow, or inconspicuous. Foot absent or present; toes absent or present 22

22a – Lorica covering clearly defined head, trunk, and foot .... **Trichotriidae**

22b – Lorica only covering trunk and occasionally foot. Foot absent or present .... **Brachionidae**

4.6.2.4 Key to families of Flosculariacea

01a – Body loricate. Free-swimming .... **Testudinellidae**
01b – Body illoricate. Free-swimming or sessile in tubes of mucus, pellets, or rigid material **02**

02a – Body with 6 arm-like appendages with fanwise arranged setae. Free-swimming .... **Hexarthridae**
02b – Body without arm-like appendages. Free-swimming or sessile **03**

03a – Apical field dome-shaped. Body with or without 2 long lateral movable setae and 1 caudal seta. Foot absent. Free-swimming .... **Trochosphaeridae**
03b – Apical field not dome-shaped. Movable setae always absent. Foot present. Free-swimming or sessile **04**

04a – Corona round, horseshoe- to U-shaped. Teeth of left uncus longer than those of right one. Free-swimming, often colonial .... **Conochilidae**

04b – Corona round, heart-shaped, or with 2–8 lobes, not horseshoe- or U-shaped. Teeth of left and right uncus equally long. Adults sessile or swimming in colonies .... **Flosculariidae**

4.6.2.5 Key to families of Collothecacea

01a – Corona funnel-shaped without lobes or cilia .... **Atrochidae**
01b – Corona with lobes, tentacles, or points bearing long setae and cilia .... **Collothecidae**

4.6.3 Characterization of families

Subclass Bdelloidea Hudson, 1884
Order Adinetida Melone & Ricci, 1995
Family Adinetidae Hudson & Gosse, 1886 (Figs. 4.49 A and 4.53 A, B)

Body fusiform to vermiform, mostly compressed dorsoventrally. Esophagus long, trophi deep, not protrusible. Stomach tube-shaped with lumen. Corona a ventral ciliated field with rake of teeth at its base (*Adineta*) or at its lateral sides (*Bradyscela*), trochi absent; rostrum terminal, not retractile. Eyespots usually absent. Foot narrow, 3 toes, 2 spurs (*Adineta*), or foot short, plump, distal foot pseudosegment disc-shaped with papillae, spurs absent (*Bradyscela*). Proximal and distal minor teeth of uncus always present. Oviparous, rarely viviparous. Gliding movement. Feeding by scraping and browsing.

Two genera: *Adineta* Hudson & Gosse, 1886 (18 spp.) and *Bradyscela* Bryce, 1910 (2 spp.).

Limnoterrestrial, in aerophytic mosses, leaf litter, soil, *Sphagnum*, hygropsammon, and littoral submerged vegetation.

Order Philodinavida Melone & Ricci, 1995
Family Philodinavidae Harring, 1913 (Fig. 4.53 C–E)

Esophagus short. Stomach tube-shaped with lumen. Corona poorly developed, reduced to small ciliated field, trochi absent or small, cheeks present, stout non-retractable rostrum, short dorsal antenna (Ricci & Melone 1998a). The trophi are close to the mouth opening, and extruded when animal is feeding. Proximal minor teeth of uncus plate reduced or absent. Foot with 4 toes, and 2 spurs. Oviparous. The aberrant carnivorous *Abrochtha carnivora* has a long pharynx that can be widened to become a large funnel, used in combination with the mouth cone to envelop the prey (rotifers); its trophi are not protrusible, and the uncus shows numerous minor teeth (Ricci et al. 2001).

Three genera: *Abrochtha* Bryce, 1910 (5 sp.), *Henoceros* Milne, 1916 (2 spp.), and *Philodinavus* Harring, 1913 (2 sp.).

Benthic-periphytic in stagnant and running waters.

Order Philodinida Melone & Ricci, 1995
Family Habrotrochidae Bryce, 1910 (Fig. 4.53 F–I)

Body fusiform to vermiform. Esophagus long, trophi deep, not protrusible. Stomach without recognizable lumen, with round pellets in its wall. Corona frontal, with small but well developed trochi, mostly elevated on pedicels. Upper lip not extending beyond ciliary disc, or hood-shaped. Eyespots present or absent. Foot with 2 spurs of variable length. Toes present (2, 3, or 4) or absent. Proximal and distal minor teeth of uncus plate always present.

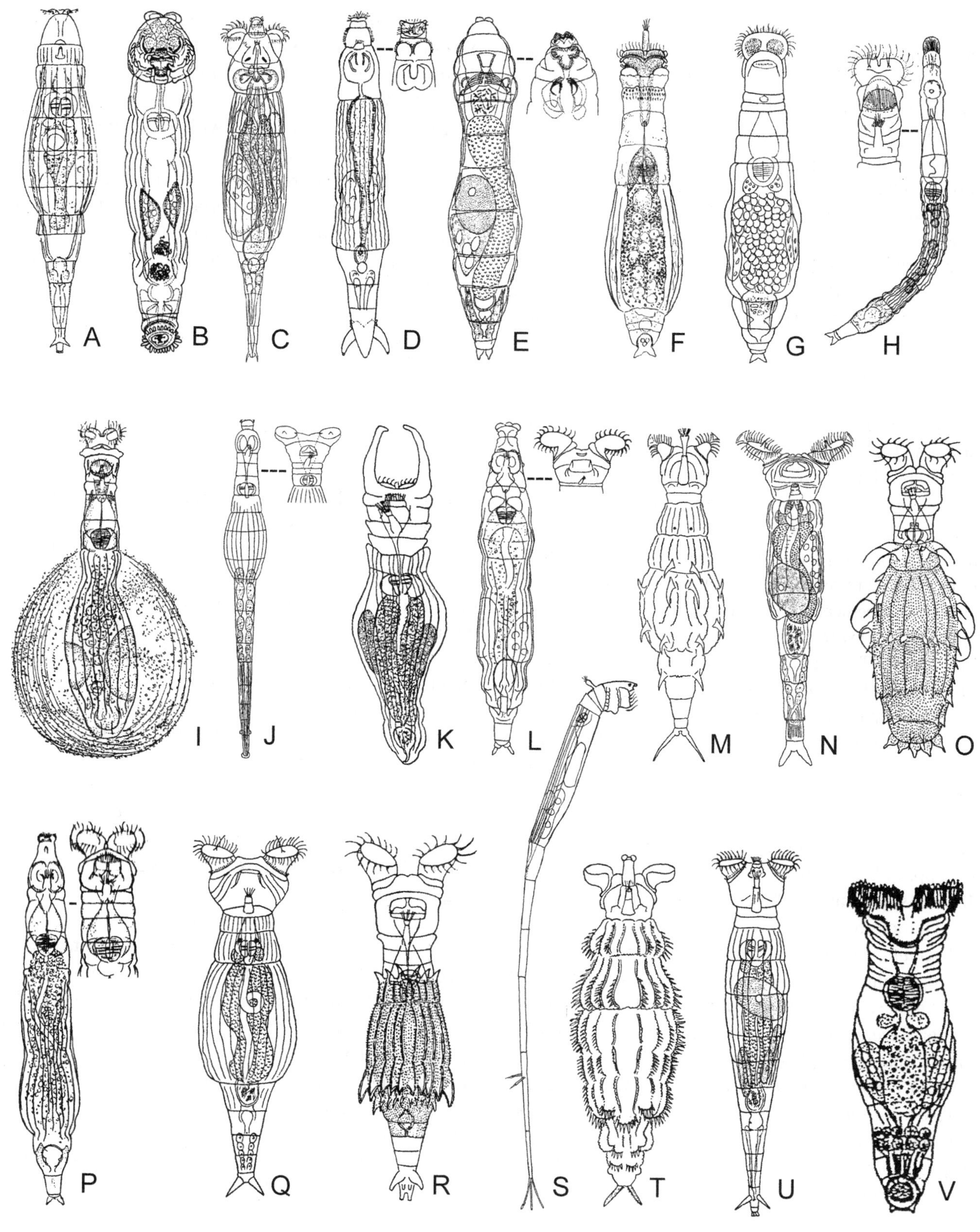

Fig. 4.53: Bdelloidea. (A) *Adineta vaga*, (B) *Bradyscela clauda*, (C) *Abrochtha intermedia*, (D) *Henoceros falcatus*, (E) *Philodinavus paradoxus*, (F) *Otostephanos monteti*, (G) *Scepanotrocha rubra*, (H) *Habrochtha serpens*, (I) *Habrotrocha pusilla textrix*, (J) *Anomopus telphusae*, (K) *Ceratotrocha cornigera*, (L) *Didymodactylos carnosus*, (M) *Dissotrocha a. aculeata*, (N) *Embata laticeps*, (O) *Macrotrachela multispinosa*, (P) *Mniobia orta*, (Q) *Philodina citrina*, (R) *Pleuretra brycei*, (S) *Rotaria neptunia*, (T) *Rotaria sordida fimbriata*, (U) *Rotaria citrina*, and (V) *Zelinkiella synaptae*. (After different authors.)

Oviparous, rarely viviparous. Vortex feeding. Some *Habrotrocha* species form secretions and more or less bottle-shaped shells or occupy shells of testate amoebae (*Centropyxis, Nebela*) or the cups (amphigastrae) under the leaflets of hepatic mosses (*Frullania, Lejeunia*); others reported from empty *Sphagnum* and plant (*Typha*) cells (Donner 1950).

Three genera: *Habrotrocha* Bryce, 1910 (128 sp.), *Otostephanos* Milne, 1916 (13 spp.), and *Scepanotrocha* Bryce, 1910 (11 spp.).

Limnoterrestrial, in aerophytic mosses and lichens, leaf litter, wet soil, *Sphagnum*, hygropsammon, and littoral submerged vegetation; occasionally epizoic on insect larvae, molluscs, etc.

Family Philodinidae Ehrenberg, 1838 (Figs. 4.49 B, C and 4.53 J–V)

Shape of body variable, fusiform, vermiform, cylindrical, etc. Integument soft or stiffened and often ornamented with grooves, spines, platelets, warts, etc. Esophagus long, trophi deep, not protrusible. Tube-shaped stomach with lumen. Corona frontal, well developed, with trochi mostly elevated on pedicels. Rostrum retractile. Eyespots present or absent. Foot with 2, 3, or 4 toes, or with adhesive disc and toes absent. Two spurs of variable length. Proximal and distal minor teeth of uncus plate always present. Vortex feeding. Oviparous and ovoviviparous.

Eleven genera: *Anomopus* Piovanelli, 1903 (2 spp.), *Ceratotrocha* Bryce, 1910 (4 spp.), *Didymodactylos* Milne, 1916 (1 sp.), *Dissotrocha* Bryce, 1910 (34 spp.), *Embata* Bryce, 1910 (5 spp.), *Macrotrachela* Milne, 1886 (97 spp.), *Mniobia* Bryce, 1910 (49 spp.), *Philodina* Ehrenberg, 1830 (50 spp.), *Pleuretra* Bryce, 1910 (14 spp.), *Rotaria* Scopoli, 1777 (27 spp.), and *Zelinkiella* Harring, 1913 (1 sp.).

Limnoterrestrial, in aerophytic mosses and lichens, *Sphagnum*, leaf litter, soil, dung; in benthos, periphyton, hygropsammon and hydropsammon of freshwaters, rarely planktonic; a few species in brackish and marine environments. Several species epizoic on crustaceans: *Mniobia branchicola* on gill plates of terrestrial isopods (*Ligidium); Embata commensalis, E. laticeps, E. parasitica, Rotaria magnacalcarata, R. murrayi, R. socialis* on freshwater isopods and amphipods, e.g., *Asellus, Gammarus; Anomopus telphusiae* and *Embata parasitica* in gill chamber of freshwater crayfish, e.g., *Astacus, Austropotamobius*, and crab (*Potamon*), and *Anomopus chasmagnathi* in gill chamber of brackish-water crab (*Chasmagnathus); Zelinkiella synaptae* on body surface and tentacles of sea cucumbers (Synaptidae) and polychaetous annelids (Terebellidae); several freshwater species have been reported epibiotic on insect larvae, molluscs, etc.

Subclass Monogononta Plate, 1889
Order Ploima Hudson & Gosse, 1886
Family Asciaporrectidae De Smet, 2006 (Fig. 4.54 A)

Illoricate. Body fusiform with offset head, trunk, and foot. Foot short to fairly long, broad. Two short toes. Trophi hemiforcipate organized for grasping, with long rod-shaped manubria bearing axe-shaped head, long fulcrum, and 2–3 large uncinal and 3–5 subuncinal teeth pivoting on the broad tips of the flat rami. Oviparous.

Three species: the free-living benthic-periphytic *Asciaporrecta hyalina* (formerly *Pleurotrocha hyalina*), and *A. difflugicola* and *A. arcellicola* inhabiting shells of live testate amoebae of the genus *Difflugia* and *Arcella*, respectively. Probably parasites, feeding on the protoplasm of their hosts (De Smet 2006).

Family Asplanchnidae Eckstein, 1883 (Fig. 4.54 B, C)

Body sac-shaped, sometimes with lateral protuberances, head differentiated, foot and toes present or absent, hyaline. Illoricate. Corona *Asplanchna* type, a single ring of cilia. Eyespot cerebral or absent. With or without intestine and anus. Vitellarium spherical, saccate, or horseshoe-shaped. Gastric glands on esophagus. Trophi incudate. Oviparous and ovoviviparous.

Three genera: *Asplanchna* Gosse, 1850 (9 spp.), *Asplanchnopus* Guerne, 1888 (4 spp.), and *Harringia* de Beauchamp, 1912 (2 spp.).

Planktonic (*Asplanchna*), semi-planktonic (*Asplanchnopus*), and benthic-periphytic (*Harringia*) species.

Family Birgeidae Harring & Myers, 1924 (Fig. 4.54 D)

Illoricate. Body plump, vase-shaped, head separated from trunk by neckfold. Foot extremely slender, 3 pseudosegments. Two lanceolate short toes. Corona frontal, circumapical band interrupted dorsally, passing laterally to auricle-like area of strong cilia, buccal field close-set with short cilia. Stomach with 10 blind sacks, stomach wall crowded with zoochlorellae. Gastric glands absent. Large eyespot ventrally on small brain. Trophi unique, highly specialized with large, hooked pseudunci expanded at their proximal ends into broad laminae; at rest hooks protrude slightly through mouth opening. Fulcrum long, rod-shaped, directed toward mouth. Rami elongate, narrow, attenuated toward tiops. Unci with 4–5 linear teeth. Manubria heart-shaped with very short cauda.

Monotypic family, with a single species: *Birgea enantia* Harring & Myers, 1922, reported from freshwater swampy pond (Wisconsin and New Jersey, USA).

Family Brachionidae Ehrenberg, 1838 (Figs. 4.50 A–C and 4.54 E–L)

Loricate, occasionally very weakly loricate. Lorica usually more or less dorsoventrally depressed, angular, rectangular, or hexagonal; anterior margins of lorica often with spines, caudally with or without spines or extensions; head and foot retractable in lorica. Foot present or absent, if present long and wrinkled or with pseudosegments; 2 small toes. Corona *Brachionus* type, frontal with reduced ciliation, pseudotrochus with 3–5 humps with short cilia on top and cirri between. Eyespots frontal, cerebral, or lacking. Trophi malleate. Oviparous.

Seven genera: *Anuraeopsis* Lauterborn, 1900 (5 spp.), *Brachionus* Pallas, 1766 (55 spp.), *Kellicottia* Ahlstrom, 1938 (2 spp.), *Keratella* Bory de St. Vincent, 1822 (45 spp.), *Notholca* Gosse, 1886 (42 spp.), *Plationus* Segers, Murugan & Dumont, 1993 (3 spp.), and *Platyias* Harring, 1913 (3 spp.).

Planktonic and semi-planktonic in littoral, temporarily attached to substrate; *Brachionus rubens* and *B. sessilis* epizoic on cladocerans, occasionally on *Corixa* sp. Freshwater, a few species in brackish and marine environments.

Family Clariaidae Kutikova, Markevich & Spirodonov, 1990 (Fig. 4.54 M)

Illoricate. Body elongate fusiform, anterior half with 16 pseudosegments, showing longitudinal striations and finely denticulate distal margin. Toes very long, weakly inflated. Trophi aberrant with thin elongate forceps-like rami, inner margin of rami lined with numerous, and loosely bound short teeth, rami with set of 4 small apical teeth. Single uncus tooth, short manubria, and long fulcrum.

Monotypic family, with a single species: *Claria segmentata* Kutikova, Markevich & Spirodonov, 1990, parasitic in earthworm *Pheretima modigliani* Rosa, 1889 (Megascolecidae).

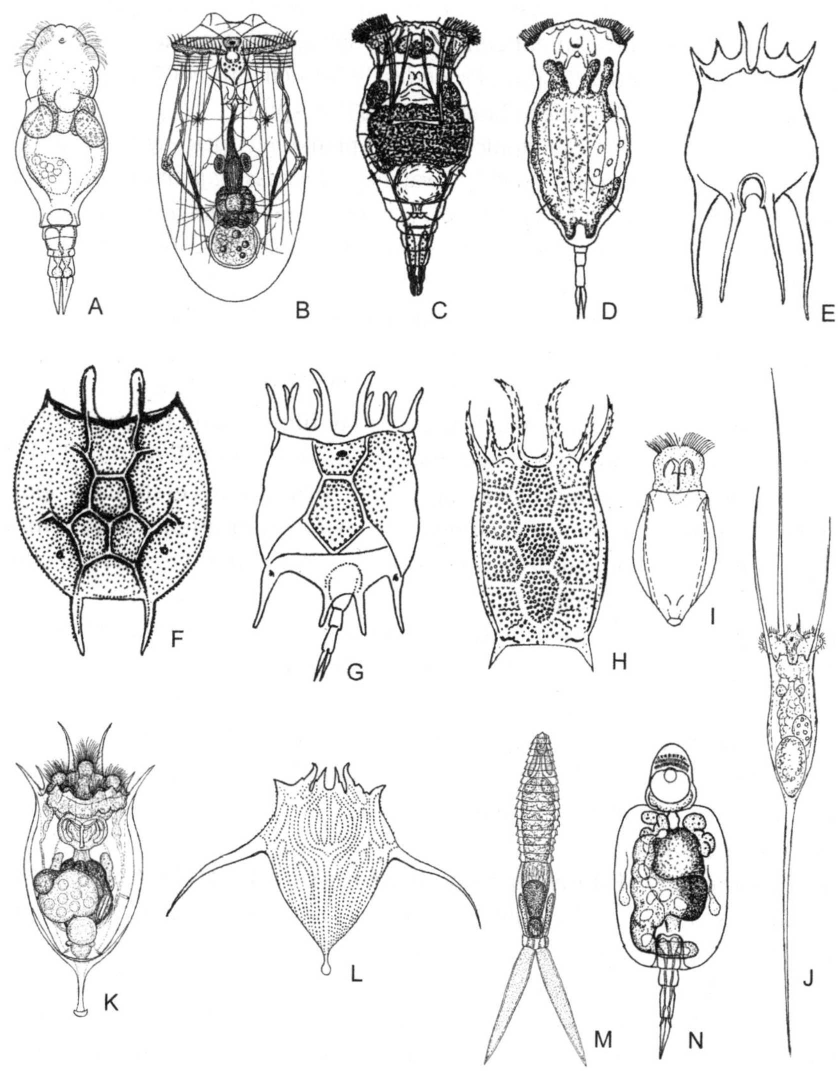

Fig. 4.54: Monogononta. (A) *Asciaporrecta arcellicola*, (B) *Asplanchna priodonta*, (C) *Harringia eupoda*, (D) *Birgea enantia*, (E) *Brachionus mirabilis*, (F) *Platyias quadricornis*, (G) *Plationus patulus*, (H) *Keratella serrulata*, (I) *Anuraeopsis fissa*, (J) *Kellicottia longispina*, (K) *Notholca kozhovi*, (L) *Notholca olchonensis*, (M) *Claria segmentata*, and (N) *Cotylegaleata perplexa*. (After different authors.)

Family Cotylegaleatidae De Smet, 2007 (Fig. 4.54 N)

Loricate. Head relatively small, covered by non-retractile head shield, offset from rectangular, and slightly dorsoventrally compressed trunk. Foot long, 4 pseudosegments, distal by one longest, bearing 2 toes, and 2 ventrolateral spurs. Corona reduced, ventral; mouth opening surrounded by large, shallow cup-shaped structure with stiffened wall. Trophi modified virgate, with small unci composed of 5–6 teeth, short manubria, long fulcrum, and 2 relatively long stilletto-shaped epipharyngeal elements.

Monotypic family, with a single species: *Cotylegaleata perplexa* De Smet, 2007, found in benthos of freshwater lake at 8–9 m depth; ectoparasite? (De Smet 2007).

Family Dicranophoridae Harring, 1913 (Figs. 4.50 E–G and 4.55 A–F)

Illoricate or semi-loricate. Body elongate cylindrical, fusiform, usually with offset head, trunk, and foot. Head usually with dorsofrontal rostrum. Trunk mostly with dorsal fold or tail, covering foot more or less. Foot and toes (2) usually short. Corona of *Dicranophorus* type, ventral or oblique, often 2 lateral ciliary tufts of longer cilia; corona absent in parasitic genus *Balatro*. Eyespots frontal, 2, rarely 4, or absent. Trophi forcipate, protrusible. Oviparous, ovoviviparous.

The family comprises 19 genera: *Albertia* Dujardin, 1838 (7 spp.), *Aspelta* Harring & Myers, 1928 (21 spp.), *Balatro* Claparède, 1867 (4 spp.), *Dicranophoroides* De Smet, 1997 (4 spp.), *Dicranophorus* Nitzsch, 1827 (52 spp.), *Donneria* De Smet, 2003 (1 sp.), *Encentrum*, Ehrenberg, 1838 (subgenera *Encentrum, Isoencentrum*, and *Pseudencentrum* De Smet, 1997, 105 spp.), *Dorria* Myers, 1933, *Erignatha* Harring & Myers, 1928 (5 spp.), *Glaciera* Jersabek, 1999 (1 sp.), *Inflatana* Kutikova, 1985 (1 sp.), *Kostea* De Smet, 1997 (1 sp.), *Myersinella* Wiszniewski, 1936 (4 spp.), *Paradicranophorus* Wiszniewski, 1929 (5 spp.), *Parencentrum* Wiszniewski, 1936 (2 spp), *Pedipartia* Myers, 1937 (1 sp.), *Streptognatha* Harring & Myers, 1928 (1 sp.), *Wierzejskiella* Wiszniewski, 1934 (2 spp.), *Wigrella* Wiszniewski, 1932 (2 spp.).

Benthic-periphytic, and psammic in freshwater, brackish, and marine environments; the most diverse rotifer family in saline waters. Several species live epizoically on freshwater crustaceans. *Encentrum grande* and *E. kulmatyckii* live on the thoracal and abdominal appendages, and the gills of *Asellus aquaticus* and *Gammarus pulex; Dicranophorus siedleckii* is also found on the gills and pleopods of *G. pulex. Dicranophorus hauerianus* and *D. cambari* inhabit the branchial cavities of severeal species of freshwater crayfish. Nearly all *Albertia* and *Balatro* species are obligatory parasites of terrestrial and aquatic oligochaetes. *Albertia* species live in the intestine of Naididae, Lumbricidae, and Lumbriculidae; *Balatro* is parasitic in the intestine or on the exterior of Lumbriculidae and Enchytraeidae. *Encentrum kozminskii* lives ectoparasitic on the skin and gills of carp (*Cyprinus carpio*).

Family Epiphanidae Harring, 1913 (Fig. 4.55 G-J)

Illoricate, occasionally weakly stiffened. Body fusiform, cylindrical, or conical to vase-shaped. Foot short to long, mostly indistinctly offset from trunk. Toes short and small, 2 or 1. Mouth set in funnel-shaped ventral buccal field with short cilia. Corona of *Euchlanis-Brachionus* type, a circumapical band of cilia; apical field with tufts of cilia, buccal field with short cilia; apical field can be elongated to form broad proboscis. Eye(s) pigmented or colorless; a single cerebral eye, or 2 eyes on proboscis. Trophi malleate. Oviparous or ovoviviparous.

Five genera: *Cyrtonia* Rousselet, 1894 (1 sp.), *Epiphanes* Ehrenberg, 1832 (6 spp.), *Mikrocodides* Bergendal, 1892 (3 spp.), *Proalides* de Beauchamp, 1907 (2 spp.), and *Rhinoglena* Ehrenberg, 1853 (4 spp.).

Planktonic and semi-planktonic, periphytic. Freshwater and brackish waters. *Epiphanes daphnicola* (formerly *Proales daphnicola*) is epibiotic on *Daphnia* spp., rarely on other cladocerans, copepods, amphipods, and oligochaetes.

Family Euchlanidae Ehrenberg, 1838 (Fig. 4.55 K, N)

Loricate. Body usually oval; trunk usually depressed, composed of 2–3 plates connected by thin membranes forming longitudinal sulci; head offset from trunk by constriction, foot well-differentiated with 2 stout, more or less long toes. Single cerebral eyespot. Corona *Euchlanis* type, with interrupted ciliary band, apical field with several tufts of cilia. Trophi malleate. Oviparous.

The family comprises 5 genera: *Beauchampiella* Remane, 1929 (1 sp.), *Dipleuchlanis* de Beauchamp, 1910 (3 spp.), *Diplois* Gosse, 1886 (1 sp.), *Euchlanis* Ehrenberg, 1832 (14 spp.), *Tripleuchlanis* Myers, 1930 (2 spp.).

Benthic-periphytic, littoral of freshwaters, rarely brackish and marine.

Family Gastropodidae Harring, 1913 (Fig. 4.55 L, M)

Loricate. Body ovate to sac-shaped, more or less compressed laterally and/or dorsoventrally. Lorica smooth, transparent, with or without longitudinal folds. Foot absent or present, more or less placed ventrally, retractable, usually annulated. Occasionally surrounded by mucus